Pediatric Head and Neck Pathology

Pediatric Head and Neck Pathology

Robert O. Greer, DDS, ScD
Professor, Departments of Pathology, Medicine and Dermatology
School of Medicine
University of Colorado Anschutz Medical Campus
Professor and Chairman
Division of Oral and Maxillofacial Pathology
School of Dental Medicine
University of Colorado Anschutz Medical Campus
Aurora, Colorado USA

Robert E. Marx, DDS
Professor, Department of Surgery
Chief, Division of Oral and Maxillofacial Surgery
University of Miami, School of Medicine
Miami, Florida USA

Sherif Said, MD, PhD
Associate Professor, Department of Pathology
School of Medicine
University of Colorado Anschutz Medical Campus
Aurora, Colorado USA
Pathologist, Denver Health Medical Center
Denver, Colorado USA

Lori D. Prok, MD
Associate Professor, Departments of Dermatology and Pathology
School of Medicine
University of Colorado Anschutz Medical Campus
Aurora, Colorado USA
Pediatric Dermatopathologist
Children's Hospital Colorado
Aurora, Colorado USA

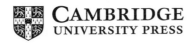

CAMBRIDGE
UNIVERSITY PRESS

CAMBRIDGE
UNIVERSITY PRESS

University Printing House, Cambridge CB2 8BS, United Kingdom

Cambridge University Press is part of the University of Cambridge.

It furthers the University's mission by disseminating knowledge in the pursuit of education, learning and research at the highest international levels of excellence.

www.cambridge.org
Information on this title: www.cambridge.org/9781316613993

© Cambridge University Press 2017

First published 2017

Printed in the United Kingdom by Clays, St Ives plc

A catalogue record for this publication is available from the British Library

Library of Congress Cataloging-in-Publication Data
Names: Greer, Robert O., editor. | Marx, Robert E., editor. | Said, Sherif, editor. | Prok, Lori D., editor.
Title: Pediatric head and neck pathology / [edited by] Robert O. Greer, Robert E. Marx, Sherif Said, Lori D. Prok.
Description: Cambridge, United Kingdom : Cambridge University Press, 2017. | Includes bibliographical references and index.
Identifiers: LCCN 2016046804 | ISBN 9781107157392 (hardback : alk. paper)
Subjects: | MESH: Head and Neck Neoplasms–pathology | Child | Infant
Classification: LCC RC280.H4 | NLM WE 707 | DDC 616.99/491071–dc23 LC record available at https://lccn.loc.gov/2016046804

ISBN 978-1-316-61399-3 Mixed media product
ISBN 978-1-107-15739-2 Hardback
ISBN 978-1-316-66194-9 Cambridge Core

Contents

Contributors

Jeffrey Schowinsky, MD
Associate Professor, Department of Pathology, School of
Medicine, University of Colorado Anschutz Medical Campus,
Aurora, CO, USA

Zenggang Pan, MD, PhD
Assistant Professor, Department of Pathology, School of
Medicine, University of Colorado Anschutz Medical Campus,
Aurora, CO, USA

Preface

Utter the phrase, "head and neck pathology" today and there will be very few healthcare practitioners who will not have some appreciation for the medical discipline that you are speaking of. It has not always been that way however. Head and neck pathology was just a glint in the eye of its many early practitioners as recently as 30 years ago; however, forward thinking pathologists like Dr. Karoly Balogh and Dr. Ronald DeLellis who taught and mentored me (ROG) as a resident; Dr. Leon Barnes who did the same for Dr. Sherif Said, and Drs. Stuart Kline and Robert P. Johnson, who helped hone the surgical skills of Dr. Robert Marx lead the way to its recognition. These are but a few of the visionary individuals who understood that surgical pathology involving the head and neck region, one of the most complex and intricate anatomic areas of the body, needed to be viewed in a comprehensive and integrated organ system fashion rather than as a set of separate and unique anatomic sites.

In the years that it has taken head and neck pathology to coalesce into a subspecialty of pathology, things have changed dramatically. Forty years ago, less than a handful of scientific journals were devoted to this anatomic region and most simply trumpeted findings related to their unique anatomic site. There are now dozens of journals worldwide devoted exclusively to pathology of the head and neck. Today, research in the area of head and neck pathology is concentrated heavily in academic institutions, where research grants designed to support the study of diseases such as cancer are concentrated. Forty years ago, however, there were no SPORE grants (specialized programs of research excellence) available to support research in head and neck cancer.

To paraphrase an old 1950s television commercial slogan, "It is not your father's Oldsmobile anymore." Things have changed in the head and neck pathology arena. Some might argue that they have changed simply because of the necessity to more intensely study cancer; but whatever the reason, pathology of the head and neck as a discipline now has global acceptance. There are now a host of textbooks that address all aspects of head and neck pathology, and indeed one might therefore take the approach: "nothing new needed here." From our perspective, however, something indeed has long been missing in the field: a comprehensive textbook devoted solely to head and neck pathology in a pediatric population.

During our lifetime, each of this book's authors has been witness to remarkable strides in medical science. Advances that have mitigated, or in fact eliminated certain diseases. In pediatric age group patients, leukemia and certain solid tumors came to mind. The cooperative multicenter approach to treating tumors in children, spearheaded by the children's oncology group (COG) has led to significant advances in the diagnosis and management of childhood tumors. Yet the problems attendant to the accurate diagnosis for and proper management of the child with a tumor or disorder of the head and neck continue to represent a substantial challenge to the clinician and pathologist.

Another thing that has changed during the professional lifetime of the authors is the answer to the question, "When is a pediatric patient no longer a pediatric patient". Melissa Reider Demer[1] addressed that very issue head on in a 2008 article in the *Journal of Pediatric Health Care*. Reider-Demer relates that with advances in the treatment of childhood diseases, 90 percent of children with severe disabilities now survive until adulthood, and because of that, the difficulties that arise in transitioning chronically ill adolescents to adult healthcare providers for primary and specialty care can be quite challenging. The same can be said for diseases and disorders other than disabilities.

For decades, the American Academy of Pediatric Medicine defined the cutoff point for patients in the pediatric age group to be 18 years of age. However, the Children Medical Services Council on Child and Adolescent Health, in 1988 defined the age limits of pediatrics to extend from fetal life until age 21. This concept has been endorsed by the National Association of Pediatric Nurse Practitioners and a host of other healthcare association providers including the American College of Physicians and the American Society of Internal Medicine.

In preparing this text we have therefore taken the position that because adult providers may be unfamiliar with the specific diagnostic course of a disease, or the expanded care that might be required for patients who would otherwise be defined as beyond the pediatric patient range, the age ranges for the disorders and disease discussed in this text and all associated illustrations will include individuals up to the age of 21.

Having established this more inclusive age range as a parameter, the principal goal of the textbook will center on discussing the disease related clinical and radiographic features, pathogenesis, diagnostic work-up and treatment rationales for pediatric disorders that involve the head and neck. This book is intended to serve as a reference source and guide for those practitioners who are involved in the care of such patients including physicians, dentists, nurses, and practitioners in related subspecialties including head and neck pathology, oral and maxillofacial pathology, oral and maxillofacial surgery, otolaryngology, pediatrics, pediatric pathology, oncology and its subspecialties and the various subspecialties of radiology and nuclear medicine. Throughout all its pages, the book is written from a clinicopathologic perspective.

Some of the names that are preferentially used for the diseases, disorders, tumors and infections that are discussed in this text are offered in an attempt to streamline and simplify terminology that has from our perspective become all too cumbersome. In concert with the first and overriding cardinal rule of medicine, "first do no harm," this book embraces the concept that in the healing arts, the practical must always trump the superfluous. Readers will therefore find that in some instances the information in this textbook is at variance with non-evidence based dogma that fails to embrace efficient and compassionate pediatric patient management. This book has been written with the expectation that it will be useful for both clinicians and scientists and that both groups will appreciate that, above all, a collaborative effort is necessary to properly manage childhood and adolescent head and neck disease.

Given the current state of science, the issue of molecular biology and genetics must of necessity be addressed in any contemporary textbook of pathology. We therefore offer an introductory chapter that discusses many of the basic molecular concepts involved in diagnosing diseases that involve the head and neck region, along with a discussion of the basic tenants routine surgical pathology from both a pathologist and surgeon's perspective. A discussion of the immunohistochemical studies and stains that are required to appropriately diagnose certain diseases, as well as a discussion of the genetic and molecular events involved in development and progression of those diseases will be found under specific disease headings in each chapter.

It is the sincere desire of the authors that this text will enable general practitioners and specialists across the numerous specialty fields that evaluate and manage pediatric patients to more effectively treat their patients. As with any attempt to be comprehensive, it becomes impossible in the end to cover every possible aspect of every possible disease, disorder or condition that one might encounter in the arena of pediatric head and neck pathology. Some specialized anatomic regions in the head and neck are therefore not a part of this text. Neuropathology, a specialty unto itself, is more appropriately addressed in the myriad of excellent textbooks on the subject, and aside from those pathologic entities that arise adjacent to, or as an adjunct to the brain, such as the encephalocele and craniopharyngioma, a discussion of the pathology of the brain is not a component of this textbook. Similarly, opthalamic pathology, a unique and specialized area of pathology, is also not included in this text. The reader is referred to a host of excellent textbooks in that specialized field.

Common syndromes with a unique or special connection to the surgical pathology of the head and neck are discussed as deemed necessary in this text; however, for a more complete discussion of childhood syndromes, the reader is referred to textbooks that deal with syndromes of the head and neck exclusively.

Reference

1. Reider-Demer M, Zielinski T, Carvajal S, et al. When is a pediatric patient no longer a pediatric patient, *J Pediatr Health Care*, 2008, 22: 267–269.

Acknowledgments

The authors would like to thank Ms. Connie Blanchard and Ms. Maria Ruiz for the significant role they played in the completion of this book. Their dedication to the typing of the manuscript, the collating of the text, and their computer expertise were absolute and yeomen. This book could not have been completed without their persistent and consistent help. We owe a great deal of gratitude to Ms. Lisa Litzenberger who helped to prepare the majority of the book's clinical photographs and photomicrographs, and to Dr. James Fitzpatrick who provided many of the soft tissue tumor photomicrographs. We thank Ms. Nisha Doshi for giving us the opportunity to author this book and for offering her editorial assistance and insights, and most of all for shepherding the book ever forward. The families of the book's four authors gave liberally of their time so that this textbook could become a reality. The time they lost can never be regained but it can and will certainly be paid forward in some important way. A book such as this could not come to fruition without the patients that the authors are called upon to diagnose and treat each day. Without them no portion of this book could be possible, and without patients, no doctor could possibly gain a fuller understanding of, or appreciation for the art and science of healing.

Diagnostic Methods and Specimen Handling Techniques in Pediatric Surgical Pathology

Robert O. Greer and Robert E. Marx

Current laboratory techniques afford pathologists and clinicians a vast array of diagnostic methods and assays that aid in the treatment of pediatric aged patients with diseases or disorders of the head and neck. These assays range from the traditional examination of routine paraffin embedded tissue that is hematoxylin and eosin stained, to sophisticated next generation genetic sequencing.

Examination of formalin-fixed tissue samples remains the most common method used to diagnose pathologic conditions involving the head and neck region in children. Immunohistochemical analysis (IHC) of tissue samples, immunofluorescence (IF) and flow cytometry are three important protein-based assays that give pathologists the ability to render a diagnosis based upon antigen–antibody recognitions. A second group of diagnostic procedures that are molecular in nature, and which depend on the identification of nucleic acids and alterations within them can also serve as important diagnostic tools. Included among those assays are polymerase chain reaction analysis (PCR), in situ hybridization assays and microarray technology.

Immunohistochemistry

Routine hematoxylin and eosin staining accompanied with IHC staining of tissue samples remain the most frequently used methods of rendering a pathologic diagnosis on a human tissue sample. IHC has as its most common application, the diagnosis of cytologically and antigen-specific abnormal cells, typically cancer cells.[1,2,3] The principal by which such IHC staining works is based on the fact that antibodies will bind, not randomly, but specifically, to certain antigens in biologic tissue samples, and that as a consequence, certain IHC staining markers will be characteristic of specific events that take place on a cellular level. IHC staining can thus easily be correlated with events such as cell proliferation and cell death.

The antigen–antibody interaction required for an IHC stain to work effectively can be visualized in multiple ways. The most widely used method to enhance any such visualization is via the use of a foreign antibody that is conjugated to an enzyme that can precipitate a reaction in the tissue that is being examined, and thereby produce a recognizable cellular-level color change in the specimen. The most common enzyme initially used to produce such a color change, which is often brown or red, was peroxide. A new generation of IHC methods emerged in the 1980s with the advent of the Avidin-biotin methods that are widely used today. One of the distinctive advantages of using IHC is the fact that the assay can be performed on formalin-fixed tissue samples, an important time and cost effective benefit when one considers that many commonly used molecular diagnostic techniques are dependent on the use of either fresh or frozen tissue, are time consuming and can be quite costly.

Since IHC can easily be performed on formalin-fixed paraffin embedded tissue and because the technique can be highly automated with a strict degree of quality control and reproducibility, IHC staining has become a mainstay of histopathology laboratories world-wide. IHC must always be used in conjunction with hematoxylin and eosin-stained tissue samples, so that morphologic and clinicopathologic correlative measures can be employed with accuracy.

Many IHC stains lend themselves to defining the origin of a tumor, including p53, p16, EGFR and cytokeratin stains (Figure 1.1). IHC staining can also be helpful in establishing or confirming the diagnosis of childhood thyroid tumors, for example, by accessing the expression of thyroid transcription factor-1(TTF-1). IHC markers can be employed as cell surface markers, intermediate filament markers, apoptotic markers and cell cycle markers. IHC can also be used to effectively

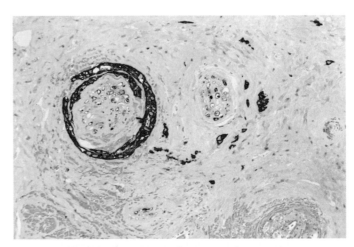

Figure 1.1 IHC stain of squamous cell carcinoma demonstrating pancytokeratin positive invasion of a S100-positive nerve.

Table 1.1 Typical tissue requirements for commonly used pathologic and molecular diagnostic procedures

Methodology	Tissue Amount	Tissue Format		
		Fresh	Frozen	FFPE
Formalin-fixed	Variable			
Flow cytometry	<1 cm³	•		
FISH/ISH*	4–10µm sections			•
Immunofluorescence	4–10µm sections		•	
Immunohistochemistry	4–10µm sections		Preferred	•
Cytogenetics	<1cm³	•	•	•
PCR**	Variable	•	•	•
Microarray	<1cm³	•	•	•

* Fluorescent in situ hybridization
** Polymerase chain reaction

access proto-oncogene expression, including oncogenes in the tyrosine kinase family, such as Ki67, which are common to various childhood salivary gland tumors.

Finally, IHC stains can be useful in the identification of pathogens, including the many viruses (i.e., human papillomavirus, herpes simplex virus) that are responsible for human disease.

Table 1.1 outlines examples of the tissue requirements that are necessary when common pathologic and molecular diagnostic procedures are used to aid in the diagnosis of pediatric head and neck tumors.

One of the limitations of IHC staining is that in a large percentage of cases, a panel of stains must be performed in order to establish a specific diagnosis, rather than a single diagnostic stain. Although this multiple panel process can be carried out rather rapidly, the process can be quite costly.

Immunofluorescence

IF is widely used as a diagnostic tool that is most often used to aid in the diagnosis of pediatric dermatologic and oral mucosal vesiculo-bullous diseases.[4,5] The technique involves the process of determining the location of an antigen or antibody in a tissue sample by demonstrating a pattern of tissue fluorescence that can be observed when that sample is exposed to a specific antigen or antibody that is labeled. IF assays are based on the premise that a standard green color change will occur in a tissue sample when an antibody is tagged to a fluorophore, most commonly fluorescein.

Indirect and *direct* IF techniques can be employed for diagnostic purposes. Indirect IF, which requires patient serum, has given way to the almost exclusive use of direct IF as a diagnostic tool. Direct IF, which is tissue dependent, mirrors the antigen–antibody recognition technique of IHC. The test involves the localization of immunoreactants in a tissue sample that is either preserved in a tissue-preserving transport medium (Michel's solution) and processed, or localized in frozen tissue (Figure 1.2). The most commonly employed IF methodology is one in which a panel of antibodies is directed against IgA, IgG, C1, C3, fibrinogen and more rarely C4d (in patients who have had renal transplants). Antibodies from the patient's serum, target antigens in a substrate and binding will occur which can be observed microscopically (Figure 1.3). Although the staining that occurs with IF is quite similar to that of standard IHC, IF uses a fluorochrome staining detection system rather than the dyes that are commonly used in IHC staining.

Cytogenetics

Karyotyping, the hallmark of cytogenetics is in the most traditional sense, a method that allows one to identify chromosomal genetic aberrations in sample cells in order to establish the genetic cause of a disease or disorder.[6] Samples for karyotyping are generally placed in a culture medium, most commonly Roswell Park Memorial Institute (RPMI) media and readied for cytogenetic evaluation. This evaluation must be done in association with a routinely prepared hematoxylin and eosin-stained tissue sample.

Tissue samples for karyotyping are disaggregated, treated and fixed to maintain chromosomal integrity, then differentially stained to identify chromosomal banding, typically G-banding (Giemsa banding). Giemsa-stained bands are numbered, using a standard reference format, and karyotypes are ultimately denoted. The process will generally yield approximately 400 genomic bands for analysis. Detection limits for G-banding are usually in the 4 mega base range, thus small amounts of DNA may at times be unidentifiable using standard karyotyping methods.

Karyotyping allows chromosomes to be examined microscopically so that chromosomal banding patterns can ultimately be compared with chromosomal pairs, and chromosomal abnormalities can be detected and accessed for aneuploidy, chromosomal damage and repair. Karyotypic *translocations*

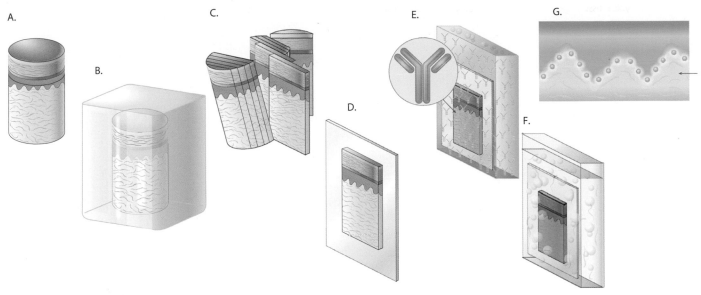

Figure 1.2 Schematic diagram depicting the various steps in direct IF processing.
A = mucosal biopsy in Michel's solution
B = frozen mucosal biopsy in OCT
C = sections of tissue while frozen
D = placement of tissue section on slide
E = placement of slide in a solution of fluorescein conjugated antihuman IgG (goat or rabbit), represented by symbol Y
F = washing of section
G = microscopic view of immunoglobulin binding site (arrow).

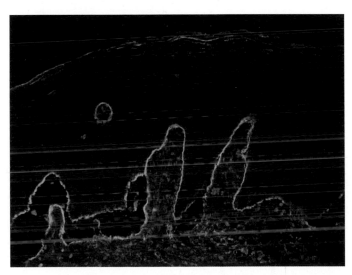

Figure 1.3 Direct immunofluorescence. Benign mucous membrane pemphigoid. Note the apple green linear band of fluorescence-tagged immune reactants bound along the epithelial basement membrane.

are common to certain childhood tumors and diseases, such as the t(8;14);q(24;q32) translocation seen in Burkitt lymphoma (Figure 1.4). Cytogenetics and karyotyping have limitations, the most significant of those being the often unpredictable amount of time it takes for cells to grow to the point that they are ready for analysis, the frequent low resolution of detection and the fact that analysis always requires fresh viable tissue.

Flow cytometry is often used to aid in the diagnosis of hematologic disorders in children. This laser-based process counts, sorts and biomarks cells by suspending target cells in a fluid stream and passing them through an electronic light detection apparatus (flow cytometer) that can analyze the chemical and/or physical characteristics of thousands of particles per second. Figures 1.5 & 1.6 show polytypic and monotypic B-cell populations in a reactive lymph node, and in a mature B-cell neoplasm respectively.

FISH and PCR are readily available and more rapid methods of analysis than cytogenetics. FISH can be employed as a cytogenetic technique to localize and detect the presence or absence of DNA sequences on chromosomes (Figure 1.7). The technique involves the use of a fluorescence microscope to identify where fluorescent probes bind to portions of chromosomes with which there is a significant degree of DNA sequence complement. FISH can detect tumor cells that are circulating as well as specific RNA targets in cells.

PCR, which can best be carried out on fresh tissue, employs a methodology that allows the pathologist or investigator to recreate and then analyze millions of copy cell numbers of a specific segment of DNA. This DNA segment or product, based upon its sequence and size, can then be analyzed and compared to other known sequences to accurately define certain diseases. Real time PCR (RTPCR), also known as quantitative PCR,[7,8,9] allows a PCR product to be visualized in real time using a computer rather than having to visualize the product after agrarose gel electrophoreses and staining. Real time PCR can detect exceedingly small amounts of target DNA, offer rapid results and minimize the risk for PCR product contamination. PCR, in either of its forms, can test for

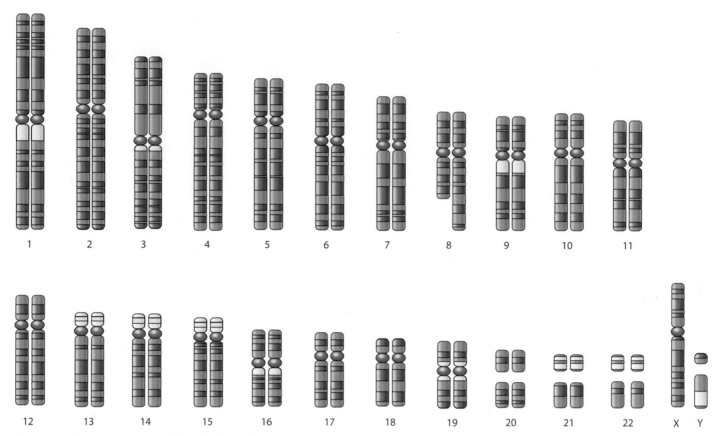

Figure 1.4 Schematic karyotype of 46 xyt (8,14) in Burkitt lymphoma.

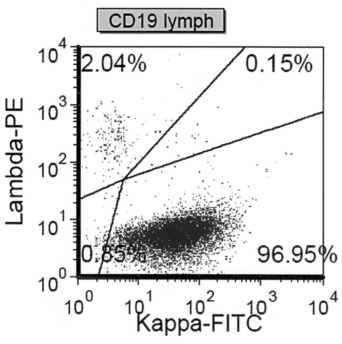

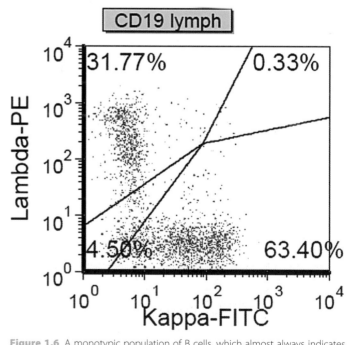

Figure 1.5 A polytypic population of B cells, which almost always indicates a reactive population. Gating on CD19-positive lymphocytes (B cells) shows a normal ratio of kappa-positive cells to lambda-positive cells of roughly 2:1.

Figure 1.6 A monotypic population of B cells, which almost always indicates the presence of a mature B-cell neoplasm. Gating on CD19-positive lymphocytes (B cells) shows nearly all B cells to be kappa-positive, with a marked elevation of the kappa:lambda ratio.

Table 1.2 Molecular testing in selected pediatric head and neck tumors

Anatomic Site	Neoplasm	Genetic Aberration	Positive Reactivity	Negative Reactivity	IHC
Head and Neck	Osteomas	May be associated with Gardner syndrome			
	Pleomorphic adenoma	FLAG 1 T(3:8) (p21:q21)	Ductal cells; cytokeratin, CEA, and EMA. Myoepithelial cells: cytokeratin, p63, S100		IHC helps identify different tumor components
	Congenital epulis			S100	S100(–) unlike other granula cell tumors
	Mucoepidermoid carcinoma	MECT1/MAML2 translocations	Cytokeratin, including CK7		
	Sinonasal papillomas		HPV, in a subset		
	Teratoma		Varies by component	AFP to rule out yolk sac tumor component	
	Nasopharyngeal angiofibroma	Some associated with APC mutations and/or FAP	β-catenin		
	Nasopharyngeal carcinoma	HLA associations	EBV/EBER; mixed cytokeratins	Cytokeratins 7 and 20	
	Adenoid cystic carcinoma	Some have t(6;9) (q21–24; p13–23); others have LOH at 6q	Ductal cells: cytokeratin, EMA, and CEA. Myoepithelial cells: cytokeratin, p63, S100		IHC helps identify different tumor components
	Salivary gland anlage tumor		Epithelial cells: cytokeratin: stromal cells: vimentin, actin and cytokeratin		
	Sialoblastoma		Ductal cells: cytokeratin; basaloid cells: S100 and actin		

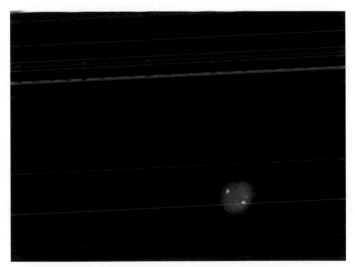

Figure 1.7 FISH in a 15-year-old with suspected Ewing sarcoma. Ewing sarcoma dual color break apart probe. Vysis LSI EWSRE1. (Abbott molecular maps to 22q12. Colorado Genetics Laboratory, Department of Pathology, University of Colorado).

genetic mutations, speciate microbes and help to identify tumor pathology. Table 1.2 depicts examples of pediatric head and neck tumors where a diagnosis can be enhanced using IHC staining techniques or various molecular markers.

Microarray Analysis

Microarrays, commonly referred to as biochips, can be employed to evaluate and interpret data generated from millions of DNA and RNA sequences. Microarrays represent an accumulation of DNA or RNA sequences that have been attached to a solid silicon wafer glass bead or glass platform surface in stepladder fashion in order to measure the expression levels of massive numbers of genes (Figure 1.8). Microarrays can also be constructed via the synthesis of oligonucleotide probes. Regardless of construction methodology, the central principle of microarray analysis is probe-target hybridization between two DNA strands.[10,11] Microarrays ensure accurate measurement of the expression levels of large numbers of RNA or DNA gene targets that have been hybridized for

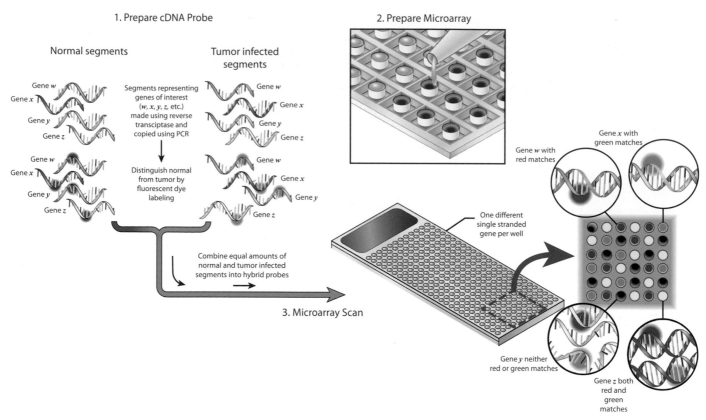

Figure 1.8 Schematic of microarray preparation and scan.

detection using a fluorescent dye (flurorophore-silver) or by chemiluminescence. Microarrays can be used to detect typical fusion transcripts in neoplasms, to identify pathogenic microorganisms or to access gene content in different cells. Microarrays are usually employed using one of two applications: 1) gene variation analysis and 2) gene expression analysis. Both forms of analysis can be used to identify gene defects in multiple forms of childhood disease.

Next Generation Sequencing

Next generation sequencing (NGS), also known as high through port sequencing, was developed in order to produce millions of DNA or RNA sequences at low cost.[12,13] Using NGS methods, as many as 500,000 synthetic sequencing operations can be run in parallel fashion. NGS sequencing can include labeling a DNA polymerase to be analyzed, nanopore DNA sequencing, sequencing by hybridization and sequencing using mass spectrometry or the electron microscope.[14,15]

Biopsy Procedures in the Pediatric Patient

Whether employed for adults or for children, the biopsy's straightforward purpose is to gain a sufficient amount of lesional tissue without tissue distortion or artifact so as to gain an accurate diagnosis. Pathologists are frequently compelled to render either a nonspecific diagnosis or describe normal appearing tissue because a biopsy specimen was too small,

did not contain lesional tissue, was not adequately fixed, or was crushed or particulated during the biopsy procedure. The clinical challenge to gaining an adequate biopsy specimen is compounded in children due to their uncertain cooperation, the smaller size of their anatomic components and the somewhat different anatomic relationships that exist in the incompletely developed maxillofacial skeletal and head and neck soft tissues. Therefore, the biopsy challenges in children must be met with appropriate clinical approaches.

Patient Cooperation: For young children and teenagers, more so than in adults, office or outpatient general anesthesia may be required. Under general anesthesia, a more direct visual inspection of any lesion or anatomic site is possible and a larger and more central biopsy specimen that is more representative of any lesion can be obtained. General anesthesia also allows more complete and direct access when a lesion is located in a remote location such as the base of tongue or the peritonsilar areas. Additionally, outpatient general anesthesia in a hospital setting can afford the clinician access to frozen section diagnosis. Frozen sections are not typically intended to render a definitive diagnosis but rather to identify that the specimen contains pathologic tissue which can be definitively diagnosed by permanent fixed tissue processing and adjuncts such as IHC. This approach lends itself to excellent parent acceptance as well as patient acceptance in the toddler to the 12-year-old child.

The American Academy of Pediatrics broadly defines a "pediatric patient" as 21 years of age or younger. The age range of 12 to 21 years lends itself to office-based intravenous sedation, a common practice in most oral and maxillofacial surgery offices and many otolaryngology offices today.

Incisional vs. Excisional Biopsy: The clinician should strive to accomplish an excisional biopsy with 2 mm to 3 mm margins of peripheral nonlesional tissue whenever possible. If the clinical/radiographic differential diagnosis for a lesion includes lesions that are primarily curable by complete removal of that lesion, then an excisional biopsy or a bony enucleation biopsy would be the procedure of choice. For instance, a well delineated mass in the midline of the oral tongue in a child might include a differential diagnosis of an epidermoid cyst, dermoid cyst, pyogenic granuloma or a nerve sheath neoplasm. (Figure 1.8) Since each of these lesions is curable by

an excisional biopsy, the suture tagged biopsy itself can be both diagnostic and curative, sparing the child a second procedure (Figures 1.10 & 1.11). Similarly, if a mixed radiolucent/radiopaque radiographic lesion in the mandible or maxilla of a child appears to have tooth-like formations or calcifications within it, suggesting a diagnosis of odontoma, ameloblastic fibro-odontoma or adenomatoid odontogenic tumor (cyst), an enucleation biopsy will likely be curative as well (Figure 1.12). Should either of these excisional biopsies identify a lesion not curable by a local excision or enucleation, the tissue that has been removed thus becomes a diagnostic incisional biopsy and the child is no further traumatized than if a smaller incisional biopsy had been taken.

Incisional biopsies are recommended when the clinical differential diagnosis of a pathologic process includes lesions that are curable only by excision, as well as lesions that might require resection, possible for adjunctive radiation or chemotherapy, or antibiotic care. For instance an expansile multilocular radiolucent lesion in a child's mandible may represent

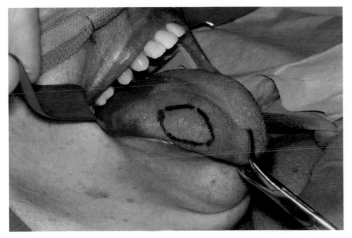

Figure 1.9 Excision of a surface lesion is guided by outlining the excision periphery with a sterile marking pen. (Reprinted from Marx R, Stern D. *Oral and Maxillofacial Pathology: A Rationale for Diagnosis and Treatment* with permission from Quintessence Publishing Company).

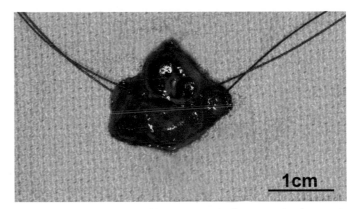

Figure 1.11 A properly tagged biopsy specimen (here tagged with sutures) can aid the pathologist identifying appropriate surgical margins. (Reprinted from Marx R, Stern D. *Oral and Maxillofacial Pathology: A Rationale for Diagnosis and Treatment* with permission from Quintessence Publishing Company).

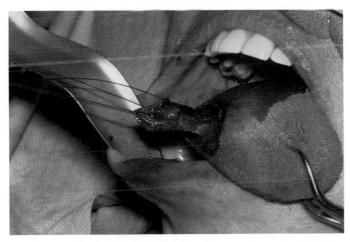

Figure 1.10 Sutures placed in a surgical specimen can be used to aid in tissue release and to identify lesional margins, and direct the pathologist to areas of concern. (Reprinted from Marx R, Stern D. *Oral and Maxillofacial Pathology: A Rationale for Diagnosis and Treatment* with permission from Quintessence Publishing Company).

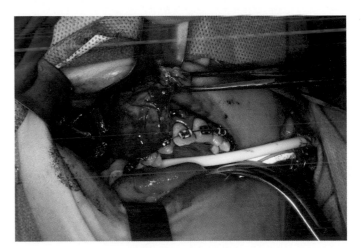

Figure 1.12 Enucleation biopsy of a radiographically mixed radiolucent and radiopaque mass involving the maxilla of a child. (Reprinted from Marx R, Stern D. *Oral and Maxillofacial Pathology: A Rationale for Diagnosis and Treatment* with permission from Quintessence Publishing Company).

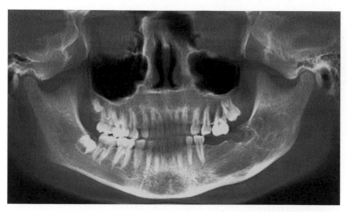

Figure 1.13 Radiograph showing an odontogenic keratocyst involving the mandible, which was managed by enucleation of the cyst. (Reprinted from Marx R, Stern D. *Oral and Maxillofacial Pathology: A Rationale for Diagnosis and Treatment* with permission from Quintessence Publishing Company).

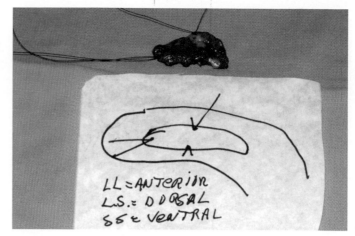

Figure 1.14 Sutures placed in an excised specimen which is accompanied by a reference drawing. (Reprinted from Marx R, Stern D. *Oral and Maxillofacial Pathology: A Rationale for Diagnosis and Treatment* with permission from Quintessence Publishing Company).

an odontogenic keratocyst or an ameloblastic fibroma, both lesions that are most often curable by enucleation (Figure 1.13). However, this same clinical/radiographic appearance might be representative of an odontogenic myxoma or an ameloblastoma, both of which are treated by a form of resection and plans for ultimate reconstruction. A definitive diagnosis using an incisional biopsy in such cases allows for adequate planning.

Adequacy of Specimens: When accomplishing an incisional biopsy in soft tissue, as much tissue should be removed as is feasible within the confines of the lesion. Since an incisional biopsy is indicated for diagnosis and not for definitive treatment, there is no gain in removing adjacent normal tissue. In fact, removing adjacent normal tissue may risk tumor implantation making any definitive surgery unnecessarily more extensive and the risks of vascular or neural injury enhanced.

Specimen Handling: Excisional biopsy specimens may require orientation to assess the excision margins. This can be accomplished using simple sutures. The recognized standard is to use silk sutures because of their durability and ease of placement. These sutures can be used to identify surgical margins by using the suture tails that are long-long, short-long, and short-short for instance (Figure 1.14). It is rare that more than three margins or anatomic areas require identification. If so, another nonresorbable suture or indelible ink can be used to identify any such margin. In the practice of head and neck surgical pathology, it is important to refrain from using dental terms such as mesial and distal. In dentistry, distal refers to the opposite direction from the facial midline. In medicine, however, distal refers to the opposite direction from the central nervous system, not a distance from midline. While oral and maxillofacial pathologists recognize the various uses of both dental and medical terms, general pathologists and medical pathology specialists may not. Therefore, it is best to use the terms anterior, posterior, superior and inferior or dorsal or ventral when referring to tongue biopsies for instance.

While it is acceptable to bisect, or cut open specimens for a gross examination before tissue fixation, the clinician should not separate the specimen into two or more pieces. In particular, bone biopsies should not be marginally curetted, since bone specimens can be difficult to diagnose due to loss of orientation.

Tissue Fixation: Most tissue specimens can be adequately fixated in neutral buffered 10 percent formalin. However, in special circumstances, as with electron microscopy, or direct IF, special fixatives are required in order to render a diagnosis, as with Langerhans Cell Histiocytosis, Pemphigus, Leukemias or Lymphomas; it is best to consult with the pathologist prior to any biopsy procedure, so that tissue samples are handled properly in order to expedite a proper diagnosis and appropriate care.

Whenever any tissue fixative is used, the clinician should place the specimen in a large volume of that fixative. A 10:1 ratio of fixative volume to specimen volume is recommended. This is critical with large specimens and with lymph node biopsies, where autolysis can quickly occur in a lesion's center due to delayed diffusion of the fixative into the specimen.

Avoiding Artifacts: The three most common artifacts to occur in biopsy specimens in pediatric age group patients are crush artifact, freezing artifact in the northern latitudes during winter and ballooning artifact due to direct injection of local anesthesia into a biopsied lesion. To avoid crush artifact, the clinician should limit the use of tissue forceps and when necessary grasp only the submucosal or dermal layer of the tissue so as to avoid implanting surface epithelium into deeper layers (Figure 1.15). To avoid freezing artifact, the clinician should be cognizant of local temperatures when mailing patient specimens to the pathology laboratory and also consider couriers or overnight/same day delivery of a specimen. To avoid ballooning artifact, the clinician should use only regional or field block local anesthesia. Injecting local anesthetic directly into a lesion will not seed cells into other locations if standard gauge dental anesthetic needles are used; however, the hydraulic pressure from a local

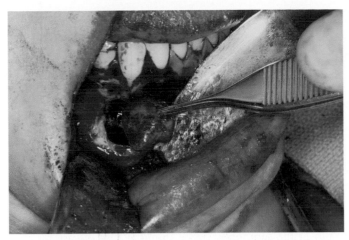

Figure 1.15 Appropriate handling of the tissue with judicious area of tissue forceps will limit crush artifact and submucosal tissue damage. (Reprinted from Marx R, Stern D. *Oral and Maxillofacial Pathology: A Rationale for Diagnosis and Treatment* with permission from Quintessence Publishing Company).

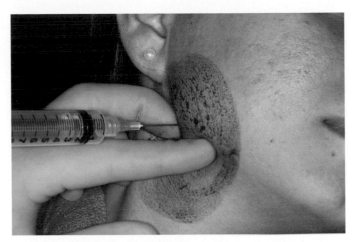

Figure 1.17 Syringe release and toggle of the mass. (Reprinted from Marx R, Stern D. *Oral and Maxillofacial Pathology: A Rationale for Diagnosis and Treatment* with permission from Quintessence Publishing Company).

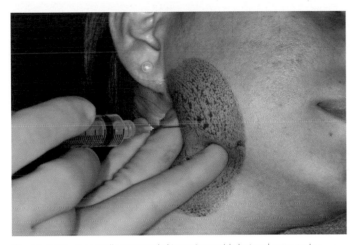

Figure 1.16 Aseptically prepared skin surface with lesional mass to be aspirated stabilized between the middle and index fingers. (Reprinted from Marx R, Stern D. *Oral and Maxillofacial Pathology: A Rationale for Diagnosis and Treatment* with permission from Quintessence Publishing Company).

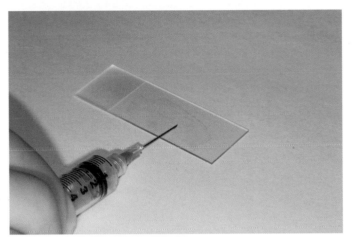

Figure 1.18 Spraying of the aspirated mass contents onto clean, dry glass slide. (Reprinted from Marx R, Stern D. *Oral and Maxillofacial Pathology: A Rationale for Diagnosis and Treatment* with permission from Quintessence Publishing Company).

anesthetic injection can disrupt tissue planes and distort cellular architecture.

Specific Biopsy Techniques

Fine Needle Aspirations: Fine needle aspiration (FNA) biopsies may be required for certain head and neck soft tissue sites in children, for parotid masses and for lymph node enlargements. Aspiration of intra bony cystic fluid from a lesion has not been shown to have any real diagnostic value and is not recommended. For FNA, a 23 to 27 gauge or smaller needle attached to a 5 ml or 10 ml syringe may be used. After an aseptic preparation of the involved surface, the mass or lesion to be aspirated should be stabilized between the middle and index finger of the nondominant hand (Figure 1.16). The syringe is typically held as one would hold a dart, with the finger tips on the syringe barrel using the dominant hand. As the needle enters the skin, a resistance will be felt that lessens as the needle passes through the dermis and into the subcutaneous fat. A second resistance will typically be felt when the needle enters the mass. Once the needle tip is within the mass, the mass should be toggled back and forth with the stabilizing nondominant hand while releasing the syringe from the dominant hand (Figure 1.17). The needle's location within the mass is confirmed if the syringe barrel moves with the mass. The plunger should be pulled back vigorously while maintaining the needle's position in the mass. The needle should be withdrawn while maintaining negative pressure in the syringe. As the needle reaches the surface, it will aspirate some air which is then used to aid in quickly spraying the aspirated contents onto a clean dry glass slide(s) (Figure 1.18). The contents are then rapidly smeared on the slide using the needle. A second glass slide can be applied to the first slide to produce surface tension before the two slides are pulled apart horizontally, leaving a thin film on both slides that can be assessed. The specimen on the glass slide is then immediately placed into a 95 percent cytorich red or Saccomanno's cytology fixative. The second slide can be air dried. After withdrawal of the needle, the process of ejecting the aspirated cells onto the glass slide (it may appear that nothing was aspirated onto the glass slide), smearing it into a thin layer, and placing it in the fixative should take less than 10 seconds so as to avoid drying and distortion of the aspirated cells. If more than one site is aspirated, a second container of fixative should be used. The cytopathology of FNAs from a spindle cell carcinoma and B-cell lymphoma are seen in Figures 1.19 and 1.20.

Bone Biopsies: The most critical aspect of a biopsy of a central osseous lesion of bone is to make certain that tissue from the marrow space or center of the lesion is obtained (Figure 1.21). Many malignancies of bone and many odontogenic and other benign tumors in children will stimulate periosteal new bone formation. A biopsy that is too superficial will result in a pathologic diagnosis of normal or "reactive bone," or often simply "a fibro-osseous proliferation," due to the fact that the actual lesional pathology beneath was not identified. Therefore, an osteome, saw or bur must be used to make certain that

the biopsy includes not simply expanded bone but also lesional tissue.

Biopsies of Mucosal Surface Lesions Suspected to be Immune-based: Immune-based diseases that occur in children, such as pemphigus and erythema multiforme, represent exceptions to the rule that mandates that a diagnostic biopsy must be within the confines of the clinical lesion. In such immune-based cases, the principal goal of the clinician is to sample clinically involved tissue that is not ulcerated, so as not to obscure a specific histologic pattern of the disease by associated nonspecific inflammation (Figure 1.22).

A regional or field block local anesthetic is typically used and an adequate large surface area of mucosa is removed to the depth of the submucosa when immune base disease biopsies are obtained. If a large enough area cannot be removed so as to separate the specimen into two distinct pieces, one for routine

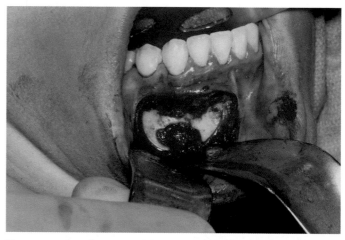

Figure 1.21 Bone biopsy in a child demonstrating deep exploration of narrow spaces. (Reprinted from Marx R, Stern D. *Oral and Maxillofacial Pathology: A Rationale for Diagnosis and Treatment* with permission from Quintessence Publishing Company).

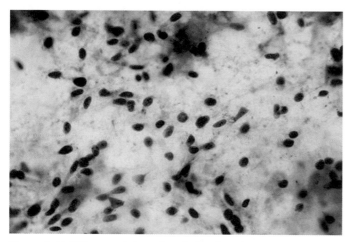

Figure 1.19 FNA cytopathology of a spindle cell carcinoma.

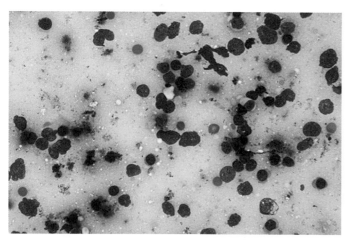

Figure 1.20 B-cell lymphoma.

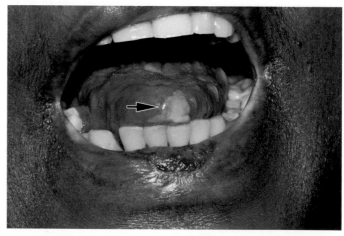

Figure 1.22 Clinically involved nonulcerated tissue (arrow) will offer the best diagnostic yield in immune-based vesiculo-bullous disorders. (Reprinted from Marx R, Stern D. *Oral and Maxillofacial Pathology: A Rationale for Diagnosis and Treatment* with permission from Quintessence Publishing Company).

formalin fixation and a second for IF evaluation, in Michel's solution, or for frozen section processing, then a second site should be biopsied as well. Before placing either specimen into its respective fixative, it is advisable to suture the specimen flat onto a template such as cardboard since thin mucosal biopsies will have the tendency to curl. Maintaining flat rigid fixation will allow for proper orientation and tissue sectioning (Figure 1.23).

Lymph Node Biopsies: Young children and teenagers often have reactive inflammatory lymph nodes that may mimic lymph node neoplasia. Enlarged lymph nodes in children or teenagers may also be representative of pathologies such as cat scratch disease, Hodgkin lymphoma or actinomycosis, for example. As in adults, open lymph node biopsies are indicated only after clinical laboratory results, a search for a primary disease location, and an FNA fail to establish a diagnosis.

Regardless of age, open lymph node biopsies are best accomplished under general anesthesia with access to electrocautery to control small bleeding vessels, largely due to the fact that lymph nodes in the neck are deep to the platysma muscle and there are robust afferent and efferent blood vessels entering and leaving the hilum of each node.

When a lymph node biopsy is contemplated, the largest and deepest lymph node in a given lymph node chain will be the most diagnostic node. When a lymph node is to be biopsied, a horizontal incision is usually made in the neck using an existing skin fold close to the lymph node targeted for biopsy. Once the superficial layer of the deep cervical fascia is exposed, a pericapsular excision is begun taking precautions to avoid the hilum of the lymph node, where the blood vessels are located (Figure 1.24) Pathologic lymph nodes are more often grossly oblong rather than the round or oral in shape (Figure 1.25) and such nodes may be adherent to adjacent nodes. The surgeon should not grasp the lymph node with a forceps as this will

macerate the soft texture of most lymph nodes. Instead, the lymph node should be maneuvered by grasping the surrounding pericapsular fat. The vessels at the hilum may be coagulated or tied off as a final portion of the harvesting procedure before delivering the lymph node to the laboratory.

Once the lymph node is delivered to the pathology laboratory, it should not be immediately placed in a fixative. Instead,

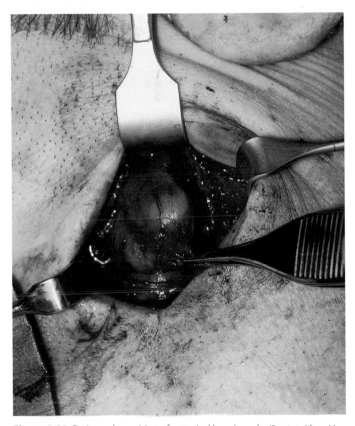

Figure 1.24 Pericapsular excision of a cervical lymph node. (Reprinted from Marx R, Stern D. *Oral and Maxillofacial Pathology: A Rationale for Diagnosis and Treatment* with permission from Quintessence Publishing Company).

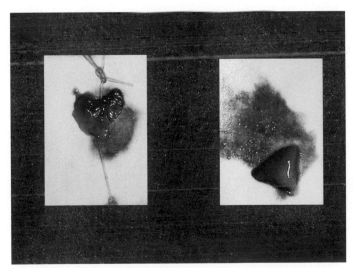

Figure 1.23 Mucosal biopsy specimen sutured to cardboard to prevent curling. (Reprinted from Marx R, Stern D. *Oral and Maxillofacial Pathology: A Rationale for Diagnosis and Treatment* with permission from Quintessence Publishing Company).

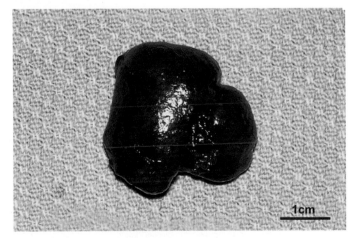

Figure 1.25 Oblong, pathologically involved lymph node. (Reprinted from Marx R, Stern D. *Oral and Maxillofacial Pathology: A Rationale for Diagnosis and Treatment* with permission from Quintessence Publishing Company).

it is recommended that the lymph node be sectioned in half in order to accomplish a touch preperatomy or "touch prep" (Figure 1.26). This procedure involves pressing the cut surface of the sectioned lymph node against a clean dry glass slide, which will produce a gross nodal imprint, before the node is placed into a fixative. The touch prep creates a monolayer of cells on the slide that can be accessed histologically for cellular organelles and other cellular details (Figure 1.27). The remaining lymph node is further sectioned into 2 mm thick sections (Figure 1.28); however, before any of these sections are placed into a fixative, one section is further cut into several pie-shaped pieces that can each be sent for aerobic, anaerobic and fungal cultures. The remaining "bread loafed" sections can then be placed in any large volume of the fixative preferred by the pathologist. This approach

ensures the most accurate identification of micro-organisms and properly fixes the friable lymph node tissue avoiding autolysis.

When scheduling a lymph node biopsy in a child, it is advisable to communicate with the pathologist to determine what type of the many available fixatives might be preferred, in order to assure that such reagents can be available at the time of the procedure. Most pathology laboratories prefer that the lymph node be sent to them fresh at which time they will accomplish the touch prep, bread loafing and fixation procedures. In the absence of such communication, formalin remains the preferred fixative for lymph node fixation, once culture specimens have been sent for assessment.

Aspiration of Radiolucent Lesions in the Jaws: As noted earlier, the aspiration of fluid contents within the jaws has little if any diagnostic value. The aspiration of radiolucencies within the jaws of a child (Figure 1.29) is therefore primarily done to clinically assess the potential bleeding nature of a lesion prior to an open biopsy and/or to assess the need for angiography.

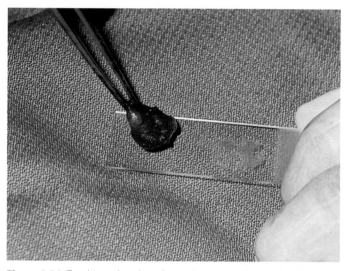

Figure 1.26 Touching a lymph node specimen to a microscopic slide to complete a gross nodal imprint. (Reprinted from Marx R, Stern D. *Oral and Maxillofacial Pathology: A Rationale for Diagnosis and Treatment* with permission from Quintessence Publishing Company).

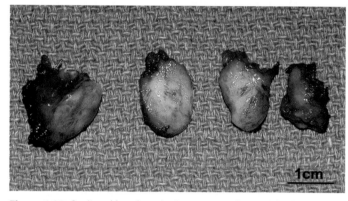

Figure 1.28 Sectioned lymph node. Specimen can be used for histologic processing and for microbiological cultures. (Reprinted from Marx R, Stern D. *Oral and Maxillofacial Pathology: A Rationale for Diagnosis and Treatment* with permission from Quintessence Publishing Company).

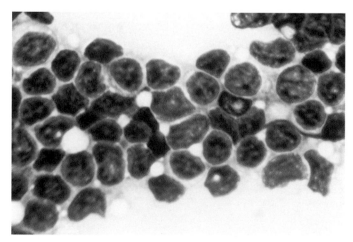

Figure 1.27 Mono layer of neoplastic cells can be seen in this stained lymphoma "touch prep." (Reprinted from Marx R, Stern D. *Oral and Maxillofacial Pathology: A Rationale for Diagnosis and Treatment* with permission from Quintessence Publishing Company).

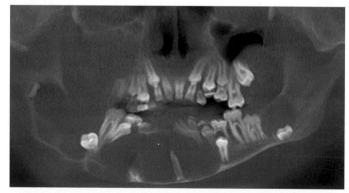

Figure 1.29 Large radiolucencies of the mandible may require aspiration to assess them for a potential bleeding risk. (Reprinted from Marx R, Stern D. *Oral and Maxillofacial Pathology: A Rationale for Diagnosis and Treatment* with permission from Quintessence Publishing Company).

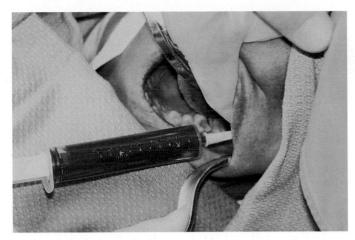

Figure 1.30 Aspiration of a hemangioma of the mandible in a child. Because the blood outflow is under low pressure, and not pulsating pressure, the risk of serious hemorrhage is low. (Reprinted from Marx R, Stern D. *Oral and Maxillofacial Pathology: A Rationale for Diagnosis and Treatment* with permission from Quintessence Publishing Company).

The most concerning childhood vascular lesion in the maxilla or mandible, and one that has the potential for exsanguination is the Arteriovenous Hemangioma (AVH). The AVH is composed of numerous large vessels under arterial pressure and it will have multiple feeding vessels. The AVH will return blood on aspiration almost routinely and the lesion must be ruled out and angiography accomplished before any extensive open surgical procedure transpires. Although idiopathic bone cavities (IBC) will also most often return blood upon aspiration, as will central giant cell tumors of the jaws and cavernous and capillary hemangiomas; their blood outflow, unlike that of an AVH, is under low pressure and tends to be oozing in nature, rather than pulsating (Figure 1.30). Thus none of these lesions represents a serious bleeding potential threat.

The specific technique for aspiration involves the use of an 18 gauge needle to puncture through the mucosa and bony cortex in a single location. If the cortex cannot be punctured

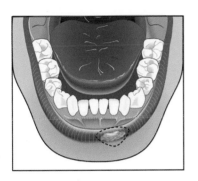

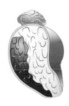

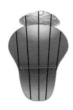

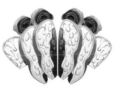

Figure 1.31 Proper sectioning of a wedge excision of the lip. Sectioning should be made perpendicular to the junction between skin and mucosa.

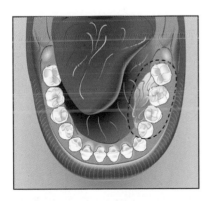

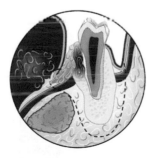

Figure 1.32 Resections that involve the mandibular gingiva and floor of the mouth require evaluation of soft tissue and bone. Sectioning should be in a buccal lingual direction and perpendicular to the mandibular long axis.

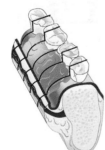

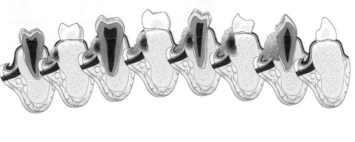

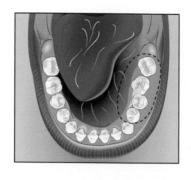

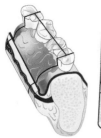

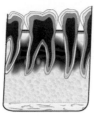

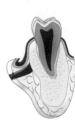

Figure 1.33 Longitudinal sectioning of the mandible will allow for assessment of resected lesions that involve medullary bone. Anterior and posterior margins can be evaluated after the resected segment has been sectioned longitudinally.

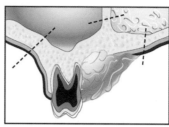

Figure 1.34 Resected specimens that involved the maxilla should be sectioned vertically and dorsally. Resected bony margins will include the hard palate the lateral nasal wall and the zygoma.

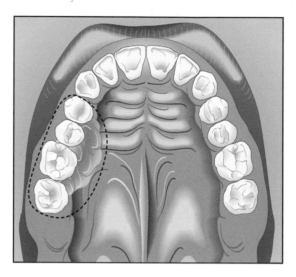

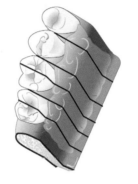

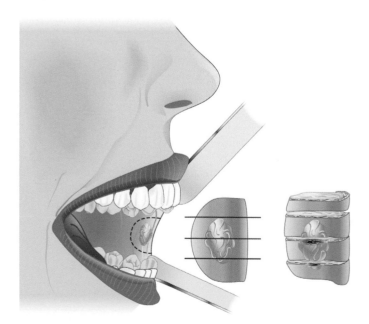

Figure 1.35 Resected specimens from the buccal mucosa should be sectioned parallel to the mucocutaneous junction.

by the needle even with malleting, then a small flap should be reflected so that the cortex can be thinned to allow the needle with a syringe attached to penetrate the cortex. The syringe should contain 1 to 2 ml of saline. As the plunger is pulled back, the first part of the return should be observed carefully. An IBC will characteristically return a few air bubbles before red blood is observed, primarily because the negative pressure in the central bony cavity from a tight needle fit will aspirate blood from the marrow space after the air has been evacuated.

Other vascular lesions, also under low pressure, may also return blood upon aspiration; however, an AVH will usually return blood immediately and push the plunger of the syringe back by its own pressure.

When accessing possible vascular lesions, the needle should be directed in three locations with the aspiration so as to assess the majority of the lesion. As a final check, the syringe should be removed, and blood flow observed at the hub of the needle. All lesions, other than an AVH, will trickle blood for a short time and stop. The AVH may actually spurt blood in a pulsating fashion and continue to bleed for much longer. If an AVH is suspected as a result of the aspiration method, bone wax can be placed in the cortex puncture site to stop any clinical

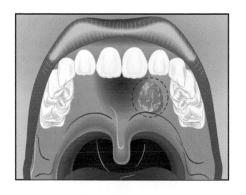

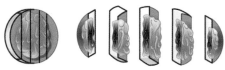

Figure 1.36 Soft palatal excisions should be sectioned parallel to the free dorsal tissue margin where the oral cavity mucosa and pharyngeal mucosa meet.

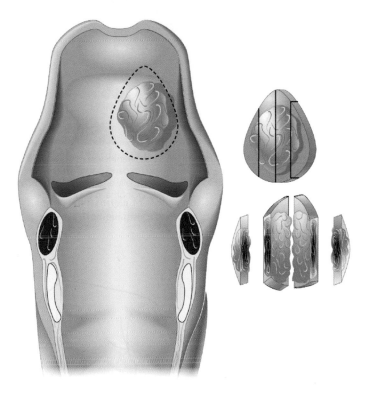

Figure 1.37 Laryngeal specimens should be sectioned in a fashion that is parallel to the long axis of the lesion. Decalcification of the specimen may be required, in which case appropriate anatomic structures (i.e. the epiglottis and cartilages) can be removed en block and serially sectioned.

bleeding and arrangements for angiography with the potential for embolization can be arranged.

Handling and Dissection of Head and Neck Tissue Surgical Specimens in Pediatric Age Patients

Head and neck tissue specimens from the child require specialized handling and sectioning largely because of the complex anatomy of the region. The seven most common anatomic areas (excluding brain and ear) from which specimens are received include tissue from; 1) the oral cavity, 2) the oropharynx, 3) the sinonasal region, 4) the larynx, 5) major or minor salivary glands, 6) the thyroid gland and rarely 7) neck dissections.

The pathologist is charged with not only evaluating tissue samples histologically and rendering a diagnosis but also with determining the extent of any lesional spread into adjacent anatomic structures. The adequacy of any surgical excision or resection as it relates to total or partial removal of pathology is the ultimate goal of the surgeon and pathologist.

Digital photography and image documentation of pre-dissection, intradissection and post-dissection specimens are mandatory, as these procedures can significantly aid in verifying tissue orientation, document the presence or absence of anatomic surfaces and record lesional or tumor association to anatomic structures.[16]

When a specimen is sectioned at the surgical bench, a corresponding description of every section, including that specimen's size and exact proportions in millimeters or centimeters of thickness must be documented. Sections of the maxilla, mandible, the various facial bones, larynx (rare in a child) and teeth will normally require either short or long-term decalcification. Large specimens can be managed by sectioning with a diamond saw that is water cooled. Decalcification of the total specimen prior to sectioning is generally inappropriate since over decalcification can occur. This author (ROG) has found that water-cooled sectioning with a dental handpiece and a diamond dental disk can be used quite effectively to section hard tissue specimens. However, any pathologist using such equipment must have the level of skill necessary to operate the handpiece and disk, and such equipment can be cost prohibitive.

When mucosal or skin surfaces are sectioned, all cuts should be made perpendicular to the skin or mucosal surface. Tissue that is handled from any anatomic area must be evaluated with an understanding of the embryology, and anatomical development of head and neck tissues. In the child, ectopic tissue of salivary gland and dental origin is often present. The surgical pathologist must recognize that such ectopic tissues have the potential to develop along cystic or neoplastic lines, and realize that the encountering of an apparent firm, cystic or partially encapsulated mass in an anatomic site that should be devoid of any structures may relate to the presence of ectopic progenitors.

Any surgical pathologist involved in the diagnosis of diseases involving the head and neck region of a child should have a familiarity with tooth development and must be aware of what teeth should or should not be present in the primary,

Two additional subtypes of fibroma that can commonly involve the head and neck region are elastofibroma and the sclerotic fibroma. Elastofibroma is a cutaneous pseudo tumor that is rarely identified in children. The elastofibroma will typically appear as soft tissue nodular growth that will be histologically composed of collagen fibers and coarse elastic fibers. The tumor's elastic fibers can readily be demonstrated with an elastin stain.[6,7] *Sclerotic fibroma* is an exceedingly rare cutaneous tumor that is most commonly identified in association with Cowden syndrome. Most sclerotic fibromas arise as solitary lesions but tumors can also be multifocal. Tumors will present as unencapsulated but well delineated masses. Histologically, the sclerotic fibroma will be composed of fibrous connective tissue that is relatively acellular and densely collagenized. The tumors will often have a storiform pattern and tumors can show clefting or spacing between collagen bundles. The sclerotic fibroma is vimentin and CD34 reactive.[6,7]

Gingival fibromatosis is a disorder that can resemble other fibrous hyperplasias that affect the oral cavity, but one that clearly deserves a separate classification. Gingival fibromatosis can be drug induced, idiopathic or hereditary. When gingival fibromatosis is either idiopathic or hereditary in origin, it typically presents as a diffuse non-inflammatory enlargement of the keratinized gingiva. Most cases of gingival fibromatosis are idiopathic and are non-painful and will result only in enlarged gingiva that can become so bulbous that it will cover the clinical crowns of teeth and erode subjacent bone. Gingival fibromatosis can be excised but often recurs rapidly.

Hereditary gingival fibromatosis is most often syndrome associated and typically linked to either Cross syndrome, Zimmerman–Laband syndrome or hypertrichosis syndrome. Children, rather than adults, represent the population most affected by the idiopathic and hereditary forms of gingival fibromatosis. When drug-induced gingival fibromatosis occurs in pediatric age group patients, it is most often associated with the use of three specific drugs, calcium channel blockers, cyclosporine and phenytoin.[8,9,10]

Gingival fibromatosis, depending on its unique subtype, is treated by surgery, scaling and root planing of the teeth or by drug discontinuance.

Juvenile Hyaline Fibromatosis

Juvenile hyaline fibromatosis (JHF) is a rare childhood autosomal recessive connective tissue disorder of undetermined origin. JHF most often involves the dermis and subcutaneous tissues to cause skin lesions that are painful enough to impair movement and cause significant disability. *Infantile systemic hyalinosis*, a disorder that overlaps with JHF clinicopathologically, will tend to present more often with visceral involvement rather than cutaneous. More significant patient symptomatology will also be present. Germ-line mutations in capillary morphogenesis gene-2 (CMG2) are considered to be responsible for both disorders.[11,12] Individuals with JHF will have significant abnormalities of collagen types three and four,[13,14] a

collagen defect that results in an underlying error in glycosaminoglycan formation and the accumulation of myelin in skin, mucosa and organs.[15]

Individuals with JHF involving the head and neck region will typically present with pearly papules and plaques of the face and posterior neck. Patients can also develop large subcutaneous nodules that affect the scalp, and a percentage of patients with JHF will display gingival hypertrophy. Largely a disorder of calcium metabolism, JHF is not classically a true neoplasm. Most individuals who develop the disorder will show signs of the process prior to the age of five. The often disfiguring masses that are associated with JHF have malignant potential.

Patients with JHF will frequently develop joint contractures and osteolytic bone lesions of the skull and jaws. Radiographically, fractures and osteoporosis may be encountered, and patients may demonstrate anemia, hypogammaglobulinemia, hypoalbuminema and electrolyte imbalance.

Clinical differential diagnostic considerations include cutaneous and oral mucosal lesions that result in nodular growths including keloids, sclerosing pyogenic granulomas of the oral cavity, hereditary gingival fibromatosis of the oral cavity, intraoral fibromas, dermatofibromas and neuromas.

Pathologic Features

Histopathologic examination of biopsies from individuals with JHF will demonstrate an amorphous, typically subepithelial, homogeneous, eosinophilic aggregation of stromal collagen. (Figures 2.6 & 2.7) The collagen will be arranged in a streaming fashion and there will be no cytologic atypia associated with proliferating fibroblasts. (Figure 2.8) Rarely, multinucleated giant cells can be identified and intracytoplasmic pink globules may be found distributed randomly throughout the amorphous ground substance. The hyaline material that is seen in JHF will stain periodic acid-Schiff positive, and be diastase resistant. The product will stain negatively with congo-red stains. Smooth muscle actin reactivity and S-100 protein reactivity will be negative in JHF.

Treatment and Prognosis

There is no definitive treatment that is curative for JHF. Oral mucosal and cutaneous lesions will sometimes have to be resected for esthetic reasons. Occasionally, intralesional injection of steroids into early lesions will result in quiescence. Physical therapy can be employed to prevent or ameliorate the symptoms that are associated with the joint contractures that patients with JHF experience.[6]

Nuchal-type Fibroma (NTF)

The NTF is an exceedingly rare benign lesion that most often arises in the posterior aspect of the neck. Tumors are of fibroblastic origin and most tumors present in individuals between the ages of 20 and 60.[17] In a review of 52 examples of NTFs analyzed from the files of the soft tissue registries of the Armed Forces Institute of Pathology, the mean age of

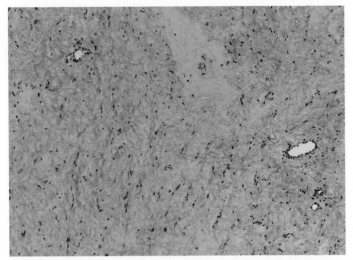

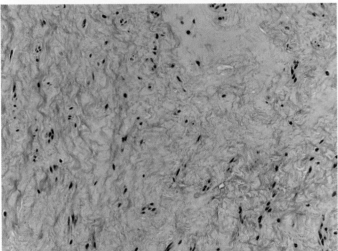

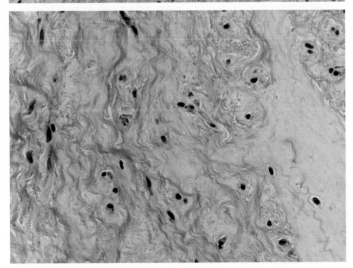

Figures 2.6 (top), 2.7 (middle) & 2.8 (bottom) JHF showing homogenous eosinophilic stromal collagen with streaming fibroblasts, at low, intermediate and high power.

patients was 40.[17] Tumors were identified in individuals as young as three years and as old as 74. Males outnumbered females significantly and the greatest dimension of most tumors at the time of diagnosis was 3.2 cm. There is a documented relationship between NTF and diabetes mellitus, and a strong association of NTF, especially those in children, to Gardner's syndrome.[18,19,20,21] Children with nuchal fibromas, however, rarely develop the colorectal adenocarcinoma associated with Gardner's syndrome.

NTFs in children can be single or multiple when they occur in the head and neck region and there is a relationship between these fibromas and the ultimate development of desmoid-type fibromas in NTF affected children.

Pathologic Features

NTFs are characterized histologically by the presence of a haphazard arrangement of dense collagen fibers that do not show cytologic atypia. The collagen fibers or bundles are most often entrapped within skeletal muscle or adipose tissue, or intertwined within peripheral nerves. From a microscopic differential diagnostic standpoint, elastofibroma, desmoid-type fibromatosis and fibrolipoma should be considered. The NTF differs from desmoid fibromatosis by virtue of the fact that desmoid fibromatosis will be composed of exceedingly long fascicles of fibro-collagen, whereas the NTF will be composed of aggregates of collagen fibers that are more attenuated blunt and foreshortened. Vascular hyperplasia is common to desmoid fibromatosis but will generally be lacking in NTF. The elastofibroma will typically contain elastic fibers and the NTF will not. NTFs are generally CD34 positive and tumors will stain strongly for vimentin, and more rarely with CD99. β-catenin reactivity can be found in approximately 66 percent of cases.[5,6]

Although the etiology of NTF remains unknown, Levesque et al. have reported a sentinel truncating mutation in *APC* in a 32-month-old child.

Treatment and Prognosis

NTFs are managed by complete surgical excision, and solitary tumors are usually cured by this single surgical procedure. Individuals with Gardner syndrome will develop desmoid-type fibromatosis in a significant number of cases, therefore additional NTFs must be excluded in those patients. Recurrence of NTFs does occur in patients with syndrome and non-syndrome associated disease, therefore close long-term follow-up of the child with NTFs or NTFs that are associated Gardner's syndrome is recommended.[21]

Nodular Fasciitis (Proliferative Fasciitis)
Clinical Findings

Nodular fasciitis, known by a host of names – including proliferative fasciitis, pseudosarcomatous fibromatosis and nodular pseudosarcomatous fasciitis – is classically a painless, benign, soft tissue lesion that most often affects superficial fascia.

21

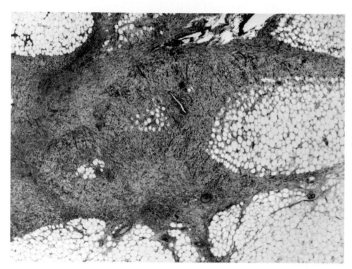

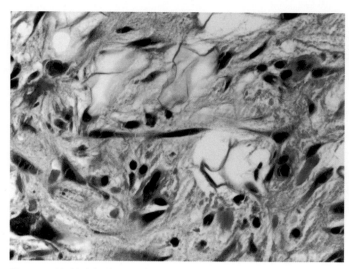

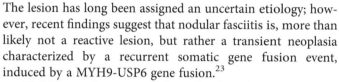

Figure 2.9 Nodular fasciitis demonstrating fascicles and bundles of collagen that can be seen extending in an infiltrative fashion into marginating submucosal adipose tissue.

Figure 2.10 Nodular fasciitis demonstrating primitive loosely arranged fibroblasts that have the appearance of cells growing in culture.

The lesion has long been assigned an uncertain etiology; however, recent findings suggest that nodular fasciitis is, more than likely not a reactive lesion, but rather a transient neoplasia characterized by a recurrent somatic gene fusion event, induced by a MYH9-USP6 gene fusion.[23]

Children and young adults will often develop nodular fasciitis in the head and neck region, along with a unique form of the disorder known as *cranial fasciitis*, which is most often identified in infants. Cranial fasciitis is limited to the scalp and can grow rapidly, and involve underlying bone. Patchefsky and Enzsinger have also identified a unique form of *intravascular fasciitis*, common in the head and neck region of children.[24]

Nodular fasciitis can occur in subfascial and subcutaneous spaces as a self-limiting myofibroblastic proliferation that can inappropriately be diagnosed as sarcoma because of its rapid growth and significant cytologic atypia. Pandian et al.[25] reviewed a large series of nodular fasciitis cases seen in children who were 18 years or younger in the Mayo Clinic study and found that the vast majority of lesions arose as rapidly enlarging mass, but without any related symptomatology in approximately 15 percent of patients. Dayan et al.[26] in a review of 36 cases of nodular fasciitis involving the oral cavity, found that most lesions affected the buccal mucosa and lips, and that their duration ranged from three days to two years.

Clinical differential diagnoses for nodular fasciitis in a child or young adult can include a host of lesions including soft tissue sarcomas, extraosseous odontogenic tumors and benign tumors of smooth muscle, salivary glands and desmoid-type fibromatosis. Since nodular fasciitis can closely resemble malignant disease clinically, biopsy is always appropriate in order to establish a definitive diagnosis. The most diagnostic area of any portion of a lesion thought to represent nodular fasciitis will be the deep tissue. Superficial biopsies can often result in a misdiagnosis.[26,27,28]

Pathologic Features

Nodular fasciitis will present grossly at the time of surgery as a soft tissue mass that will often be slightly gelatinous. There is a tendency for subfascial lesions to be well circumscribed, if not encapsulated, whereas lesions that are within fascia tend to appear less well circumscribed.

Microscopically, nodular fasciitis will consist of a proliferation of spindle type cells that are organized in a fascicular pattern as they extend into collagen or fat. (Figure 2.9) That pattern of growth will often be that of a loose arrangement of tumor cells that will cause the cells to appear as if they are cells growing in tissue culture. (Figure 2.10) The tumor may show areas of myxoid degeneration, extensive fibrosis, hyalinization, granulation tissue formation and microhemorrhage. The cell cytology seen in what is essentially a myofibroblastic proliferation will be typically bland, and tumor cells will not display the cytologic atypia that is characteristic of a malignant neoplasm, although mitoses can be common. Multinucleated type giant cells will often be identified with the tumor, and cells that appear neurogenic in origin or ganglion-like in appearance will also be seen within the tumor mass. It is not unusual for nodular fasciitis in pediatric age group patients to show areas of necrosis. Such zonal necrosis should not be interpreted as representing malignant neoplasia.

Since the cells that make up nodular fasciitis are in fact myofibroblasts, they will stain positively with not when calponin, smooth muscle actin and muscle specific actin.[29] β-catenin will not be expressed by nodular fasciitis tumor cells, an IHC finding that helps to separate nodular fasciitis from desmoid-type fibromatosis, which will show positive expression of β-catenin. Nodular fasciitis will not usually demonstrate desmin, CD34 or CT68 reactivity. The so-called *inflammatory myofibroblastic tumor* that can be seen in children can be distinguished from nodular fasciitis by virtue of the fact that the

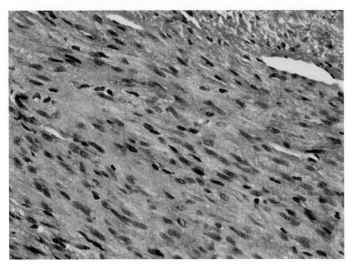

Figure 2.11 Myofibroma demonstrating plump spindle cells and rare oval myofibroblasts. Sparse, slightly irregularly shaped vessels can also be identified.

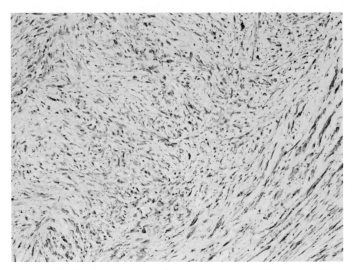

Figure 2.12 Myofibroma tumor cells stain moderately positive for smooth muscle actin.

inflammatory myofibroblastic tumor will be characterized by an ALK gene arrangement that is not seen in nodular fasciitis.[30]

Nodular fasciitis in the pediatric age group patient must be differentiated from malignant spindle cell neoplasms such as fibrosarcoma. Fibrosarcoma will generally arise deeper in its anatomic location than nodular fasciitis, and fibrosarcomas will tend to be larger in size than nodular fasciitis. Fibrosarcoma will typically demonstrate a herringbone pattern histologically that will not be seen with nodular fasciitis, and most fibrosarcomas are of a longer duration than any of the forms of nodular fasciitis that occur in childhood.

Treatment and Prognosis

Nodular fasciitis is treated by conservative surgical excision, and regardless of their site of origin, tumors rarely re-occur.[31] When assessing soft tissue lesions of the head and neck in children in an attempt to determine whether a spindle cell lesion might be benign or malignant on clinicopathologic grounds, the following features should be considered. The absence of cytologic atypia, atypical mitotic figures, a small tumor size, a short lesional history and a superficial anatomic location would favor a benign process such as nodular fasciitis. Although various forms of nodular fasciitis have been described, including fascial, subcutaneous and intradermal subtypes, none of these tumor subtypes have shown any form of aggressive behavior and all tumor subtypes appear to be self-limiting.[32]

Infantile Myofibromatosis and Solitary Myofibroma

Infantile myofibromatosis is a proliferative disorder of infants and children that is characterized by the development of single or multiple nodular lesions that arise in cutaneous, subcutaneous or submucosal tissues, muscle, bone or viscera. Solitary lesions are clinically classified as solitary myofibromas, while multiple lesions are defined as myofibromatosis. Lesions arising in adults will always be solitary in nature.[33,34,35]

In the head and neck region, lesions can involve any soft tissue site but most often affect the soft tissue of the tongue, lips and buccal mucosa. Tumors of the dermal soft tissue and fascia are less common. Tumors can also arise centrally within bones.[36] Tumors will usually present as nodular soft tissue masses. Lesions that involve bone will usually present as well demarcated radiolucent lesions that show peripheral enhancement on CT. Boys are more often affected than girls regardless of whether the lesions are solitary or multiple. Ninety-two percent of individuals who have multiple myofibromas will present with lesions at birth.

Pathologic Features

Myofibromas grow as nodular lesions that are usually well demarcated, firm and non-painful. Tumors that are richly vascularized can often take on the appearance of a hemangioma when inspected grossly. Tumors will typically be composed of two relatively distinctive components histologically. A peripheral marginating aggregation of fusiform or spindle shaped cells that are arranged in fascicles, and a central tumor zone that will be composed of round, often pericyte-like cells. (Figure 2.11) The peripheral marginating tumor cells may demonstrate hyalinoid or chondroid differentiation, while the central portion of the tumor may show necrosis. Tumors in pediatric age patients will most often display the fusiform pattern of cell proliferation.

Tumors will stain immunohistochemically positive for smooth muscle actin (Figure 2.12) and vimentin, while S-100 protein and desmin stains will be negative. The biphasic histologic pattern that is seen in myofibroma, should allow one to distinguish the lesion from more monophasic tumors such as desmoid-type fibromatosis, odontogenic myxoma, fibrosarcoma and spindle cell neoplasms, including neurofibroma, leiomyoma and myoepithelial neoplasms of salivary gland origin.[37,38,39,40]

Treatment and Prognosis

Most infantile myofibromas in the head and neck region of pediatric age patients will be solitary lesions and local surgical excision will affect a cure.[40] Rare spontaneous regression of tumors has been reported. However, when multicentric infantile lesions occur, the prognosis is less favorable, and with visceral involvement the prognosis for the patient is quite poor. Twenty percent of patients with multicentric visceral involvement will die during the first days of life. Recurrence is common in patients with multicentric disease. Up to three years after surgery, the relapse rate is reported to be 7 to 9 percent.[40] Individuals with multicentric infantile myofibromatosis can present with up to 100 myofibromas. In such cases surgical abstinence may be appropriate. Chemotherapy and radiation therapy have not been proven effective for this disorder.

Myositis Ossificans

Myositis ossificans (MO) arises as ectopic or heterotopic form of bone formation in soft tissue and skeletal muscle.[41] Three specific forms of MO have been identified; 1) a severe and aggressive progressive form of the disease that is generalized and hereditary, which can be precipitated by trauma, 2) a non-traumatic form of MO in which there is no history of trauma and 3) MO circumscripta, a non-aggressive form of MO that occurs in concert with direct trauma.[42] The progressive form of the disease originates as a result of connective tissue maldevelopment and affects tendons, aponeuroses, muscle fascia and muscle. This form of the disease which is transmitted as an autosomal dominant trait is rare in children. The most common form of MO to occur in children is the circumscripta form of the disease, which accounts for 60 to 75 percent of all cases in children.[42,43,44]

MO circumscripta, most commonly affects the arms, legs, shoulders and hands. Rarely is the head and neck region involved. When affected, the most common site of occurrence in the head and neck is the masseter muscle. When MO circumscripta will present as a painful doughy soft tissue mass, it may be misconstrued in a child to represent some form of soft tissue sarcoma. Imaging studies, including MRI imaging will typically show a strongly enhanced soft tissue lesion with a central irregular hypointense area. The enhancement may also be diffuse throughout the muscle or poorly delineated. Plain film radiographs can also often delineate MO.[43,44] MO cirsumscripta will be typically developed in three distinct zonal patterns, in which the disease begins as a fibrous cellular proliferation that progresses through stages of endochondral ossification to ultimately transition to mature lamellar bone. MO circumscripta can develop following bone fracture, joint dislocation and even after minor contusions. In the wake of such traumatic episodes, inflammation ensues, and on the heels of the inflammatory process a fibro-proliferative response occurs that ultimately leads not to normal repair, but to ossification.

The genetic cause of progressive or aggressive MO is thought to be caused by a recurrent missense mutation in the GS activation domain of activin receptor LA/activin-like kinese 2(ACVR1/ALK2). These genetic alterations have not been identified in the traumatic form of the disease.[45,46]

Pathologic Features

The histologic findings in MO circumscripta, closely parallel the lesion's hallmark radiographic findings of zonal proliferation. Initially, MO circumscripta will be characterized by a central zonal proliferation of fibroblasts set in a richly vascularized mesenchymal stroma.[47,48] Fibroblasts within the stroma will demonstrate a high mitotic rate and they will be associated with significant hemorrhage. A secondary intermediate or middle zone will be dominated histologically by a proliferation of osteoblasts, an immature osteoid product with occasional areas of cartilage formation. Finally, a marginating or peripheral zone that is largely composed of mature bone will be identified. At full maturity a densely realized margin of mature compact bone will surround a core of lamellar bone. From a differential diagnostic perspective, MO can resemble Garre's osteomyelitis, osteoid osteoma, a fracture callus, parosteal osteosarcoma, fibrosarcoma, osteomyelitis or a childhood mesenchymal malignancy.[49,50] It is therefore exceedingly important to attempt to identify a history of antecedent trauma when establishing a clinicopathologic differential diagnosis.

Treatment and Prognosis

The progressive and aggressive hereditary form of MO represents a severe generalized form of the disease that is difficult to eradicate. In fact, with this form of the disease, areas of surgical excision can re-ossify and limit mobility following a surgical procedure. The progressive form of the disease can proceed to immobility and even respiratory failure.[47] Steroids and Accutane have been used in the management of the progressive disease with little effect. In rare instances, the progressive form of the disease has been managed by radiotherapy.

Most forms of the far more common MO circumscripta are managed by an initial biopsy in which the disease is appropriately diagnosed. Eventual resolution of the traumatically induced lesion occurs in most instances.

Calcifying Fibrous Tumor (Calcifying Fibrous Pseudotumor)

Originally described as a childhood fibrous tumor with psammoma bodies, the calcifying fibrous tumor represents a form of fibrous hyperplasia with associated calcifications that can affect the trunk, the neck, the medistenium, the extremities, the paratesticular region and the oral cavity.[51,52] When the lesion occurs in the head and neck region the most common location is the neck.[53] The etiology of the tumor is unknown. Lesions tend to be painless and most patients will not give a history of trauma or surgery in the affected area. CT scans may show a well delineated soft tissue mass with calcifications, while plain film radiographs will typically show a non-calcified tumor that is well marginated. MRI images tend to give a mottled tumor signal that resembles that of muscle or adipose tissue. Tumors can range in size from 1 cm to 15 cm in diameter.

Pathologic Features

Grossly, tumors will be marginated by collagen but not encapsulated. Microscopically, hyalinized fibro-sclerotic tissue with zones of calcification that are psammomatoid or dystrophic will be identified within the tumor mass in high percentage of cases. Inflammatory cells are common to the tumor stroma. Mitotic activity is generally low and cytologic atypia will be absent. Most of the tumor will be composed of spindle cells that are histologically uniform and that are of fibroblastic origin. Spindle cells will express vimentin, smooth muscle actin, desmin and factor 8A. S-100 protein IHC stains, and stains for CD31 stains will be negative. Histologically, the tumor can resemble desmoid-type fibromatosis, solitary fibrous tumor (SFT) and infantile fibrosarcoma. Evaluation of tumor cells for atypical mitotic activity is important in order to rule out malignant neoplasia. The ALK reactivity and chromosome 2p22-24 abnormalities that can be observed in inflammatory and myofibroblastic tumors are absent in the calcifying fibrous tumors.[54,55]

Treatment and Prognosis

The calcifying fibrous tumor is most often managed by complete surgical excision to a margin of normal tissue and recurrence is rare.[56]

Desmoid-type Fibromatosis (Aggressive Fibromatosis, Desmoid Tumor)

Desmoid-type fibromatoses represent a group of locally aggressive non-metastasizing tumors of mesenchymal origin that are considered to be of intermediate or borderline malignancy.[57] Considered to be a neoplasm of unpredictable biologic behavior, desmoid-type fibromatoses occur throughout most anatomic regions of the body, and as a group, will affect muscle, adipose tissue and bone. Approximately 10 percent of all cases occur in the head and neck region.[58] The natural history of desmoid tumors in the head and neck region as elsewhere, is somewhat unpredictable and the precise etiology of the disorder has not been determined, although Flucke et al.[57] have shown that in a group of seven childhood desmoid-type fibromatoses, mutations in the CTNNB1 gene could be demonstrated.

Most desmoid-type fibromatoses in the head and neck of pediatric age patients will present as solitary, painless, rapidly enlarging growths or masses. Tumors that arise in individuals from birth up to five years are generally termed infantile fibromatosis of the desmoid type. These tumors are more common in girls than boys.[59] Desmoid tumors that affect the oral and maxillofacial region tend to appear in individuals

who range from 5 to 20 years of age. Lesions in this site are somewhat more infiltrative and faster growing than the desmoid-type fibromatoses that occur in other head and neck sites. Lesions that arise within the nasal sinuses tend to emerge rapidly over a one to two month period, and they often show a central destructive pattern involving medullary bone. Although lesions that involve the soft tissues of the neck usually manifest as a painless neck swelling, patients may at times complain of otitis media or a chronic tonsillar infection. As tumors grow, regardless of their site of origin, they can infiltrate nerves and cause pain and muscle dysfunction. Desmoid-type tumors of the head and neck region tend not to be encapsulated and tend to blend into surrounding tissues as they grow. *Fibromatosis colli* is a rare form of fibromatosis that is typically identified within the first two weeks of life. In nearly all instances, fibromatosis colli will involve the sternocleidomastoid muscle. The vast majority of cases will undergo regression within the first year of a child's life.

Pathologic Features

On gross inspection, desmoid tumors will generally present as a firm rubbery soft tissue mass. Histologically, desmoid-type fibromatosis will present as a circumscribed mass that will be composed of interlacing fascicles of collagen and aggregates of spindle shaped fibroblasts. Tumors tend to be infiltrative, but tumor cells will not appear atypical cytologically. Most tumors will consist of interlacing collagen fascicles that have incorporated within them a large number of small vascular channels. Inflammation is common to desmoid-type fibromatosis, as are areas of myxoid degeneration and zones of dense collagenation resembling scar. Tumors can contain aggregates of multinucleated giant cells, generally at their periphery, and tumor necrosis is rare. (Figure 2.13)

Desmoid tumors are phenotypically fibroblastic or myofibroblastic and tumor cells will tend to stain positively for smooth muscle actin, and β catenin.

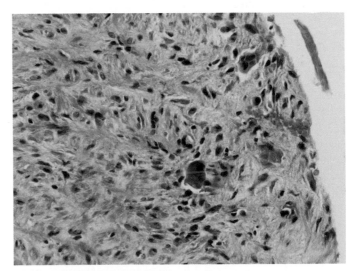

Figure 2.13 Desmoid-type fibromatosis shows primitive collagen fascicles marginated by multinucleated giant cells.

Differential Diagnoses

Desmoid-type fibromatosis can resemble juvenile or infantile fibrosarcoma; however, it can be distinguished from fibrosarcoma based upon the uniformity of its growth pattern, the relative maturity of its cells, the tumor's general lack of atypical mitotic figures and its lack of invasion into surrounding structures. Desmoid-type fibromatosis can also resemble peripheral nerve tumors and nodular fasciitis microscopically. Tumors of nerve sheath origin will be S-100 protein reactive, unlike desmoid fibromatosis. Nodular fasciitis tends to be a much smaller tumor than most desmoid-type fibromatoses, and nodular fasciitis will also demonstrate a primitive cell culture appearance with myxoid stromal change. Although desmoid-type fibromatosis can closely resemble scar tissue or a keloid, desmoid tumors tend to arise as much deeper lesions than keloids or scar, and they will demonstrate a more infiltrative pattern of growth than either scar or a keloid.

Treatment and Prognosis

Desmoid-type fibromatoses in the head and neck region are treated by wide local excision regardless of whether they arise in soft tissue or bone. A surgical margin of 1 to 1.5 cm and frozen section control at the time of surgery are mandatory. Although surgery remains the treatment of choice for desmoplastic type fibromatosis, some tumors have been treated using radiotherapy. However, radiation therapy is usually reserved for lesions that are large and unresectable, for recurrent tumors or for tumors that have been incompletely excised. Rare radiation induced sarcomas have been reported to arise from previously treated desmoid fibromatoses. Chemotherapy, employing Adriamycin cyclophosphamide and actinomyocin-D have been used to treat tumors where residual lesion remains following surgery.[60,61,62,63]

Solitary Fibrous Tumor

The SFT, considered to be a component of the hemangiopericytoma spectrum of neoplasms, was originally described by Klemperer and Rabin in 1931.[64] Since that original description, the tumor has been assigned a host of names, ranging from sclerosing hemangioma to subplural fibroma.

The vast majority of SFTs occur in adults and affect the plura. Tumors in children are quite rare. In a 2013 review, Noriko et al.[65] were able to identify only 12 reported cases of SFT in the head and neck region of children.[65,66]

Most SFTs that have been described in the head and neck region have occurred in the nasal cavity.[66] This author (ROG) has diagnosed only one SFT of the head and neck, (a lesion of the tongue) in a pediatric age patient over the course of more than 40 years of practice as a pathologist. Clinically most tumors will present as a soft tissue nodule or mass. MRI imaging will tend to reveal a well circumscribed hypointense mass. The most common clinical differential diagnoses for SFT in the head and neck area of a child include sheath tumors, salivary gland neoplasms and the fibromatoses.

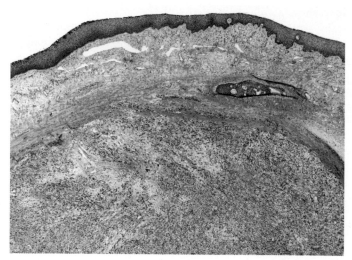

Figure 2.14 Solitary fibrous tumor composed of a nodular aggregate of spindle cells.

Pathologic Features

Grossly, the SFT will present as a firm often hemorrhagic nodular mass. The tumor will be composed largely of spindle-shaped cells that lack cytologic atypia. (Figure 2.14) These spindle cells are often described as having a "patternless" orientation. Ramifying throughout the tumor's spindled parenchyma will be numerous branching vessels that often take on a hemangiopericytoma-like, stage horn type of appearance. Separation of collagen fibrils and myxoid change are common. (Figures 2.15 & 2.16) Tumors will tend not to show areas of necrosis, but will demonstrate collagen hyalinization. On IHC examination, tumor cells will be immunoreactive to CD34 and vimentin, and reactive, although weakly, to CD50 and CD99. Tumors will be epithelial membrane antigen (EMA) negative, S-100 protein negative, smooth muscle actin negative, desmin negative and β-catenin negative immunohistochemically. The most significant IHC finding to be seen in association with the SFT is its strong CD34 reactivity. Tumor cells strongly recognize this single chain transmembrane glycoprotein which is associated with vascular progenitor cells, which points to a fibrovascular origin for the tumor.[67,68]

Treatment and Prognosis

SFTs are managed by complete surgical excision to a margin of normal tissue. Tumors have little potential for recurrence. However, the pathobiology of these tumors in the head and neck region remains poorly understood and long-term follow-up is necessary for all pediatric age patients.

Benign Fibrohistiocytic Tumors

Benign Fibrous Histiocytoma

Benign fibrohistiocytic tumors of the head and neck can be classified as cutaneous lesions, deep and non-cutaneous, or osseous lesions. The vast majority of benign fibrous histiocytomas

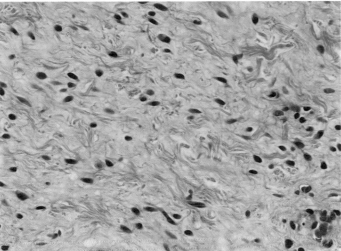

Figures 2.15 (top) & 2.16 (bottom) The myxoid change characteristic of the solitary fibrous tumor and the separation of collagen fibrils common to the tumor can be seen in these low and high power photomicrographs.

arise as cutaneous lesions and are discussed more completely in Chapter 3 of this text. Regardless of subclassification, most benign fibrous histiocytomas will affect males between the ages of 25 and 40.[69] Deep and non-cutaneous benign histiocytomas of the head and neck account for 30 percent of all tumors.[69,70] The most commonly affected head and neck sites are the buccal mucosa, the submandibular triangle, the tongue, the larynx, the nasal cavity, the mandible and the supra follicular fossa.[69,71] Benign fibrous histiocytomas are exceedingly rare in children with most pediatric cases reported in the literature occurring in the nasal sinuses and the oral cavity.[72,73,74,75,76]

Benign fibrous histiocytomas that involve the nasal sinuses, most commonly result in initial symptoms of nasal obstruction, epistaxis, dysphasia and dysphonia. Patients who present with lesions involving the oral cavity will typically present with a complaint of a swelling. If a lesion occurs posteriorly in the tongue, patients will occasionally complain of dysphasia, dysphonia or snoring.[75]

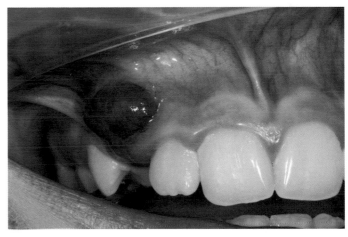

Figure 2.17 Benign fibrous histiocytoma presenting as a hemorrhagic soft tissue mass that involves the maxillary alveolar mucosa. (Courtesy of Dr. Thomas Borris).

Tumors will generally present clinically as a soft tissue mass, ranging in size from 2–12 cm in diameter (Figure 2.17). Lesions of the oral soft tissue will tend to present as red nodular masses that are often ulcerated and have the appearance of a pyogenic granuloma. Differential diagnoses can include pyogenic granuloma, irritation fibroma, dermatofibroma, hemangioma, traumatic eosinophilic granuloma, SFT and verruciform xanthoma, among other tumors. Central bony lesions will appear as a well circumscribed radiolucency on plain films.

Pathologic Features

Grossly, the benign fibrous histiocytoma will present as rubbery mass, whether in soft tissue or in bone, and tumors will tend to have a cut surface that is white and fibroelastic in consistency. Microscopic examination will reveal a storiform admixture of collagen fibers with interlacing scattered aggregates of proliferating fibroblasts and foamy histiocytes. (Figures 2.18 & 2.19). Collagen bundles that appear hyalinized are common to the tumor and individual tumor cells will appear lightly eosinophilic. A mixed inflammatory cellular infiltrate is common to the tumor and tumors will frequently contain multinucleated and Touton-type giant cells.

A storiform pattern of tumor cells tends to be more common to lesions that have been classified as *cellular benign fibrous histiocytomas*. The cells that make up the more classic benign fibrous histiocytoma will consist of a relatively heterogeneous non-storiform proliferation of both spindled fibroblastic appearing cells, and aggregates of tumor cells that are more oval. These secondary oval cells will be less oval than those seen in dermatofibrosarcoma proturberans. Cellular benign fibrous histiocytomas will tend to demonstrate a greater degree of cytologic atypia than classical lesions and in fact they may show cellular necrosis.

Benign fibrous histiocytomas typically demonstrate tumor cell CD68 reactivity when stained immunohistochemically. Tumor cells will also stain positively for vimentin.

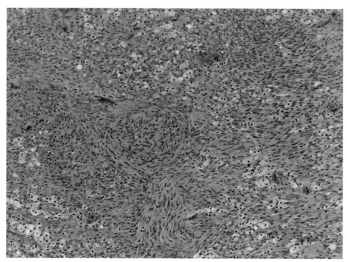

Figure 2.41 Schwannoma composed of well organized spindle cell aggregates (Antoni A tissue) and loosely arranged spindle and epithelioid cells (Antoni B tissue).

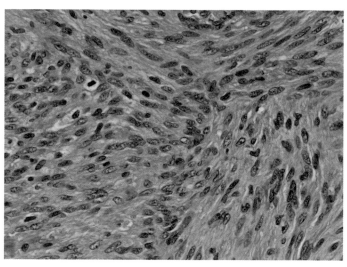

Figure 2.43 Loosely arranged spindle to epithelioid cells with occasional vacuoles between them characterize Antoni B type tissue is a Schwannoma.

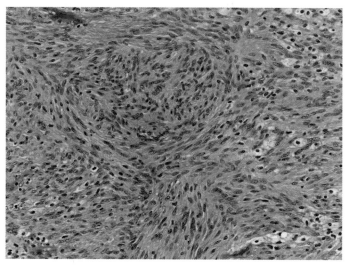

Figure 2.42 Palisaded clusters of Antoni A tissue are seen in this Schwannoma.

do neurofibromas. Thus Schwannomas are more easily excised. Complete surgical excision is usually curative. The prognosis for the patient is excellent and recurrence is rare.

Granular Cell Tumor

Clinical Findings

Granular cell tumors are benign tumors of Schwann cell origin. Although granular cell tumors have been reported to arise in the skin, breast and lungs, the majority of all tumors will arise in the head and neck region. The tongue is by far the most common site of occurrence.[169,170] Tumors are most commonly identified in individuals in the second through fourth decades of life, and although tumors do occur in children and adolescents, they are rare. Granular cell tumors show a predilection for women and are somewhat more common in African Americans than other ethnic groups.[171,172,173] Tumors can present as multifocal lesions, and as many as 20 percent of granular cell tumors will arise in more than one anatomic site in an individual. Most lesions will be less than 2 to 3 cm in diameter at the time of their diagnosis and in pediatric age group patients, as a rule, lesions will be poorly circumscribed nodules (Figure 2.44) that have been growing for six months to one year prior to their recognition.

Clinically, the granular cell tumor can resemble rhabdomyoma, lipoma, RMS, sclerosing hemangioma, pyogenic granulomas and other benign and reactive tumors of fibrous connective tissue origin.

Pathologic Features

Grossly, the granular cell tumor will present as a poorly circumscribed non-encapsulated infiltrative mass. Tumors tend to be somewhat fibrotic in appearance and they are histologically characterized by the proliferation of large polygonal, round or oval cells with small hyperchromatic nuclei and cytoplasm that is richly granular. The coarse cytoplasm of tumor cells is most often quite eosinophilic and the tumor cells will tend to be arranged in clusters, or sheets that are separated by fibrous connective tissue. (Figure 2.45) Approximately 30 percent of granular cell tumors will show some relationship to a nerve. Rarely, tumor cells show a minimal degree of pleomorphism.

One of the most characteristic features of granular cell tumors of the oral cavity and pharyngeal areas will be the association of tumor cells with marked pseudoepitheliomatous hyperplasia of any overlying surface epithelium. (Figure 2.46) This hyperplasia will be seen in approximately 50 percent of oropharyngeal tumors.[174,175] The granular cells seen within the tumor are typically strongly and diffusely positive for S-100 protein, vimentin, calretinin, NKI/C3 and inhibin-alpha.[1]

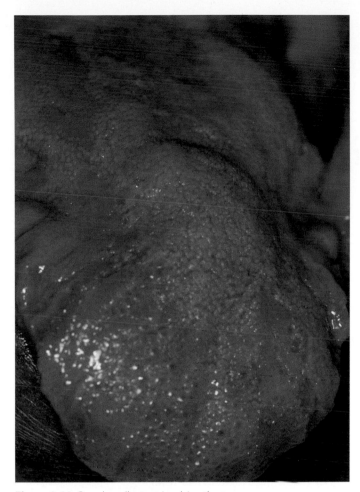

Figure 2.44 Granular cell tumor involving the tongue.

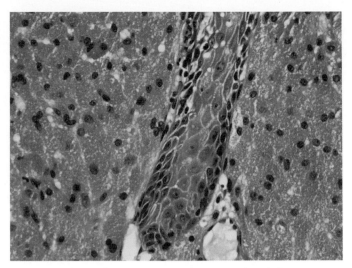

Figure 2.46 Granular cell tumor demonstrating pseudoepitheliomatous hyperplastic epithelium knifing its way between granular cells.

tumor cells that show altered nuclear cytoplasmic ratios, significant mitotic and cytologic atypia, a prominent fascicular growth pattern and necrosis.[8] No such tumors have been reported in children, although some degree of cellular pleomorphism may be evident in the typical granular cell tumor of a child.

It is, above all, important for the surgical pathologist to be able to separate a squamous epithelial malignancy of oral or pharyngeal epithelium from the cancer mimicking pseudoepitheliomatous hyperplasia that can be seen in association with the granular cell tumor.

Treatment and Prognosis

Granular cell tumors are usually treated by local excision of the tumor to a margin of normal tissue. In most instances such surgery is curative. However, 7 percent of granular cell tumors recur.[170] The recurrence rate may be related to the fact that the tumors can grow in an infiltrative-type pattern with associated satellite tumor nodules, which may give rise to recurrent disease. There are documented cases in which the lesions have undergone spontaneous regression, but such occurrences are quite rare.

Congenital Granular Cell Tumor (Congenital Epulis)

The congenital tumor is a rare tumor that affects newborns. Present at birth, the congenital granular cell tumor will present as a nodule or a mass that will arise most often from the anterior maxillary or mandibular gingiva. Once referred to as "congenital epulis of the newborn," tumors will vary in size from as small as several millimeters in diameter to as large as 10 cm in diameter. Lesions are painless and they typically arise from a stalk-like process. Instances in which multiple lesions arise from the maxilla or mandible have been documented.[177] Schwann cells have long been considered by many investigators to be the source of origin for the congenital granular cell tumor; however, the true histogenesis of the tumor remains

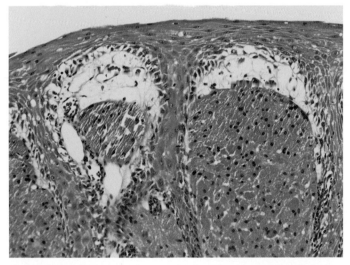

Figure 2.45 Large polygonal to round cells with richly granular cytoplasm characterize this granular cell tumor.

Malignant granular cell tumors have been reported; however, they are exceedingly rare and there is considerable debate in the literature as to whether or not such tumors truly represent a granular cell neoplasm. These rare tumors are characterized by

unclear, largely because ultrastructural and IHC findings suggest that tumors may be of mesenchymal origin, and that some tumor cells have features that suggest a histiocytic or fibroblastic or orgin.[178] It is also possible that the tumors arise from vascular pericytes or even from smooth muscle as opposed to Schwann cells.[179] Lesions will tend to appear clinically as relatively vascular lesions. The stalk on which they arise can be rich in blood supply and the tumors can bleed quite readily.

Clinically, the congenital granular cell tumor can closely resemble the melanotic neruorectodermal tumor of infancy. However, the melanotic neuroectodermal tumor typically occurs two months to eighteen months following birth, and the lesion will characteristically appear dark blue, or black. While neuroblastoma and RMS can resemble a congenital granular cell tumor clinically, those tumors tend to be quite destructive of underlying bone and will grow quite rapidly as malignant rather than benign processes. One of the most common classes of tumors to resemble the congenital granular cell tumor is the broad group of angiomatous lesions that can arise in pediatric age patients. These vascular tumors tend to arise as sessile solitary growths, however, and rarely arise from a stalk.[179,180]

Pathologic Features

The congenital granular cell tumor, on gross inspection will usually demonstrate a homogenous tan cut surface. Histologically, the tumor will be composed of sheets, nests, cords and clusters of polygonal cells with round to oval nuclei and abundant granular cytoplasm. (Figure 2.47) The histological appearance of the tumor is identical to that of the granular cell tumor of adults; however, the congenital granular cell tumor will not demonstrate the common surface pseudoepitheliomatous hyperplasia seen in the adult tumor. Congenital granular cell tumors will stain positively for S-100 protein, vimentin, actin and desmin. Interestingly, electron microscopic examination of tumor cells will show granular cells that contain heterogeneous electron-dense granules, lysosomes and cytoplasmic lipid droplets, features that do not support a Schwann cell derivation for the tumor.

Treatment and Prognosis

The congenital granular cell tumor is treated by surgical excision. Tumors rarely recur, and there are reports of tumors spontaneously regressing.[181]

Neuromas

Neuromas are a class of neurogenic tumors that can affect all anatomic regions of the body including the head and neck. Most head and neck neoplasms in children will affect the skin, or the oral/pharyngeal mucosa. Eighty-five percent of all neuromas, regardless of subtype, will be benign. Three types of neuromas can be seen in the soft tissues of the head and neck of children; 1) traumatic neuroma, 2) neuromas that arise as a component of multiple endocrine neoplasia syndrome 2B and 3) palisaded encapsulated neuroma. The *palisaded encapsulated neuroma*, which will usually present as a subcutaneous or submucosal nodule, is, however, exceedingly rare in children. The tumor will be composed of an encapsulated nodular admixture of spindle cells with wavy nuclei and mature Schwann cells with rare axons. (Figure 2.48) The palisaded encapsulated neuroma may be continuous with the perineurium of a peripheral nerve.[1] Tumors are of Schwann cell origin, and they will be S-100 reactive immunohistochemically. Tumors show little tendency to recur.

The multiple mucosal neuromas that are a component of *multiple endocrine neoplasia syndrome 2B* present as multiple nodular lesions that can affect the oral mucosal (most often the tongue), the eyelids and the intestinal tract. The vast majority of syndrome associated neuromas are identified within the first

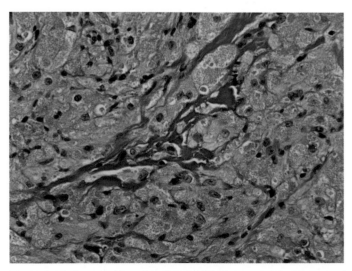

Figure 2.47 Congenital granular cell tumor showing an aggregation of round to polygonal cells with granular cytoplasm.

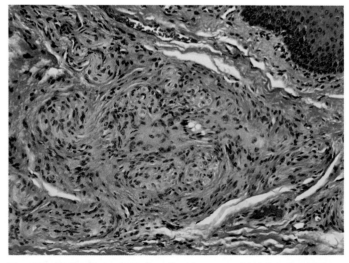

Figure 2.48 An admix of spindle cells with wavy nuclei and mature Schwann cells make up this palisaded encapsulated neuroma.

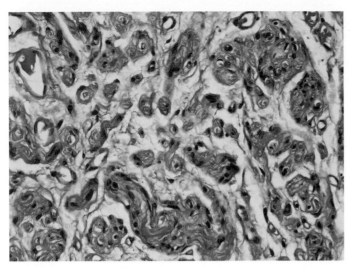

Figure 2.49 Neuroma of the tongue in a child with MEN 2B syndrome. Note the hyperplasia of nerve bundles that can be seen in a loosely arranged connective tissue stroma.

year of life and will histologically be characterized by hyperplasia of nerve bundles with a loose connective tissue stroma (Figure 2.49) nerve bundles that have a marginating prominent perineurium. Syndromic neuromas are associated with medullary carcinoma or hyperplasia of the thyroid gland, adrenal phenochromocytomas that are bilateral and hyperplasia of the parathyroids.[183] A more complete discussion of this syndrome can be found in Chapter 18.

Traumatic neuromas, sometimes referred to as amputation neuromas, are quite rare in children. These lesions in fact represent nodular C-fiber neuromas in most cases. Most lesions arise in response to nerve injury and they most often result in pain although patients may complain of numbness as well. The pain associated with true C-fiber neuromas tends to be constant whereas the pain associated with an amputation neuroma will tend to fluctuate. Most head and neck lesions will be found within the oral cavity (tongue, lips and gingiva) and most lesions arise as a result of trauma or injury that ranges from self-induced to injury from dental treatment, to jaw fracture.[184,185] Histologically, traumatic neuromas will be typical nodular lesions that are composed of nerve bundles that attempt to aggregate or coalesce. Nerve bundles will be surrounded by either loosely arranged or dense collagen.

Neurogenic Malignancies

Malignant Peripheral Nerve Sheath Tumor

Malignant peripheral nerve sheath tumors (MPNSTs) are tumors that arise from the peripheral nerve sheath, most commonly from Schwann cells.[186,187] MPNSTs as solitary lesions and are quite rare; however, the incidence escalates precipitously in individuals who have neurofibromatosis (NF-1). Patients who are afflicted with that disorder will have a Schwannoma or a benign neurofibroma transform into an MPNST, 10 percent of the time. MPNSTs are thought to

account for as high as 10 percent of all soft tissue sarcomas of the head and neck, and in children, they represent the most common malignancy of soft tissue after RMS.[188,189,190] In patients who are 20 years of age or less, MPNSTs account for as high as 20 percent of all soft tissue sarcomas.[188,189,190,191,192]

Most MPNSTs in the head and neck region will present as a nodular, rapidly enlarging cervical mass. Occasionally, patients will have hoarseness, recurrent laryngeal nerve palsy or nasal obstruction. Seventy percent of cases will demonstrate a nerve origin for the tumor and tumors occasionally arise within bone. Solitary non-NF1 associated MPNSTs do occur but are quite rare in both adults and pediatric age patients. There is an apparent latency period of 10 to 20 years during which an NF1 associated neurofibroma undergoes malignant transition. This lengthy gestation period may explain why MPNSTs are uncommon in children. Since NF1 shows this well documented transition, caution should be exercised when irradiating any patient with neurofibromatosis,[1] especially a child.[193]

When MPNSTs arise within bones in the head and neck region, the jaws are most often affected, and paresthesia or anesthesia to regional nerve distribution can occur. Jaw lesions will appear as irregular radiolucencies that cause marked expansion of the maxilla or mandible. A percentage of tumors that are seen in pediatric patients will be located at the lateral skull base and may actually originate from the vagus nerve. MRT and CT scans can be used effectively to identify the anatomy and extent of tumor involvement.

Pathology Features

On gross inspection, MPNSTs are generally rubbery, fleshy or sometimes gelatinous masses. In some instances, tumors may be directly attached to a nerve. Histologically, tumors are composed of aggregates of spindle cells that grow in a fascicular pattern. This spindle cell component dominates most tumors; however, 5 to 10 percent of tumors will show an epithelioid component.[194,195,196] Tumor cells tend to grow in long streaming aggregates, and nuclear pleomorphism and atypical mitotic figures are common to the tumor cells, which will have wavy to often comma shaped nuclei. (Figure 2.50) Tumors can show a wide range of cellular differentiation, such that portions of any tumor may resemble a neurofibroma, while other portions may be rich in giant cells and histiocytic appearing cells that cause the MPNST to resemble undifferentiated pleomorphic sarcoma.

Rare epithelioid MPNSTs will tend to contain nests of cells with prominent eosinophilic cytoplasm; round to oval nuclei and a degree of cellular differentiation that can make them appear to be of skeletal muscle or epithelial origin. On occasion, MPNSTs will contain mucous secreting cells, and bone or cartilaginous material. Pleomorphism of tumor cells is quite common to MPNSTs; however, such pleomorphism is generally associated with tumors that show a characteristic background of neurogenic appearing spindle cells, and not with epithelioid variants of the tumor. MPNSTs will be focally

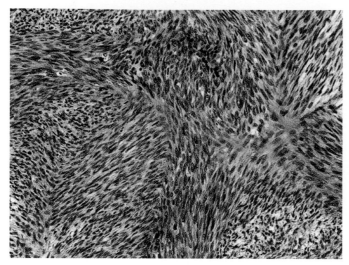

Figure 2.50 MPNST composed of a fascicular arrangement of spindle cells with marked nuclear pleomorphism.

CD34 protein reactive and S-100 protein positive when stained immunohistochemically. Tumors that have a skeletal muscle appearing component, and which look rhabdomyoblastic, may stain immunohistochemically positive for myogenin, desmin and MyoD1. This variant of MPNST will also tend to be more strongly S-100 protein reactive than tumors that are primarily spindle in character. Glandular appearing tumors that are cytokeratin reactive do occur rarely.

Differential Diagnosis

Diagnosis of the MPNST can be difficult in pediatric age group patients, and diagnoses of RMS, fibrosarcoma and undifferentiated pleomorphic sarcoma must often be entertained. Molecular studies may be necessary to confirm a diagnosis. Although no definitive genetic aberrations are associated with MPNST, a t(X:18) has been reported.[197]

Soft tissue *perineurial tumors* can be confused with MPNSTs histologically, as can pleomorphic anaplastic sarcomas, and SFTs. Perineurial tumors tend to demonstrate a so-called shredded or horsehair spiraling type of proliferation of tumor cells and these tumors will lack the cytologic atypia of MPNSTs. In addition, perineurial tumors will be S-100 protein and CD34-negative on IHC. SFTs will be strongly CD34-reactive and they are generally much less myxoid in appearance or loosely arranged as MPNSTs.

Treatment and Prognosis

The principal mode of treatment for MPNSTs in children is wide excision of the tumor. Any involved neurovascular tissue or bony structures, including fascial spaces and their contents should be removed in continuity with the tumor.[194] Although MPNSTs have long been considered to be radioresistant, radiation therapy has been employed more recently to treat local recurrences and as a principal mode of therapy for lesions that are unresectable.[192,197]

Chemotherapy has not been employed to routinely treat MPNSTs in children and most tumors are not responsive to this form of therapy.[198] Adjuvant chemotherapy as a whole has proven to be most efficacious in tumors that do not involve the head and neck region.[198] The best overall response rate for MPNSTs to chemotherapy in children has been with those regimens that contain ifosfamide.[192] Overall recurrence rates for the tumor are around 60 percent and five-year survival rates approach 50 percent. Less differentiated tumors have a poorer prognosis than those that are better differentiated.

Olfactory Neuroblastoma (Esthesioneuroblastomas)

Olfactory neuroblastomas are rare, biologically aggressive malignant neoplasms of the nasal cavity and paranasal sinuses. First described in 1924,[199] the olfactory neuroblastoma accounts for approximately 10 percent of all malignant neoplasms that are not squamous in origin and that affect nasal and paranasal anatomic sites.[199] Tumors can be further subclassified as either nasal, neurologic, oral/facial, cervical or ophthalmologic. Most esthesioneuroblastomas will be nasal in their presentation,[200] and symptoms will generally include nasal obstruction, epistaxis, headaches, nausea, tooth mobility, facial swelling anesthesia and trismis. Unlike neuroblastoma, which generally occurs from infancy up to three years of age, olfactory neuroblastoma tends to occur in individuals after the age of ten. Esthesioneuroblastomas are estimated to occur in 0.1 per 100,000 children up to 15 years of age.[201] From a clinical differential diagnostic perspective, RMS, nasopharyngeal angiofibroma and fibrosarcoma may be considered. The chromosomal translocation t(11;22) (q24;q12) with a *EWS/FL11* gene fusion has been proposed as a possible cause for rare olfactory neuroblastomas; however, definitive causation has not been proven.[202]

Pathologic Features

The tumor will be composed of nests or sheets of small but uniform cells with round nuclei, chromatin that is punctuate and indistinct cell membranes. (Figure 2.51) Nuclear pleomorphism will be moderate. Tumors will display a prominent fibrillary stroma and Homer–Wright rosettes will surround central aggregates of fibrils. (Figures 2.52 & 2.53) The histopathology and management of esthesioneuroblastoma is discussed in more detail in Chapter 14.

Neuroblastoma

Neuroblastomas represent high grade malignant neoplasms of neural crest derivation. Most often recognized in children, these tumors usually arise within the adrenal gland or from sympathetic ganglia, as the second most common solid tumor to occur in childhood. Most neuroblastomas are diagnosed by five years of age. A congenital form of the disease occurs in one quarter of all patients. Neuroblastoma displays a significant ethnic predilection, with tumors occurring less frequently in

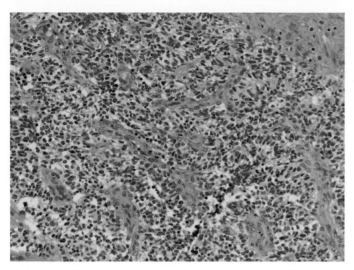

Figure 2.51 Olfactory neuroblastoma. The tumor is characterized by nests and clusters of uniform small round cells with indistinct cell membranes.

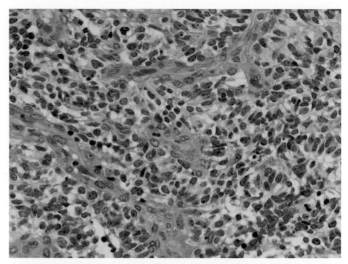

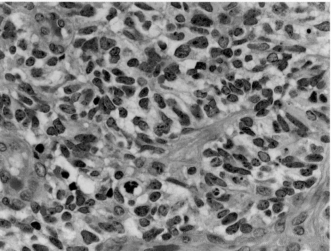

Figures 2.52 (top) & 2.53 (bottom) A fibrillary stroma and Homer–Wright rosettes that surround central aggregates of fibrils characterize this olfactory neuroblastoma at low and high power.

Blacks and Asians than in Caucasians. Those tumors that involve the head and neck region of children most often affect the cervical region. Tumors of the oral and maxillofacial region are exceedingly rare.[206]

Neuroblastomas that occur in children in the head and neck region will most often present as a nodular mass or masses that will frequently give a bluish ecchymotic appearance to the overlying skin. Patients may have constitutional symptoms of fever, weight loss and fatigue. Tumors that involve the orbit will often extend to the superior orbital fissure and displace the eye.[206]

Radiographic surveys, including CT scans and PET scans can be used to determine the extent of tumor in the head and neck region and to identify any associated metastases. Metastases frequently occur to the femur, skull, humerus and lung.[207,208] Children who are thought to have a neuroblastoma should be assessed for catecholamine levels. Elevated vanillyl mandelic acid as well as other catecholamine metabolites, including HVA and MHPG, can be seen in more than 90 percent of neuroblastoma cases.

Pathologic Features

Grossly, neuroblastomas present as lobular tumor masses that are fleshy or rubbery in appearance. On microscopic examination, tumors are composed of sheets and aggregates of small, round, blue cells with atypical mitoses, extremely high nuclear/cytoplasmic ratio and markedly hyperchromatic nuclei. (Figures 2.54 & 2.55) Cells that are more highly differentiated will often demonstrate zones of Homer–Wright pseudorosette formation. Occasionally, tumor cells can differentiate to become quite eosinophilic. Tumors can also differentiate to form ganglion cells and necrosis within the tumor may be seen.

Immunohistochemical stains can be helpful in establishing a diagnosis of a neuroblastoma. Neuron-specific enolase (NSE), Vimentin, CD56, MIB-1 and synaptophysin stains will be positive in neuroblastoma. Tumor cells will stain negatively for epithelial membrane antigen, desmin, cytokeratin and CD99. S-100 protein stains will also be negative. These IHC staining patterns can be helpful in distinguishing neuroblastoma from embryonal RMS, Ewing's sarcoma/PNET and malignant lymphomas.

Neuroblastomas will stain positively for NSE whereas Ewing sarcoma (PNET) will not. Ewing's sarcomas also tend to be CD99 positive whereas neuroblastomas tend to be CD99 negative. RMSs will be desmin reactive and will stain positively for glycogen whereas neuroblastomas will react negatively with both of those IHC markers. RMSs will also demonstrate CD45 positivity whereas neuroblastomas will stain negatively for that marker. Neuroblastomas, unlike Ewing's sarcoma/PNET will tend not to show an MYCN gene amplification.[209] Interestingly, germline mutations in *ALK* and *PHOX2B* genes have been identified in neuroblastomas.[210]

Treatment and Prognosis

The most common forms of treatment for those neuroblastomas that involve the head and neck region and craniofacial complex include surgery and radiation therapy. Tumors can be graded as 1, 2, 3 or 4 stage tumors.[206] Stage 1 tumors involve only one organ; stage 2 tumors will involve 1 organ with some peripheral extension, without a midline crossing; stage 3 tumors are tumors that cross the midline, and stage 4 tumors will demonstrate distant metastases. Most stage 1 and stage 2 tumors are treated by local excision with a 2 cm margin of normal tissue. Stage 3 tumors are most often managed using local excision and radiation therapy, and stage 4 tumors are treated using radiation therapy at primary and metastatic sites. Neonatal tumors in the head and neck are treated in a less aggressive fashion, with stage 1 tumors often being treated with a regimen of chemotherapy that includes vincristine,

cyclophosphamide and pirarubicin.[206] Rare cases have also been treated using stem cell transplants.[211]

Vascular Tumors

Benign and Reactive Vascular Formations

Pyogenic Granuloma

Pyogenic granulomas are common lesions in pediatric age group patients. These tumors represent benign vascular lesions with an inflammatory component, and do not represent true epithelioid granulomas as might be seen in tuberculosis, nor do they produce a necrotic pus-like product as the name implies. Therefore the nomenclature for the lesions is somewhat inappropriate; however, long-term usage of the term pyogenic granuloma continues. Lesions in the head and neck region can be solitary or multiple. The most common head and neck soft tissue sites of occurrence are the skin and oral cavity although the sinonasal region, larynx and other soft tissue sites within the head and neck can be affected.[212,213,214,215,216]

Sixty percent of pyogenic granulomas that occur in the head and neck region will be related to irritation or trauma. Lesions that involve oral and pharyngeal sites are somewhat unique in that they may be related to poor oral hygiene, dental plaque development or pregnancy, in which estrogen levels are altered, resulting in a form of localized hyperplastic hormonal induced gingivitis.

Most pyogenic granulomas will present clinically as pedunculated or nodular mucosal or soft tissue growths that will appear hemorrhagic. (Figure 2.56) The lesions are frequently ulcerated and most pyogenic granulomas range in size from 2 to 5 cm in diameter. Lesions can grow quite rapidly and they may undergo localized necrosis.

Pathologic Features

Pyogenic granulomas are richly vascularized lesions that are composed of a proliferation of dilated vascular channels,

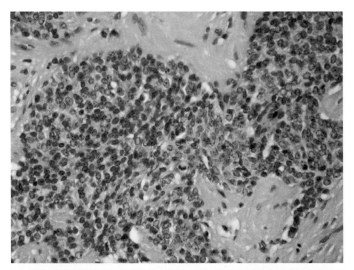

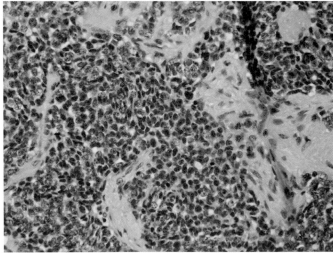

Figures 2.54 (top) & 2.55 (bottom) Small round blue cells arranged in sheets and with atypical mitoses characterize this neuroblastoma. (Figure 2.55) Note the hyperchromatic nuclei and high nuclear cytoplasmic ratios that are seen in the tumor at high power magnification.

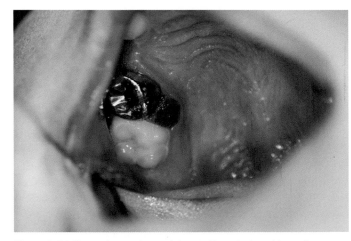

Figure 2.56 Pyogenic granuloma of the maxillary gingiva arising adjacent to a stainless steel crown that is likely causal.

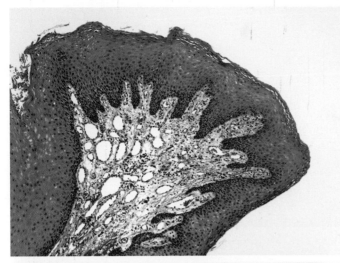

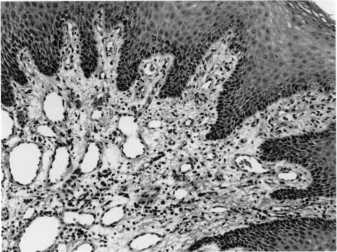

Figures 2.57 (top) & 2.58 (bottom) Low and high power photomicrographs of a pyogenic granuloma that is rich in endothelial cells, fibroblasts and vascular channels.

endothelial cells, plump fibroblasts, histiocytes, other inflammatory cells and mature collagen. (Figures 2.57 & 2.58) Lesions will generally be marginated by epidermis or mucosal epithelium, and their associated inflammatory cellular infiltrate is often dominated by plasma cells. Ulcerated epithelium can undergo pseudoepitheliomatous hyperplasia, and scattered eosinophilia may be seen within tumors, especially those that are ulcerated. Distinction of a pyogenic granuloma from a chronic ulcer with eosinophilia (traumatic ulcer with stromal eosinophilia) can be difficult sometimes.

Distinguishing pyogenic granuloma from hyperplastic gingivitis is important. Hyperplastic gingivitis that is hormonally induced, caused by irritation from calculus or debris or that is hereditary in nature is most often a generalized process and not a localized one as with pyogenic granulomas. Pyogenic granulomas can also resemble Kaposi sarcoma (KS) and true hemangiomas. KS will, however, be characterized histologically by a proliferation of spindle cells that are cytologically atypical. Intracellular hyaline goblets and aggregates are also

characteristic of KS, and not of pyogenic granuloma. Hemangiomas in pediatric age patients can resemble pyogenic granulomas; however, hemangiomas typically have either a dominant capillary and endothelial cell proliferative component or a histiocytic component without other cellular inflammation that will be lacking in the typical diffusely inflamed pyogenic granuloma.

Pyogenic granulomas of the oral cavity can resemble the *peripheral giant cell granuloma* or *peripheral ossifying fibroma*, and in concert these three tumors account for 80 percent of the isolated reactive lesions that affect the gingiva in both adults and children. Peripheral giant cell granuloma and peripheral ossifying fibroma have a significantly higher recurrence rate than pyogenic granuloma. Histologically, the lesions are easily separated. Peripheral giant cell granulomas will be dominated by an accumulation of multinucleated giant cells microscopically, while 70 percent of peripheral ossifying fibromas will contain reactive bone formation and a prominent proliferating fibrous stroma. Neither of the aforementioned features are common to the pyogenic granuloma. The so-called *pregnancy tumor, a hyperplastic gingival lesion seen during pregnancy* is in fact a pyogenic granuloma.

Treatment and Prognosis

Most pyogenic granulomas in the head and neck region are treated by conservative surgical excision with a margin of normal tissue or by cautery.[218] The recurrence rate for lesions that are surgically excised is generally in the 10 to 15 percent range in children, but can range as high as 30 percent. The pulsed-dye laser can be used to remove pyogenic granulomas and this modality has shown good cosmetic results in children.[219]

Hemangioma and its Variants

Hemangiomas, vascular malformations and vascular anomalies are common in pediatric age group patients. This group of lesions can be as common place as birthmarks or represent true vascular neoplasms. The most common vascular tumors seen in children in the head and neck region are lymphangiomas and capillary/venous or arteriovenous malformations.[220] Regardless of whether such lesions are classified as malformations or tumors, they will be characteristically composed of vessels that appear otherwise histologically normal in all respects. Vascular lesions may also represent hamartomatous growths that may not emerge until after birth. Characteristically, however, vascular malformations will be present at birth, whereas hemangiomas tend to appear rapidly during the first months of life.[220] Richter et al. have proposed a simplified clinicopathologic classification for benign vascular anomalies and tumors in children (Table 2.1). Although childhood hemangiomas have long been classified as either cavernous, capillary or strawberry-type hemangiomas, Richter et al. have further suggested modifying that classification so that hemangiomas are staged on a clinical level as either superficial, deep or compound lesions.

Table 2.1 Classification of benign vascular anomalies by Richter and Friedman[220]

Vascular tumors	Vascular malformations
Infantile hemangioma	Slow flow
Congenital hemangioma	• Capillary malformations
Tufted angioma	• Venus malformations
Kaposiform hemangioendothelioma	• Lymphatic malformations
	Fast flow
	• Arteriovenous malformations

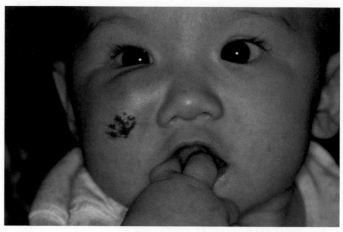

Figure 2.59 Lobular-appearing hemangioma of the face in an infant.

Capillary Hemangioma and Compound Hemangioma

Capillary and compound hemangiomas as defined by Richter et al.[220] represent the most common form of hemangioma seen in infants and children, and are broadly known as infantile hemangiomas. The vast majority of head and neck lesions will involve the oral mucosa and skin, but tumors can occur in other sites in the head and neck, including the nasal cavity, viscera and bones. Capillary hemangiomas, the most common form of infantile hemangioma, are typically present at birth or develop shortly after birth, as either solitary multifocal lesions that can either involute or grow rapidly over a brief period of time. Infantile hemangiomas are thought to most likely arise from progenitor stem cells that are of hematopoietic origin. These stem cells develop and proliferate when there are associated abnormal levels of matrix metallo proteinases (MMP-9) and the proangiogeneic factors VEGF, b-VFG and TGF-beta. In the presence of genetic alterations and altered cytokine levels, hemangiomas and vascular malformations commonly occur.[221,222,223]

Infantile capillary hemangiomas, in both mucosal and cutaneous sites, tend to present clinically as red patches, nodules or macules all of which will be fairly well demarcated. Lesions can appear multinodular and lobular, (Figure 2.59) and most hemangiomas that affect children will undergo a developmental growth phase that will extend from an initial proliferative phase to progress to a phase of quiescence and ultimately, in a large percentage of cases, to a phase of involution. Lesions can be superficial within affected tissues, deep within anatomic structures or compound in their clinical presentation. While lesions that are superficial or capillary, tend to be red and nodular and usually lack a subcutaneous component,[220] more deeply located (cavernous) hemangiomas, will often have a bluish tint. Compound hemangiomas, which can have both superficial and deep component, can appear either bluish or telangiectatic.[220]

Although both capillary hemangiomas and cavernous hemangiomas will most often occur shortly after birth, and eventually involute, deep hemangiomas tend to be much larger and more diffuse lesions that will often persist into adulthood.

From a clinical differential diagnostic standpoint, deep (cavernous) hemangiomas often present as diffuse and sometimes quite large multilobular lesions that may resemble neurofibromas or lipomas except for their characteristic purple, red or bluish hue. While deep hemangiomas can also clinically resemble lymphangiomas, lymphangiomas will tend to be less purple or bluish in color, especially when they affect mucosa or skin. Deep hemangiomas that involve bone can simulate odontogenic tumors, or odontogenic cysts if they appear radiolucent, or they can resemble ossifying fibroma or an odontoma if they are more radiodense in their presentation. Hemangiomas of the head and neck will often arise along the distribution of the trigeminal nerve, while subglottic lesions will often have a beard-like anatomic distribution.[224]

PHACE syndrome is a segmental infantile hemangiomatous process that manifests as a disorder with posterior fossa brain malformations, arterial cerebral vascular anomalies, cardiovascular anomalies or eye malformation, associated hemangiomas of the face and sternal defects or clefting.[225]

Regardless of their assigned clinical subtype, hemangiomas tend to involute in as high as 70 percent of cases, with most involutions occurring before nine years of age.[226]

Pathologic Features

Superficial hemangiomas, deep hemangiomas and compound hemangiomas will display distinctly different histopathologies. *Superficial hemangiomas* and compound hemangiomas will, upon gross inspection, be composed of red nodular or macular-like blue to violet growths. Histologically, capillary hemangiomas will consist of a proliferation of endothelial cells that form capillaries. Tumors may be extremely cellular and will be composed almost entirely of endothelial cells, or they can be relatively acellular and consist of only a minimal number of endothelially lined vessels (Figures 2.60 & 2.61). Tumor cell mitoses may be present, but they do not dominate lesional histopathology. Mast cells will often be seen in the intervening, and often thin fibrillar fibrous connective stroma of tumors. It is not uncommon to see myxoid change within a superficial or capillary hemangioma.

Deep or *cavernous hemangiomas* are less common than superficial (capillary) hemangiomas. Microscopically, deep

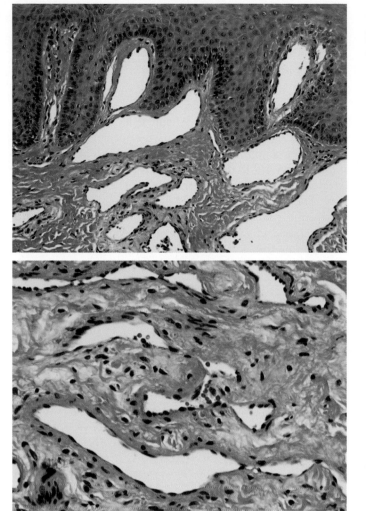

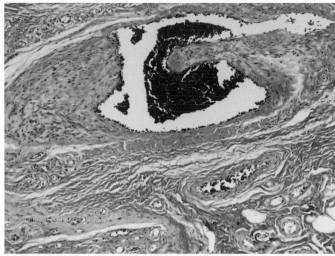

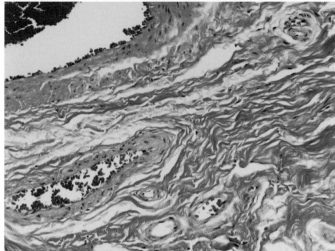

Figures 2.60 (top) & 2.61 (bottom) Low and high power photomicrographs of a hemangioma composed of a limited number of endothelially lined vessels.

hemangiomas will be composed of numerous, large dilated vascular channels that will be lined by flattened endothelial cells. Deep hemangiomas often contain areas of dystrophic calcification, organizing thrombi and fibrosis. The supporting tumor stroma will tend to be relatively mature, and if a cavernous hemangioma arises within bone, bone resorption and reactive bone formation will typically be seen at the tumor's periphery.

Compound hemangiomas will be composed of an admixture of both superficial and deep hemangiomatous elements and may therefore contain an abundance of dilated capillary sized vascular channels that will be lined by endothelial cells, as well as large dilated vascular channels lined by flattened endothelial cells (Figures 2.62, 2.63 & 2.64). Stromal dystrophic calcification may also be seen.

A host of syndromes tend to be associated with cavernous or deep hemangiomas, including Kasabach–Merritt syndrome, Maffucci syndrome and blue rubber bleb nevus syndrome.

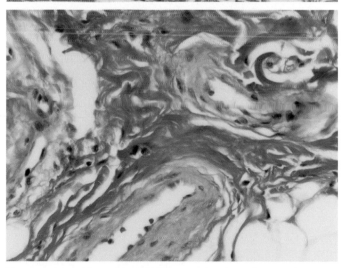

Figures 2.62 (top), 2.63 (middle) & 2.64 (bottom) Compound hemangioma made up of capillary sized as well as larger vascular channels can be seen in these low, medium and high power photomicrographs.

The *juvenile capillary hemangioma*, is a distinctive lesion that occurs in the superficial skin area of the chin. Also known as a "strawberry nevus," the lesion is simply a superficial hemangioma with a distinctive anatomic site of presentation. The histopathology of the lesion is similar to that of other superficial (capillary) hemangiomas that occur in the head and neck, although the juvenile capillary hemangioma can tend toward being extremely cellular, with only minimal vascular channelization when viewed microscopically.

The *tufted angioma* or *angioblastoma* is a relatively uncommon subtype of hemangioma that usually presents as a macule, papule or nodule in infancy or childhood. The neck region and the upper trunk are the most frequent sites of occurrence.[226] The tufted angioma will be composed histologically of circumscribed capillary aggregates, the capillaries of which will be lined by plump endothelial cells that will in turn be surrounded by spindle shaped pericytes. (Figures 2.65 & 2.66) Aggregated tumor capillaries will typically not contain red blood cells and the tumor's dilated vascular spaces will appear lymphatic-like as they arise in association with vascular tufts that have a characteristic "cannon ball-like" appearance.

Treatment and Prognosis

Superficial, deep and compound hemangiomas, whether congenital or infantile, are most often managed by long-term clinical observation of the patient.[227] Even with long-term scrutiny, it is estimated that 40 percent of children with any of the three common forms of hemangioma seen in the head and neck region will require some form of medical or surgical intervention, largely due to the fact that lesions in this anatomic area can potentially bleed, ulcerate, cause some form of visual impairment or produce airway obstruction.[228] In the vast majority of cases, aggressive intervention involving a hemangioma that is asymptomatic is inappropriate. For those lesions that are problematic, cryosurgery, sclerosing agents and surgical excision may be employed. However, scaring and disfigurement may result from such interventions.

Cortical steroids, interferon and the chemotherapeutic use of vincristine have all been employed to manage hemangiomas in pediatric age group patients.[229,230,231] Propranolol has been used more recently to treat infantile hemangiomas. This non-selective β adrenergic antagonist does carry with it some risk, however, including drug-associated hypoglycemia and lethargy.[232] Even after a hemangioma involutes, the pediatric patient may still require cosmetic surgery in which skin flaps and tissue extenders may, of necessity, be employed in order to obtain normal cosmesis.

Vascular Tumors of "Borderline" Malignant Potential

Kaposiform Hemangioendothelioma

The Kaposiform hemangioendothelioma (KH), a tumor of vascular endothelial cell origin, arises most commonly in the head and neck region. The majority of tumors will present in the first year of life as either solitary or multifocal lesions of the oral mucosa or skin.[233,234,235] KH is reported to occur in association with Kasabach–Merritt syndrome in as many as 20 percent of infantile cases.[236] The overall mortality rate for this consumptive coagulopathy and thrombocytopenic driven syndrome can range as high as 30 percent.[235] Most KHs will manifest as bluish red, irregular, superficial and rapidly growing bruises or nodules.[235] Rarely, lesions will originate within bone. Most lesions will not involute on their own. Tachycardia and shock represent the most life threatening components of the KH associated syndrome.

Kaposiform hemangiomas that undergo angiography will generally demonstrate feeder vessels that must be identified appropriately if embolization is considered as a treatment modality. Doppler ultrasonography or MRI can be used to enhance the image of the tumor and show the extent of the lesion or lesions.[237]

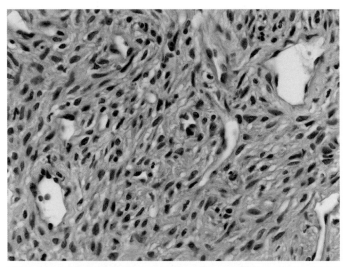

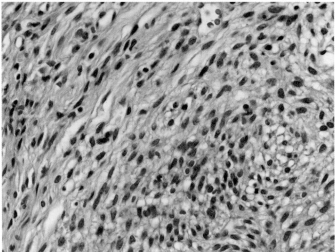

Figures 2.65 (top) & 2.66 (bottom) Tufted angioma composed of capillaries lined by plump endothelial cells, which are marginated by spindle shaped pericytes, are seen in these two photomicrographs.

Pathologic Features

On gross inspection, most KHs will be red macules, papules or nodules. Larger, deeper lesions tend to appear as multi-lobulated blue masses on gross examination.

Histologically, tumors will be composed of islands of tumor cells that are endothelial in origin, but which will often appear epithelioid. Vascular channels and endothelial cells will aggregate into glomeruloid islands. Vascular channels within these islands will be lined by so-called hobnail appearing endothelial cells. Hobnail cells will project into the vascular lumen in a spur-like fashion, causing vascular spaces to appear quite papillary. Individual cells lining vascular spaces can range from mitotically inactive bland cells to cells that show significant cytologic atypia. The tumor stroma will usually be chronically inflamed and is often hyalinized. The typically compressed vessels that are part of the tumor histology will demonstrate CD31, CD34 and FLI1 reactivity. Tumor cells will stain negatively for GLUT1 and LeY. CD61-positive fibrin thrombi may be found within the tumor and typically characterize areas of platelet consumption.[238] The so-called *retiform hemangioendothelioma* can resemble KH microscopically. However, retiform lesions occur more commonly in adults than children and also differ from KH by virtue of their commonly associated lymphedema and lymphatic hyperplasia. KH must, of necessity, be distinguished from KS. While KS will demonstrate human herpes virus 8 (HHV8) transcripts by RTPCR, KH will not. KH can generally be separated from juvenile hemangiomas on the basis of negative GLUT-1 and LeY immunostaining in KH.

KH will also typically demonstrate vessels with microthrombi, and a characteristic glomeruloid pattern, whereas KS will be composed of vascular spaces that are often back-to-back, and which are much larger and more cytologically atypical in their lining cells than those seen in KH.

Epitheloid-like hemangioendothelioma, spindle cell hemangioendothelioma and retiform hemangioendothelioma can all resemble KH clinically and microscopically. The characteristic finding that separates these three entities from KH is that KH is predominantly a tumor of infants and young children, while infantile hemangioendotheliomas will be located in the liver in nearly all instances, even though the age demographic may be similar to KH.

Treatment and Prognosis

KH is treated in one-third of cases by high dose steroid therapy,[239] and with vincristine therapy in cases where there is steroid resistance.[240] Lesions have also been treated with cyclophosphamide and interferon.[240] KHs are considered to be vascular tumors of intermediate grade malignancy, and they are associated with a significant mortality rate. Locally aggressive lesions have the potential for distant metastasis. It is therefore exceedingly important to separate KH from the less aggressive and benign infantile forms of hemangioma, with which it can be confused, both clinically and microscopically.

Dabska-type Hemangioendothelioma (Retiform Hemangioendothelioma)

The retiform or Dabska-type hemangioendothelioma (DH) is a vascular and endothelial cell proliferative neoplasm that most often involves the skin or subcutaneous tissues of infants and children. The lesion, which has a low incidence in adults, shows no ethnic or racial predilection and the etiology is unknown.[241,242,243] Lesions are exceedingly rare in the head and neck region and will often be diagnosed simply as hemangiomas. Clinically, tumors will present as slow growing, pink, blue or black nodules that can reach 2 to 3 cm in diameter. The surface of the DH can become ulcerated, and differential diagnoses include intravascular papillary endothelial hyperplasia, capillary hemangioma, angiosarcoma, hemangioendothelioma and pyogenic granuloma.

Pathologic Features

Grossly, tumors tend to represent a hemorrhagic subcutaneous nodule or nodules. Histologically, tumors will be composed of vascular spaces that are lined by endothelial cells, which proliferate with hobnail excrescences extending into vascular lumena. The tumor cells will often be marginated by perivascular lymphocytic infiltrate and the tumor stroma may be hyalinized. Factor 8-related antigen, CD31, CD34 and vimentin will be variably expressed in the tumor. The highly specific lymphatic endothelial marker, D2–40 will also be reactive. Hemangioendothelioma, angiosarcoma and benign intravascular endothelial hyperplasia will all also mark positively for CD31, CD34 and vimentin. However, these three tumors will less commonly express D2–40, and they do not express vascular endothelial cell growth factor receptor type 3, as will the DH.[244]

Treatment and Prognosis

DH is treated by surgery and/or radiation therapy.[244] The tumor is considered to be a lesion of borderline malignancy by some investigators and a true malignant neoplasm by others. Clearly, the tumor has the ability to metastasize and result in the death of the patient. However, the overall prognosis for most patients is quite favorable.[242] Because so few of these tumors have been recorded in children in the head and neck region, a standard approach to therapy has not been determined. Thus head and neck tumors should be approached with the understanding that local tumor invasion with lymph node metastasis can occur.

Malignant Vascular Tumors

Kaposi Sarcoma

Kaposi sarcoma (KS) is a malignant vascular neoplasm that occurs most frequently in the head and neck region. The tumor, which favors the scalp and oral cavity is commonly classified into four subtypes: 1) *sporadic or classic disease*, 2) *African or endemic disease*, 3) *disease associated with acquired immune deficiency syndrome (AIDS)* and 4) *iatrogenic disease*, seen primarily in transplant patients.

The classic form of the disease was first described in 1872 as a cutaneous disorder that primarily affected the lower extremities of elderly men of Jewish, European or Mediterranean descent.[245] The much later recognized African endemic form of the disease can be cutaneous or lymphadenopathic. The African cutaneous form of the disease occurs most commonly in patients who are in the 30 to 40 year age-range, and therefore tends to present two to three decades earlier than in patients with the classic form of KS. Lymph node involvement is rare in the African cutaneous form of the disease; however, the African (endemic) form of the disease can be associated with significant lymphadenopathy.

The endemic lymphadenopathic form of the disease, most often identified in African children, represents a non-AIDS-related KS that is usually seen in the head and neck region. Children with this form of the disease will present with generalized lymphadenopathy and head and neck tumors that affect the nose, eyes, ears, larynx and the oral cavity. Boys with the lymphadenopathic African endemic form of KS are affected more often than girls. The most common site in the head and neck for this form of the disease will be the hard and soft palate and the oropharynx region. Salivary glands and the scalp are rarely affected.[246,247,248]

AIDS-related KS was initially most often identified in homosexual men. The incidence of KS in that population is now nearly equal to its incidence in the heterosexual population.

Whether endemic in nature or epidemic, KS is associated etiologically with infection with HHV8,[249] which encodes homologes of human cellular proteins involved in cell cycle regulation, cell proliferation, apoptosis, angiogenesis and immune regulation.[246]

A small percentage of KSs are identified in immune compromised individuals, and represent a non-AIDS-associated disseminated form of the disease. This form of iatrogenic KS rarely affects the mucous membranes of the soft tissues in the head and neck region. The vast majority of affected patients will have undergone renal transplantation. However, iatrogenic disease can be seen in patients who have had other forms of transplantation including liver and cardiothoracic transplants. Most patients who develop this form of KS are in the fourth or fifth decade of life, and men outnumber women. Rare cases of this subset of KS have been documented in children, however.

Since the vast majority of KSs to occur in children will involve the head and neck region and will represent the African endemic lymphadenopathic form of the disease, most pediatric age patients will present with nodular or ulcerated, scalp or oral/oropharyngeal tumor masses and generalized lymphadenopathy. From a differential diagnostic perspective, vascular lesions such as hemangioma, mucoepidermoid carcinoma, lymphangioma, pyogenic granuloma, RMS and nerve sheath neoplasms have to be considered. CT scans can be used to demonstrate the extent of lesions in the head and neck area and a test for HIV antibodies should always be undertaken.

Pathologic Features

Histologically, KS will tend to progress from an early stage polyclonal reactive inflammatory angiogenic process to a true monoclonal sarcomatous process in late stages.[246] The immunosuppression that occurs in association with transplantation tends to support HHV8 KS progression. Thus, iatrogenic or immunosuppressed transplantation associated KS tends to be a more biologically aggressive form of the disease than other KS forms, even when it occurs in children.[250]

KS can be divided into three clinical stages: a patch stage, a plaque stage and a nodular stage or tumor stage. These clinical stages can be closely correlated with the histopathology of the disease. Lesions that are patch-like in their clinical presentation will tend to be composed of numerous intersecting small dilated thin-walled vascular channels that are lined by endothelial cells. The endothelial lining of the vascular spaces in patch stage KS tends not to be cytologically atypical and generally there is only a mild inflammatory infiltrate in the supporting tumor stroma. Early patch-like lesions will often show extravasated red cells and hemosiderin, and the neoplastic spindle cell aggregation of tumor cells that is common to the plaque and nodular phases of the disease will be minimal.

The plaque-like stage of the disease will begin to demonstrate an accumulation of malignant spindle cells that will be transected by numerous dilated vascular channels that interlace and intersect. These vascular channels tend to be quite jagged in their appearance and in many instances the cells lining vascular spaces will be cytologically atypical, demonstrating a significant number of atypical mitoses, and altered nuclear cytoplasmic ratios.

The nodular stage of KS will be dominated by a malignant spindle cell component that will override the vascular component of the tumor to proliferate as intersecting bands of malignant cells. These individual brands of tumor cells will show significant cytologic atypia and tumor cells will be densely packed. (Figure 2.67) Mitotic activity in this stage of the disease, which is often multifocal nowadays, does not necessarily have to be prominent.

Regardless of the stage of progression, KS will mark for CD31, CD34 and FL1–1 protein histochemically. D2–40 and endothelial growth factor receptors, which are markers for lymphocytic endothelial differentiation, will also be positive. Most KSs will also express HHV8 as a latency associated nuclear antigen. This finding will tend to distinguish KS from angiosarcoma and other spindle cell malignancies such as fibrosarcoma, which will not demonstrate such expression. Tumor cell HHV8 positivity (Figure 2.68) also will allow one to distinguish KS from a simple inflammatory process, such as pyogenic granuloma, and from hemangioendothelial and hemangiopericytic lesions, which will be non-expressive for HHV8.[251]

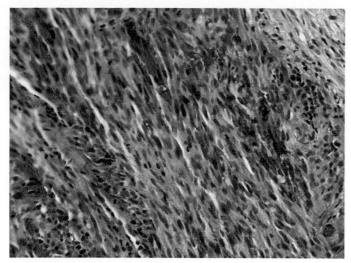

Figure 2.67 KS demonstrating intersecting bands of malignant cytologically atypical endothelial cells and significant hemorrhage.

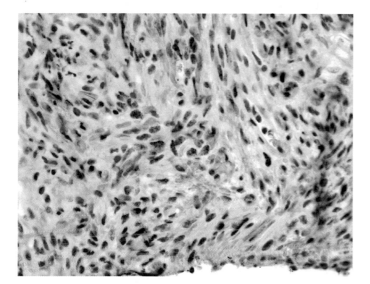

Figure 2.68 HHV8 positive staining of a KS.

Treatment and Prognosis

Kaposi sarcoma has been treated by a wide variety of modalities including local surgical therapy, radiation therapy, chemotherapy and immunotherapy. Immunotherapy for isolated lesions may include intralesional injections of drugs such as vinblastine. Low-dose radiation therapy up to 2400 cGy has also been employed to treat isolated lesions.

Disseminated forms of the disease are managed with other chemotherapeutic regimens that include the liposomal group of drugs such as liposomal doxorubicin, vinblastine, bleomycin and etoposide. Interferon is less commonly used due to its significant side effects. Interleukin-12 can be used as a biologic, and antiviral drugs, including HAART along with interferon has been used to treat KS. Angiogenesis inhibitors, antisense oglionuclotides that are directed against angiogenesis growth factors and HIV protease inhibitors have all been employed in the management of KS.[252]

The most frequently employed AIDS-related treatment for KS of the oral cavity, common to children, is radiation therapy, and remission rates of 85 percent have been reported.[246] Individuals who have either classic KS or the African cutaneous form of KS have a relatively good prognosis, although a large percentage of the patients in that group will die from a secondary, disease-related malignancy. AIDS-related forms of KS have shown a progressively better prognosis, as knowledge of the disease and the refinement and appropriate use of antiretroviral drugs and immunotherapy have improved. Children who have transplant-associated KS will often show tumor regression after immunosuppressive drugs are discontinued. Nonetheless, the overall mortality rate for this form of KS in children approaches 30 percent.

Angiosarcoma

Angiosarcoma will affects pediatric age patients as either a malignant hemangioendothelioma or as a lymphangiosarcoma. Both tumors, however, are poorly studied in children, and little is known about their biology, or natural history in this age group.[253,254,255] Tumors tend to show a slight male predilection and generally when angiosarcomas occur in the head and neck region, the deep soft tissues of the head and neck or the mediastinum are the favored sites. Radiographically, tumors will show a destructive pattern, and MRI will demonstrate the presence of a lobulated mass with increased signal intensity or hemodynamic flow characteristics.[253,254]

Angiosarcomas in children can present as flat ecchymotic appearing lesions, or as lesions that are firm and indurated, or ulcerated, nodular or fleshy. Angiosarcomas of the oral and maxillofacial region tend not to be associated with edema. However, lesions in other sites of the body are frequently associated with massive accumulations of edema. Clinically, tumors can resemble melanoma, squamous cell carcinoma and adnexal tumors of skin.

Pathologic Features

Grossly, most angiosarcomas will be firm hemorrhagic masses that will be multinodular. Tumors will tend to have ill-defined margins and will usually range in size from 5 to 7 cm in diameter, although lesions have been reported of up to 13 cm in diameter.[253] Histologically, tumors will be composed of an accumulation of spindle cells and epithelioid appearing cells. (Figure 2.69) Tumor cells will be cytologically atypical, displaying hyperchromatic nuclei and atypical mitoses as they often proliferate in a fascicular pattern as they attempt to form vascular channels. (Figures 2.70 & 2.71) Papillary endothelial projections may be seen within the lumena of vascular spaces. The cytoplasm of tumor cells is generally eosinophilic and hyaline globules and hemorrhage will be common to the tumor stroma.

Angiosarcomas can be graded histologically as low, intermediate or high grade tumors. Most angiosarcomas that occur

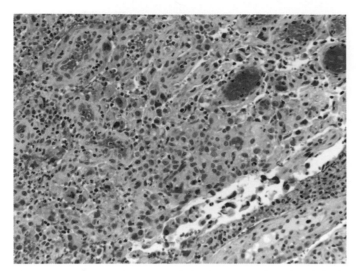

Figure 2.69 Angiosarcoma composed of malignant spindle and epithelioid appearing cells.

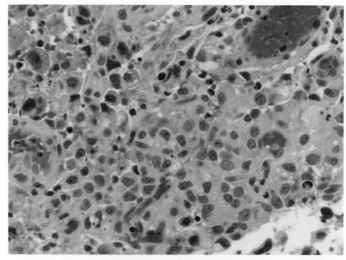

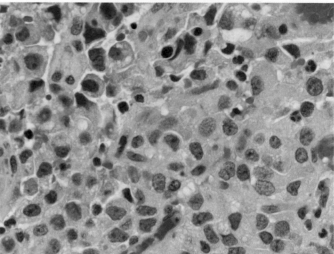

Figures 2.70 (top) & 2.71 (bottom) Malignant cells of endothelial origin with marked cytologic atypia including hyperchromatic nuclei and atypical mitosis are seen in this angiosarcoma at low and high power.

in children are high grade neoplasms. Since angiosarcoma can histologically resemble other forms of undifferentiated sarcoma, IHC assessment is important in establishing a proper diagnosis. Angiosarcoma will stain positively with endothelial markers including CD31, CD34 and CD144, and focally positive for factor 8 related antigen.[256] Epithelial membrane antigen S-100 protein and HHV8 will be immunohistochemically negative.

Differential Diagnosis

Soft tissue angiosarcomas in children must be differentiated from KS, hemangioendothelioma, hemangiopericytoma and spindle cell hemangioendothelioma. The malignant spindle cells in KS unlike those of angiosarcoma, will be factor 8 negative. The vessels seen in angiosarcoma will tend to be more cavernous than those seen in KS.[256] The staghorn histologic pattern typical of the vascular channels seen in hemangiopericytoma can help to distinguish that tumor from angiosarcoma, which will lack such staghorn channels.[255] Hemangiopericytomas will tend to be more uniformly cellular and less vascular than angiosarcomas. The tumor cells of hemangiopericytoma will not stain for agglutinin 1 as will the tumor cells of angiosarcoma. Immunostaining for factor 8 will be weak or absent in hemangiopericytoma.[255]

Treatment and Prognosis

Angiosarcomas in pediatric patients tend to invade perineural tissue and metastasize readily.[257] Treatment modalities are variable and often will depend on the size of the tumor. Tumors that measure 5 cm or more in diameter generally represent a high surgical risk, while tumors that are less than 5 cm in diameter are of lower risk, and thus are associated with a higher rate of survival.[258]

Childhood angiosarcomas have been treated with paclitaxel with some degree of success.[259] Radiation can also play a role in the management of the patients, but the long-term risk to

children can be quite high.[258,259] Pediatric age group angiosarcomas tend to be more aggressive than angiosarcomas in adults and all such tumors are classified as either intermediate or high grade. A large percentage of patients will succumb to their disease within 15 months of their diagnosis, and metastasis is primarily to lymph nodes regionally and to lungs distantly.[260]

Tumors of Muscle Origin

Benign Tumors of Smooth Muscle Origin

Leiomyoma

Leiomyomas are benign tumors that arise from smooth muscle, the vast majority of which will arise in middle aged women from the myometrium, from the gastrointestinal tract or skin. Tumors in the head and neck region are thought to arise from pilar smooth muscle, from vascular smooth muscle that is either dermal or subcutaneous or from the vessels in the lamina propria and submucosa of the oral cavity, larynx or nose.[261] Oral leiomyomas will most often involve the lips, the buccal mucosa, the palate, the gingiva and the mandible.[261]

Leiomyomas in the head and neck region are quite rare in children.[262] Veeresh et al.[261] reported finding only two leiomyomas in pediatric age patients in an extensive institutional review of leiomyomas. Wang assessed 21 head and neck leiomyomas seen at the National Taiwan University Hospital and documented only one case occurring in a child, a preauricular lesion.[263]

Head and neck tumors in children as well as adults will generally present as a nodular, solitary, subdermal or submucosal growth that rarely attains a size of greater than 2 cm in diameter. Tumors tend to be firm with well defined margins.

Although leiomyomas can occur as multiple lesions, this presentation is exceedingly rare in children. Tumors that arise as multifocal growths are typically pilar leiomyomas and in many instances such lesions are painful. Solitary leiomyomas of the head and neck tend to be more deeply seated and less painful than multifocal lesions. From a clinical differential diagnostic perspective, leiomyoma can resemble pyogenic granuloma, lymphangioma, tumors of nerve sheath origin, such as neurofibroma and Schwannoma, or even juvenile fibromatosis. Leiomyosarcoma, dermatofibroma and soft tissue cysts such as dermoid cysts can also resemble leiomyoma clinically.[264]

Leiomyomas in children can occur as central osseous lesions of the jaws or bones of the skull.[262] These central osseous lesions will typically present as radiolucencies with associated bony expansion.

Pathologic Features

Leiomyomas can be histologically classified as: 1) solid leiomyomas, 2) vascular leiomyomas and 3) epithelioid leiomyomas.[265] Vascular leiomyoma, the most common of the three histologic subtypes, which occur in the head and neck region[266] can be further subclassified into capillary, solid or cavernous subtypes. Vascular leiomyomas, which arise from vascular smooth muscle, tend to be well circumscribed lesions microscopically. These lesions will be composed of streaming spindle cells. Tumor cells will tend to have rounded elongated cigar-shaped nuclei and cytoplasm that is eosinophilic. (Figures 2.72 & 2.73) Smooth muscle proliferation around vessels will be quite prominent. Solid leiomyomas tend to be better circumscribed than those that are pilar in origin, but the spindle cell proliferative component of the tumor will be identical in both tumor subtypes. Regardless of subtype, leiomyomas tend not to be mitotically active. Epitheloid leiomyomas will contain plump cells that can appear epithelial or even histiocytic as they ramify among the tumors spindle cell component. Leiomyomas of deep soft tissue, regardless of their subtype, are rare and these tumors may show zones of calcification.

Differential Diagnosis

Leiomyomas will mark strongly for smooth muscle actin while desmin expression will be variable. Leiomyomas can be

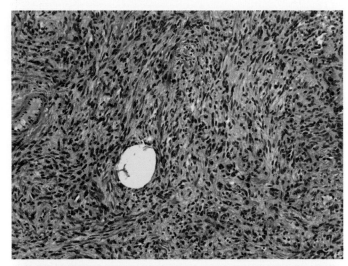

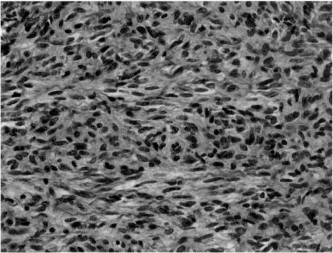

Figures 2.72 (top) & 2.73 (bottom) Vascular leiomyoma composed of streaming spindle cells. The elongated cigar shaped nuclei characteristic of the tumor cells can be seen in Figure 2.73.

differentiated tumors of nerve sheath origin, such as Schwannoma in that leiomyomas will lack Antoni A and B type tissue and verocay bodies. In addition, nerve sheath tumors will be S-100 protein reactive, whereas leiomyomas will not be. Neurofibroma can simulate leiomyoma histologically; however, the spindle cells in a neurofibroma will tend to have wavy nuclei with pointed ends rather than the blunt round ended nuclei that are typical of leiomyoma. Fibromas can resemble leiomyomas histologically; however, the "irritation" fibromas that are common to the oral cavity of children will be composed of dense vascular collagen, and trauma will routinely be identified as the causative agent.

Juvenile fibromatosis can resemble leiomyoma; however, juvenile fibromatosis is a more highly cellular lesion than leiomyoma, and juvenile fibromatoses tend to be infiltrative and biologically aggressive lesions, unlike leiomyoma. Mitotic figures and cytologic atypia will also be more common in juvenile fibromatosis than leiomyoma. Unlike leiomyomas, leiomyosarcoma will tend to show cellular atypia, hypercellularity, pleomorphism and necrosis, all of which are histologic features that support a diagnosis of a malignant neoplasm, rather than a benign one. Recognition of more than ten mitoses per ten high power fields in a suspected leiomyoma would tend to suggest either a malignant tumor such as leiomyosarcoma or perhaps undifferentiated pleomorphic sarcoma, rather than leiomyoma.

Pilar leiomyomas must be distinguished from DFSP, a cutaneous tumor with a monotonous storiform pattern. DFSP, unlike leiomyoma, will be CD34 reactive and stain negatively for smooth muscle actin.

Treatment and Prognosis

The treatment for leiomyomas occurring in the head and neck region is surgical excision with an adequate margin of normal tissue. Recurrence following complete excision of the tumor is exceedingly rare.[267]

Malignant Tumors of Smooth Muscle Origin

Leiomyosarcoma

Predominantly a disease of adults, leiomyosarcoma occurs only rarely in pediatric age group patients. Tumors in children most commonly involve the trunk region.[268] The head and neck, the lower limbs and the upper limbs are the next most frequently involved sites in children. Tumors arising in the head and neck region in children tend to be quite small, and most tumors will measure less than 2.5 cm in diameter at the time of diagnosis and, on the whole, tumors in the head and neck area tend to be much smaller than those that arise from somatic soft tissues.[268] Tumors can sometimes have a corrugated or papillary appearance. Oral cavity and cutaneous tumors tend to be well elevated above the surface.

Although leiomyosarcomas typically arise from the smooth muscle cells of blood vessels, they tend not to form vascular channels histologically. Tumors can also arise from undifferentiated mesenchymal cells or from benign leiomyomas. Most tumors will be fixed within the submucosa or dermis, and although leiomyosarcomas can arise wholly within bone, a bony origin for tumors is rare. CT scans and MRI scans will most often demonstrate a tumor that is infiltrative and invasive of the surrounding normal anatomic structures.[269]

Leiomyosarcoma can clinically resemble other soft tissue tumors, including benign or malignant salivary gland tumors, skin appendage tumors, tumors of fibrous connective tissue origin, leiomyoma, DFSP and benign fibrous histiocytoma.

Pathologic Features

On gross inspection, leiomyosarcomas tend to be unencapsulated lesions that have a tan to white homogenous cut surface. The neoplasm will be composed of fascicles of spindle cells with centrally placed blunt ended, elliptical or cigar-shaped nuclei. The cytoplasm of tumor cells is typically eosinophilic and myofibrils may be seen running the length of tumor cells.

The tumor will be composed of fascicles of spindle cells that demonstrate nuclear pleomorphism, significant mitotic activity and focal necrosis. (Figure 2.74 & 2.75) Tumor cells will often feature perinuclear vacuoles, and depending on the degree of differentiation of the tumor, tumor cells may not resemble smooth muscle at all. (Figures 2.76 & 2.77) Tumors can also become quite hyalinized, to the point that they can resemble scar. Many histologic variants of leiomyosarcoma are recognized, including giant cell rich leiomyosarcoma, epithelioid leiomyosarcoma, inflammatory leiomyosarcoma, granular cell leiomyosarcoma, dedifferentiated leiomyosarcoma and the rare pleomorphic leiomyosarcoma.[270] While these tumor variants may contain granular cells, a myxoid component with giant cells, or epithelioid or histiocytoma-like components, the typical storiform pattern of leiomyosarcoma will always be evident.[271,272]

IHC will demonstrate leiomyosarcomas will be smooth muscle actin reactive, while desmin expression tends to be

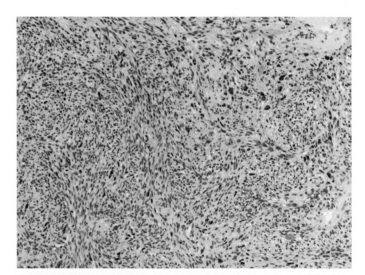

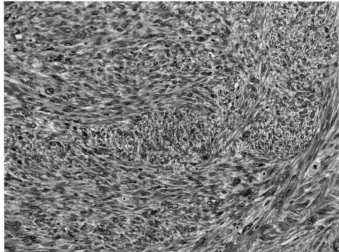

Figures 2.74 (top) & 2.75 (bottom) Low and medium power photomicrographs of leiomyosarcoma, showing fascicles of spindle cells with eosinophilic cytoplasm. Nuclear pleomorphism and significant mitotic activity are evident.

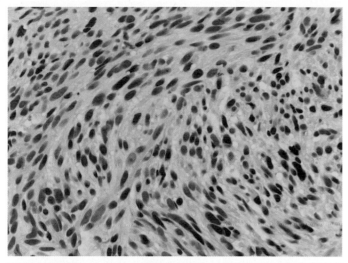

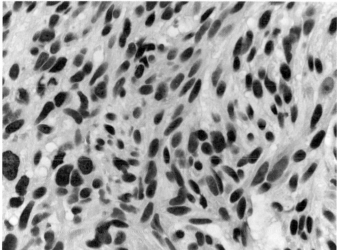

Figures 2.76 (top) & 2.77 (bottom) Low and medium power photomicrographs of leiomyosarcoma demonstrating the individual tumor cell cytologic atypia and the swirling pattern that is common to tumor histopathology.

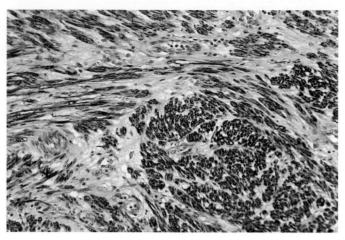

Figure 2.78 Leiomyosarcoma demonstrating muscle specific actin IHC reactivity.

somewhat variable. Muscle-specific actin stains will be positive. (Figure 2.78) These IHC findings are similar to those of leiomyoma.

Differential Diagnosis

Leiomyosarcoma can resemble fibrosarcoma and neurogenic tumors histologically, and all three neoplasms can show a palisading storiform pattern of their tumor cells. Thus, IHC is mandatory for separation of the three entities. Leiomyosarcoma can also sometimes resemble RMS or benign fibrous histiocytoma. Benign fibrous histiocytoma will, however, tend to be a somewhat more hyalinized tumor, made up of tumor cells with cytoplasm that is not as eosinophilic as that seen in leiomyosarcoma. Nerve tumors will tend to show streaming fascicles of cells with sharper ended nuclei than the blunt nuclei seen in leiomyosarcoma. IHC staining for MyoD1 and myogenin, the transcriptional regulatory proteins expressed early in skeletal muscle formation, can help one to distinguish RMS from leiomyosarcoma.

Finally, the juvenile fibromatoses that occur in the head and neck region, particularly those that involve the oral cavity and jaw bones, can resemble leiomyosarcoma. These tumors, however, tend not to show the degree of necrosis that one finds with leiomyosarcoma, and the fascicles of tumor cells seen in juvenile fibromatosis will tend to be more elongated and lengthy than those seen in leiomyosarcoma. Chronic inflammation is also more common to juvenile fibromatosis and the tumor vascularity that will be seen in juvenile fibromatosis will generally be greater than that seen in leiomyosarcoma.

Treatment and Prognosis

Leiomyosarcomas that occur in the head and neck region of children represent low to intermediate grade malignancies. Most tumors are treated by surgical excision using 2 cm margins of normal tissue. Leiomyosarcoma will recur in 25 to 40 percent of cases following surgical excision. Recurrences are most often treated by re-excision and adjuvant chemotherapy and radiation therapy.

Tumors of Muscle

Benign Tumors of Striated Muscle Origin
Rhabdomyoma

Rhabdomyomas are uncommon tumors that are thought to arise from primitive striated muscle fetal rests. Three forms of rhabdomyoma occur: *fetal rhabdomyoma*, *adult rhabdomyoma* and *genital rhabdomyoma*. The fetal rhabdomyoma, common to pediatric age group patients, is most often seen in boys, and will generally arise between birth and three years of age. Most fetal rhabdomyomas will occur in the head and neck region.[274,275]

Cardiac rhabdomyomas, which also occur in the pediatric age group, will usually develop in utero.[274] Patients with cardiac rhabdomyomas will commonly present with a history of shortness of breath, and cardiac rhabdomyomas can be associated with tuberous sclerosis. Adult and genital type rhabdomyomas have a histopathology that is quite different from that of fetal type rhabdomyomas, neoplasms that will commonly display a myxoid component histologically.

Most fetal rhabdomyomas will present as a painless mass that will be identified within musculature subjacent to skin or mucosa. The vast majority of fetal type rhabdomyomas that arise in the head and neck region will present in the retro-auricular area or posterior triangle of the neck.[273,274,275] Fetal rhabdomyomas are only rarely multifocal, unlike adult rhabdomyomas, which tend to be multifocal frequently.

Reciprocal translocation of chromosomes 15 and 17, and abnormalities involving chromosome 10 have been reported in adult rhabdomyomas. These findings have not, however, been duplicated in fetal rhabdomyomas.[276] A *TSC2* gene missense mutation has been reported in cardiac rhabdomyomas that are associated with tubular sclerosis[277] but not in fetal tumors. However, fetal rhabdomyomas in the head and neck region can also result in progressive disease that can cause difficulty in breathing and swallowing as well as nasal obstruction.

Clinically, a fetal rhabdomyoma in the head and neck region can appear similar to a hyperplastic lymph node, early RMS, vascular malformations, a granular cell tumor or hibernoma. Embryonal RMS would be the most significant differential diagnosis to be considered in such instances.

Pathologic Features

Fetal rhabdomyomas are unencapsulated tumors that will be composed of elongated spindle cells, (so-called spider cells) and aggregates of skeletal muscle fibers that are immature. There may be intracytoplasic cross striations within tumor cells. Nuclei will be prominent at the periphery of tumor cells. Although unencapsulated, the tumor will be marginated by collagen and show no invasion of surrounding tissue. Immunohistochemically, the fetal rhabdomyoma will be desmin positivity and be reactive to muscle specific actin, myoglobin and myogenin. Tumors will stain negatively for S-100 protein. Tumors that are subclassified as *myxoid* will tend to show a significant myxoid matrix, whereas tumors that are classified as *intermediate* will tend to show numerous differentiated aggregates of skeletal muscles and very little evidence of a myxoid stromal component. Tumor cells can be mildly pleomorphic.

Differential Diagnosis

Embryonal rhabdomyosarcoma will generally be poorly circumscribed, clinically invasive and destructive of the surrounding tissues unlike fetal rhabdomyoma. From a differential diagnostic perspective, fetal rhabdomyoma will not demonstrate the atypical cytologic feature of an RMS.

Hibernomas will usually show numerous multivacuolated cells and some univacuolated cells with nuclei that are centrally located, a feature that differs from fetal rhabdomyoma. Granular cell tumors will tend to show pseudoepitheliomatous hyperplasia in a high percentage of cases, as well as granular cells with markedly eosinophilic cytoplasm and dense nuclear

chromatin, features that are less common to fetal rhabdomyomas. In addition, granular cell tumors are S-100 protein reactive, which helps to separate that tumor from not only the S-100 negatively reacting rhabdomyoma, but from tumors that are histiocytic, fibroblastic and smooth muscle in origin.

Treatment and Prognosis

The fetal rhabdomyoma is treated by surgical excision of the tumor to a margin of normal tissue. Recurrences are rare. Rhabdomyomas of the head and neck can become quite large, and as such they can cause significant medical compromise. Rare instances of malignant transformation of a fetal rhabdomyoma have been reported in the gastrointestinal tract.[278]

Malignant Tumors of Striated Muscle Origin

Rhabdomyosarcoma

Rhabdomyosarcoma is a malignant soft tissue tumor composed of primitive mesenchymal cells, which ultimately mature to striated muscle as tumor cells differentiate along a rhabdomyoblastic course. RMS, is the most common soft tissue sarcoma to occur in pediatric age patients, and accounts for 20 percent of all malignant soft tissue tumors in children.[279] Two percent of RMSs will be present at birth and 5 percent will occur in individuals younger than one year of age. Nearly 30 percent of all RMSs in children will arise in the head and neck region. The most common sites of occurrence will be the parameningeal region, orbit, oral cavity, nasal pharynx, sinuses, ear and neck.[280] Head and neck RMSs can be subclassified into parameningeal and non-parameningeal forms of disease. Males develop RMSs more often than females and tumors tend to show two distinctive age peaks; one at approximately four years of age and another at about 17 years.[281,282]

RMSs that arise in the oral cavity, nasal cavity or cheeks as well as other head and neck soft tissue sites will typically present as a rapidly growing fleshy mass, while tumors that arise in close proximity to bone (orbit, maxilla, mandible) will generally result in bony destruction and symptoms of swelling and pain, paresthesia or paresis.

The current World Health Organization classification of RMS recognizes *embryonal*, *alveolar*, *spindle cell/sclerosing* and *pleomorphic* forms of the neoplasm in adults.[283] A *botryoid* histopathologic subtype is not recognized in the WHO classification. The international classification of RMS does, however, include a botryoid tumor subtype.[284]

Embryonal RMS accounts for 70 percent of all RMSs seen in children. Alveolar RMS accounts for nearly all remaining neoplasms in children. Rudzinski et al.[283] recently reviewed nine consecutive children's oncology group clinical trials in an attempt to determine if the WHO RMS classification is applicable to pediatric age group patients and concluded that the four histopathologic forms of the neoplasm recognized by the WHO are appropriate for a pediatric population.

Most investigators involved in pediatric head and neck pathology continue to consider the botryoid and pleomorphic subclasses of RMS seen in the pediatric population to be variants of embryonal RMS.[285,286]

Tumor Cytogenetics

Embryonal RMSs will typically show an allelic loss at chromosome 11p15.5. This loss of heterozygosity tends to alter a number of tumor suppressor genes including *IGF-2*, *H19*, and *CDKNIC*.[287,288]

Alveolar RMSs will demonstrate a characteristic t(2;13) or t(1;13) translocation, which results in a PAX3-FOX 01 fusion transcription. These fusions are thought to result in a phenotypic transformation that ultimately results in an alveolar RMS histopathologic subtype.[289] Many investigators also believe that the tumor suppressor gene p53, which is responsible for the control of cell proliferation at the G1/S checkpoint in the cell cycle, mutates in RMS, losing its regulatory function, which allows primitive tumor precursor cells to undergo neoplastic differentiation and growth.[290]

Pleomorphic RMSs do not show the definitive genetic alterations that are seen in embryonal RMS and alveolar RMS.

Pathologic Features

Embryonal Rhabdomyosarcoma

Embryonal rhabdomyosarcoma will be composed of aggregates of primitive basophilic small round or oval cells. (Figures 2.79, 2.80 & 2.81) These small round cells will be identified in concert with a proliferation of spindle-type cells and primitive muscle strap-like cells that will have eosinophilic cytoplasm (Figures 2.82 & 2.83) and may show cross-striations. Rhabdomyoblasts that are ganglion-like may also be seen within the tumor cell, sheets or nests. Tumor cells will tend to show significant mitotic activity and cytologic atypia as they proliferate throughout a scant connective tissue stroma. Myxoid stromal change is quite common in embryonal RMSs, and tumors which are submucosal in their location, will often show a polypoid myxoid proliferative pattern that has in the past been referred to as the "botryoid variant" of embryonal RMS. Tumors that arise subjacent to epithelium often demonstrate a so-called cambium zone, in which there is a linear proliferation of tumor cells subjacent to the overlying mucosa. In tumors that are well differentiated, elongated tadpole shaped rhabdomyoblasts can be demonstrated. Giant cells may occasionally be seen within the tumor, and thus tumors can demonstrate a pattern that is reminiscent of fibrosarcoma or undifferentiated pleomorphic sarcoma.

Immunohistochemically, embryonal RMSs will show MyoD1 expression, and diffuse desmin reactivity. Myogenin expression can be quite variable. Smooth muscle actin and muscle specific actin will generally be positive, and on occasion, S-100 protein reactivity can be observed.[291]

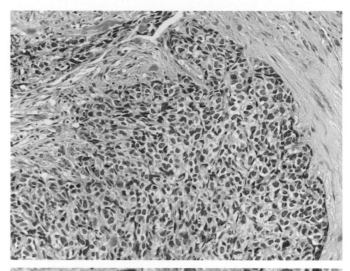
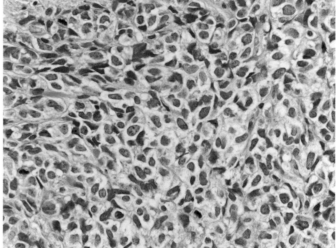
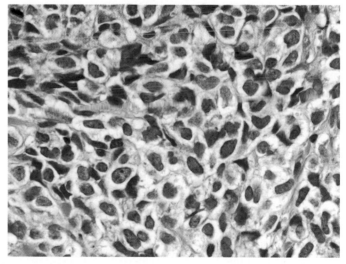

Figures 2.79 (top), 2.80 (middle) & 2.81 (bottom) Low, medium and high power photomicrographs of embryonal RMS composed of loosely arranged aggregates of primitive small round and oval shaped basophilic tumor cells. Note the marked pleomorphism of tumor cells in Figures 2.80 and 2.81.

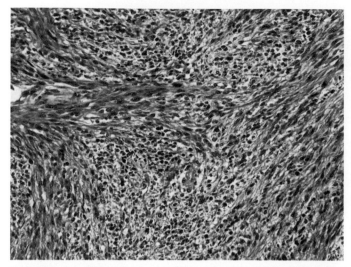

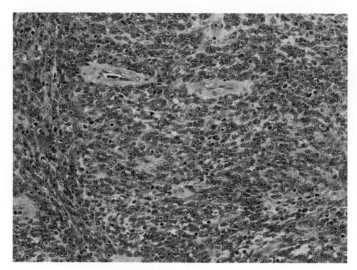

Figure 2.84 Alveolar RMS composed of cytologically atypical small round tumor cells that are both diffusely arranged, as well as arranged in a pattern that resembles lung alveoli.

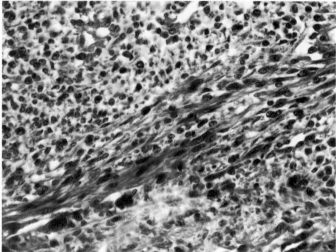

Figures 2.82 (top) & 2.83 (bottom) Primitive spindle and strap cells with streaming eosinophilic cytoplasm characterize this embryonal RMS at low and medium power.

Differential Diagnosis

From a differential diagnostic standpoint, embryonal RMS can be misinterpreted to represent other small round cell malignancies including Ewing sarcoma/PNET, lymphoblastic lymphoma, rhabdomyoma and leiomyoma. Embryonal RMS will be more cytologically atypical and far more pleomorphic in its appearance histologically than Ewing sarcoma/PNET, or even lymphoblastic lymphoma. Leiomyomas and rhabdomyomas will also not demonstrate the cytologic atypia of embryonal RMS.

Nerve tumors, including neurofibroma and Schwannoma can resemble embryonal RMS histologically; however, neither tumor will show the cytologic atypia of embryonal RMS. Finally, infantile fibrosarcoma, a tumor that is seen in the same age group as embryonal RMS, can appear quite histologically similar to it. Infantile fibrosarcoma will not, however, demonstrate myogenic expression immunohistochemically. In all pediatric age patients in which embryonal RMS is a

clinicopathologic diagnostic consideration, IHC markers for striated muscle, including myogenin and MyoD1 should be employed before rendering a diagnosis of any other spindle cell neoplasm.

Alveolar Rhabdomyosarcoma

Alveolar rhabdomyosarcoma will be characterized histologically by an accumulation of nests of small primitive-appearing round cells that grow within a thin connective tissue stroma to produce a pattern that resembles that of lung alveoli. (Figure 2.84) The stromal component of the tumor will tend to be richly hyalinized, highly vascular and markedly eosinophilic. The tumor cells in alveolar RMS will be small round cells in 90 percent of cases, and only rarely will strap cells with cross striations be identified. (Figure 2.85) The nesting or alveolar pattern that is typical of this form of RMS may only be focally present. As with embryonal RMS, alveolar RMSs will mark for desmin, myogenin and MyoD1. However, IHC muscle markers tend to be less strongly positive than in an embryonal RMS. As with embryonal RMS, other small round cell malignancies should be excluded including, lymphoblastic lymphoma, neuroblastoma, Ewing sarcoma/PNET and even melanoma. The only other tumor that commonly demonstrates the alveolar pattern seen in alveolar RMS is alveolar soft part sarcoma. However, the tumor cells that make up alveolar soft part sarcoma tend to be quite large and eosinophilic, rather than the typical small round cells that one generally observes in alveolar RMS.

Pleomorphic Rhabdomyosarcoma

Pleomorphic rhabdomyosarcoma is exceedingly rare in pediatric age group patients and remains, almost exclusively, a tumor of adults. Histologically, the neoplasm will consist of streaming interlacing aggregates of spindle cells that will contain highly anaplastic tadpole shaped hyperchromatic tumor

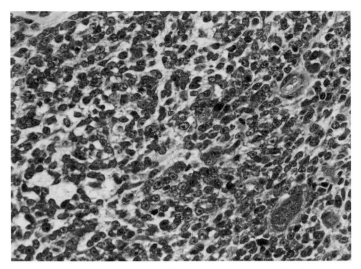

Figure 2.85 Alveolar RMS tumor cells are predominately small and round, and lack strap cell cross striations.

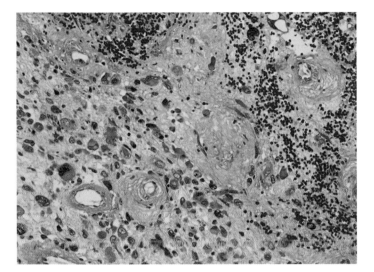

Figure 2.86 Pleomorphic RMS characterized by tadpole-like tumor cells and giant cells that are highly anaplastic.

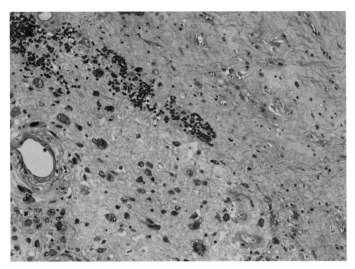

Figure 2.87 Pleomorphic RMS displaying tumor cells with marked nuclear atypia. Note the loosely arranged fibrillary to myxoid stromal component of the tumor.

IHC skeletal muscle differentiation markers can be helpful in separating pleomorphic RMS from undifferentiated pleomorphic sarcoma.

Treatment and Prognosis

Rhabdomyosarcomas are treated by a combination of therapeutic protocols that include surgery, chemotherapy and combined radiation and chemotherapy. The Intergroup Rhabdomyosarcoma Study Group (IRSG), also known as The Soft Tissue Sarcoma Committee of the Children's Oncology Group was formed in 1972 to investigate the biology of RMS and to try and improve treatment for the disease. Over the course of more than four decades and as a result of combined therapies, five-year survival rates for pediatric age group patients with RMS have improved greatly.

During a more than 40-year period, tumors have been assigned to four specific treatment groups in order to assess treatments and outcomes. Group 1 patients have included individuals with localized disease and microscopically free tumor margins; group 2 patients have included patients with grossly negative disease, but microscopically positive tumor margins; group 3 patients have included patients with grossly visible disease present, and left behind at the time of surgery and group 4 patients have included patients with distant metastasis, regardless of what tumor resection margins showed microscopically. Patients have routinely been treated with chemotherapy, most often vincristine, Adriamycin and cyclophosphosmide, and radiation therapy up to 6,000 c Gy. Five-year survival rates for patients in group 1 are commonly above 80 percent; group 2 survival is approximately 70 percent; group 3 survival is just over 50 percent and group 4 survival is 20 percent.[290]

Even with the aforementioned improvements in the management of disease, and with the knowledge that children now live into adult life with RMS, complications from therapy can

cells. (Figure 2.86) Nuclear atypia is common to nearly all tumor cells, and tumor cells will have abundant eosinophilic cytoplasm and a myxoid or fibrillary stromal component (Figure 2.87). Tumor necrosis will also be common. As with other forms of RMS, the connective tissue component of the tumor will be quite sparse. Pleomorphic RMS will be desmin, myogenin and MyoD1 reactive.

In assessing pleomorphic RMS from a microscopic differential diagnostic standpoint, one must, of necessity, consider undifferentiated pleomorphic sarcoma. Pleomorphic RMS will, however, tend to show large numbers of racket-shaped cells, tadpole shaped cells and strap cells in addition to the multinucleated giant cells that are common to undifferentiated pleomorphic sarcoma. The cells of pleomorphic RMS will also tend to be somewhat more eosinophilic in their appearance than the cells of an undifferentiated pleomorphic sarcoma.

been successful in rare cases. Appropriate treatment is indicated for defects of other organ systems involved in cases of Epidermal Nevus Syndrome, including seizures, ocular defects, and bony abnormalities.

Nevus Sebaceus

Clinical Features and Pathogenesis

Nevus sebaceus is a benign, congenital hamartoma comprised of an aggregate of enlarged sebaceous glands. At birth, patients present with a solitary, well-demarcated, hairless, pink-yellow plaque on the scalp or, more rarely, the face, trunk, or oral cavity (Figure 3.3). During puberty and hormonal stimulation, the lesion may become verrucous, scaly, or more raised.

A risk of secondary neoplasia, both benign and malignant, has been reported in multiple studies at between 10 and 15

percent. The risk of malignant transformation is likely less than 5 percent. [5] Numerous follicular and adnexal tumors have been reported to develop within nevus sebaceus, including basal cell carcinoma (BCC), trichoblastoma, syringocystadenoma papilliferum, apocrine cystadenoma, leiomyoma, and others. [6] These changes, if they occur, are usually noted in adulthood, but the risk of their development increases during puberty.

In rare cases of diffuse, large, or extensive nevus sebaceus, the Epidermal Nevus Syndrome should be suspected. Affected patients have associated abnormalities of other ectodermal tissues, including bone, eye, and central nervous system, and may have hamartomas of other body systems.

The exact cause of nevus sebaceus is unknown. Postzygotic mutations give rise to a local overgrowth of cutaneous sebaceous glands. As such, many authors consider nevus sebaceus to occur on a spectrum with epidermal nevus and other cutaneous hamartomas.

Pathologic Features

Nevus sebaceus is characterized by a proliferation of enlarged sebaceous glands present within the papillary dermis. Many are unassociated with normal hair follicles, and open directly to the epidermal surface. Clear spaces or "holes" are often present in the sebaceous lobules. There is frequently a surrounding chronic lymphocytic infiltrate. Ectopic glandular structures, including enlarged apocrine and eccrine glands, are present beneath the sebaceous proliferation. There is characteristic alopecia within the lesion. The overlying epidermis demonstrates papillomatosis (Figure 3.4).

Treatment and Prognosis

Management strategies for nevus sebaceus vary. Given the risk of malignant transformation in later life, most clinicians recommend prophylactic excision of nevus sebaceus at puberty.

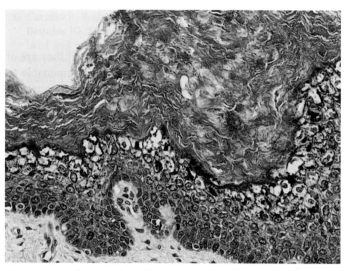

Figure 3.2 Epidermolytic hyperkeratosis in an epidermal nevus, with reticular degeneration of the granular and spinous layers of the epidermis.

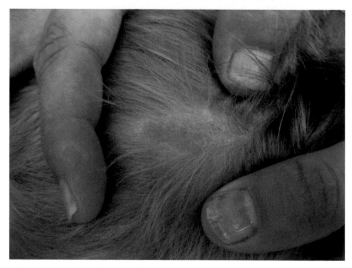

Figure 3.3 Nevus sebaceus of the scalp.

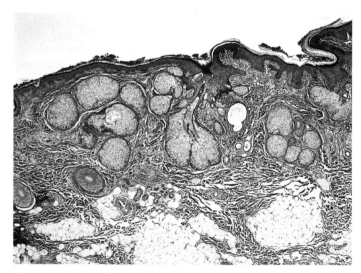

Figure 3.4 Nevus sebaceus demonstrating enlarged sebaceous glands and alopecia.

However, there is controversy in the literature regarding the risk of malignant change; some clinicians and families may opt for careful clinical observation only.

Accessory Tragus

Clinical Features and Pathogenesis

An accessory tragus represents a developmental anomaly of the dorsal portion of the first branchial arch. As such, it may arise anywhere from the tragus to the corner of the mouth or anterior to the sternocleidomastoid muscle. It presents as a fleshy, exophytic papule; firm cartilage may be palpated. Two or more lesions may be present (Figure 3.5). Accessory tragi most often occur sporadically, although they may be a marker for Goldenhar, Treacher–Collins, VACTERL, and other cranio-facial syndromes. [7]

Pathologic Features

Accessory tragi are readily recognizable by their polypoid architecture, often with a central core of cartilage. The epidermis may be rugated or slightly papillomatous. Vellus hair follicles are present in the papillary dermis, and line the periphery of the lesion. In the center is a core of collagen, telangiectatic vessels, and lipocytes (Figure 3.6).

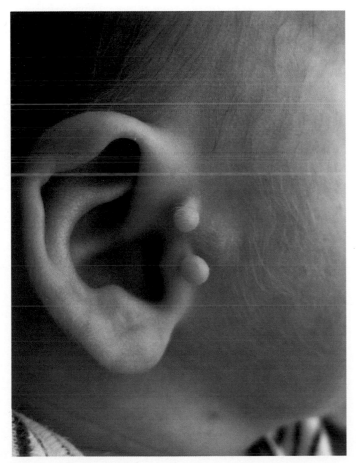

Figure 3.5 Accessory tragi in a neonate.

Treatment and Prognosis

Accessory tragi do not require treatment. Simple excision is required if the lesion is of cosmetic concern.

White Sponge Nevus

Clinical Features and Pathogenesis

White sponge nevus (WSN) is a rare disorder that affects the mucosal surfaces of the oral cavity (buccal, labial, gingival, and floor of mouth in decreasing order of frequency). In rare instances it has also been reported on the ano-genital mucosa and skin. It presents in childhood, and may be noted at birth. WSN is characterized clinically, as the name implies, by white, "spongy," velvety, or corrugated plaques of the mouth. The lesions are painless, but patients may report anesthesia or irritation at the affected site. WSN may mimic oral candidiasis, traumatic hyperkeratosis from bite or dental appliances, lichen planus, and inherited dermatologic conditions with mucosal involvement (including Darier's disease, pachyonychia congenital, and dyskeratosis congenita). [8]

WSN is inherited in an autosomal dominant fashion with variable penetrance; cases where multiple family members are affected are rare. Keratins 4 and 13, which are specifically expressed in the spinous layer of the oral mucosa, are defective, leading to the characteristic clinical and histologic features.

Pathologic Features

Marked hyper and parakeratosis are present, with acanthosis and vacuolization of the spinous layer (Figure 3.7). The basement membrane zone will be intact, and the lesions are generally non-inflammatory.

Treatment and Prognosis

WSN is a benign entity, with no reported malignant transformation, and persists throughout life. Biopsy is indicated to

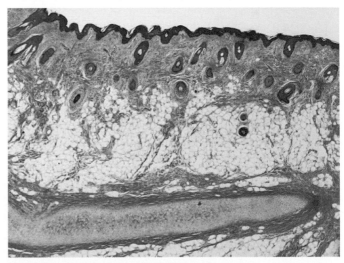

Figure 3.6 Accessory tragus demonstrating peripheral vellus hairs, central fatty tissue, and a cartilage fragment.

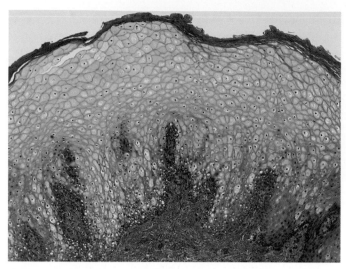

Figure 3.7 White sponge nevus showing epithelial acanthosis and pallor.

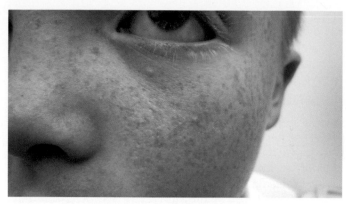

Figure 3.8 Several small basal cell carcinomas in child with Gorlin syndrome.

confirm the clinical diagnosis and exclude malignant, infectious, or other inherited causes of white mucosal plaques.

Basal Cell Carcinoma

Clinical Features and Pathogenesis

Basal cell carcinoma is the most common cancer in humans. Its occurrence in childhood is rare, but often associated with genetic syndromes which predispose to its development. Genodermatoses in which BCC is a prominent feature include Gorlin, Bazex–Dupré–Christol, Rombo, and xeroderma pigmentosum. [9] Diagnosis of BCC in a child should prompt investigation for an underlying genetic cause. [10]

BCC presents as a discrete, pink, pale, translucent or red, flat or raised papule, which may be ulcerated, hemorrhagic, or scaly. Pigmented variants occur. The lesions are generally asymptomatic, although patients may complain of bleeding with minor trauma. BCCs are slow-growing and metastasize only rarely (less than 0.5 percent). In children with predisposing genetic disorders, these tumors occur on both sun-exposed and sun-protected skin. In both children and adults, the anatomic distribution of BCC correlates with embryonic fusion planes [11].

BCCs develop from pluripotent cells in the basal layer of the epidermis or hair follicle. The exact cause is unknown, and multiple genetic and environmental factors likely play a role (including genetic mutations, immunosuppression, infection, skin type, radiation, and environmental exposures). However, the patched/hedgehog intracellular signaling pathway is a well-studied model for development of BCC in both sporadic BCCs and in the most common genetic syndrome predisposing to the development of childhood BCC, Gorlin syndrome.

Gorlin syndrome ("nevoid basal cell carcinoma syndrome") is an autosomal dominant inherited defect in the PTCH1 tumor suppressor gene (chrom 9q22.3). PTCH1 encodes patched protein, a ligand-binding component of the hedgehog receptor complex in the cell membrane. [12] This complex is crucial in cell proliferation and regulation. Smoothened (SMO), another protein member of the receptor complex, is also responsible for transducing hedgehog signaling. When sonic hedgehog protein (SHH) is present, it binds PTCH, which then releases and activates SMO. When SHH is absent, PTCH binds to, and inhibits, SMO. Mutations in PTCH gene prevent binding to SMO, stimulating the presence of SHH, leading to unregulated cellular proliferation and, ultimately, BCC. Gorlin syndrome is thus characterized clinically by the development of multiple cutaneous BCC early in life (Figure 3.8). Other cutaneous manifestations include palmar/plantar pits, facial milia, cysts (dermoid, sebaceous, and meibomian cysts of the eyelid), and acrochordons. Patients also develop odontogenic keratocysts, skeletal abnormalities of the ribs and vertebrae, and intracranial calcifications. Cardiac and ovarian fibromas occur, and 5 percent of patients will develop childhood medulloblastoma.

Pathologic Features

BCCs are characterized by well-differentiated tumor cells that resemble the basal layer keratinocyte. The cells demonstrate high nuclear-to-cytoplasmic ratios, minimal pleomorphism, and often scattered apoptotic or necrotic cells. Mitoses are rare to absent. The tumor cells are usually arranged in nodules or aggregates that demonstrate peripheral palisading of deeply basophilic cells at the periphery. Retraction artifact, caused by loss of peritumoral mucin during tissue processing, is a common finding histologically. Connection to the overlying epidermis is common but not required for diagnosis.

Multiple histologic subtypes of BCC have been described. The nodular and micronodular variants are most common in the rare cases seen in childhood. Superficial variants demonstrate tumor islands that maintain continuity with the epidermis throughout the specimen, and invade only into the superficial dermis (Figure 3.9). Morpheaform or infiltrative types are characterized by thin tumor strands embedded in a dense collagenous stroma. There is often minimal to absent palisading and retraction. This latter subtype may be difficult to distinguish histologically from desmoplastic trichoepithelioma, syringoma, microcystic adnexal carcinoma,

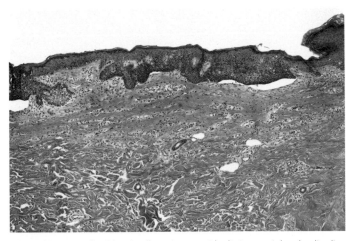

Figure 3.9 Superficial basal cell carcinoma with distinct peripheral palisading of basophilic tumor cells and retraction artifact.

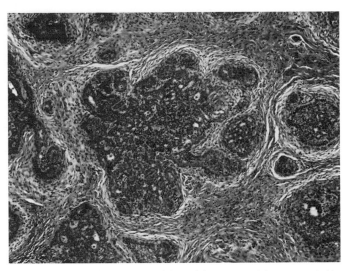

Figure 3.10 Trichoepithelioma with basophilic tumor nodules surrounded by an eosinophilic stroma and a rudimentary papillary mesenchymal body.

merkel cell carcinoma, and other basophilic follicular and ductal tumors.

BCC tumor cells express keratin markers, Ber EP4, and bcl-2. P53 shows increased and aberrant staining. EMA positivity is rare. PHLDA-1 is negative, helping distinguish BCC from desmoplastic trichoepithelioma. [13]

Treatment and Prognosis

BCCs may be managed surgically, with local excision or Mohs micrographic surgery. Very large or aggressive tumors may require adjuvant radiation. Topical immunomodulator therapy with imiquimod is also effective for some tumors. For patients with widespread tumors or underlying genetic disorders, photodynamic therapy, systemic retinoids, or the recently approved systemic hedgehog pathway inhibitor vismodegib may be useful. [14]

Hair Follicle Tumors

Trichoepithelioma
Clinical Features and Pathogenesis

Trichoepitheliomas are benign, slow-growing adnexal tumors. They most commonly present on the face or scalp as small, flesh-colored, firm papules. They may present as solitary sporadic lesions, or as multiple central facial papules in the autosomal dominant familial form. Their incidence is difficult to estimate in children and adolescents, although they may present in childhood as a component of several genetic syndromes, including Brooke–Spiegler and Rombo syndrome. Patients with these disorders develop other associated cutaneous tumors, including cylindroma, spiradenoma, BCC, milia, and fibromas.

The cause of sporadic trichoepitheliomas is unknown. Some familial cases and those associated with known genetic syndromes have been linked to abnormalities in a tumor suppressor gene on chromosome 9 and/or the CYLD oncogene on chromosome 16.

Pathologic Features

Trichoepitheliomas are characterized by basophilic nodules centered on the superficial dermis (Figure 3.10). An epidermal connection is present in approximately one-third of cases. Peripheral palisading is present. There is a distinct eosinophilic stroma surrounding the tumor nodules. Formation of papillary mesenchymal bodies is a unique diagnostic feature (foci resembling abortive follicular papillae). [15] Keratinizing structures and calcification are often present. Peritumoral mucin and retraction artifact are absent, and the tumors do not demonstrate significant cytologic atypia, necrosis, or mitotic activity. These latter features help distinguish trichoepithelioma from BCC.

Immunohistochemistry can also be used to help distinguish these two tumors. [16] Trichoepitheliomas express outer root sheath cytokeratins (5, 6, 7, 17), transforming growth factor beta, and contain merkel cells (demonstrated by cytokeratin 20 and chromogranin positivity). Dendritic stromal cells mark with CD34. Androgen receptor, which marks many BCCs, is not expressed in trichoepitheliomas. Conversely, CD10 has been shown to mark stromal cells in trichoepitheliomas, but is negative in most BCCs.

Treatment and Prognosis

Surgical excision is the treatment of choice for patients desiring removal. Dermabrasion, laser therapy, and topical immunomodulators have been employed with varying success.

Trichilemmoma
Clinical Features and Pathogenesis

Trichilemmomas are benign follicular tumors that present as discrete, smooth, solitary papules. While they most commonly present in adulthood, their importance to the pediatric provider lies in their association with other cutaneous tumors that may present in childhood, including nevus sebaceus and

The sporadic and inherited forms of both tumors have been linked to defects in and around the CYLD gene.

Pathologic Features

Cylindroma: The tumor is centered on the superficial to mid-dermis, and is comprised of multiple aggregates of basophilic epithelial cells with focal ductal differentiation. Two cell types are present. Cells at the periphery of the nodules are small and deeply basophilic, and may demonstrate palisading. Cells in the center of the aggregates are larger with more abundant, pale cytoplasm. An eosinophilic hyaline stromal band surrounds the nodules, and they often demonstrate a molded or "jigsaw-pattern" configuration. Inflammation is minimal to absent (Figure 3.14).

Spiradenoma: The tumor is centered on the deep dermis, and is characterized by large, well-circumscribed, deeply basophilic

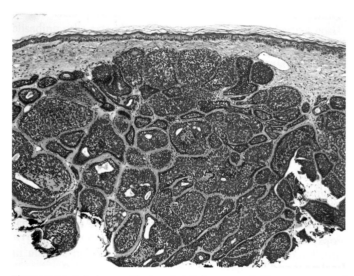

Figure 3.14 Cylindroma with characteristic jigsaw-puzzle-like arrangement of basophilic tumor nodules.

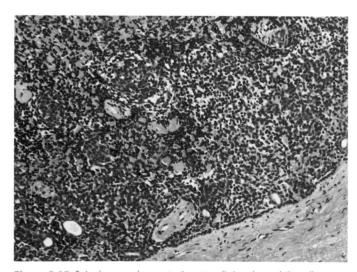

Figure 3.15 Spiradenoma demonstrating two distinct basophilic cell types and eosinophilic globules.

"balls" of epithelial cells and ductal elements. Two cell types, similar to those described in cylindromas, are present. Unlike cylindromas, lymphocytic inflammation is common within and around the tumor nodules (Figure 3.15).

Treatment and Prognosis

For painful, large, or disfiguring tumors, excision and ablative laser therapy may be employed. Malignant variants of cylindroma and spiradenoma have been rarely reported; in these cases, surgical excision and/or adjuvant radiation or chemotherapy is necessary.

Fibrous and Fibrohistiocytic Tumors

Juvenile Xanthogranuloma

Clinical Features and Pathogenesis

Juvenile xanthogranuloma (JXG) presents as an asymptomatic, discrete, pink-yellow or brownish-orange, broad-based papule, commonly on the head and neck (Figure 3.16). Ulcerated and

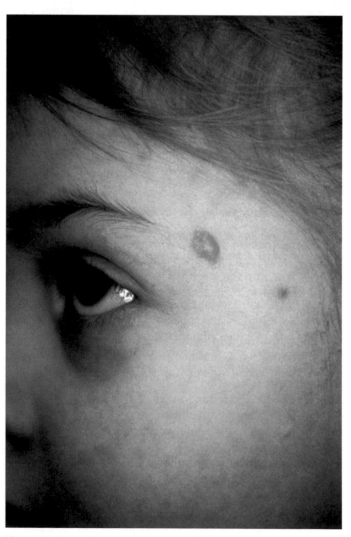

Figure 3.16 Juvenile xanthogranuloma with characteristic orange color.

hemorrhagic variants are rare. Solitary lesions are most common, although multiple may be present in some patients. Other organ systems may be affected, with the eye being the most common extracutaneous site of involvement. [25] The etiology is unknown; most authors consider JXG to represent an abnormal macrophage response to tissue injury, and thus a reactive, rather than neoplastic, process.

Pathologic Features

The lesion is well-circumscribed but unencapsulated, and centered on the papillary dermis. There is usually attenuation of the overlying epidermis. Early lesions show plump densely packed histiocytes (Figure 3.17). Eosinophils are common in the surrounding infiltrate, and lymphocyte emperipolesis by histiocytes is present. There are often numerous dilated vessels present. In more established lesions, Touton giant cells may be abundant (Figure 3.18). These are characterized by multinucleate

histiocytes with wreath-like peripheral nuclei and lipidized cytoplasm. Touton cells are common in JXG, but not specific for this entity. Mitoses may be present. [26] Lesional cells in JXG mark with factor XIIIa, CD68, and CD163. In contrast to Langerhans cell histiocytoses, they are CD1a negative. Of note, surrounding dendritic stromal cells may mark with S-100.

Treatment and Prognosis

JXG resolves spontaneously in most cases, and clinical observation is appropriate. Patients under age two with multiple cutaneous lesions should undergo ophthalmologic evaluation, as intraocular JXG can cause visual impairment and other ocular complications if not managed appropriately.

Dermatofibroma

Clinical Features and Pathogenesis

The dermatofibroma generally presents as a solitary firm dermal nodule, with a predilection for the lower extremities of women. It may occur more rarely on the upper extremities or head/face. Approximately 20 percent of tumors develop in children and adolescents. Lateral palpation of the lesion produces as a central "dimple" or "Fitzpatrick's sign." The lesion may be painful.

The cause of dermatofibromas is unclear. There is evidence for both a reactive or inflammatory etiology, and a true neoplastic origin. The lesional cells in a dermatofibroma are a mixture of skin fibroblasts, dendritic cells, and a variable number of histiocytes [27].

Pathologic Features

Dermatofibromas are centered on the superficial and mid-dermis, and are characterized by a poorly defined aggregate of spindled or stellate shaped fibrohistiocytic cells (Figure 3.19). Lesional cells may show a haphazard, fascicled, or storiform

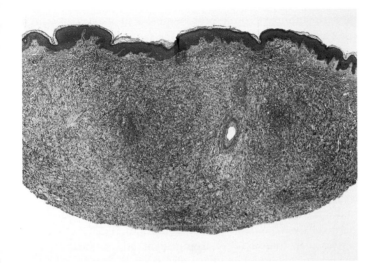

Figure 3.17 Juvenile xanthogranuloma, low power architecture.

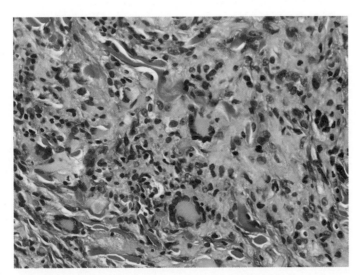

Figure 3.18 Touton giant cells in juvenile xanthogranuloma.

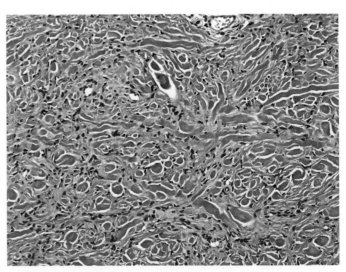

Figure 3.19 Dermatofibroma showing characteristic spindled cells and "trapped" dermal collagen bundles.

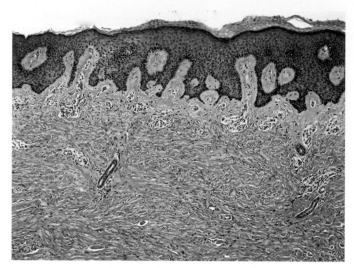

Figure 3.20 Dermatofibroma with epidermal induction.

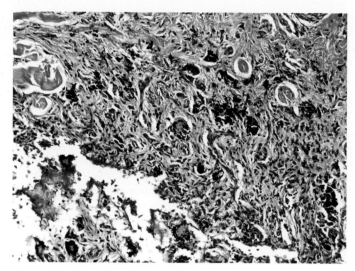

Figure 3.21 Hemosiderotic dermatofibroma.

arrangement. There is trapping of dense, eosinophilic bundles of collagen at the periphery of the lesion (so-called "collagen balls.") The lesional cells may push or infiltrate into the subcutis; however, extensive involvement of the subcutis should alert the pathologist to a potential diagnosis of dermatofibrosarcoma protuberans. The overlying epidermis often shows characteristic induction, with acanthosis, flattening and hypermelanosis of the rete, and increased basaloid or follicular differentiation of the basal layer (Figure 3.20). This latter finding may be mistaken for a superficial BCC or other adnexal neoplasm. The hemosiderotic variant of the tumor demonstrates multinucleate cells and abundant hemosiderin (Figure 3.21).

Lesional cells in dermatofibromas mark with factor XIIIa, CD-10, and stromelysin-3. [28] CD-34 and nestin positivity are more common in dermatofibrosarcoma protuberans, and can help distinguish the two lesions.

Treatment and Prognosis

No treatment is required for this benign lesion. However, some tumors may be painful or unsightly. In such cases, complete excision is curative. Large and densely cellular dermatofibromas, particularly those on the head or neck, have been reported to show an increased risk of rapid recurrence and enlargement after incomplete excision. [29]

Giant Cell Fibroblastoma
Clinical Features and Pathogenesis

Original reports of the lesion now termed "giant cell fibroblastoma" described a cutaneous fibroblastic tumor with a low potential for local recurrence, but no metastasis, occurring in male children [30]. The lesion presents as a cutaneous nodule, palpable in the deep dermis and subcutis, with predilection for the head, neck, trunk, or extremities. Giant cell fibroblastoma is thought to have pathophysiologic and histologic similarities

to dermatofibrosarcoma protuberans, and may represent a spectrum or histologic variant of the same process.

Histologic and electron microscopy suggest a fibroblastic origin for this tumor, but the exact etiology is unknown. Molecular studies of both giant cell fibroblastoma and dermatofibrosarcoma protuberans demonstrate the chromosomal translocation t(17,22)(q22;q23).

Pathologic Features

The lesion is centered on the deep dermis and subcutis. Original reports described parallel fascicles of wavy spindled cells associated with dense, wiry collagen, sclerosis, and peripheral multinucleate giant cells. Ectatic spaces lined by floret-like giant cells were noted. A honeycomb pattern, myxoid areas, perivascular "onion-skin" arrangement of lymphocytes, and intralesional hemorrhage have also been reported. Storiform areas, a characteristic feature in dermatofibrosarcoma protuberans, are often present. Mitoses are rare or absent. Lesional cells mark with CD34 and, in some reports, CD99. [31] CD31 and S-100 are negative, distinguishing giant cell fibroblastoma from vascular tumors (hemangioma, angiosarcoma) and neural tumors, respectively. Pleomorphic lipomas may show similar floret cells, but lack the collagenous stromal matrix and contain more abundant lipocytes.

Treatment and Prognosis

Giant cell fibroblastomas are considered to be of intermediate or unknown malignant potential. They may recur locally after incomplete excision, but metastasis has not been reported.

Myofibroma
Clinical Features and Pathogenesis

Cutaneous myofibroma is the most common fibrous tumor of infancy. Over 50 percent are present at birth; the remainder develop within the first two years of life. There is a slight male predominance. The cutaneous lesions are usually solitary, with a predilection for the head and neck. They have been reported in the in the skin, orbit, mandible, cranial vault, and airway. These tumors can also occur as myofibromatosis, characterized by multiple lesions with visceral or bony involvement. [32], [33], [34], [35]

The solitary cutaneous lesions present as pink to purple papules or nodules. They may be large (> 2cm) and ulcerated (Figure 3.22). If the vascular component is prominent, they may be mistaken clinically for a vascular neoplasm or malformation. [36]

Myofibromas show differentiation toward myofibroblasts with a variable vascular component. The exact etiology is unknown.

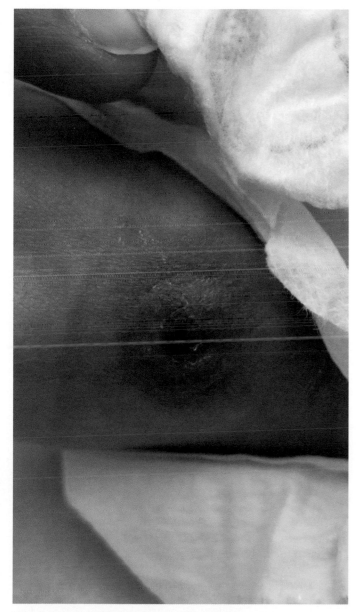

Figure 3.22 Congenital myofibroma with ulceration.

Pathologic Features

Myofibromas show biphasic or zonal histology. In the tumor's center is a dense proliferation of round, polygonal, or spindled cells. These cells are often hyperchromatic with a high nuclear-cytoplasm ratio, but mitoses are rare to absent. Branching ectatic vessels akin to those seen in hemangiopericytomas are also present centrally. At the tumor's periphery, plump myofibroblastic cells with spindled, tapered nuclei are arranged in short fascicles and whorls. A surrounding chondroid stroma with mucin is characteristic.

The central cells mark with smooth muscle actin; the peripheral myofibroblasts are variably positive with smooth muscle markers. Colloidal iron highlights the myxoid stroma.

Treatment and Prognosis

Rarely, solitary myofibromas spontaneously regress. More commonly, they are biopsied or conservatively excised for diagnostic purposes. Complete excision is curative and few recur after incomplete excision. In cases of myofibromatosis with extensive soft tissue or visceral involvement, prognosis varies in relationship to the involved anatomy, and the condition may be very difficult to treat or fatal. Chemotherapy and interferon have been employed in these cases.

Angiofibroma
Clinical Features and Pathogenesis

In the head and neck region, angiofibromas present as solitary, smooth, pink papules. Angiofibromas are common on the nasal ala ("fibrous papule of the nose"), but also occur on the cheek, forehead, or chin. They most frequently present as solitary lesions in young to middle-aged adults. Multiple angiofibromas in childhood is a marker for Tuberous Sclerosis, an autosomal dominant disorder characterized by facial angiofibromas, hypopigmented macules of the skin ("ash leaf macules"), and hamartomas of the brain, kidneys, lungs, eyes, and other organ systems.

Pathologic Features

Angiofibromas are characterized histologically by a dome-shaped papule which demonstrates a triad of thickened papillary dermal collagen, telangiectasia, and stellate shaped fibroblasts (Figure 3.23). Cellular, clear cell, pigmented, and pleomorphic variants have been described. [37]

Management

Solitary angiofibromas do not require treatment, although shave biopsy or excision is curative. Numerous angiofibromas in the setting of Tuberous Sclerosis have shown response to laser therapy and topical rapamycin. [38]

Fibrous Hamartoma of Infancy
Clinical Features and Pathogenesis

Fibrous hamartoma of infancy (FHI) presents as a solitary, asymptomatic, deep subcutaneous nodule in infants, usually

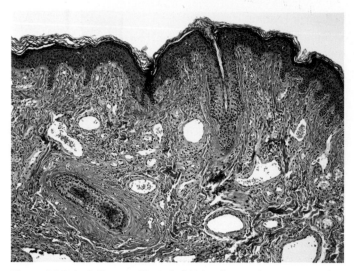

Figure 3.23 Angiofibroma with triad of thick collagen, telangiectasia, and scattered fibroblasts.

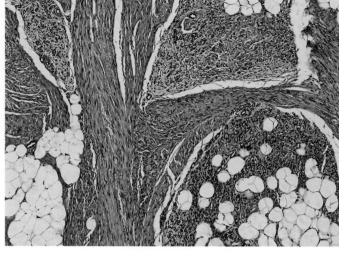

Figure 3.24 Fibrous hamartoma of infancy with triad of thickened collagen, mesenchymal "balls," and aggregates of lipocytes.

before the age of two years. The lesion may be present at birth (approximately 25 percent). Parents or caregivers often report rapid development over days to weeks, causing alarm, although the lesion is benign. FHI shows predilection for the limb girdle (axilla, shoulder, hip, inguinal area), and has rarely been reported on the scalp. The cause is unknown. [39]

Pathologic Features

FHI is a subcutaneous tumor which shows a characteristic triphasic histologic pattern. Lobules of mature fat (1) are intermixed with thick bundles of fibrocollagenous tissue (2). Mesenchymal cells, characterized stellate or wavy nuclei, are arranged in aggregates within a myxoid stroma (3) (Figure 3.24). Cytologic atypia and mitoses are not present. Immunohistochemistry is usually not required in the evaluation.

Treatment and Prognosis

Non-aggressive surgical removal is the treatment of choice for this benign tumor. There is a low recurrence risk after complete excision.

Neural Tumors

Neurofibroma and Schwannoma

Clinical Features and Pathogenesis

The neurofibroma is a benign tumor composed of neural cells. It presents as a discrete, soft, flesh-colored, broad-based papule anywhere on the skin. The lesion often demonstrates a "button-hole" sign upon palpation, as the center of the lesion can be depressed into the dermal tissue, to ultimately rebound upon release. Diffuse cutaneous neurofibromas arise in the deep dermis and fat, and most commonly present as swelling on the head or neck. Lesions in the oral cavity have also been described. Plexiform neurofibromas are large dermal nodules or plaques that follow the course of a peripheral nerve. Their

presence is a diagnostic criterion for neurofibromatosis (NF). Schwannomas (neurilemmomas) are clinically indistinct, but present deeper in the subcutis and may be painful. They show a predilection for the head and neck. The psammomatous melanotic variant of schwannoma is strongly associated with Carney complex, an inherited disorder of lentigines, cardiac myxomas, and endocrine overreactivity. Carney complex is discussed further in Chapter 4 (Lentigines and related syndromes).

Both neurofibromas and schwannomas may arise as solitary spontaneous lesion in adults and children. However, in the pediatric age group or when multiple lesions are present, their appearance should prompt further evaluation for NF. This autosomal dominant inherited neurocutaneous disorder is divided into three types. NF1 is characterized by cutaneous neurofibromas, café-au-lait macules, axillary or groin freckling, optic glioma, iris hamartomas, and bony dysplasia. Nevus anemicus is frequent, and has recently been suggested as a new diagnostic criterium. [40], [41] NF2 presents with acoustic neuromas and hearing loss. Schwannomatosis describes a syndrome of painful tumors on cranial, spinal, and peripheral nerves. [42]

Neurofibromas develop from Schwann cells that demonstrate homozygosity of the inactive version of the NF1 gene. The pathophysiology of schwannomas is unclear, although alteration of the NF2 gene ("merlin") may be responsible.

Pathologic Features

Neurofibromas are centered on the papillary and mid-dermis, and are comprised of a fairly well-circumscribed but unencapsulated proliferation of delicate, cytologically bland cells with wavy, spindled, tapered nuclei and scant cytoplasm (Schwann cells). These are arranged in a haphazard manner within a loose or pale collagenous stroma (Figure 3.25). Myxoid variants are common. Other cellular components of peripheral

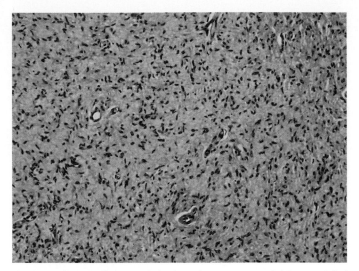

Figure 3.25 Neurofibroma with haphazard arrangement of delicate spindled cells in a loose stroma.

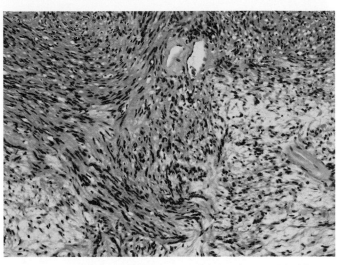

Figure 3.26 Schwannoma with Antoni A (cellular) and Antoni B (pale) areas.

nerve are also present, including mast cells, axons, fibroblasts, and nerve corpuscles.

Plexiform neurofibromas demonstrate thickened nerve bundles, often with a prominent myxoid component and nodular areas. In cases of diffuse cutaneous neurofibroma, lesional cells extend into the fat and often trap adnexal structures.

Schwannomas are centered on the subcutis or, rarely, the deep dermis. An EMA positive capsule is present. Antoni A and Antoni B areas are a characteristic feature; this describes alternating areas of compact spindled cells arranged in short fascicles (Antoni A) and less cellular areas of loose matrix and inflammation (Antoni B) (Figure 3.26). Verocay bodies are composed of tightly packed rows of Schwann cell nuclei adjacent to fibrillar pink aggregates of cytoplasmic processes. They are characteristic of the Antoni A area of the tumor. The psammomatous melanotic variant demonstrates psammoma bodies (concentric calcified bodies) and melanin pigment.

The lesional Schwann cells of neurofibromas and schwannomas mark with S-100. Mast cells in the surrounding stroma are CD117 positive. Schwannomas mark with cytokeratins and glial fibrillary acid protein in most cases; there is cross-reactivity of the two proteins. [43]

Treatment and Prognosis

Solitary neurofibromas and schwannomas do not require treatment, but excision is curative. In cases of NF, lesions may be removed for cosmesis or comfort. NF and related syndromes must be managed with a multidisciplinary team.

Palisaded Encapsulated Neuroma
Clinical Features and Pathogenesis

Palisaded encapsulated neuroma (PEN), also referred to as a solitary circumscribed neuroma, presents as a solitary, firm, pink, dome-shaped, or exophytic papule on the face or oral mucosa. The tumor is most common in adults but has been

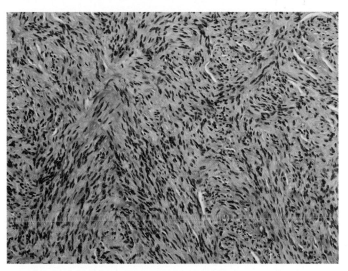

Figure 3.27 Palisaded encapsulated neuroma, high power.

reported in children. PEN is a benign lesion which occurs sporadically, and is not associated with NF, multiple endocrine neoplasia, or other known syndromes. [44]

Pathologic Features

PEN is centered on the papillary dermis, and is characterized by a well-circumscribed aggregate of cytologically bland, densely packed spindled Schwann cells and axons arranged in fascicles (Figure 3.27). The term "thumbprint sign" has been used to describe its characteristic thumbprint-like low-power architecture (Figure 3.28). There is a surrounding perineural capsule in most cases. The location of the tumor in the superficial dermis helps distinguish PEN from schwannoma, and the surrounding capsule and presence of distinct fascicles distinguish it from neurofibroma.

Lesional cells mark with S-100. The surrounding capsule is derived from perineurium, and thus expresses EMA. The

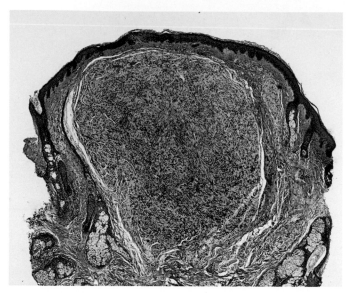

Figure 3.28 Palisaded encapsulated neuroma, low power "thumbprint sign."

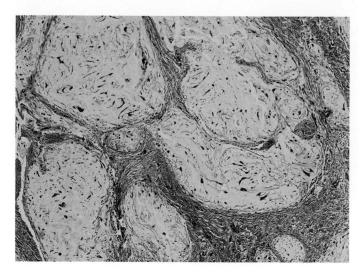

Figure 3.29 Neurothekeoma (nerve sheath myxoma) with thequed cells and abundant mucin.

intralesional fascicles do not demonstrate EMA at their periphery, a feature which helps differentiate PEN from traumatic neuroma. [45]

Treatment and Prognosis

PEN is a benign lesion; no treatment is required.

Neurothekeoma

Clinical Features and Pathogenesis

Neurothekeoma and nerve sheath myxoma likely represent entities on a spectrum, with the term "neurothekeoma" used to describe the more cellular neoplastic variant, and "nerve sheath myxoma," the more mucinous tumor type. The lesion presents as a solitary indistinct papule or nodule on the head or neck. [46] It is most common in young adults, with several reports in younger children. The etiology is unknown. It is generally accepted that the myxoid variant is of neural derivation, but more controversy exists regarding the etiology of the cellular variant. Some investigators have suggested that the tumor may represent an epithelioid variant of a dermatofibroma. [47]

Pathologic Features

Cellular subtypes of the tumor are poorly circumscribed lesions centered on the mid-dermis. Plump epithelioid cells are arranged in nests and fascicles within a myxoid stroma. Sclerotic collagen and multinucleate cells are rarely present. There may be nuclear pleomorphism and an increased mitotic rate. In the myxoid subtype, there are larger fascicles and lobules of spindled and epithelioid cells associated with abundant mucin (Figure 3.29). S-100 shows variable positivity, and is often negative. [48] CD10 and KBA 62 are more reliable markers. [49] The myxoid component is strongly positive with colloidal iron or other mucin stains.

Treatment and Prognosis

Neurothekeomas are considered benign lesions, and histologic atypia does not appear to correlate with aggressive clinical behavior. There is no definitive standard therapy. However, given the confusion over the exact cell of origin and because recurrence is reported after incomplete excision, most clinicians choose to conservatively but completely excise neurothekeomas.

Granular Cell Tumor

Clinical Features and Pathogenesis

Granular cell tumor (GCT) most often presents as a solitary, indistinct nodule on the head, neck, trunk, or extremities. Intraorally, the tongue is a frequent site of involvement, and a variant also occurs on the alveolar ridge of newborns (granular cell epulis). [50] Blacks are more frequently affected. [51] GCT is a neoplastic process of neural derivation, and modified lysosomes are responsible for the granules seen histologically. [52] The lesion is generally considered benign, although malignant GCT has been reported.

Pathologic Features

The tumor is frequently associated with prominent epidermal acanthosis and pseudoepitheliomatous hyperplasia, which can be mistaken for infection or an atypical squamous process. Nodules of large, homogenous, pink, polyhedral or angulated cells fill the dermis. They demonstrate abundant cytoplasm with coarse PAS-positive granules and central pyknotic nuclei (Figure 3.30). Angulate bodies, which may be noted, represent enlarged lysosomes which are extruded and phagocytosed by histiocytes. These cells are readily visible on electron microscopy. Necrosis, nuclear pleomorphism, and the presence of numerous or atypical mitoses are features of malignancy. Lesional cells mark with S-100. The "primitive non-neural granular cell tumor" shows identical histologic features, but

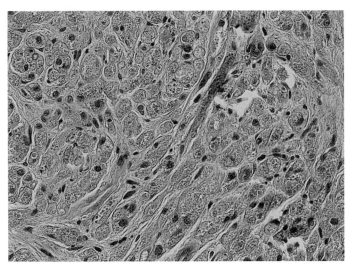

Figure 3.30 Granular cell tumor showing large cells with coarse pink intracytoplasmic granules.

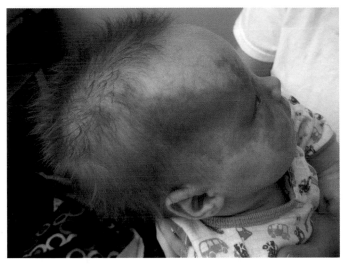

Figure 3.31 V1 distribution of capillary malformation in Sturge-Weber syndrome.

is S-100 negative in all reports [53]. The lesion marks with NKI-C3, and variably with CD68 and NSE. The exact line of differentiation of this unique tumor is unknown.

Treatment and Prognosis

GTC is treated with conservative local excision, and rarely do tumors recur.

Nasal Glioma and Encephalocele

Clinical Features and Pathogenesis

Both nasal glioma and encephalocele are congenital malformations.

Nasal gliomas are rare, and their designation as a neoplasm is a misnomer, as they actually represent hamartomatous ectopic neural tissue. Over half are extranasal; the remainder are intranasal or combined. The extranasal form presents on the midline dorsal nose as a firm, non-compressible, smooth, blue-red lesion. It may be mistaken for a dermoid cyst or hemangioma. The intranasal variant is usually seen protruding from a nostril as a polyp, or may present with epistaxis or difficulty with nasal breathing. Accurate diagnosis is crucial, as intracranial connection is present in approximately 20 percent, leading to potential cerebrospinal fluid leakage and meningeal infection. [54] Untreated lesions may also induce distortion of the nasal bone.

Ectopic neural tissue can also rarely be present in other locations of the midline scalp. All forms of ectopic neural tissue represent failure of embryologic fusion and sequestration of neural tissue [55].

Encephaloceles are more common, reported in 1/4000 live births. They represent a direct cutaneous connection from the underlying cranium, and thus demonstrate pulsation and enlargement with crying or valsalva. They can present on the midline frontal scalp, but are most common on the occiput.

Pathologic Features

Both gliomas and encephaloceles are characterized by the presence of glial tissue in the skin, and they may be histologically indistinguishable. Ependymal and leptomeningeal tissue, when present, are more specific for an encephalocele.

Treatment and Prognosis

Excision is the treatment of choice for large nasal gliomas, those with intracranial connections, and encephaloceles. All midline facial or scalp lesions should be imaged prior to biopsy or excision.

Vascular Malformations and Tumors

Capillary Malformation (Port Wine Stain, Nevus Flammeus)

Clinical Features and Pathogenesis

A port wine stain is a congenital malformation of capillary development. The vast majority occur on the head and neck, followed by the trunk and distal extremities. Lesions are present at birth and appear as flat, pink to dark purple vascular patches. They do not regress, but grow with the child and are persistent into adulthood. Over time they may thicken, darken, or develop nodules within. Other vascular malformations of arteries, veins, or lymphatics may also be present. The cause of capillary malformations is unknown. Vascular endothelial growth factor is strongly expressed in these lesions, and a neural role for development has been postulated.

Facial capillary malformations may be associated with local complications and several syndromes, particularly when the V1 dermatome is involved (Figure 3.31). These patients are at increased risk for glaucoma and disorders of the central nervous system. Sturge–Weber syndrome describes the triad of capillary malformation of the face (involving the V1 distribution), ipsilateral leptomeninges, and ipsilateral cerebral

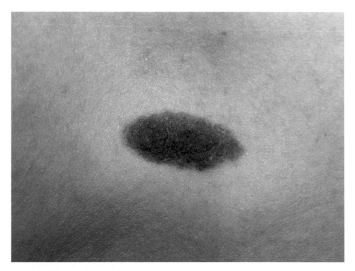

Figure 4.2 Small congenital melanocytic nevus.

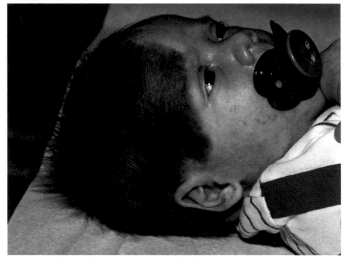

Figure 4.3 Large congenital melanocytic nevus and neurocutaneous melanosis.

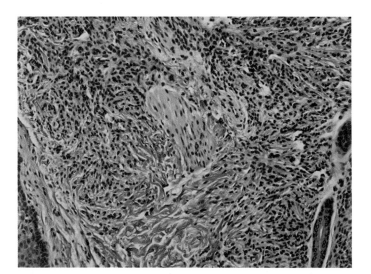

Figure 4.4 Congenital melanocytic nevus showing nevus cell entrapment smooth muscle bundles.

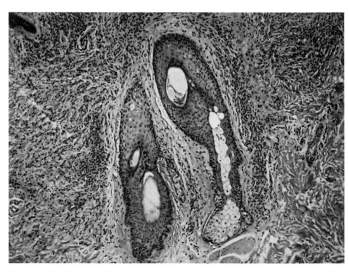

Figure 4.5 Congenital melanocytic nevus showing nevus cells entrapping hair follicles.

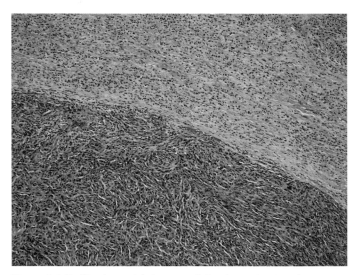

Figure 4.6 Proliferative nodule in congenital melanocytic nevus, low power.

appropriate maturation. Larger nodules present as sharply demarcated aggregates of large epithelioid cells with abundant cytoplasm (Figure 4.6, 4.7). In both types, there is no junctional component, no necrosis, and mitoses are rare to absent. These features distinguish proliferative nodules from melanoma. Of note, proliferative nodules with spindled, neural, mesenchymal, and hamartomatous lineages have also been described. For these types, the term "tumoral dermal or subcutaneous nodule" has been suggested. The lesion known as "neurochristic hamartoma" demonstrates neural and melanocytic derivation, extension into the fat, and may be mitotically active.

Treatment and Prognosis

The lifetime risk of melanoma development in small congenital nevi is not clear, but consensus data suggests it is quite low, and likely similar to that of an acquired nevus. Most small congenital nevi are followed clinically over the long term.

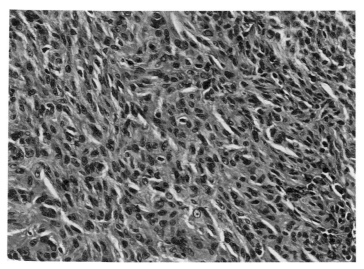

Figure 4.7 Proliferative nodule in congenital melanocytic nevus, high power.

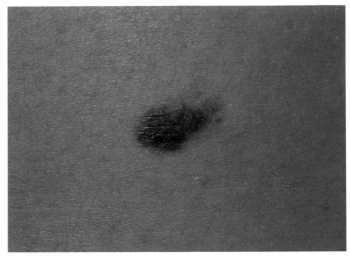

Figure 4.8 Atypical (dysplastic) compound nevus.

Risk of melanoma development in large congenital nevi is increased, but management is complicated by several factors. Excision is difficult given the large size of these lesions. In addition, prophylactic excision has not been shown to significantly decrease risk, as the nevus often involves underlying muscle or the central nervous system, and cannot be removed in full. Perhaps most importantly, dermal melanomas, the most common type to arise within large congenital nevi, are difficult to detect clinically. Current management recommendations vary widely. Dermal ultrasound monitoring may be an option for some patients. Most lesions require ongoing frequent clinical examination and biopsy of any concerning foci.

Acquired Melanocytic Nevi

Clinical Features and Pathogenesis

Junctional, Compound, and Intradermal Nevi. Acquired melanocytic nevi are benign hamartomas composed of pigment-producing melanocytes. By definition, they are not present at birth, but develop in childhood or beyond. Junctional and compound nevi present as small, discrete brown macules (junctional) or papules (compound). Nevi may also be very dark brown or pink-red. Intradermal nevi are often exophytic, pink, and fleshy. The pathophysiology of nevus development is poorly characterized; however, the number of nevi in a child is thought to be related to genetic factors (including the inherited "Dysplastic Nevus Syndrome"), skin type, and sun exposure [14].

Dysplastic or atypical nevi represent a special problem in evaluation of the pediatric patient. Several criteria are used to characterize nevi which are clinically atypical or show features of increased risk of malignant change (see section on "melanoma") (Figure 4.8). As discussed below, many of these clinical features are also seen in pediatric Spitz nevi, and the distinction between Spitz nevi, dysplastic nevi, and melanoma remains a clinical and histologic challenge [15].

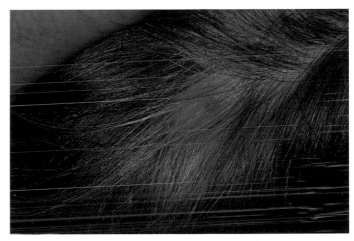

Figure 4.9 Halo nevus with associated depigmented hair (poliosis).

Halo Nevus. The halo nevus presents as a central brown or pink macule or papule surrounded by a larger depigmented patch (Figure 4.9). Intense lymphocytic inflammation destroys melanocytes in the basal epidermis, resulting in the white color seen clinically. Nevi often completely regress after the appearance of a halo. Halo nevi can be seen as a presenting feature in children with vitiligo, and may herald onset of the disease. [16] In adults, halo nevi may indicate host response to an atypical melanocytic lesion or melanoma; in childhood, halo nevi rarely show significant histologic atypia or malignant clinical behavior.

Clonal Nevus. Clonal nevi are also referred to as "fried egg nevi," which alludes to their clinical appearance of a darker (brown or blue-brown) clone of cells within a larger pigmented lesion (Figure 4.10). Some investigators consider clonal nevi to be a superficial variant of deep penetrating nevi (discussed below) [17].

Pigmented Spindle Cell Nevus. This nevus presents as a very dark brown to black, well-demarcated lesion with a

Pathologic Features

STKs will occur directly in the area of tobacco placement. The vast majority of the STKs will be identified in the labial mandibular mucobuccal folds, the most common site of tobacco placement in nearly all pediatric age patients. The lesion will most frequently develop between the alveolus and buccal or labial mucosal surface. [34] Other anatomic sites that can be affected include the maxillary alveolar mucosa and the buccal mucosa. A characteristic and consistent histopathologic pattern can be identified in individuals who develop STKs lesions. Lesions will demonstrate varying degrees of hyperkeratosis ranging from mild to severe (Figures 6.13 & 6.14). The lesions tend to have a relatively standard pattern of presentation in which the oral epithelial surface becomes parakeratinized, with or without vacuolization, and develops an ocean wave, undulating, chevron-like or church spiral appearance (Figures 6.15 & 6.16). The chevron streaks are lattice-like and are often pyramidal. Cells between the chevrons will often demonstrate vacuolated cytoplasm with koilocytes (Figure 6.17), and keratohyalin granules tend to be prominent in these areas. The epithelium of STKs will

rarely if ever demonstrate cytologic atypia. However, basal layer hyperplasia, a form of altered epithelial cellular maturation can become quite prominent in smokeless tobacco lesions. Histologic changes in the connective tissue of STKs

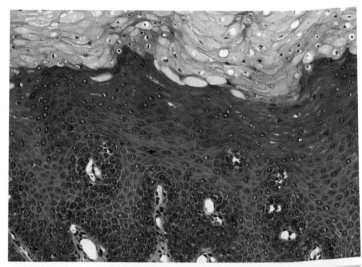

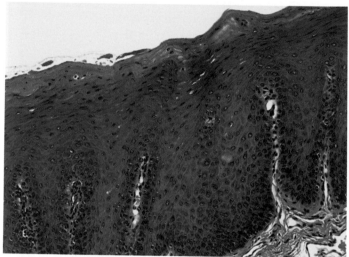

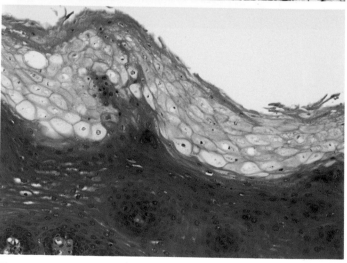

Figures 6.13 (top) & 6.14 (bottom) Grade I STKs displaying minimal hyperkeratosis and marked hyperkeratosis and parakeratosis.

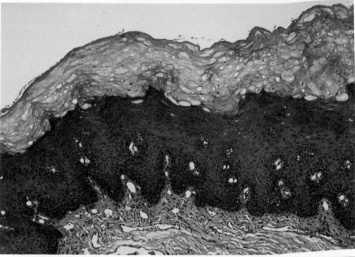

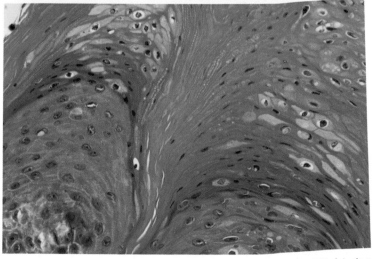

Figures 6.15 (top), 6.16 (middle) & 6.17 (bottom) Grade III STK showing classic chevron keratinization, marked generalized hyperkeratosis and vacuolated cytoplasm with koilocytes.

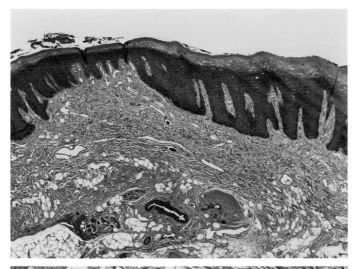

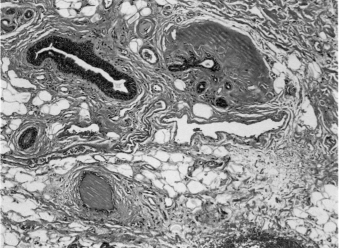

Figures 6.18 (top) & 6.19 (bottom) Grade III STK in a teenager, showing salivary gland fibrosis and hyalinization, and marked periductal fibrosis respectively.

can include focal collagen sclerosis of the salivary gland lobular architecture (salivary gland fibrosis) (Figure 6.18), chronic sialadenitis, collagen sclerosing and dilated excretory ducts (Figure 6.19). These changes in the connective tissue tend to be most commonly identified in grade III STKs when seen in teenagers.

Greer and colleagues identified a series of classic histologic features that can be seen STKs in patients ranging in age from 16 to 25. [35, 36, 37, 38, 39, 50] (See Table 6.1.) These investigators identified a host of epithelial changes and connective tissue changes ranging from dark cell keratinocytes to koilocytosis. However, they did not find dysplastic atypia to be a feature associated with smokeless tobacco lesions in any of the lesions they reviewed in teenagers.

STK Associated Oral Cancer

A meta-analysis of the relationship between European and American SLT users and oral cancer was completed by Weitkunat and colleagues in 2007. [51] These investigators reviewed the literature and completed an analysis of 32 epidemiologic studies published between 1920 and 2005 in an attempt to identify a linkage between oral cancer and SLT use. Their study included tests for homogeneity and publication bias. [51] They concluded that the oral cancer risk in individuals using SLT products is relatively minor and that any risk that was present was significantly decreased in studies that were adjusted for the elimination of smoking and alcohol. Rodu [29] has reported that SLT use has a very low potential for initiating oral cancer in any population, especially in the pediatric population. Dry snuff especially, according to the studies of Rodu, shows very little risk for oral cancer initiation. Nonetheless, the neoplastic risk, although exceedingly minimal, is in fact considered to be real.

The biggest flaw in those studies that have been performed concerning SLT use, and that have attempted to identify a relationship to oral cancer progression, relates to the fact that most studies have not controlled for cigarette smoking, alcohol usage or HPV infection, the three most important confounding factors that would most likely facilitate such a neoplastic transition. Therefore, what clinical and histologic or molecular features would allow the pathologist to identify a high risk STK lesion, remains the significant unanswered question. Few studies have addressed this issue; however, Greer and collagues [52] and Palefsky and colleagues [53] have suggested that the highest risk STK patients are those with grade III STKs that harbor HPV. Overexpression of the enzyme telomerase, a key marker of cellular immortalization, and a marker that has been documented to be present in precancerous verrucous hyperplasia as well as in STKs, may in fact be a significant predictor of such potential neoplastic transition as well. [52]

There are also certain clinical features that can be recognized in pediatric associated STKs that may indicate whether or not a lesion is a high risk STK lesion. Lesions that tend to show a marked papillary or velvety appearance or texture have a higher risk for possible neoplastic transformation than lesions that are flat with a homogeneous surface. This clinical feature tends to be a high risk feature regardless of the clinical grade of the lesion. [54]

The International Head and Neck Cancer Epidemiology Consortium reported in a 2009 study that a substantial proportion of head and neck cancers cannot be attributed to tobacco or alcohol use among young onset cases. [55] It will therefore be important in the future to determine what percentage, if any, of oral epithelial cancers in pediatric age group patients can be linked to SLT use.

Oral Epithelial Dysplasia

Oral epithelial dysplasia is a condition in which the oral mucosa undergoes preneoplastic transition. [56] Lesions that represent oral epithelial dysplasia can appear red, white or some other variation of color since there is no uniformly characteristic color change associated with the condition. Epithelial dysplasia can

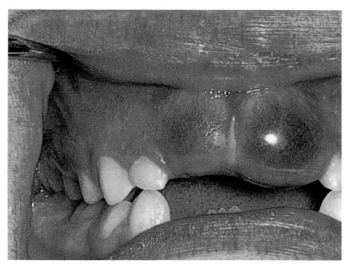

Figure 7.11 Eruption cyst causing thinning of the overlying oral mucosa and a resultant bluish hue. (Reprinted from Marx R, Stern D. *Oral and Maxillofacial Pathology: A Rationale for Diagnosis and Treatment* with permission from Quintessence Publishing Company).

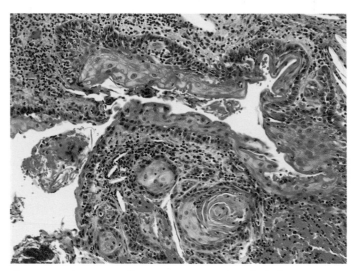

Figure 7.13 Squamous cell carcinoma arising in the wall of a dentigerous cyst.

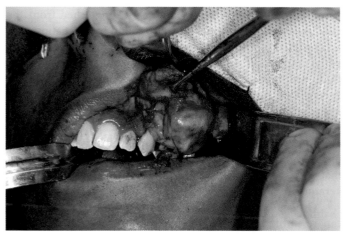

Figure 7.12 Surgical enucleation of a dentigerous cyst. (Reprinted from Marx R, Stern D. *Oral and Maxillofacial Pathology: A Rationale for Diagnosis and Treatment* with permission from Quintessence Publishing Company).

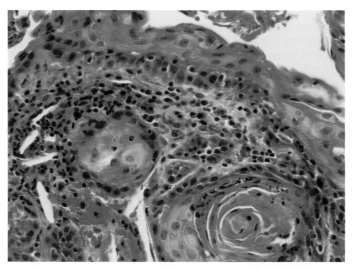

Figure 7.14 High power photomicrograph showing well differentiated, acanthotic squamous epithelial tumor nests invading the cysts connective tissue wall.

appreciable radiographic findings. In most instances, the eruption cyst will rupture and the tooth will erupt on its own. However, on occasion, excision of the roof of the cyst (marsupialization) will be required, so that the confining cyst epithelium, which may be confluent with overlying gingival epithelium is displaced, enabling tooth eruption.

Treatment and Prognosis

Most dentigerous cysts are managed by complete removal of the lesion from its bony cavity, which entails enucleating the cyst and extraction of the involved tooth (Figure 7.12). Recurrence rates for dentigerous cysts are reported to range from as low as 5 percent to as high as 50 percent.[22,23,24] If a large portion of cyst epithelial lining remains following after surgery, then recurrence tends to be higher. Since most

dentigerous cysts arise from reduced enamel epithelium, which in terms of embryonic development represents a relatively mature epithelial form, the recurrence potential for dentigerous cysts in children is relatively low. However, the OKC (keratocystic odontogenic tumor [KCOT]), which can present clinically and radiographically as dentigerous cyst, generally develops from the more primitive dental lamina cells – cells which are biologically and molecularly programed to invaginate their way into oral epithelium and bone. Therefore one must recognize that any OKC that arises in association with an impacted tooth, will have a more biologically aggressive behavior potential, than the common dentigerous cyst. Finally, squamous cell carcinoma can rarely arise from the epithelial lining of a dentigerous cyst in pediatric age group patients (Figures 7.13 & 7.14).[35]

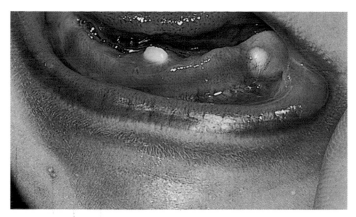

Figure 7.15 Gingival cysts in a newborn. Nodular white growths filled with keratin can be seen along the mandibular alveolar ridge. (Reprinted from Marx R, Stern D. *Oral and Maxillofacial Pathology: A Rationale for Diagnosis and Treatment* with permission from Quintessence Publishing Company).

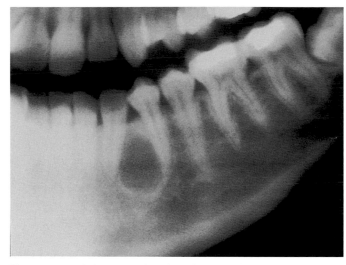

Figure 7.17 Radiolucent teardrop-shaped LPC in a child.

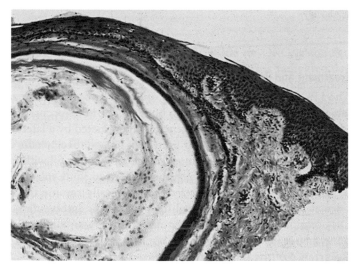

Figure 7.16 Keratin filled gingival cyst of the newborn. The cyst is lined by squamous epithelium and the cyst lumen is filled with keratin. (Reprinted from Marx R, Stern D. *Oral and Maxillofacial Pathology: A Rationale for Diagnosis and Treatment* with permission from Quintessence Publishing Company).

Gingival Cyst

The gingival cyst is a soft tissue cyst that can occur in two distinct demographics. The *gingival cyst of the adult* is a rare alveolar mucosal lesion which represents the soft tissue counterpart of a biologically more aggressive intraosseous lesion, known as the *lateral periodontal cyst (LPC)*.

Gingival cysts of the newborn represent a second demographic. These cysts typically present within three to six weeks of birth, as either single or multiple small white pearl-like nodules (Figure 7.15) that string their way along the crest of the alveolar ridge mucosa of the jaws.[36,37,38,39] Once referred to as *Bohn's nodules* or *Epstein's pearls*,[36,37,38] gingival cysts of the newborn are no more than soft tissue out growths of dental lamina tissue that has undergone cystic degeneration.

Microscopically, the gingival cyst of a newborn will present as a cystic cavity within connective tissue lamina propria that lies just beneath the oral mucosa. The cyst will generally be lined by a thin 1 to 2 cell layer thickness of stratified squamous epithelium that tends to most often be parakeratinized (Figure 7.16). The lumen of the cyst will contain proteinaceous debris or keratin and the basal epithelial layer of the lining epithelium will be quite flattened.[40] Gingival cysts of the newborn typically involute or rupture by three months of age, rarely if ever requiring excision.[41]

Lateral Periodontal Cyst

The LPC is a developmental primordial cyst of odontogenic origin believed to develop from residual epithelium of the dental lamina or from displaced rests of Serres.[42] The LPC, considered by most investigators to be an intraosseous unicystic counterpart of the adult gingival cyst, will typically present as a unique unilocular process that occurs between, rather than at, the apex of teeth. The polycystic variant of the LPC, known as rather *botryoid odontogenic cyst* (BOC) will be discussed under a separate heading in this chapter.

LPCs are extremely rare in children. Telang et al.[43] and de Souza et al.[44] in their extensive reviews of cysts of odontogenic origin that occur in children – studies that included in toto 1077 odontogenic cysts – found the LPC to represent less than 1 percent of all cases. Manor et al.[45] in a clinicopathological study of 322 odontogenic cysts which included 95 lesions in the age group from 1 month to 16 years, found that LPCs also represented less than 1 percent of the cysts they studied.

Most LPCs present as painless asymptomatic lesions that represent an incidental radiographic finding. The vast majority of such cysts arise as a well circumscribed radiolucency in the mandibular canine or premolar region (Figure 7.17). The teeth adjacent to the cyst are typically vital without evidence of root resorption, although there may be occasional splaying of the roots of adjacent teeth due to expansion of the cyst. Buccal and lingual expansion of the cortical bone is frequently identified,

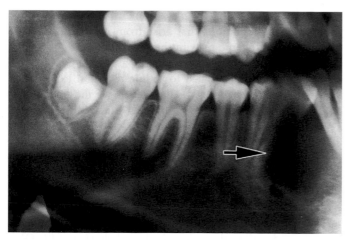

Figure 7.34 SOC presenting as a unilocular radiolucency of the mandible (arrow).

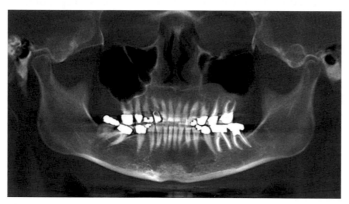

Figure 7.35 Large multilocular SOC of the mandible. (Reprinted from Marx R, Stern D. *Oral and Maxillofacial Pathology: A Rationale for Diagnosis and Treatment* with permission from Quintessence Publishing Company).

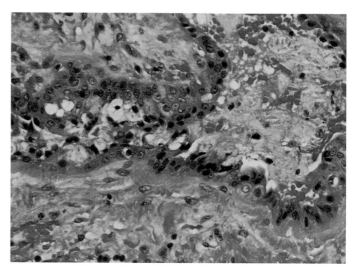

Figure 7.36 SOC showing a lumen filled with mucin and inflammatory cells. The cyst lumen is lined by mucous secreting cells and columnar epithelial cells.

Differential Diagnosis

Clinical differential diagnoses for a possible SOC in a child can include central mucoepidermoid carcinoma, BOC, OKC, COC (CCOT), central giant cell granuloma and ameloblastic fibroma. All of these lesions can demonstrate a unilocular or multilocular expansile radiographic pattern similar to an SOC.

Pathologic Findings

Grossly, the SOC will be composed of multiple saccular or cyst-like fragments of soft tissue. A thin cystic epithelial lining may be identified grossly. Nodular luminal excrescences and a mucinous product may also be discernible.

Microscopically, the SOC cyst will consist of a cyst or fragments thereof, display an epithelial lining of variable thickness. That epithelium is typically non-keratinized squamous epithelium with intermingled aggregates of cuboidal or columnar cells that may have cilia (Figure 7.36). Nodular epithelial excrescences are common to the cyst lining epithelium and small micro cysts containing mucin can often be seen within these excrescences (Figure 7.37). Mucin can be found within the central lumen of the cyst as well. Mucicarmine positive staining cells will be a prominent component of the cyst lining epithelium (Figure 7.38). The epithelial plaques or nodules that extend into the cyst lumen, or into the connective tissue wall of the cyst are similar to those plaques that can be seen in an LPC or BOC, and except for the fact that there is typically a mucous secreting cellular component to the plaques in an SOC, the three lesions can appear quite similar microscopically.

Tosios et al.[104] accessed a series of SOCs immunohistochemically and found that the lesions were immunoreactive to bcl-2 protein in the basal and suprabasalar epithelial layers of the cyst's epithelial lining. These investigators also report finding a lower percentage of Ki-67 or p53 positive cells in SOCs than in dentigerous cysts, with which SOCs were compared in the study. The biologic behavior of the SOC is therefore

that can be either unilocular or multilocular in their radiographic presentation (Figures 7.34 & 7.35). The SOC has only rarely been reported in the maxilla.[101,102,103]

Marx[98] has proposed that there are three possibilities by which the SOC might develop: (1) as a true cyst of glandular origin that arises from entrapped salivary gland primordial or undifferentiated primitive epithelial odontogenic rests that differentiate into glandular epithelium; (2) as a lesion in which the epithelial lining of the cyst undergoes either metaplastic or neoplastic differentiation to ultimately eventuate into a glandular neoplasm or (3) as a compartmentalized low-grade mucoepidermoid carcinoma that forms as an initial single cystic space instead of developing in a more classic multicystic fashion. Krishnamurthy et al.[99] in a recent comprehensive review of glandular odontogenic cysts, could only glean 111 cases from the literature. Therefore until larger numbers of SOCs are documented, and accessed and their molecular mechanisms and biologic behavior examined, especially in children, the true source of their development will remain open to speculation.

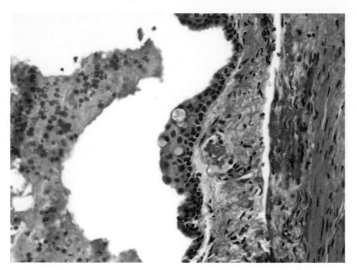

Figure 7.37 A portion of the lumen of an SOC showing mucous cells with clear cytoplasm admixed with epidermoid cells.

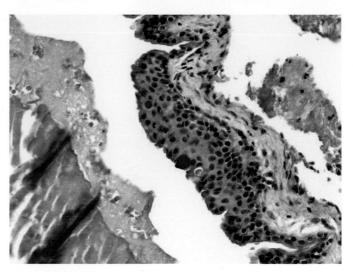

Figure 7.38 SOC demonstrating cyst lining cells that stain positively for mucous with a mucicarmine stain.

assuredly associated with immunologic deregulation of cell death in the epithelial cells that line the cyst.[104,105]

The most important histopathologic diagnostic consideration for the pathologist contemplating a diagnosis of glandular odontogenic cyst in a child is to separate SOC from the more commonly occurring low-grade central osseous mucoepidermoid carcinoma. Sialo-odontognic cyst can demonstrate mucous secreting cells and epidermoid cells similar to those seen in mucoepidermoid carcinoma, however, central osseous mucoepidermoid carcinoma will generally demonstrate solid neoplastic clusters of epidermoid and mucous secreting cells microscopically, rather present as a cyst. Central osseous mucoepidermoid carcinoma will also lack the epithelial plaques or nodular spherical aggregates of epithelial cells that extend from the cyst lining of an SOC and typically into the cyst lumen or connective tissue wall. The presence of cilia or mucous secreting cells alone as a component of the lining of the SOC does not warrant a diagnosis of SOC, since the LPC and even more rarely a dentigerous cyst can display similar histologic features.

Treatment and Prognosis

SOCs have most often been treated by enucleation and curettage. Recurrence rates can range as high as 30 percent and some investigators have suggested that marginal resection may be an appropriate management modality in some cases.[103,105,106] All patients diagnosed with an SOC should be placed on a long-term follow-up. Given the experience of two of the authors of this text, (ROG and REM), such follow-up is key, since a diagnosis of low-grade mucoepidermoid carcinoma may not be appropriately rendered until five to six years after the initial diagnosis of SOC. Any patient follow-up protocol should therefore be similar to that recommended for malignant neoplasia, which would include four month follow-up intervals for three years, and six month follow-up intervals thereafter. Should a diagnosis of low-grade mucoepidermoid carcinoma be rendered in association with a previously enucleated SOC, resection of the jaw with 1 to 1.5 cm margins that includes a segment of overlying mucosa is recommended.

Calcifying Odontogenic Cyst (Calcifying Cystic Odontogenic Tumor)

The COC is a rare and unique lesion of odontogenic origin, with a histopathology that can mimic that of a cutaneous pilomatrixoma. The lesion accounts for less than 1 percent of all jaw cysts and tumors. First described in 1962 by Gorlin and associates,[107] the COC generally presents as a slow growing, asymptomatic, central osseous lesion. Rare soft tissue variants have also been reported,[108,109,110] and the COC has been reported to occur in association with other odontogenic tumors, most often, an odontoma.[109,110]

The WHO has recently classified the COC as a neoplasm, preferring the name CCOT to that of COC. As with the OKC, however, most practicing surgical pathologists and oral and maxillofacial surgeons find such terminology to be impractical, unnecessary and confusing, largely due to the fact that the classic type of COC occurs in 80 to 90 percent of all cases,[109] and because there are no definitive molecular studies that support the concept that the COC, particularly those in children, is a true neoplasm.

COCs are indeed quite rare in children. The cyst has been reported in individuals that range in age from 1 year to 82 years. COC also shows a bimodal age distribution.[111] In a review of 215 COCs Buchner et al.[112] found that the diagnosis of lesions showed peaks in patients in the second or the sixth and seventh decades of life. Pindborg et al.[110] found that as high as 24 percent of COCs they reviewed were associated with a co-existing odontoma, an association that tended to occur in older patients[110,111,112] rather than children.[7]

Servato et al.[114] in an analysis of 431 odontogenic tumors in children and adolescents, found 18 COCs (4.2 percent) of

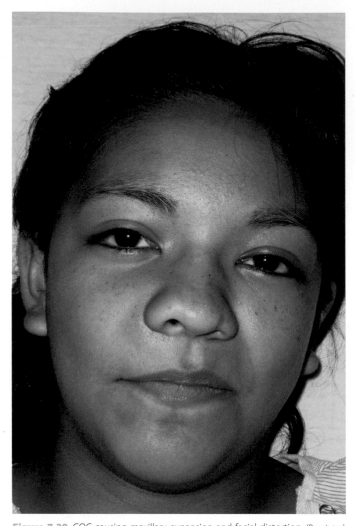

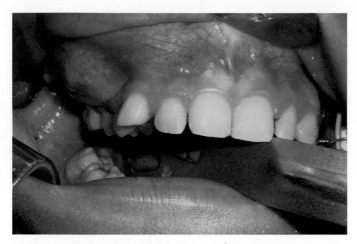

Figure 7.40 COC showing nodular expansion of the maxilla.

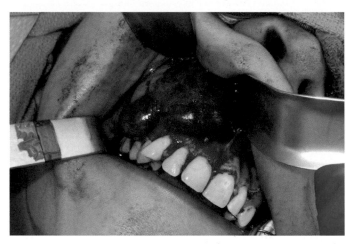

Figure 7.39 COC causing maxillary expansion and facial distortion. (Reprinted from Marx R, Stern D. *Oral and Maxillofacial Pathology: A Rationale for Diagnosis and Treatment* with permission from Quintessence Publishing Company).

Figure 7.41 COC showing buccal expansion of the maxilla with cortical perforation. (Reprinted from Marx R, Stern D. *Oral and Maxillofacial Pathology: A Rationale for Diagnosis and Treatment* with permission from Quintessence Publishing Company).

the lesions studied. The COCs were nearly evenly distributed between males and females and patients ranged in age from 7 to 18. Guerrisi et al.[115] in a retrospective study of 146 odontogenic tumors in children, found that six cases – 3.9 percent of their study sample – were COCs. The COC is most common in the anterior maxilla when found in children. However the cyst tends to be more evenly distributed throughout the posterior maxilla and mandible when found in both children and adults.[112,113,114] The COC can be associated with other odontogenic tumors, most often an odontoma, when seen in children.[116] Biologically aggressive variants of the COC have been documented in adults; however, they are exceedingly rare in children. Extraosseous examples of COC have been documented; however, such lesions are also exceedingly rare in children.[113,114]

Most COCs in children will present radiographically as a unilocular well marginated radiolucent lesion that may contain calcifications. Lesions can also be multilocular, and the COC may be associated with an unerupted tooth. The radiographic margins of a COC can be either well defined or poorly

demarcated. Uchiyama et al.[117] in a study that evaluated CT images of so-called CCOTs, found root resorption and lesional radiopacities in over half the tumors that were studied. These authors also found that CT evaluation was superior to conventional radiographic evaluation in detecting 1) buccal/lingual bony expansion, and 2) the association of a CCOT with an odontoma.

The COC is usually an asymptomatic lesion that shows no apparent gender predilection. Most COCs will be identified anterior to the first molar region of the jaws, with 75 percent of cases reported to occur in the incisor/canine region. Swelling and bony expansion of the jaw with facial distortion can occur, (Figure 7.39) but rarely is lingual expansion of the bone encountered. COC's have been reported to expand (Figure 7.40) and perforate the bony cortical plate of the mandible or maxilla (Figure 7.41) and to cause tooth displacement as well as root resorption of teeth (Figure 7.42). Interestingly, 25 to 35 percent of COCs are reported to occur in association with an impacted tooth, most often a canine tooth.[108]

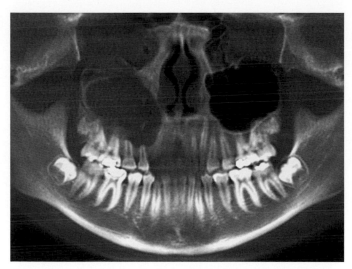

Figure 7.42 COC of the maxilla. Note root resorption of the teeth and tooth displacement. (Reprinted from Marx R, Stern D. *Oral and Maxillofacial Pathology: A Rationale for Diagnosis and Treatment* with permission from Quintessence Publishing Company).

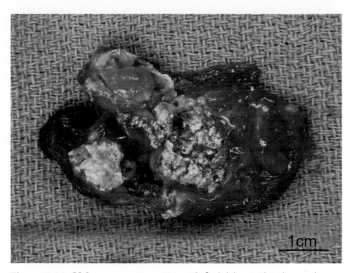

Figure 7.44 COC, gross specimen. Note calcified debris within the cyst lumen. (Reprinted from Marx R, Stern D. *Oral and Maxillofacial Pathology: A Rationale for Diagnosis and Treatment* with permission from Quintessence Publishing Company).

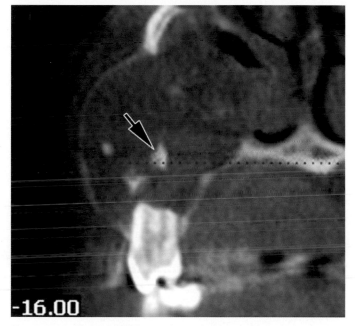

Figure 7.43 CT scan of COC. Note the cyst's thin marginating rim of calcification, and central zones of luminal calcification (arrow). (Reprinted from Marx R, Stern D. *Oral and Maxillofacial Pathology: A Rationale for Diagnosis and Treatment* with permission from Quintessence Publishing Company).

Radiographically, the COC will present as a unilocular or multilocular cystic appearing lesion with margins that are typically well demarcated. Calcified bodies of various sizes may be seen within larger COCs (Figure 7.43). Since the COC can present grossly as either a cyst or a solid mass, radiographic patterns can be quite varied.

Differential Diagnosis

From a radiographic differential diagnostic aspect, the COC can have an appearance that is similar to that of an adenomatoid odontogenic tumor, a calcifying epithelial odontogenic tumor or an odontoma (especially in children). Ameloblastic odontoma and ameloblastic fibro-odontoma can also resemble the COC radiographically. One feature that tends to separate the latter two entities from COC is the fact that ameloblastic odontoma and ameloblastic fibro-odontomas tend to grow and expand the jaws quite rapidly when compared with the COC.

Pathologic Findings

The COC can present grossly as either a sack-like cystic lesion or as a solid tumor mass (Figure 7.44). In either instance, calcified foci may be identified within the specimen grossly. Histologically, the COC will most often have a fibrous peripheral capsule that marginates a central cystic lumen, which will be lined by columnar or cuboidal epithelium of odontogenic origin. The basal layer of the cyst's epithelial lining will stain strongly basophilic and this layer of cells may resemble ameloblasts (Figure 7.45). Above the basal epithelial layer, loosely arranged aggregates of epithelial cells that simulate the stellate reticulum of the enamel organ will be identified. Interspersed among these stellate cells, accumulations of eosinophilic cells that are devoid of nuclei will be prominent. These cells, which tend to retain their peripheral cell outline, have been termed "ghost cells" (Figure 7.46). Ghost cells frequently calcify to form dense sheets of a calcified or keratin-like product. The entire lumen of the cyst may contain such ghost cells. These cells are considered by most investigators to represent epithelial cells that have undergone coagulative necrosis, dystrophic calcification or abnormal keratinization.

Freedman[108] and Sauk[118] have reported that the basal epithelial layer of the COC may demonstrate prominent budding which can extend into the supporting connective tissue wall. This epithelial budding can be associated with the induction of aggregates of dentin, enamel and even melanin within the lumen or the walls of COCs.[108,114,115,116]

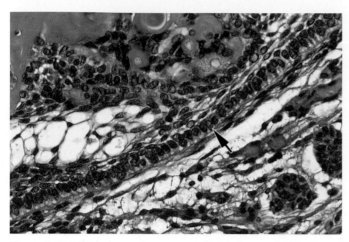

Figure 7.45 COC displaying characteristic columnar lining cells (arrow) with cell nuclei that are polarized away from the basement membrane.

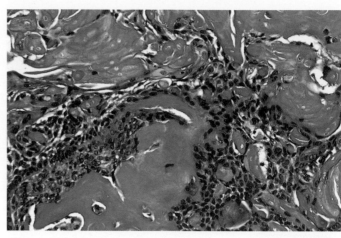

Figure 7.46 Globular eosinophilic "ghost cell" aggregates of keratin can be seen above the epithelial lining in this COC.

Oliveria et al.[113] have described four specific histologic COC subtypes: 1) a cystic non-proliferative form of the lesion, which is a predominantly cystic lesion which may contain eosinophilic dentinoid-like material; 2) a cystic proliferative subtype that is ameloblastomatous in nature, and in which there are satellite cysts in the supporting cyst wall, along with odontogenic epithelial rests, or epithelial odontogenic proliferations that resemble an ameloblastoma; 3) an odontoma-associated COC, which will have odontoma-like or dentical-like structures in the cyst wall and 4) an epithelial odontogenic ghost cell tumor, which contains aggregates of eosinophilic material along with associated eosinophilic epithelial cells that appear to be ghost-like keratin cells. These ghost cells may be seen in association with strands of epithelium that resembles that seen in ameloblastoma. The term *odontogenic ghost cell tumor* has been applied to this fourth variant of the COC.[119] Instances of true ameloblastoma arising in conjunction with the COC have been reported as well.[120] Locally aggressive COCs and even malignant COCs or so-called ghost cell odontogenic carcinomas have been reported,[118] but no such tumors have been appropriately documented in children.

Differential Diagnosis

The ghost cells in a COC can resemble the concentric calcifications that are seen in craniopharyngiomas as well as the ghost cells that are present in the pilomatrixoma of skin. The anatomic location of the three lesions should allow for separation of the three entities.

The often contradictory histopathologic findings that have been reported in association with the COC have led seasoned investigators including Gnepp and Marx[121,122] to take the position that the exuberant and unnecessary over-classification of the COC (because such classification is not predictive of clinical outcome) is largely unwarranted. Therefore, until appropriate, well designed, longitudinal and long-term studies that include molecular findings and management outcomes are carried out on a significant number of cases of COC, such excessive subclassification, especially in pediatric age group patients is deemed inappropriate.

Treatment and Management

COCs occurring in the pediatric age group tend to be non-aggressive lesions biolgoically. The treatment of choice for such COCs is enucleation. In those rare cases in which a COC shows either concomitant ameloblastomatous proliferation or ghost cell differentiation in association with an ameloblastoma, more aggressive surgery may be warranted. It is the position of two authors of this text, (ROG and REM) that in pediatric age group patients, neither the term *odontogenic ghost cell tumor* nor CCOT should be used to replace the term COC. Whenever an ameloblastoma or extensive ghost cell proliferation within an ameloblastoma is identified in concert with a COC's cystic histologic component, the biologic behavior of that lesion should be considered to be that of an ameloblastoma. We can find no data in the literature that supports assigning such tumors a name other than ameloblastoma, and certainly lumping two entities together, or otherwise assigning the lesion a new name does not seem to benefit the patient. Although there are clearly reported cases of COC occurring in association with ameloblastic fibro-odontoma and ameloblastoma,[123] such lesions do not represent true COCs, but are more likely simply cystic change or cystic degeneration within the primary odontogenic tumor. Close scrutiny of all such lesions by the pathologist and the clinician, and appropriate clinicopathologic correlation is mandatory if proper management of such lesions is to ensue, especially in light of the fact that rare malignancies have been reported to occur in association with the COC.[124]

Primary Intraosseous Squamous Cell Carcinoma Arising in Odontogenic Cysts

Primary intraosseous squamous cell carcinoma is a distinctly rare entity, in both adults and individuals in the pediatric age group.[125] Bodner et al.[126] reviewed 116 cases of intraosseous squamous cell carcinoma arising from odontogenic cysts and recorded only two instances of such a transition occurring in patients who were either in the first or second decades of life. The youngest patient in the Bodner series was two years old. In a more recent review of the literature by Manish et al. no children with primary intraosseous squamous cell carcinoma were found.[127]

The pathogenesis of primary intraosseous squamous cell carcinoma arising from an odontogenic cyst is unclear.[128] Some authorities suggest that long-term chronic inflammation in the cyst wall is the primary predisposing factor. This would seem to be an unlikely causation since such a lesion arising in a child would, almost of necessity, have been associated with inflammation over a much shorter term than in an adult. Carcinogenesis can occur, nonetheless when there is long-standing inflammation caused by, or related to, DNA damage to proteins and cell membranes, and/or loss of the protective influence of enzymes that modulate carcinogenesis, a long-standing inflammation can also affect cell division, differentiation and apoptosis, as well as alter immune surveillance through the mechanism of immunosuppression. Even so, it is just as likely that some genetic mechanism may favor the development of carcinoma in an odontogenic cyst, via the up or down regulation of genetic events that might trigger malignant neoplastic differentiation of odontogenic rests in the cyst wall. Although such molecular events can be postulated, such transition remains exceedingly rare in children. Metastasis of carcinoma arising from an odontogenic in cyst is also quite rare in children.[128,129,130,131]

Pathologic Findings

Most squamous cell carcinomas that arise from odontogenic cysts have been reported to be either well or moderately differentiated neoplasms. The lesions occasionally present in a fashion similar to ameloblastic carcinoma. However, primary intraosseous squamous cell carcinoma will lack the nuclear reverse polarity and basilar palisading of the tumor cells seen at the margins of islands. Matsuzaki et al.[132] have divided primary intraosseous squamous cell carcinoma into solid, KCOT and odontogenic cyst subtypes. Only the latter two subtypes are seen with any frequency in children.

Treatment and Prognosis

In order to accurately diagnose primary intraosseous squamous cell carcinoma that is arising from an odontogenic cyst, preoperative biopsy is mandatory, and a thorough gross and microscopic examination of the cyst lining is required. Therapy may include minimally invasive procedures, such as enucleation, if the lesion is in-situ or intramural. More commonly however, resection, radiation therapy and chemotherapy are required. The overall survival rate for intraosseous squamous cell carcinoma arising from an odontogenic cyst, regardless of the patient's age, has been reported by Bodner to be 62 percent at two years and 38 percent at five years.[125] Interestingly, those

primary intraosseous squamous cell carcinomas that have been reported to arise from odontogenic cysts in children have most often arisen from "inflammatory" odontogenic cysts such as radicular cysts, rather than from "developmental" odontogenic cysts, such as a dentigerous cyst.

Surgical Approaches to Odontogenic Cysts

Soft Tissue Cysts: The rare gingival cyst and eruption cysts are treated with a marsupialization of the cyst lining to the gingival mucosa in a straightforward fashion. The cyst lining becomes part of the gingival-papilla complex.

Cysts in Bone

Marsupialization: To reduce food ingress, the incision is best made in the vestibule rather than the ridge crest, unless it is done for the purpose of erupting a permanent tooth. A large (2 cm) window is made through the bone cortex while keeping the cyst lining intact. A portion of the cyst lining is then excised for a biopsy and the remaining cyst lining sutured to the oral mucosa. At this point, the contents of the cyst lumen should be evacuated with irrigation and an exploration of the cyst lumen conducted with either direct vision or an endoscope to rule out luminal proliferations or suspicious thickenings of the cyst lining that might indicate that an enucleation would be preferred. Initially, it is helpful to suture a shortened nasopharyngeal airway in place so as to allow the opening to mature (Figure 7.47).

Since the oral vestibular opening has a tendency to close, an acrylic plug is often required after the opening matures (Figure 7.48). This can be made in the postoperative course. The cavity is then followed clinically and radiographically for several months until either sufficient bone regenerates radiographically or the lining is seen to become flush with the adjacent mucosa. In some cases of particularly large cysts, a delayed enucleation is accomplished when the cystic cavity has reduced sufficiently in size so that the secondary enucleation surgery is more straightforward (Figure 7.49).

Enucleation and Curettage: A transoral enucleation and curettage requires a wide access, full thickness, mucoperiosteal

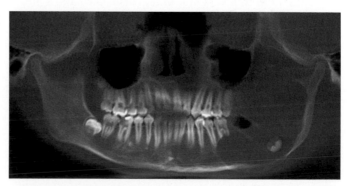

Figure 7.47 Marsupialization of a large cyst with shortened nasopharyngeal airway tube in place. (Reprinted from Marx R, Stern D. *Oral and Maxillofacial Pathology: A Rationale for Diagnosis and Treatment* with permission from Quintessence Publishing Company).

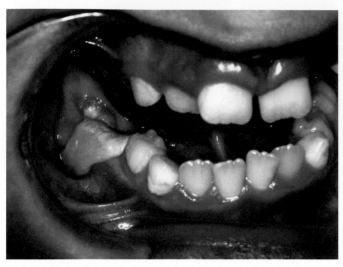

Figure 7.48 Acrylic plug maintaining an opening to the cyst's lumen. (Reprinted from Marx R, Stern D. *Oral and Maxillofacial Pathology: A Rationale for Diagnosis and Treatment* with permission from Quintessence Publishing Company).

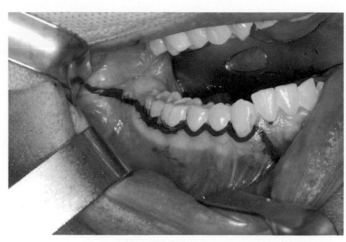

Figure 7.50 Incision design for the wide access required to completely enucleate a cyst. (Reprinted from Marx R, Stern D. *Oral and Maxillofacial Pathology: A Rationale for Diagnosis and Treatment* with permission from Quintessence Publishing Company).

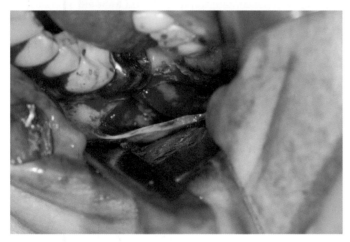

Figure 7.49 Delayed enucleation of a smaller cyst after several months of a marsupialization. (Reprinted from Marx R, Stern D. *Oral and Maxillofacial Pathology: A Rationale for Diagnosis and Treatment* with permission from Quintessence Publishing Company).

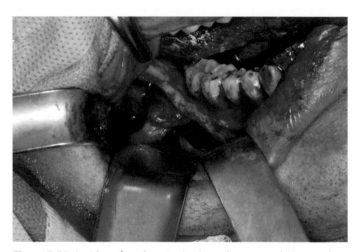

Figure 7.51 A wide surface decortication is used to curette the cyst under direct vision. (Reprinted from Marx R, Stern D. *Oral and Maxillofacial Pathology: A Rationale for Diagnosis and Treatment* with permission from Quintessence Publishing Company).

flap. The incision is best initiated about the necks of associated teeth so as to access cyst lining about their roots and is carried well beyond the cyst location for a releasing incision (Figure 7.50). Similarly, a wide surfaced decortication is recommended so as to directly visualize the majority of the cyst lining and avoid curetting in a blind fashion (Figure 7.51). The author (REM) prefers to thin the cortex with an acrylic or round bur to visualize a small portion of the cyst wall lying against the inner wall of the cortex. A periosteal elevator can then be inserted between the cyst wall and the inner wall of the cortex to protect the cyst as further cortex is removed. In some cases, the cyst will have perforated the cortex allowing the same maneuver to be accomplished without removing an initial portion of the cortex (Figure 7.52).

Once sufficient bony access has been gained, the cyst can be separated from the bony cavity under direct vision using the

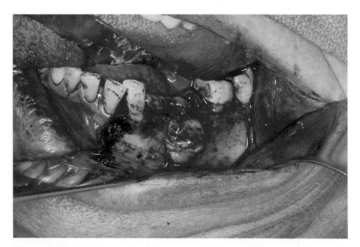

Figure 7.52 This cyst resorbed the cortex of the mandible. (Reprinted from Marx R, Stern D. *Oral and Maxillofacial Pathology: A Rationale for Diagnosis and Treatment* with permission from Quintessence Publishing Company).

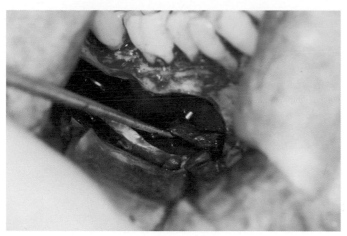

Figure 7.53 Inferior alveolar neurovascular bundle separated from a mandibular cyst. (Reprinted from Marx R, Stern D. *Oral and Maxillofacial Pathology: A Rationale for Diagnosis and Treatment* with permission from Quintessence Publishing Company).

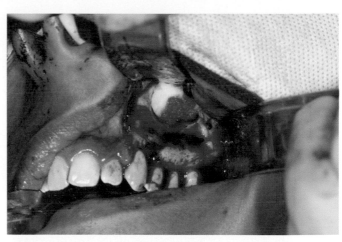

Figure 7.55 Caldwell Luc access used to remove a cyst in the maxilla. (Reprinted from Marx R, Stern D. *Oral and Maxillofacial Pathology: A Rationale for Diagnosis and Treatment* with permission from Quintessence Publishing Company).

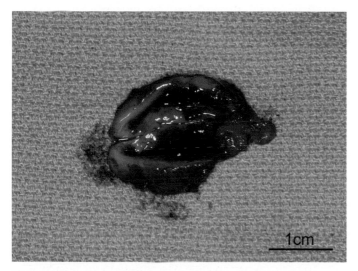

Figure 7.54 Excised cyst with lumen opened for a direct examination. (Reprinted from Marx R, Stern D. *Oral and Maxillofacial Pathology: A Rationale for Diagnosis and Treatment* with permission from Quintessence Publishing Company).

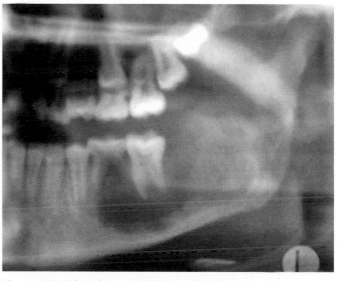

Figure 7.56 Defect of the mandible immediately after cyst removal. (Reprinted from Marx R, Stern D. *Oral and Maxillofacial Pathology: A Rationale for Diagnosis and Treatment* with permission from Quintessence Publishing Company).

back end of a molt curette or periosteal elevator. The use of a Kitner sponge or moistened cotton may assist in separating the lining from the bony cavity. The cyst should also be separated from the inferior alveolar neurovascular bundle and roots of teeth (Figure 7.53). There is no reason to remove one neurovascular bundle or to accomplish root canal treatments on associated teeth. Curetting about the apices of teeth deinnervates them for about one year, but does not devitalize the pulp due to collateral blood vessels within the entire periodontal ligament up to the furcation of multirooted teeth. On occasion, the cyst may extend lingually or palataly so as to prevent access to the cyst from a facial approach. In such cases, a root canal treatment will not improve the access. In those cases, removing some teeth becomes necessary, or, if feasible, approach the cyst from both a labial and lingual/palatal approach simultaneously.

Upon removal of the cyst, it should be examined grossly for complete removal (Figure 7.54). If the surgeon finds or suspects an area of cyst lining remaining, it is best to physically curette the area. Use of Carnoy's solution, cryotherapy or phenol to sterilize residual cyst lining has not been shown to reduce recurrences and has potential complications and risks. Neither is recommended.

Odontogenic cysts in the maxilla are approached in a similar manner. However, those that expand close to or into the maxillary sinus, require a thorough entry and removal of the sinus membrane as a barrier using a wide Caldwell Luc access (Figure 7.55). The maxillary sinus membrane will regenerate completely after such an entry.

The resultant bony cavity in either the mandible or maxilla can be expected to regenerate the lost bone radiographically, especially in children (Figures 7.56 & 7.57). There is no need to

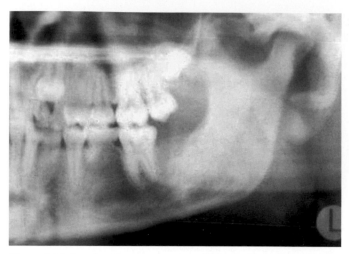

Figure 7.57 Complete bone regeneration of defect in Figure 7.10 by six months. (Reprinted from Marx R, Stern D. *Oral and Maxillofacial Pathology: A Rationale for Diagnosis and Treatment* with permission from Quintessence Publishing Company).

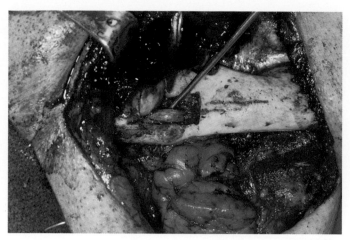

Figure 7.59 Decortication of the mandible to isolate and preserve the inferior alveolar neurovascular bundle. (Reprinted from Marx R, Stern D. *Oral and Maxillofacial Pathology: A Rationale for Diagnosis and Treatment* with permission from Quintessence Publishing Company).

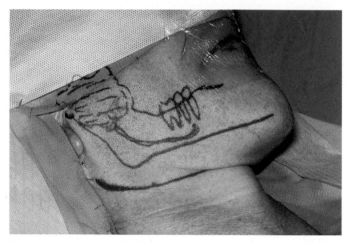

Figure 7.58 Extraoral approach incision design to hide scar in a natural skin fold. (Reprinted from Marx R, Stern D. *Oral and Maxillofacial Pathology: A Rationale for Diagnosis and Treatment* with permission from Quintessence Publishing Company).

graft such defects unless in the late teenage patient a dental implant reconstruction is planned. In such cases a graft will retain a better bucco-lingual width for implants than a post-surgical native bone regeneration. Although autogenous cancellous marrow grafts are effective in large defects and allogeneic grafts can be effective in small defects, the author (REM) prefers to use an in-situ tissue engineering concept of cancellous allogeneic bone, platelet rich plasma and rhBMP-2/ACS, which will regenerate bone in all sized defects without the morbidity of a donor site.

Resections: Resections of cysts are reserved for cysts that recur repeatedly, large ones in which an enucleation would result in a continuity defect, and those in which a malignant histopathology of the lining is confirmed. Most cysts that require resection are OKCs.

Those rare cysts that require a resection of the mandible are mostly accomplished via a transcutaneous approach. The incision should be placed in a natural skin fold in the neck or if none exists in the child, the incision is placed parallel to the inferior border of the mandible, 2 to 3 cm below it following the natural curvature of the mandible (Figure 7.58). In this fashion a minimal scar and a maximal cosmetic outcome can be gained. Straight line incisions, vertical swings in the incision line and chin-lip splits incision should be avoided as these are unnecessary and create a more noticeable scar.

Once the mandible is accessed, a periosteal reflection is accomplished. If the cyst is adherent to the periosteum, then inclusion of the cyst and periosteum in a sub periosteal surgical plane may be necessary. The author (REM) prefers to decorticate the buccal cortex to gain access to the inferior alveolar neurovascular bundle and displace it with nerve hooks so as to preserve it while the resection of the remaining mandible is accomplished (Figure 7.59). This has resulted in 95 to 100 percent preservation of sensation to the lip and chin. The resultant defect is best stabilized with a titanium reconstruction plate (Figure 7.60). If the cyst has not caused a significant buccal expansion, the titanium plate should first be placed on the intact mandible, then removed to accommodate the resection and then replaced using the same screws and screw holes. In this fashion, the position of the condyle and the occlusion are regained precisely. If the buccal expansion is significant, this method would result in an over-contoured plate. Therefore, the jaws are placed in centric occlusion via arch bars, the resection accomplished and the titanium plate placed with manual positioning of the condyle. In children 12 years and under, the mandibular defect can be expected to regenerate the entire defect with native bone regeneration (Figures 7.61 & 7.62). This becomes less predictable in ages beyond 12 years. In such cases, the author (REM) prefers to wait one year at which time a second surgery may only need to remove the titanium plate, or to remove the plate and accomplish a bone graft of smaller size, or in cases where no native bone regeneration has occurred, a full bone graft can be

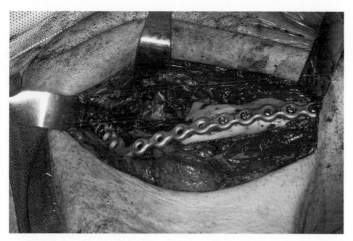

Figure 7.60 A rigid titanium plate is used to stabilize the continuity defect of the mandible. (Reprinted from Marx R, Stern D. *Oral and Maxillofacial Pathology: A Rationale for Diagnosis and Treatment* with permission from Quintessence Publishing Company).

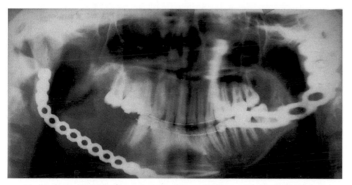

Figure 7.61 Continuity defect of the mandible after resection. (Reprinted from Marx R, Stern D. *Oral and Maxillofacial Pathology: A Rationale for Diagnosis and Treatment* with permission from Quintessence Publishing Company).

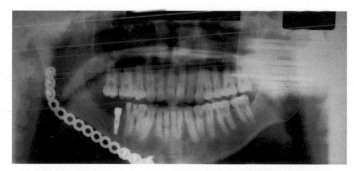

Figure 7.62 Complete natural bone regeneration suitable for a dental implant in the defect. (Reprinted from Marx R, Stern D. *Oral and Maxillofacial Pathology: A Rationale for Diagnosis and Treatment* with permission from Quintessence Publishing Company).

accomplished. In children and adolescents, the in-situ tissue engineering grafts of rhBMP-2/ACS, platelet rich plasma and crushed cancellous allogeneic bone is very predictable if a complete bone graft reconstruction is required (Figures 7.63, 7.64 & 7.65). However, if the surgeon does not have access to these materials, autogenous cancellous marrow grafts will also

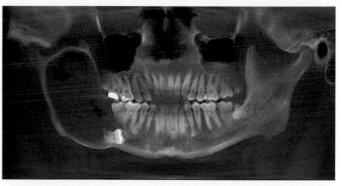

Figure 7.63 Large cyst of the mandible. (Reprinted from Marx R, Stern D. *Oral and Maxillofacial Pathology: A Rationale for Diagnosis and Treatment* with permission from Quintessence Publishing Company).

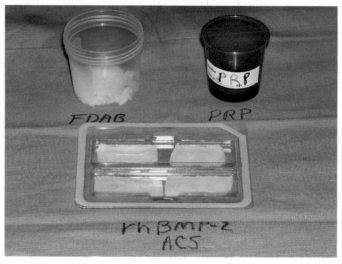

Figure 7.64 In-situ tissue engineering for bone regeneration is accomplished with Platelet Rich Plasma, recombinant human bone morphogenetic protein and freeze dried allogeneic bone particles. (Reprinted from Marx R, Stern D. *Oral and Maxillofacial Pathology: A Rationale for Diagnosis and Treatment* with permission from Quintessence Publishing Company).

predictably regenerate the lost bone. Microvascular free osteo-cutaneous grafts from donor sites such as the fibula should be discouraged. The small straight anatomy of the fibula and the morbidity of harvest are inappropriate for children.

Non-Odontogenic Cysts of the Jaws

Nasopalatine Duct Cyst (Incisive Canal Cyst)

The nasopalatine duct cyst, first described by Meyer in 1914[133] is an uncommon cyst that arises from epithelial remnants of the two embryonic nasopalatine ducts. Also known as *incisive canal cyst*, the lesion generally develops in the midline of the anterior maxilla, near the incisive foramen, although it can arise anywhere along the original course of the embryonic ducts, to extend posteriorly along the palate. The cyst can also develop wholly within soft tissue in the premaxillary anatomic region. Such soft tissue cysts have been classified as *cysts of the incisive papilla*.

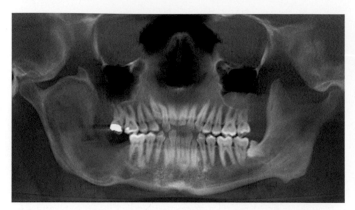

Figure 7.65 Rapid bone regeneration is seen with in-situ tissue engineered grafts. (Reprinted from Marx R, Stern D. *Oral and Maxillofacial Pathology: A Rationale for Diagnosis and Treatment* with permission from Quintessence Publishing Company).

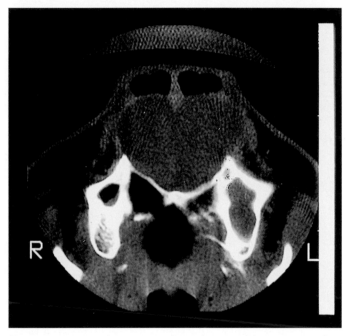

Figure 7.66 CT scan showing nasopalatine duct cyst of the anterior maxilla in a young child. (Reprinted from Marx R, Stern D. *Oral and Maxillofacial Pathology: A Rationale for Diagnosis and Treatment* with permission from Quintessence Publishing Company).

Cysts that occur in a more posterior location in the bony palatal midline have sometimes been referred to as median palatine cysts; a term that has appropriately been dropped from the literature. Most nasopalatine duct cysts occur between the fourth and sixth decades of life, and the lesions are more common in males than females, the ratio of occurrence being 3:1.[134] In a comprehensive review of 334 nasopalatine duct cysts, Swansonks et al. found the mean overall age of patients in their study to be 42.5 years.[135] Most reports in the literature also document an adult predilection for the cyst. However, Ely et al. have reported nasopalatine duct cysts in patients who were ten and eight years of age respectively,[136] and Scolozzi et al.[137] Rahul et al.[138] and Nortje et al.[139] have also reported cases in children.

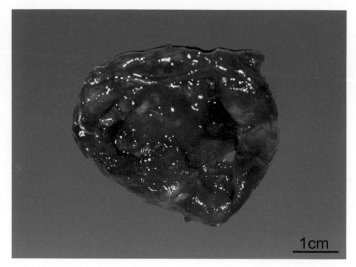

Figure 7.67 Nasopalatine duct cyst, gross surgical specimen showing hemorrhagic thin walled cyst. (Reprinted from Marx R, Stern D. *Oral and Maxillofacial Pathology: A Rationale for Diagnosis and Treatment* with permission from Quintessence Publishing Company).

Radiographically, most nasopalatine duct cysts will present as a heart or pear-shaped radiolucency in the anterior maxillary midline. (Figure 7.66) Lesions tend to be unilocular and have smooth, regular borders. The cyst may cause resorption of the roots of the central incisor teeth, but lesions do, of necessity, cause cortical expansion. In order to confirm a diagnosis of nasopalatine duct cyst, it is mandatory that the clinician determine the vitality of teeth in the area of the suspected cyst, especially the maxillary incisor teeth, since from a radiographic differential diagnostic perspective, a periapical granuloma, radicular cyst, LPC or primordial OKC – all of which generally result in the associated teeth becoming non-vital-can produce the same radiographic appearance. Since nasopalatine cysts can become infected, resulting in drainage from the anterior maxilla, patients may complain of a salty taste in the mouth.

The etiology of the nasopalatine duct cyst has not been determined, although infection, trauma to the nasopalatine duct and mucous retention of adjacent salivary glands have all been proposed as causative factors.[140] The lesion may also simply develop from spontaneous cystic degeneration of remnants of the nasopalatine duct.

Pathologic Findings

The nasopalatine duct cyst will most often be submitted to the laboratory as saccular or cystic fragments of soft tissue (Figure 7.67). Microscopically, the cyst will be composed of an epithelially lined cavity that is marginated by squamous or pseudostratified columnar epithelium that may or may not be ciliated (Figures 7.68). Mucous grands may be present in the cyst lining epithelium. The collagenous supporting wall of the cyst will generally contain an abundance of thick walled blood vessels, fibroadipose tissue and scattered mucous secreting cells. One feature that tends to aid in the microscopic diagnosis

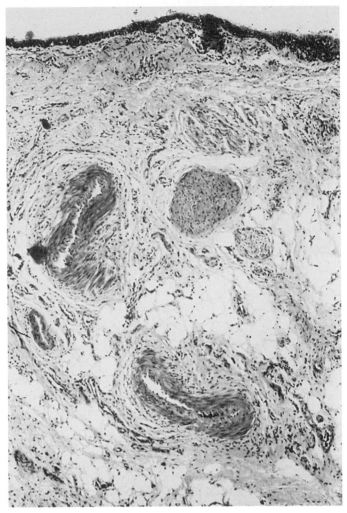

Figure 7.68 Nasopalatine duct cyst characterized by a thin epithelial lining and nerve aggregates in the cyst wall. A higher power photomicrograph demonstrates that the lining is focally ciliated. (Reprinted from Marx R, Stern D. *Oral and Maxillofacial Pathology: A Rationale for Diagnosis and Treatment* with permission from Quintessence Publishing Company).

of a nasopalatine duct cyst is the identification of small nerve aggregates in the cyst's supporting connective tissue wall. This microscopic feature, while common to the nasopalatine duct cyst is rare in inflammatory cysts, OKCs or LPCs. Bone and cartilage are also common to the wall of nasopalatine duct cysts.

Treatment and Prognosis

Nasopalatine duct cysts are treated by enucleation and have little potential to recur.

Nasolabial Cyst (Nasoalveolar Cyst)

The nasolabial cyst is an extraosseous slow growing lesion of soft tissue that typically presents as a locally expansile growth below the nasal ala and medial nasal labial fold. Nasolabial cysts are usually painless round growths that are reported to comprise approximately 0.6 percent of all jaw cysts. Patients in

the 30 to 50 age range are most commonly affected; however, nasolabial cysts have been documented in children as young as ten.[141] Females tend to be affected more frequently than males, at a ratio of at least 3:1.[141] Most nasolabial cysts will generally present as unilateral lesions, although bilateral lesions have been documented.[142] Individuals of East Asian descent are reported to have a higher incidence of nasolabial cyst development than other populations.[141] The nasolabial cyst is thought to arise from invaginations of the nasal mucosa responsible for nasolacrimal duct formation.[143]

Most patients with a nasolabial cyst will complain of a painless swelling that may be associated with nasal drainage, difficulty in nasal breathing, rhinorrhea and even numbness or loosening of the maxillary incisor teeth. On occasion, the cyst can compromise lacrimal drainage as well. Most nasolabial cysts are less than 3 cm in diameter, but much larger lesions have been reported.

Periapical plain radiographic films and occlusal films are typically not diagnostically informative, although occasionally a nasolabial cyst may produce a localized radiolucency that can be seen adjacent to the apices of the incisor teeth. CT scans, which are more appropriate diagnostically, will demonstrate a soft tissue cyst that is oval, well circumscribed and clearly extraosseous. The lesion will generally appear lateral to the piriforme aperture and alar base. Although nasolabial cysts do not typically involve bone, they may cause underlying bony destruction because of pressure resorption. When lesions are injected with a contrast agent for better visualizations, they will generally be seen as an egg-shaped radiopaque mass.

From a clinical differential diagnostic standpoint, a localized infection and other soft tissue cystic lesions should be considered. The mucous retention cyst, epidermoid cyst, periapical cyst, nasopalatine duct cyst and the oral heterotopic gastrointestinal cyst can closely resemble a nasolabial cyst clinically. The heterotopic gastrointestinal cyst, which is a foregut duplication disorder, can easily be distinguished on the basis of its unique histology. The dermoid cyst can simulate a nasolabial cyst clinically; however, dermal appendage structures will be seen in that cyst's wall. Inflammatory cysts of dental origin can typically be distinguished clinically from a nasolabial cyst because in the case of a nasolabial cyst, the teeth in the area, rather than being non-vital, will retain their vitality. A thorough dental examination and careful pulp testing of the teeth for vitality are mandatory in order to separate the nasolabial cyst from a cyst of possible odontogenic origin or from an odontogenic infection.

Pathologic Findings

Most nasolabial cysts grossly present as an oval, rubbery, firm mass that when sectioned will reveal a central cystic cavity. The cyst lumen will frequently contain mucinous or viscous material along with hemorrhage. Histologically, the nasolabial cyst will be lined by cuboidal or columnar epithelium that will often contain focal aggregates of mucinous secreting goblet cells (Figure 7.69). The goblet cells will typically stain

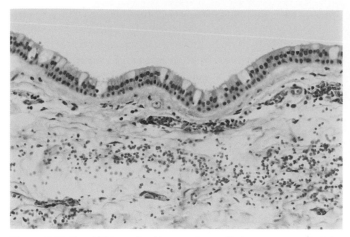

Figure 7.69 Nasolabial cyst lined by pseudo stratified squamous epithelial cells and intermittent mucous secreting cells. (Reprinted from Marx R, Stern D. *Oral and Maxillofacial Pathology: A Rationale for Diagnosis and Treatment* with permission from Quintessence Publishing Company).

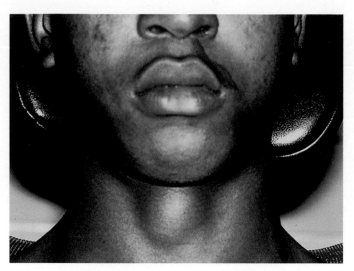

Figure 7.70 TTC arising in the neck midline of a teenager. (Reprinted from Marx R, Stern D. *Oral and Maxillofacial Pathology: A Rationale for Diagnosis and Treatment* with permission from Quintessence Publishing Company).

mucicarmine positive, and the supporting cyst wall will generally be composed of reticular collagen that is well vascularized and chronically inflamed. Occasionally, skeletal muscle bundles can be seen at the depth of the cyst wall. Cyst lining epithelium will stain strongly positive for various cytokeratins and for p53 when stained immunohistochemically.[144]

Treatment and Prognosis

Nasolabial cysts are typically treated by complete excision using a transoral, sublabial approach,[145,146] or by transnasal marsupialization.[147] Recurrence is exceedingly uncommon, and the long-term esthetic outcome for patients is excellent.

Thyroglossal Tract Cyst (Thyroglossal Duct Cyst)

The thyroglossal tract cyst (TTC), the most common cyst of the neck, will arise most often in the midline of the neck over the thyroid membrane, at or just below the hyoid bone level. The TTC can also occur slightly off the midline, and may rarely present in the tongue.[148,149,150,151] (Figure 7.70) TTC is reported to occur in between 5 and 7 percent of the population and the lesion accounts for as high as 70 percent of all neck cysts that are congenital.[152,153] Arising from thyroglossal duct remnants, most TTCs present as palpable, doughy asymptomatic masses. Upon swallowing, the mass will move, or if it is deep within the tongue, it may protrude from the tongue base. Occasionally, patients will have neck or throat pain or dysphasia. TTC does not occur in the lateral neck and not surprisingly most cysts will be found to be connected to the hyoid bone at surgery.

Developmentally, the TTC will originate as an anomaly associated with migration of the thyroid gland during the fourth through eighth weeks of gestation, to ultimately present as a cystic remnant that will be found along the tract of the thyroglossal duct as it extends from the foramen cecum of the tongue base to the base of the thyroid gland. Fifty percent of TTCs occur before 20 years of age, with the average age of presentation being from 6 to 10 years.[149,150,151,152] Fifteen to twenty percent of TTCs present in patients over 50 years of age.[148,149,150]

Uba et al.[152] reviewed a series of 36 TTCs in children and found the age range of patients to be between 4 and 14 years, with a median age of eight. Twenty-seven of the cysts in the Uba et al. study were in boys. Samuel et al.[153] have reported the occurrence of TTCs in infants as young as 10 weeks of age. TTCs are considered to be twice as common as branchial cleft cysts.

The TTC can generally be diagnosed using ultrasound or CT imaging, and both modalities can prove useful in determining the extent of any lesion and for accessing the relationship of the cyst to adjacent structures and the hyoid bone. Lesions typically present as round or egg-shaped cavitated appearing growths. The most common complication of the TTC in a child is infection, while malignancy is the most significant complication in adults.[154]

Pathologic Findings

Grossly, the TTC will present as a thin walled cystic sac that may contain mucinous fluid. (Figure 7.71) TTCs tend to range in size from 1 to 2 cm in diameter and they typically do not contain purulent material unless they are infected. Histologically, the TTC will be lined by respiratory-type epithelium, pseudostratified columnar epithelium or on occasion, especially if the lesion is infected or inflamed, squamous epithelium. The supporting collagenous wall of the cyst will generally contain acute and chronic inflammatory cells, and in 25 to 60 percent of cases, thyroid tissue will be identified. (Figure 7.72) Thyroid tissue can appear histologically normal, hyperplastic or even neoplastic. Mucous glands may be identified in the wall of TTCs along with cholesterol granulomas. Fibrosis and scarring are common in cysts of long-standing duration. Follicular thyroid adenomas and papillary and follicular thyroid

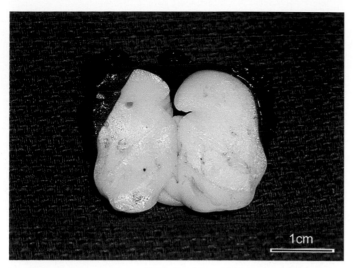

Figure 7.71 Gross specimen of TTC. The thin epithelial lining is supported by an injectable product placed in the cyst lumen at the time of resection. (Reprinted from Marx R, Stern D. *Oral and Maxillofacial Pathology: A Rationale for Diagnosis and Treatment* with permission from Quintessence Publishing Company).

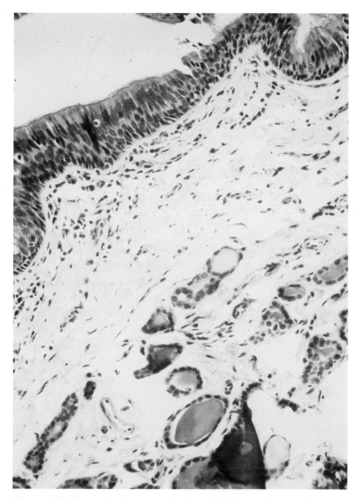

Figure 7.72 Thin walled TTC. Note the thyroid follicles in the cyst wall and the cyst's columnar epithelial lining. (Reprinted from Marx R, Stern D. *Oral and Maxillofacial Pathology: A Rationale for Diagnosis and Treatment* with permission from Quintessence Publishing Company).

carcinoma as well as squamous carcinoma have been reported to arise from TTCs.[154,155]

The branchial cleft cyst, cervical thymic cyst and metastatic cystic thyroid papillary carcinoma can all resemble the TTC histologically. The branchial cleft cyst will, however, be located in the lateral neck, and not in the midline. Histologically, that cyst will lack thyroid follicles. The cervical thymic cyst will contain thymic tissue, lack thyroid follicles and will have no hyoid bone association. Metastatic cystic thyroid papillary carcinomas, which are exceedingly rare in children, will display readily apparent and diagnostic cytologic atypia.[156,157] Rare adenosquamous and papillary follicular carcinoma which can arise from TTCs in adults have not been reported in children.[158,159]

Treatment and Prognosis

The treatment of choice for the TTC is enblock surgical resection of the cyst to include the middle third of the hyoid bone and the associated suprahyoid cystic tract up to the foramen cecum at the tongue base. This surgical procedure known as s Sistrunk procedure is generally curative.[160,161,162] In many instances, the TTC is initiated by a lengthy case of pharyngitis. In such instances, the use of antibiotics, primarily penicillin, over the course of ten days can prove beneficial. The body of the hyoid bone can be preserved in most instances of childhood TTC and the tract remnant tied off. Although a high level of postoperative wound infections, hematomas and recurrence has been reported in Nigerian children with TTC, these complications appear to be far less common in studies outside of Africa.

Non-Odontogenic Cysts in Children

Branchial Cyst (Cervical Lymphoepithelial Cyst, Branchial Cleft Cyst)

Branchial cleft anomalies, including cysts represent the second most common congenital head and neck lesions to be seen in children. These anomalies can present as cysts, fistulas, sinuses and occasionally as cartilaginous remnants. They arise from the five sets of ectodermal clefts, and the five associated endodermal branchial pouches that separate the six branchial arches.[163]

The etiology of the branchial cyst is unknown, but partial or incomplete obliteration of the branchial clefts and pouches during embryogenesis is thought by most authorities to be the most likely cause.[164] Branchial anomalies, which account for 20 percent of all cervical masses in children, arise from the associated clefts in a disproportionate fashion. Second branchial cleft lesions account for 95 percent of all lesions, while first branchial cleft anomalies account for 1 to 4 percent of lesions. Third and fourth pouch anomalies are quite rare and generally involve the larynx, resulting in laryngeal lesions.[165]

Some investigators have suggested that branchial cleft anomalies arise from salivary gland epithelium that becomes

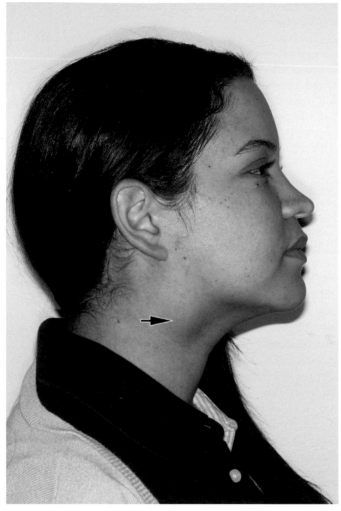

Figure 7.73 (Branchial) Lymphoepithelial cyst of the right lateral neck in a teenage girl. (Reprinted from Marx R, Stern D. *Oral and Maxillofacial Pathology: A Rationale for Diagnosis and Treatment* with permission from Quintessence Publishing Company).

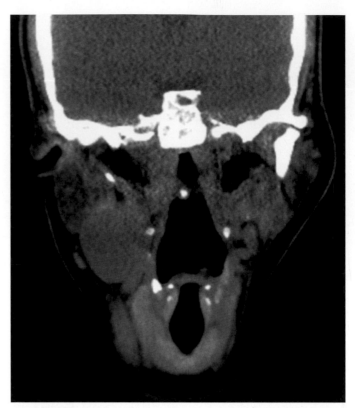

Figure 7.74 Branchial cyst deep to the sternocleidomastoid muscle and superficial to the carotid sheath. (Reprinted from Marx R, Stern D. *Oral and Maxillofacial Pathology: A Rationale for Diagnosis and Treatment* with permission from Quintessence Publishing Company).

embryonically entrapped within cervical lymph nodes. This entrapped epithelium is then thought to undergo cystic degeneration at some stage in the patient's development. Lymphoid elements, however, are common in the head and neck region on an embryonic basis, and any association that links branchial cleft anomalies with lymphoid aggregation or salivary gland aggregation may simply be a result of the anatomic development of the region and not a truly a causal factor in the initiation of a branchial cyst.

The benign lymphoepithelial cyst, (BLEC), a lesion that is identical histopathologically to the branchial cleft cyst, can occur in the parotid gland and in the floor of the mouth. The BLEC rarely attains a size of more than 4 cm in diameter, and it can typically be managed quite successfully by complete surgical excision.

Branchial cysts tend to have a bimodal age presentation, and a nearly equal gender distribution. Although many branchial cleft cysts are identified in patients before the fifth year of age, 75 percent of all BCCs are found in patients in the

20 to 40 year age-range. Less than 1 percent of all BCCs will occur in patients over 50 years of age. Bilateral instances of branchial cysts have been reported, but they are rare.[165]

Most branchial cysts will present as a lateral neck mass along the anterior border of the sternocleidomastoid and muscle, anywhere between the hyoid bone to the suprasternal notch. (Figure 7.73) Lesions of long-standing duration can become painful, especially when they become infected. One clinical feature common to the branchial cyst is its tendency to expand and decompress over its lifetime. This characteristic feature is often a result of fistulation. The branchial cyst, if fistulated, will frequently extrude or express mucous, a feature that can be seen in both children and adults. Squamous cell carcinoma or metastatic disease to the neck, common differential diagnostic considerations the adult, is a far less frequent consideration in the pediatric age group.

In any diagnostic evaluation of a child or adolescent for a suspected branchial cyst, especially if there has been a rapid or progressive growth pattern that might simulate that of a squamous cell carcinoma, a fine needle aspiration (FNA) biopsy should be the initial recommended diagnostic procedure. Following FNA, a more complete diagnostic biopsy can always be obtained.

MRI scanning will typically demonstrate a fluid-filled cyst, as will CT scans (Figure 7.74).

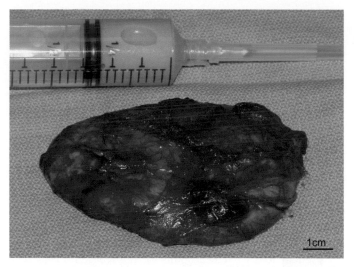

Figure 7.75 Gross surgical specimen of a thin walled branchial cyst, and the tan colored cystic fluid contents. (Reprinted from Marx R, Stern D. *Oral and Maxillofacial Pathology: A Rationale for Diagnosis and Treatment* with permission from Quintessence Publishing Company).

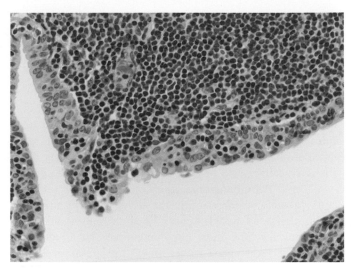

Figure 7.77 High power photomicrograph demonstrating a benign lymphocytic infiltrate in the cyst's connective tissue wall.

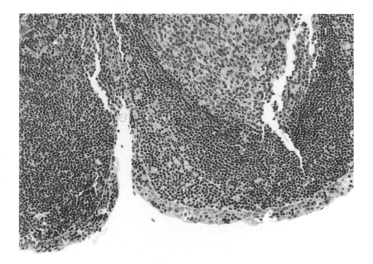

Figure 7.76 Branchial cyst lined by squamo-columnar epithelial lining. The connective tissue wall contains a dense lymphoid infiltrate with a germinal center.

Branchial cysts are generally located deep to the sternocleidomastoid muscle, but superficial to the carotid sheath;[166,167] however, on occasion, the branchial cysts can present clinically as a parotid mass, an odontogenic tumor or as an odontogenic infection. These categories of lesions and disorders should therefore be included in the clinical differential diagnosis of a branchial cyst.

Although reactive lymphadenopathy and lymphoma can also resemble a branchial cyst clinically, the most common differential diagnostic consideration for a branchial cleft cyst in a child is TTC. Histologically, branchial cleft cysts can easily be distinguished from a TTC because thyroid tissue will be identified in the latter lesion histologically, and the hyoid bone will typically be involved clinically as well. The cervical thymic

cyst, lymphangioma, dermoid cyst and bronchogenic cyst may also be considered in the differential diagnosis of branchial cleft cyst.[168] Endoscopic evaluation is frequently carried out on patients suspected of having a branchial cleft cyst in order to rule out other cystic lesions of the head and neck.

Pathologic Findings

The branchial cyst will present grossly as a unilocular cystic cavity that may contain clear fluid, tan or brown fluid, granular material or a gelatinous substance (Figure 7.75). Lesions rarely attain a size greater than 8 to 10 cm. Microscopically, the cyst will most often be lined by stratified squamous epithelium, (Figure 7.76) although 10 to 15 percent of lesions are lined by respiratory-type epithelium. The cyst lumen may be filled with inflammatory cells, keratinaceous or proteinaceous debris or a mucinous product. The supporting collagenous cyst wall is typically chronically inflamed and it will contain lymphoid aggregates (Figure 7.77). The lymphoid aggregates generally are arranged in a normal anatomic pattern and the lymphoid architecture is usually maintained such that germinal centers are readily recognizable. On occasion, multinucleated giant cells can be seen in the supporting collagenous cyst wall of a branchial cyst, most often in cysts that are long-standing or in cysts that have ruptured or developed a drainage tract. In some instances, salivary gland tissue can be identified in the cyst wall and in a small percentage of cases, cartilage may also be identified. Cellular atypical and pleomorphism of the epithelial lining cells of the cyst will typically not be present.

FNA of a branchial cyst, if employed, will demonstrate respiratory-type epithelial cells with an accumulation of lymphoid tissue, macrophages and, in some instances, micro-abscess formation.

Immunohistochemical studies tend to demonstrate the cyst lining epithelium that is positive for a host of cytokeratins. If squamous cell carcinoma is suspected in the microscopic differential diagnosis, glucose transporter 1 (GLUT-1) assessment can be helpful in separating the branchial cleft cyst from a cystic squamous cell carcinoma that is metastatic. GLUT-1 reactivity will be negative in a branchial cleft cyst, but positive in a squamous epithelial malignancy.[169]

Differential Diagnosis

The *cervical thymic cyst* can resemble a branchial cyst both clinically and microscopically. Unlike a branchial cyst, however, identifiable thymic tissue and Hassall corpuscles along with calcifications will be identified in the wall of a cervical thymic cyst. Lymphangioma, another microscopic differential diagnostic consideration in the child, will typically show an abundance of lymph spaces lined by endothelial cells microscopically, and most lymphangiomas will involve the posterior cervical space rather than the lateral neck. On occasion, *laryngeoceles* and *dermoid cysts* can resemble a branchial cyst. Dermoid cysts however, unlike branchial cysts, will lack lymphoid elements, cartilage or nerve. The laryngeocele, unlike the branchial cyst, is generally a midline lesion similar to the thyroglossal duct cyst, and it will lack lymphoid aggregates in its connective tissue wall. Finally, a bronchogenic cyst can resemble a branchial cyst microscopically. The bronchogenic cyst, however, presents low in the neck, and it will always be lined by respiratory epithelium that is supported by a collagenous wall that contains smooth muscle and bronchial glands.

Treatment and Prognosis

Branchial cysts are treated by complete excision with ligation of any residual cystic tract. Repeated incision and drainage of the lesion is not an acceptable mode of therapy, and may result in high recurrence. The cyst can be treated surgically by approaching it with a horizontal neck incision in the closest natural skin crease area overlying the prominence of the mass.[170] The cyst will be found deep to the sternocleidomastoid muscle and superficial to the layer of the cervical fascia, where it can be separated from surrounding tissue via a pericapsular dissection. The cyst may perforate and deflate at the time of surgery. In those instances where a branchial cyst perforates surrounding muscle and fascia, the cavity can be injected with a soft tissue liner in order to maintain cyst contour, and then removed by pericapsular dissection.[170] Intravenous or oral antibiotics, most often penicillin, can be used as ancillary support in those instances where patients present with an infected cyst. Infected lesions have a recurrence rate that is much higher than those cysts that are non-infected prior to initial surgery. An increased risk of complications in children less than eight years of age has been reported for branchial cleft cysts.[167] Bajay et al.[165] Goff et al.[167] and Nicoucar et al.[171] report that in the future, endoscopic excision and cauterization[171] may prove to be more effective therapies for branchial cleft cysts in children rather than complete surgical excision, although surgery currently remains the treatment of choice.[172]

Epidermoid Cyst (Infundibular Cyst)

Epidermoid cysts account for just over 13 percent of all developmental cysts that occur in the head and neck region of pediatric patients.[173] Males are more frequently affected than females and the lesions most often involve the facial skin or skin of the neck, with the mid-cheek being the most common site. Epidermoid cysts can occasionally occur in the oral cavity but are quite uncommon in that site, accounting for 0.01 percent of all oral cavity cysts.[173] Most epidermoid cysts present as subcutaneous lumps, although in some instances cysts may present as an abscess. Lesions tend to be freely movable within the skin or oral mucosa. However, if they have been present for an extended period of time, they may become fibrosed and occasionally become fixed to underlying tissues. Hair follicles represent the source for epidermoid cysts, and it is these hair follicles that account for the sebaceous cells that give rise to the epithelial lining of the cyst. Accumulation of these sebaceous cells accounts for the plugging restriction of the gland by sebum. The vast majority of epidermoid cysts are multifocal and are associated with a history of acne.

From a differential diagnostic standpoint, the epidermoid cyst can resemble a pilomatrix tumor, dermoid cyst, TTC or even a parotid tumor.[173,174] Among the five most common head and neck cysts seen in children (dermoid cyst, pilomatrixoma, epidermoid cyst, TTC and branchial cleft cyst), the epidermoid cyst is the least common, accounting for only 13.3 percent of all such lesions.[174]

Epidermoid cysts tend to present clinically as firm, round, mobile lesions that are covered by normal overlying skin or mucosa. The lesions, which can ulcerate, are frequently described clinically as having a pearly or a shiny appearance.

Pathologic Findings

Epidermoid cysts are nodular in appearance and tend to appear waxy if intact (Figure 7.78). If ruptured, cysts can take on a cavity-like appearance. Frequently, the cyst will be submitted as tissue fragments due to rupture of the lesion at surgery. The cysts are most often lined by squamous epithelium that is orthokeratinized and which will be supported by a chronically inflamed connective tissue wall. The lumen of the cyst will typically contain desquamated debris consistent with keratin, proteinaceous material or cholesterol or lipid-like material (Figure 7.79). Cystic rupture may result in the proliferation of a foreign body giant cell reaction in the cyst wall. *Epidermoid inclusion cysts* represent cysts that involve skin only and although epidermoid inclusion cysts can resemble epidermoid cysts clinically, they are generally solitary rather than multifocal and not associated with acne and they generally arise due to traumatic implantation of epithelium into the dermis. From a differential diagnostic standpoint, and because of their solitary nature, epidermoid inclusion cysts can mimic HIV-related lymphadenopathy, cat scratch disease, reactive lymphoid hyperplasia or a salivary gland tumor or infection. Depending on their anatomic location, the epidermoid inclusion

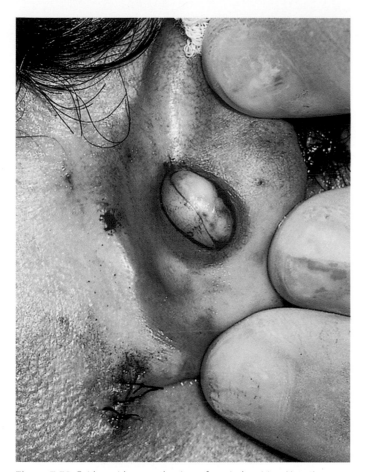

Figure 7.78 Epidermoid cyst at the time of surgical excision. Note the encapsulation and the cyst's yellow/white waxy appearance. (Reprinted from Marx R, Stern D. *Oral and Maxillofacial Pathology: A Rationale for Diagnosis and Treatment* with permission from Quintessence Publishing Company).

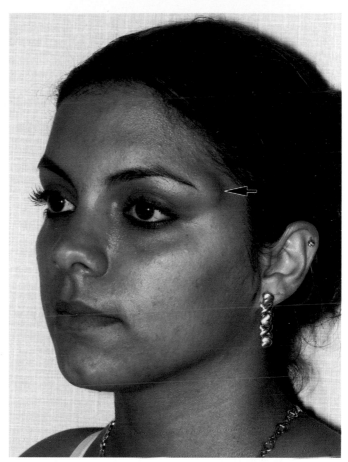

Figure 7.80 Tricholemmal cyst arising with the eyebrow of a teenager (arrow). (Reprinted from Marx R, Stern D. *Oral and Maxillofacial Pathology: A Rationale for Diagnosis and Treatment* with permission from Quintessence Publishing Company).

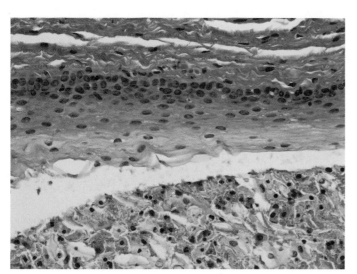

Figure 7.79 High power photomicrograph of an epidermoid cyst showing epithelial lining and keratin within the cyst lumen.

cyst can also clinically resemble a branchial cleft cyst or a TTC. The epidermoid inclusion cyst will be lined by a thin layer of keratinizing squamous epithelium and the cyst lumen will often contain keratinaceous and proteinaceous debris.[177] Lymphoid or thyroid tissue will be absent.

Tricholemmal cysts are cutaneous cysts that rarely arise in children. These cysts, also known as pilar cysts, show a marked female predilection (Figure 7.80), and when they arise in children, they most often involve the scalp. This cyst, along with pilomatrixoma, is discussed in detail in Chapter 3 of this text.

Treatment and Prognosis

Epidermoid cysts, epidermoid inclusion cysts and tricholemmal cysts are treated by complete surgical excision of the lesion.[178] Surgical excision can sometimes prove to be quite difficult because epidermoid cysts are so often secondarily infected, causing the cysts to become fibrotic and adhesive as they extend into supporting anatomic structures. Management with antibiotic therapy for up to two weeks following excision is recommended because of the high incidence of staphylococcal infection associated with these lesions. Dicloxicillin, cephalexin or doxycycline can be employed. It is important for the clinician to recognize that because epidermoid cysts are often multifocal, new lesions may arise in the same patient in adjacent or in distant sites.

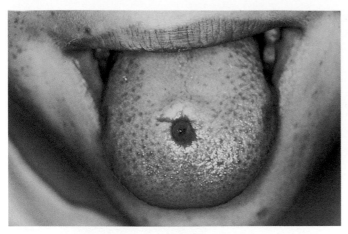

Figure 7.81 Dermoid cyst of the tongue at the time of pericapsular surgical excision. (Reprinted from Marx R, Stern D. *Oral and Maxillofacial Pathology: A Rationale for Diagnosis and Treatment* with permission from Quintessence Publishing Company).

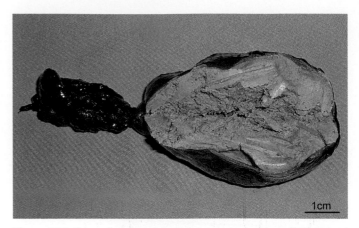

Figure 7.82 Thin walled dermoid cyst that contains keratin and compressed hair. The attached hemorrhagic tissue fragment represents a tract to the tongue. (Reprinted from Marx R, Stern D. *Oral and Maxillofacial Pathology: A Rationale for Diagnosis and Treatment* with permission from Quintessence Publishing Company).

Dermoid Cyst

Dermoid cysts represent ectodermally and mesodermally derived developmental lesions that are uncommon in patients in the pediatric age group. Most dermoid cysts arise in young adults. Approximately 7 percent of all dermoid cysts affect the head and neck region, with the periorbital region being the most common site, followed by the neck, nasal sinuses, submental region, tongue, orbit and cranial suture lines.[179,180] Dermoid cysts in the pediatric age group are exceedingly uncommon in the oral cavity. Oral lesions tend to be identified as a compressible mass in the submental triangle, external to the mylohyoid muscle or in the floor of the mouth or tongue (Figure 7.81). Pryor et al.[179] reported only a single case of a dermoid cyst in a review of 49 pediatric patients with dermoid cysts of the head and neck who were diagnosed at the Mayo Clinic between 1980 and 2002. The median age at diagnosis for patients in the Pryor series was 22 months, and the most common presenting symptom was a palpable mass. Marx and Stern[181] have reported similar findings, noting that only 2 percent of all dermoid cysts in the head and neck region affect the oral cavity. Patients with dermoid cysts in the head and neck region can present with a host of symptoms, including swelling, pain or even ptosis, if the lesion involves the periorbital region.[179,180,181,182] Imaging studies are indicated when intraorbital extension or intracranial extension of a dermoid cyst is suspected. *Craniofacial dermoid cysts* are congenital developmental cysts that are histologically similar to dermoid cysts found elsewhere in the body. Craniofacial dermoid cysts tend to be midline in their presentation, occasionally familial, and may be seen in conjunction with other congenital malformations.

Differential Diagnosis

The differential diagnoses for a dermoid cyst in a child is largely based upon the lesion's anatomic location in the head and neck, and may include epidermal inclusion cyst, glioma, teratoma, thyroglossal duct cyst, branchial cleft cyst, meningomyelocele, pilomatrixoma or epidermoid cyst.

Pathologic Findings

Dermoid cysts tend to present grossly as dilated relatively thick walled cavitations that contain "buttery or cheese-like" material[183] (See Figure 7.82.) Microscopically, the cyst lumen is typically lined by keratinizing squamous epithelium. Respiratory epithelium can also line the cyst, especially in the case of nasal dermoid cysts. The connective tissue wall of the cyst will contain dermal derivatives including hair follicles, sweat glands and sebaceous glands. Adipose tissue, smooth muscle and dystrophic calcifications may also be seen in the cyst wall. The dermoid cyst lumen will most often contain lipid-like material derived from sebaceous secretions.

Treatment and Prognosis

Dermoid cysts are treated by complete surgical excision.[184] Cysts are generally excised in order to prevent subsequent infection or to manage a developing cosmetic deformity. Recurrence is quite rare after complete excision of the lesion. Nasal dermoid cysts may require lateral rhinotomy, and rhinoplasty.[185,186,187] Subcranial approaches to nasal dermoid cysts can give the surgeon excellent exposure to lesions and reduce the risk of frontal lobe retention of cyst epithelium or contents.

Teratoma (Teratoid Cyst)

Teratomas in the head and neck region in children develop as congenital extragonadal growths of diploid origin that require a mixture of chromosomes from both parents. These lesions arise from pluripotential embryonic stem cells in the branchial arches and differentiate along any cell line from all three germ cell layers. One to two percent of all teratomas involve the head and neck region,[188] which is the second most common location for teratomas in early infancy, exceeded only by teratomas in the sacrococcygeal region.[189] Although the majority of head and neck teratomas are identified during the first year of life, nearly all teratomas involving the orbits and most intracranial teratomas will manifest at a slightly later age (mean age 2.5 years).[190] Teratomas in the oral cavity tend to most often resemble dermoid cysts, although they tend to be firmer, denser or harder lesions than dermoid cysts, largely because they frequently contain bone or teeth. The calcifications within oral teratomas generally appear as amorphous radiopacities with no definitive anatomic appearance, and can thus resemble anything from a jawbone to teeth.

Clinical differential diagnostic considerations for a suspected teratoma in the head and neck region can include salivary gland tumor, malignancies of skeletal muscle (congenital rhabdomyosarcoma), branchial cleft cyst, TTC, epidermal inclusion cyst, mucous retention cyst, dermoids cyst, encephalocele and glial heterotopia.

Orbital teratomas are extremely rare, and typically present radiographically as calcified orbital or periorbital masses that are marginated by unilocular or multilocular cystic appearing zones. The differential diagnosis for an orbital mass, thought to represent a teratoma, can include hemangioma, lymphangioma, epidermoid cyst, meningoencephalocele, coloboma and congenital cystic eye. On CT scans, hemangiomas and vascular lesions, as well as solid tumors, will generally show dense tomographic enhancement, whereas the enhancement seen with a dermoid cyst will tend to be ring-like, and the enhancement patchy. Congenital teratomas in the head and neck region can be quite problematic clinically because of their ability to cause airway obstruction, facial disfigurement and blindness.

Teratomas of the neck, nasopharynx, pharynx and oral cavity generally present as bulky masses that are identified by imaging studies prior to birth. Such a lesion will be identified as a multicystic mass showing high signal intensity on CT and weighted MRI imaging. Head and neck teratomas, in contrast to unicystic dermoid cysts and epidermoid inclusion cysts in this region tend, to be not simply multiloculated, but centrally calcified masses.

Pathologic Findings

Teratomas have a varied and heterogenous histologic appearance. As with teratomas in adults, childhood teratomas contain derivatives from all three embryonic germ cell layers; however, neuroectodermal elements tend to be exceedingly prominent in childhood teratomas, with as high as 95 percent of all head and neck teratomas in children showing neuroectodermal elements histologically.[191] Childhood teratomas containing neuroectodermal elements fortunately tend not to be associated with malignancies, unlike their adult teratoma counterparts.

As a whole, teratomas of the head and neck region in children will tend to show a markedly diverse gross anatomic and histologic pattern, which can include the gross or histologic presence of skin, neural tissue, muscle, teeth or primitive odontogenic structures, including teeth and bone, as well as brain, glial tissue, choroid plexus and fat (Figure 7.83).

Treatment and Prognosis

Teratomas are treated by complete surgical excision. Incomplete excision of the lesion can result in recurrence. Those

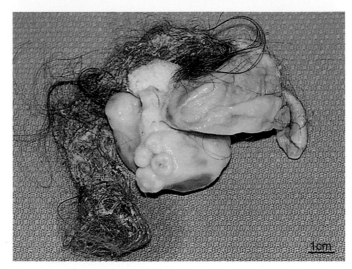

Figure 7.83 Teratoma composed of teeth, hair, skin, mucosa and bone. All three germ layers are thus present. (Reprinted from Marx R, Stern D. *Oral and Maxillofacial Pathology: A Rationale for Diagnosis and Treatment* with permission from Quintessence Publishing Company).

lesions that involve the jaw bones may require resection with reconstruction, making certain that the surgery does not interfere with or displace developing tooth buds. Oral cavity lesions, nasal lesions and nasopharyngeal lesions in neonates often require immediate surgery to avoid airway obstruction.[192] Rare instances of malignant teratomas in children in the head and neck region have been reported.[193,194,195,196]

Heterotopic Oral Gastrointestinal Cyst

Heterotopic gastrointestinal cysts are cysts of developmental origin that can occur throughout the entire course of the gastrointestinal tract. The vast majority of heterotopic gastrointestinal cysts occur in the small intestine. Those cysts that occur in the head and neck region most often involve the tongue or the floor of the mouth.[198,199,200] Most children diagnosed with oral heterotopic gastrointestinal cysts are males and most cysts will occur before two years of age, although cysts have been reported in neonates.[201] Also known as gastric mucosal choriostoma, these lesions in fact represent gastrointestinal duplication cysts. Lesions can be solid or cystic and typically range in size from less than 1 cm to 10 cm. Most cysts are 2 to 4 cm in size. Pediatric patients tend to present with symptoms ranging from difficulty with feeding and swallowing to respiratory difficulty. The heterotopic gastrointestinal cyst is thought to arise due to entrapment of undifferentiated endodermal cells within the oral cavity during the third or fourth week of fetal life.[201] Residual fetal mucosa retained at the point where the gastrointestinal tract develops a lumen may account for these lesions as well.

Heterotopic gastrointestinal cysts can be found in the upper one-third of the esophagus and a rare mixed heterotopic gastrointestinal cyst with combined oral cavity mucosa extranasal glial tissue has been reported in a child with a cleft palate.[202]

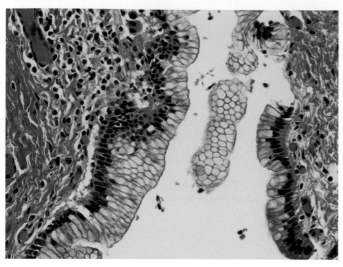

Figure 7.84 Heterotopic gastrointestinal cyst lined by intestinal mucosa, and supported by a chronically inflamed connective tissue wall.

CT scans will show a relatively well defined cystic structure without loculation or septation. Heterotopic gastrointestinal cysts typically lack an infiltrative pattern and most lesions simply present as a well defined nodular firm mass within the body of the tongue or the floor of the mouth.

Clinical differential diagnoses include epidermoid cyst, dermoid cyst, teratoma, mucous retention cyst, odontogenic cyst and rarely rhabdomyosarcoma. Patients who have symptoms of obstruction or drainage often require additional CT scans or a gastrointestinal tract workup.

Grossly, the heterotopic gastrointestinal cyst will present as a cystic appearing mass with a peripheral marginating capsule. The cyst is typically lined by epithelium that can be gastric, respiratory, squamous or intestinal in type (Figure 7.84). The supporting cyst wall will be composed of collagen that is typically marginated by alimentary smooth muscle. Immunohistochemical studies have shown that the mucin in the heterotopic gastrointestinal cyst contains lectin binding galactose, suggesting a high degree of cellular differentiation influenced by oral ectoderm.[203,204]

Treatment and Prognosis

The heterotopic gastrointestinal cyst is treated by complete surgical excision or marsupialization and recurrence is rare.

References

Introduction and Cyst Development

1. Barnes L, Everson JW, Richart P, Sidransky D. (eds) *World Health Organization Classification of Tumours. Pathology and Genetics. Head and Neck Tumours.* The International Agency for Research on Cancer (IARC) Press, Lyon, 2005.

2. de Souza LB, Gordon-Nunez MA, Nonaka GFW, et al. Odotogenic cysts: demographic profile in a Brazilian population over a 38-year period. *Med Oral Pathol Cir Bucal*, 2010, 15: 3: 583–590.

3. Manor E, Kachko L, Puterman MB, et al. Cystic lesions of the jaws: a clinicopathological study of 322 cases and review of the literature. *Int J Med Sci*, 2012, 9: 20–26.

4. Telang A, Lahari K, Shetty P. Odontogenic cysts in children: a 19 year institutional review. *Latin Am J Ortho Ped Dent*, 2011, 7: 1–4.

5. Nunez-Urrutia S, Figueiredo R, Gay-Escoda C. Retrospective clinicopathologic study of 418 odontogenic cysts. *Med Oral Pathol Oral Cir Bucal*, 2010, 15: 767–773.

6. Salako NO, Talwo EO. A retrospective study of oral cysts in Nigerian children. *West Afr J Med*, 1995, 14: 246–248.

7. Meningaud JP, Oprean N, Pitak-Arnnop P, et al. Odontogenic cysts: a clinical study of 695 cases. *J Oral Sci*, 2006, 48: 59–62.

8. Tortorici S, Amodio E, Massenti M, et al. Prevalence and distribution of odontogenic cysts in Sicily: 1986–2005. *J Oral Sci*, 2008, 50: 15–18.

9. Pechalova P, Bakardjiev AG, Beltcheva AB. Jaw cysts at children and adolescence: a single retrospective study of 152 cases in Southern Bulgaria. *Med Oral Pathol Oral Cir Bucal*, 2011, 1: 867–771.

10. Lima GS, Fontes ST, deAraujo LM, et al. A survey of oral and maxillofacial biopsies in children: a single-center retrospective study of 20 years in Pelotas Brazil. *J Appl Oral Sci*, 2008, 16: 397–402.

11. Bodner L. Cystic lesions of the jaws in children. *Int J Pediatr Otorhinolaryngol*, 2002, 62: 25–29.

12. Lapthanasupkul P, Juengsomjit R, Klanrit P, Taweechaisupapong S, Poomsawat S. Oral and maxillofacial lesions in a Thai pediatric population: a retrospective review from two dental schools. *J Med Assoc Thai*, 2015, 98: 291–297.

13. Ha WN, Kelloway E, Dost F, Farah CS. A retrospective analysis of oral and maxillofacial pathology in an Australian pediatric population. *Aust Dent J*, 2014, 59: 221–225.

Inflammatory Odontogenic Cysts
Radicular Cyst

14. de Souza LB, Gordon-Nunez MA, Nonaka GFW, et al. Odontogenic cysts: demographic profile in a Brazilian population over a 38-year period. *Med Oral Pathol Cir Bucal* 2010, 15: 3: 583–590.

15. Manor E, Kachko L, Puterman MB, et al. Cystic lesions of the jaws – a clinicopathological study of 322 cases and review of the literature. *Int J Med Sci*, 2012, 9: 20–26.

16. Telang A, Lahari K, Shetty P. Odontogenic cysts in children: a 19-year institutional review. *Latin Am J Ortho Ped Dent*, 2011, 7: 1–4.

17. Stockdale CR, Chandler NP. The nature of the periapical lesion: a review of 1108 cases. *J Dent*, 1988, 16: 123–129

18. Rushton MA. Hyaline bodies in the epithelium of dental cysts. *Proc R Soc Med*, 1955, 48: 407–409.

19. Alcantara BA, Carli ML, Beijo LA, Pereira AA, Hanemann JA. Correlation between inflammatory infiltrate and epithelial lining in 214 cases of periapical cysts. *Braz Oral Res*, 2013, 27: 490–495.

20. Parmar RM, Brannon RB, Fowler CB. Squamous odontogenic tumor-like proliferations in radicular cysts: a clinicopathologic study of 42 cases. *J Endod*, 2011, 37: 623–626.

Dentigerous Cyst and Eruption Cyst

21. Shear M. *Cysts of the Oral Regions*. Ed 3. Oxford, UK,1992.

22. Manor E, Kachko L, Puterman MB, et al. Cystic lesions of the jaws: a clinicopathological study of 322 cases and review of the literature. *Int J Med Sci*, 2012, 9: 20–26.

23. Telang A, Lahari K, Shetty P. Odontogenic cysts in children: a 19-year institutional review. *Lat Am J Ortho Ped Dent*, 2011, 7: 1–4.

24. de Souza LB, Gordon Nunez MA, Nonaka GFW, et al. Odontogenic cysts: demographic profile in a Brazilian population over a 38-year period. *Med Oral Pathol Cir Bucal*, 2010, 15: 583–590.

25. Martinez-Perez D, Varela-Morales M. Conservative treatment of dentigerous cysts in children. A report of 4 cases. *J Oral Maxillofac SLurg*, 2001, 59: 331–334.

26. Bonder L, Woldenberg Y, Bar-Ziu J. Radiographic features of large cysts of the jaws in children. *Pediatr Radiol* 2003, 33: 3–6.

27. MacDonald D, Jankowski D, Chan KC. Clinical presentation of dentigerous cysts. Systematic review. *Asian J Oral and Maxillofac Surg*, 2005, 17: 109–120.

28. Weir JC, Davenport WD, Skinner RL. A diagnostic and epidemiologic survey of 15,783 oral lesions. *J Am Dent Assoc*, 1987, 115: 439–442.

29. Fusetti F, Cordioli G, Miotti A. Clinico-statistical study of 1014 cases of odontogenic cysts of the jaws. *G Stomatol Orthognathodonzia*, 1983, 2: 141–146.

30. Stanley HM, Alattar M, Collett WK, et al. Pathological sequelae of neglected impacted third molars. *J Oral Pathol*, 1988, 17: 113–117.

31. Li N, Gao X, Xu Z, Chen Z, Shu L, Wang J, Liu W. Prevalence of developmental odontogenic cysts in children and adolescents with emphasis on dentigerous cyst and odontogenic keratocyst (keratocystic odontogenic tumor). *Acta Odontol Scand*, 2014, 72: 795–800.

32. Shear M. *Cysts of the Oral Regions*. Ed 3. Oxford, UK, 1992, 99–101.

33. Seward MH. Eruption cyst. An analysis of its clinical features. *J Oral Surg*, 1973, 31: 31–35.

34. Kuczek A, Beikler T, Herbst H, et al. Eruption cyst formation associated with cyclosporine. *Am J Clin Periodontal*, 2003, 30: 462–466.

35. Gulbranson SH, Wolfrey JD, Raines JM, et al. Squamous cell carcinoma arising in a dentigerous cyst in a 16-month-old girl. *Otolaryngol, Head and Neck Surg*, 2002, 127: 463–464.

Gingival Cysts

36. Ritchey B, Orban B. Cysts of the gingiva. *Oral Surg Oral Med oral Pathol*, 1953, 6: 765–768.

37. Gardner DG, Sapp JP. Odontogenic and fissural cysts of the jaws. Part 1. *Pathol Annu*, 1978, 13: 177–200.

38. Cataldo E, Berkman MD. Cysts of the oral mucosa in newborns. *Am J Dis Child* 1968, 116: 44–48.

39. Monteagudo B, Labandeira J, Cabanillas M, et al. Prevalence of milia and palatal and gingival cysts in Spanish newborns. *Pediatr Dermatol*, 2012, 29: 301–305.

40. Paula JO, Dezan CC, Frossard WT, et al. Oral and facial inclusion cysts in newborns. *J Clin Pediatr Dent*, 2006, 31: 127–129.

41. Moda A. Gingival cyst of newborn. *International J of Clin Pediatr Dent*, 2011, 4: 83–84.

Lateral Periodontal Cyst

42. Standish, SM Shafer WG. The lateral periodontal cyst. *J Peridontal*, 1958, 29: 27–33.

43. Telang A, Lahari K, Shetty P. Odontogenic cysts in children: a 19-year international review. *Lat Am Ortho and Ped Dent*, 2011, 7: 1–14.

44. de Souza LB, Nunez-Gordon MA, Nonaka CFW. Odontogenic cysts: demographic profile in a Brazilian population over a 38-year period. *Med Oral Pathol Oral Cir Bucal*, 2010, 15: 583–590.

45. Manor E, Kachko L, Puterman MB, et al. Cystic lesions of the jaws – a clinicopathological study of 322 cases and review of the literature. *Int J Med Sci* 2012, 9: 20–26.

46. Telang A, Lahari K, Shetty P. Odontogenic cysts in children: a 19 year institutional review. *Latin Am J Ortho and Ped Dent*, 2011, 7: 1–4.

47. Ramer M, Valauri D. Multicystic lateral periodontal cyst and botryoid odontogenic cyst. Multifactorial analysis of previously unreported series and review of literature. *N Y State Dent J*, 2005, 71: 47–51.

48. Borgonovo AE, Rigaldo F, Censi R, Conti G, Re D. Large buccal bifurcation cyst in a child: a case report and literature review. *Eur J Paediatr Dent*, Jul 2014, 15: 2 suppl: 237–240.

49. Siponen M, Neville BW, Vamn DD, et al. Multifocal lateral periodontal cysts: a report of 4 cases and review of the literature. *Oral Surg Oral Med Oral Pathol Oral Radiol Endod*, 2011, 111: 225–244.

50. So F, Daley TD, Jackson L, et al. Immunohistochemical localization of fibroblast growth factors FGF-1 and FGF-2 and receptors FGFR-2 and FGFR-3 in the epithelium of human odontogenic cysts and tumors. *J Oral Pathol Med*, 2001, 30: 428–833.

Botryoid Odontogenic Cyst

51. Telang A, Lahari K, Shetty P. Odontogenic cysts in children: a 19-year institutional review. *Lat Am Ortho and Ped Dent*, 2011, 7: 1–4.

52. de Souza LB, Nunez-Gordon MA, Nonaka CFW. Odontogenic cysts: demographic profile in a Brazilian population over a 38-year period. *Med Oral Pathol Oral Cir Bucal*, 2010, 15: 583–590.

53. Weathers DR, Waldron CA. Unusual multilocular cysts of the jaws (botryoid odontogenic cysts). *Oral Surg*, 1973, 36: 235–241.

54. Kaugars GE. Botryoid odontogenic cyst. *Oral Surg Oral Med Oral Pathol*, 1986, 62: 555–559.

55. Greer RO, Johnson M. Botryoid odontogenic cyst: clinicopathologic analysis of ten cases with three recurrences. *J Oral Maxillofac Surg*, 1988, 46: 574–579.

56. Gurol M, Burkes EJ Jr, Jacoway J. Botryoid odontogenic cyst: analysis of 33 cases. *J Periodontol*, 1995, 66: 1069–1073.

57. AA, UU, Srinivas GV, Deviramisetty S, Hk P. Boyryoid odontogenic cyst: a diagnostic chaos. *J Clin Diagn Res*, 2014, 8: 11–13.

58. Ramer M, Valauri D. Multicystic lateral periodontal cyst and botryoid odontogenic cyst. Multifactorial analysis of previously unreported series

and review of literature. *N Y State Dent J*, 2005, 71: 47–51.

59. Siponen M, Neville BW, Vamn DD, et al. Multifocal lateral periodontal cysts: a report of 4 cases and review of the literature. *Oral Surg Oral Med Oral Pathol Oral Radiol Endod*, 2011, 111: 225–244.

60. Maisu J, Sankalp M, Gupta DK, et al. Primary intraosseous squamous cell carcinoma arising in odontogenic cysts: an insight into pathogenesis. *J Oral and Maxillofac Surg*, 2013, 71: 7–14.

Odontogenic Keratocyst

61. Phillipsen HP. Um keratocyst (Kalesteatomer) I Kaeberne. *Tandlaegebler*, 1956, 60: 963.

62. Pindborg JJ, Hansen J. Studies on odontogenic cyst epithelium, 2, Clinical and roentgenologic aspects of odontogenic keratocysts. *Acta Pathol Microbiol Scand*, 1963, 58: 283–294.

63. Barnes L, Everson JW, Reichart P, Sidransky D. (eds) *World Health Organization classification of Tumours. Pathology and Genetics. Head and Neck Tumours.* The International Agency for Research on Cancer (IARC) Press, Lyon, 2005.

64. Eryilmaz T, Ozmen S, Findikcioglu K, Kandal S, Aral M. Odontogenic keratocyst: an unusual location and review of the literature. *Ann Plast Surg*, Feb 2009, 62: 2: 210–212.

65. Shear M. The aggressive nature of the odontogenic keratocyst: is it a benign cystic neoplasm? Part 1. Clinical and early experimental evidence of aggressive behavior. *Oral Oncol*, 2002, 38: 219–226.

66. Shear M. The aggressive nature of the odontogenic keratocyst: is it a benign cystic neoplasm Part 2. Proliferation and genetic studies. *Oral Oncol*, 2002, 38: 323–331.

67. Shear M. The aggressive nature of the odontogenic keratocyst: is it a benign cystic neoplasm? Part 3. Immunocytochemistry of cytokeratin and other epithelial cell markers. *Oral Oncol*, 2002, 38: 407–415.

68. Agaram NP, Collins BM, Barnes L, et al. Molecular analysis to demonstrate that odontogenic keratocysts are neoplastic. *Arch Pathol Lab Med*, 2004, 128: 313–317.

69. Henley J, Summerlin DJ, Tomich C, et al. Molecular evidence supporting the neoplastic nature of odontogenic keratocyst: a laser capture micro dissection study of 15 cases. *Histopathology*, 2005, 47: 582–586.

70. Pavelić B, Levanat S, Crnić I, Kobler P, Anić I, Manojlović S, Sutalo J. PTCH gene altered in dentigerous cysts. *J Oral Pathol Med*, 2001, 30: 569–576.

71. Madras J, Lapointe H. Keratocystic odontogenic tumour: reclassification of the odontogenic keratocyst from cyst to tumour. *J Can Dent Assoc*, 2008, 74: 165–165.

72. Ide F, Shimoyama T, Horie N. Peripheral odontogenic keratocyst: a report of 2 cases. *J Periodontol*, 2002, 73: 1079–1081.

73. Stoelinga PJW, Peters JH. A note on the origin of keratocysts of the jaws. *Int J Oral Surg*, 1973, 2: 37–44.

74. Telang A, Lahari K, Shetty P. Odontogenic cysts in children: a 19 year institutional review. *Latin Am J Ortho and Ped Dent*, 2011, 1–4.

75. de Souza LB, Gordon-Nunez MA, Nonaka CFW, et al. Odontogenic keratocyst: demographic profile in a Brazilian population over a 38 year period. *Med Oral Pathol Oral Cir Bucal*, 2010, 15: 583–590.

76. Chi AC, Owings JR Jr, Muller S. Peripheral odontogenic keratocyst: report of two cases and review of the literature. *Oral Surg Oral Med Oral Pathol Oral Radiol Endod*, 2005, 99: 1: 71–78.

77. Ide F, Mishima K, Saito I, Kusama K. Rare peripheral odontogenic tumors: report of 5 cases and comprehensive review of the literature. *Oral Surg Oral Med Oral Pathol Oral Radiol Endod*, 2008, 106: 4: e22–e28.

78. Hyun HK, Hong SD, Kim JW. Recurrent keratocystic odontogenic tumor in the mandible: a case report and literature review. *Oral Surg Oral Med Oral Pathol Oral Radiol Endod*, 2009, 108: 2: e7–e10.

79. Bakaeen G, Rajab LD, Sawair FA, Hamdan MA, Dallal ND. Nevoid basal cell carcinoma syndrome: a review of the literature and a report of a case. *Int J Paediatr Dent*, 2004, 14: 4: 279–287.

80. Gonzalez-Alva P, Tanaka A, Oku Y, et al. Keratocystic odontogenic tumor: a retrospective study of 183 cases. *J Oral Sci*, 2008, 50: 2: 205–212. (Medline)

81. Evans DG, Ladusans EJ, Rimmer S, Burnell LD, Thakker N, Fardon PA. Complications of the nevoid basal cell carcinoma syndrome: results of a population based study. *J Med Genet*, 1993, 30: 6: 460–464.

82. Kimonis VE, Goldstein AM, Pastakia B, et al. Clinical manifestations in 105 persons with nevoid basal cell carcinoma syndrome. *Am J Med Genet*, 1997, 69: 3: 299–308. (Medline)

83. Reisner KR, Riva RD, Cobb RJ, Magidson JG, Goldman HS, Sordill WEC. Treating nevoid basal cell carcinoma syndrome. *J Am Dent Assoc*, 1994, 125: 7: 1007–1011.

84. Maish J, Sankup M, Gupta DK, et al. Primary intraosseous squamous cell carcinoma arising in odontogenic keratocysts. An insight into pathogenesis. *J Oral Maxillofac Surg*, 2013, 71: 7–14.

85. Crowley TE, Kaugars GE, Gunsolley JC. Odontogenic keratocysts: a clinical and histologic comparison of the parakeratin and orthokeratin variants. *J Oral Maxillofac Surg*, 1992, 50: 1: 22–26.

86. Dong Q, Pan S, Sun LS, et al. Orthokeratinized odontogenic cyst. A clinicopathologic study of 61 cases. *Arch Path Lab Med*, 2010, 134: 271–275.

87. Gurgel CA, Ramos EA, Azevedo RA, et al. Expression of Ki-67, p53, and p63 proteins in keratocyst odontogenic tumours: an immunohistochemical study. *J Mol Histol*, 2008, 39: 3: 311–316.

88. Lo Muzio L, Santarelli A, Caltabiano R, et al. p63 expression in odontogenic cysts. *Int J Oral Maxillofac Surg*, 2005, 34: 6: 668–673.

89. Cavalcante RB, Pereira KM, Nonaka CF, et al. Immunohistochemical expression of MMPs 1, 7 and 26 in syndrome and nonsyndrome odontogenic keratocysts. *Oral Surg Oral Med Oral Pathol Oral Radiol Endod*, 2008, 106: 1: 99–105.

90. Vered M, Peleg S, Taicher A, Buchner A. The immunoprofile of odontogenic keratocyst (keratocystic odontogenic tumor) that includes expression of PTCH, GLI-1 and bcl-2 is similar to ameloblastoma but different from odontogenic cysts. *J Oral Pathol Med*, 2009, 38: 597–604.

91. Da Silva T, Batista AC, Mendonca EF. Comparative expression of RANK,

RANKL, and OPG in keratocystic odontogenic tumors, ameloblastomas, and dentigerous cysts. *Oral Surg Oral Med Oral Pathol Oral Radiol Endod*, 2008, 105: 333–341.

92. Marx RE, Stern D. *Oral and Maxillofacial Pathology: A Rationale for Diagnosis and Treatment.* Ed 2, Quintessence Publishing Company, Chicago, 2012, 621–662.

93. Sulabha AN, Choudhari S, Kenchappa U, et al. Massive keratocystic odontogenic tumor of mandible crossing the midline in 11 year old child. *Dent Hypotheses*, 2013, 4: 28–32.

94. Morgan TA, Burton CC, Qian F. A retrospective review of treatment of odontogenic keratocyst. *J Oral Maxillofac Surg*, 2005, 63: 635–639.

95. Allon DM, Allon I, Anavi Y, Kaplan I, Chaushu G. Decompression as a treatment of odontogenic cystic lesions in children. *J Oral Maxillofac Surg*, 2015, 73: 649–654.

96. Sánchez-Burgos R, González-Martin-Moro J, Pérez-Fernández E, Burgueño-Garcia M. Clinical, radiological and therapeutic features of keratocystic odontogenic tumours: a study over a decade. *J Clin Exp Dent*, 2014, 1: e259–264.

Sialo-Odontogenic Cyst (Glandular Odontogenic Cyst)

97. Gardner DG, Kessler HP, Morency R, et al. Glandular odontogenic cyst. An apparent entity. *J Oral Pathol*, 1988, 17: 359–366.

98. Marx RE, Stern D. *Oral and Muxillofacial Pathology: A Rationale for Diagnosis and Treatment.* Ed 2, Quintessence Publishing Company, Chicago, 2011, 643.

99. Krishnamurthy A, Sherlin HJ, Ramalingam, K, et al. Glandular odontogenic cyst: report of two cases and reviews of the literature. *Head and Neck Pathol*, 2009, 3: 153–158.

100. Cohen-Kerem R, Campisi P, Bo-Yee N. Central mucoepidermoid carcinoma of the mandible in a child. *Int J Pediatric Otorhin*, 2004, 68: 1203–1207.

101. Salehinejad J, Saghafi S, Zare-Mahmordabadi R, et al. Glandular odontogenic cyst of the posterior maxilla. *Arch Iran med*, 2011, 14: 416–418.

102. Gunzi HJ, Horn H, Vesper M, et al. Diagnosis and differential diagnosis of sialo-odontogenic (glandular odontogenic cyst). *Pathologep*, 1993, 14: 346–350.

103. Koppang HS, Johannessen S, Haugen K, et al. Glandular odontogenic cyst (sialo-odontogenic cyst): report of two cases and literature review of 45 previously reported cases. *J Oral Pathol Med*, 1998, 9: 455–462.

104. Tosios K, Kakarantza-Angelopoulou E, Kapranos N. Immunohistochemical study of bcl-2 protein Ki-67 antigen and p53 protein in the epithelium of glandular odontogenic cysts and dentigerous cysts. *J Oral Pathol Med*, 2000, 29: 139–144.

105. Kaplan I, Anavi Y, Manor R, et al. The use of molecular markers as an aid in the diagnosis of glandular odontogenic cyst. *Oral Oncol*, 2005, 41: 895–902.

106. Shah M, Kale H, Ranginwala A, et al. Glandular odontogenic cyst: a rare entity. *J Oral Maxillofac Pathol*, 2014, 18: 89–92.

COC Calcifying Odontogenic Cyst

107. Gorlin RJ, Pindborg JJ, Clausen FP, et al. Calcifying odontogenic cyst- a possible analogue of the cutaneous calcifying epithelioma of Malherbe (an analysis of fifteen cases). *Oral Surg Oral Med Oral Pathol*, 1962, 15: 1235–1240.

108. Freedman PD, Lumerman H, Gee JK. Calcifying odontogenic cyst. A review and analysis of seventy cases. *Oral Surg*, 1975, 40: 93–106.

109. Keszler A, Gugliemotti NB. Calcifying odontogenic cyst associated with odontoma: report of two cases. *J Oral Surg*, 1987, 45: 457–459.

110. Pindborg JJ, Kramer IR, Torlont H. Histological typing of odontogenic tumors, jaw cysts and allied lesions. *Geneva Switzerland WHO*, 1971, 28–35.

111. Rajkumar K, Kamai K, Sathish MR, et al. Calcifying odontogenic cyst. *J Oral Maxillofac Pathol*, 2004, 8: 99–103.

112. Buchner A, Merrel PW, Carpenter, WM, et al. Central (intraosseous) calcifying odontogenic cyst. *Int J Oral Maxfacial Surg*, 1990, 19: 260–265.

113. Oliveria JA, da Salva CJ, Costa IM, et al. Calcifying odontogenic cyst of infancy: report of a case associated with compound odontoma. *AS DC J Dent Child*, 1995, 62: 70–73.

114. Servarto JPS, de Souza PEA, Horta DC, et al. Odontogenic tumors in children and adolescents. A collaborative study of 431 cases. *Int J Oral Maxillofac Surg*, 2012, 44: 768–773.

115. Guerrisi M, Piloni MJ, Keszler A. Odontogenic tumors in children and adolescents. A 15-year retrospective study in Argentina. *Med Oral Pathol Oral Cir Bucal*, 2007, 12: 180–185.

116. Hirshberg A, Kaplan I, Buchner A. Calcifying odontogenic cyst associated with odontoma: a possible separate entity (odontocalcifying odontogenic cyst). *J Oral Maxillofac Surg*, 1994, 52: 555–558.

117. Uchiyama Y, Akiyama H, Murakami S, et al. Calcifying cystic odontogenic tumor: CT imaging. *Br J Radiol*, 2012, 85: 548–554.

118. Sauk JJ. Calcifying and keratinizing odontogenic cyst. *J Oral Surg*, 1972, 30: 893–897.

119. Colmenero C, Patron M, Colemnero B. Odontogenic ghost cell tumors. The neoplastic form of a calcifying odontogenic cyst. *JJ Craniomaxillofac Surg*, 1990, 18: 215–218.

120. Hong SP, Ellis GL, Hartman KS. Calcifying odontogenic cyst. A review of ninety-two cases with re-evaluation of their nature as cysts or neoplasms, the nature of ghost cells and sub-classification. *Oral Surg Oral Med Oral Pathol*, 1991, 72: 56–64.

121. Marx RE, Stern D. *Oral and Maxillofacial Pathology: A Rationale for Diagnosis and Treatment.* Ed 2, Quintessence Publishing Company, Chicago, 2011, 630–638.

122. Gnepp DR. *Diagnostic Surgical Pathology of the Head and Neck.* Ed 2, 2009, Saunders Elsevier, Philadelphia.

123. Toida M. So-called calcifying odontogenic cyst: review and discussion on terminology and classification. *J Oral Pathol Med*, 1998, 27: 49–52.

124. Habibi A, Saghravanian N, Salehinejad J, et al. Thirty years clinicopathological study of 60 calcifying cystic odontogenic tumors in Iranian population. *J Contemp Dent Pract*, 2011, 1: 171–173.

Primary Intraosseous Squamous Cell Carcinoma Arising in Odontogenic Cysts

125. Bodner L, Manor E, Shear M. Primary intraosseous squamous cell carcinoma arising in an odontogenic cyst – clinicopathologic analysis of 116 reported cases. *J Oral Pathol Med*, 2011, 40: 733–738.

126. Barr C, Leong I, Ngan BY, et al. Primary intraosseous malignancy originating in an odontogenic cyst in a young child. *J Oral Maxillofac Surg*, 2008, 66: 813–819.

127. Manish J, Sankalp M, Gupta DK. Primary intraosseous squamous cell carcinoma arising in odontogenic cysts. *J Oral Maxillofac Surg*, 2013, 19: 7–14.

128. Bodner L, Manor E. Cystic lesions of the jaws – a review and analysis of 269 cases. *Eur J Plastic Surg*, 2010, 33: 277–282.

129. Kavin M, Greten FR, Kappab NF. Linking inflammation and immunity to cancer development and progression. *Nat Rev Immunol*, 2005, 5: 749–759.

130. Kuper H, Adami HO, Trichopoulos D. Infections as a major probable cause of human cancer. *J Int Med*, 2000, 248: 171–183.

131. Hold GL, Elomar ME. Genetic aspects of inflammation and cancer. *Bichem J*, 2008, 410: 225–235.

132. Matsuzak H, Katase N, Matsumura T. Solid-type primary intraosseous squamous cell carcinoma of the mandible. A case report with histopathological and imaging features. Oral Surg, Oral Med, Oral Pathol, *Oral Rad*, 2012, 114: 71–77.

Nasopalatine Duct Cyst

133. Meyer AW. A unique supernumerary paranasal sinus directly above the superior incisors. *J Anato MY*, 1914, 48: 118–129.

134. Hegde R, Shetty R. Nasopalatine duct cyst. *J Indian Soc Pedod Prev Dent*, 2006, 24: 31–32.

135. Swansonks KS, Kaugars GE. Nasopalatine duct cyst: an analysis of 334 cases. *J Oral Maxillofac Surg*, 1991, 49: 268–271.

136. Ely N, Sheehy E, McDonald F. Nasopalatine duct cyst. A case report. *Int J Ped Dent*, 2001, 11: 135–137.

137. Scolozzi P, Martinez A, Richter M, et al. A nasopalatine duct cyst in a 7 year old child. *Pediatr Dent*, 2008, 30: 530–534.

138. Rahul J, Hegde R, Shetty R. Nasopalatine duct cyst. *J Indian Soc Pedod Prev Dent*, 2006, 24: 31–32.

139. Nortje CJ, Farman AG. Nasopalatine duct cyst. An aggressive condition in adolescent Negros from South Africa. *Int J Oral Slurg*, 1978, 7: 65–72.

140. Staretz L, Brian B. Well defined radiolucent lesion in the maxillary anterior region. *J Am Dent Assoc*, 1990, 12: 335–336.

Nasolabial Cyst

141. Toribio Y, Roehre M. The nasolabial cyst: non-odontogenic cyst related to nasolacrimal duct epithelium. *Arch Path Lab Med*, 2011, 135: 1499–1503.

142. Marcoviceanu MP, Metger MC, Deppe H, et al. Report of rare bilateral nasolabial cysts. *J Cranio Maxillofac Surg*, 2009, 37: 83–86.

143. Yuen HW, Julian CY, Samuel CL. Nasolabial cysts: clinical features diagnosis and treatment. *Br J Oral Maxillofac Surg*, 2007, 45: 293–297.

144. Wagner Y, Filippi A, Kirschner H, et al. Cytokeratin and p53 expression of odontogenic cysts. *Mund Kiefer Gesichtsehir*, 1999, 3: 263–269.

145. Choi JH, Cho JH, Kang HJ, et al. Nasolabial cyst: a retrospective analysis of 18 cases. *Ear Nose Throat J*, 2002, 8: 94–96.

146. Roed-Petreson B. Nasolabial cysts: a presentation of five patients with a review of the literature. *Br J Oral Surg*, 1969, 7: 84–95.

147. Lee JY, Back BJ, Byun JY, et al. Comparison of conventional excision via a sublabial and transnasal marsupialization for treatment of nasolabial cysts: a prospective randomized study. *Clin Exp Otorhinolaryngol*, 2009, 2: 85–89.

Thyroglossal Tract Cyst

148. Dedivitis RA, Camargo RA, Peixoto GC. Thyroglossal duct: a review of 55 cases. *J Am Col Surg*, 2002, 194: 274–277.

149. Allard R. The thyroglossal cyst. *Head and Neck Surg*, 1982, 5: 134–146.

150. Ahuja AT, Wong KT, King AD, et al. Imaging for thyroglossal duct cyst: the bare essentials. *Clin Radiol*, 2005, 60: 141–148.

151. Solomon J, Rangecroft L. Thyroglossal-duct lesions in childhood. *J Pediatr Surg*, 1984, 19: 555–561.

152. Uba, AF, Chiroan LB, Jya D, et al. Thyroglossal duct lesions in childhood – a review of experience in Nigerian children. *South African J Surg*, 2004, 42: 125–127.

153. Samuel M, Freeman NV, Sajwang MJ. Lingual thyroglossal duct cyst presenting in infancy. *J Pediatr Surg*, 1993, 28: 891–893.

154. Boswell WC, Zoller M, Williams JS, et al. Thyroglossal duct carcinoma. *Am Surg*, 1994, 60: 650–655.

155. Fernandez JR. Thyroglossal duct carcinoma. *Surgery*, 1991, 110: 928–935.

156. Kate AD, Hachigian M. Thyroglossal duct cysts: a thirty-year experience with emphasis on occurrence in older patients. *Am J Surg*, 1988, 155: 741–743.

157. Falvo L, Giacomelli L, Vanni B, et al. Papillary thyroid carcinoma in thyroglossal duct cyst: case reports and literature review. *Int Surg*, 2006, 91: 141–146.

158. Borger JA, Bercu BB. Papillary follicular carcinoma arising in a thyroglossal duct cyst in a 12 year old child. *J Pediatr Surg*, 1988, 23: 362–363.

159. Kinoshita N, Abe K, Sainoo Y. Adenosquamous carcinoma arising in a thyroglossal duct cyst. Report of a case. *Surt Today*, 2011, 41: 533–536.

160. Marx RE, Stern D. *Oral and Maxillofacial Pathology: A Rationale for Diagnosis and Treatment*. Ed 2, Quintessence Publishing Company, Chicago, 2012, 652–653.

161. Pastore V, Bartoli F. Extended Sistrunk procedure in the treatment of recurrent thyroglossal duct cysts: a 10 year experience. *Int J Pediatr Otorhinolaryngol*, 2014, 78: 1534–1536.

162. Hong P. Is drain placement necessary in pediatric patients who undergo the Sistrunk procedure? *Am J Otolaryngol*, 2014, 35: 628–630.

Branchial Cyst

163. Mitroi D, Dumitrescu C, Simionesal C, et al. Management of second branchial cleft anomalies. *Rom J Morphol Embroyol*, 2008, 49: 69–74.

164. Waldhansen JHY. Branchial cleft and Arch anomalies in children. *Semin Pediatr Surg*, 2006, 15: 64–69.

165. Bajaj Y, Ifeacho S, Tweedie CG, et al. Branchial anomalies in children. *Int J Pediatr Otorhinolaryngol*, 2011, 75: 1020–1023.

166. Zatouski T, Inglot J, Krecicki T, et al. Branchial cleft cyst. *Pol Merkur Lekarski*, 2012, 32: 341–344.

167. Goff CJ, Allred C, Glade RS. Current management of congenital branchial cleft cysts, sinuses and fistulae.

Curr Opin Otolaryngol Head and Neck Surg, 2012, 20: 533–539.

168. Harnsberger HR, et al. Branchial cleft anomalies and their mimics: computed tomographic evaluation. *Radiology*, 1984, 152: 739–748.

169. Weiner MF. Diagnostic value of GLUT-1 immunoreactivity to distinguish benign from malignant squamous lesions of the head and neck in fine needle aspiration biopsy material. *Diagn Cytopathol*, 2004, 31: 294–299.

170. Marx RE, Stern D. *Oral and Maxillofacial Pathology: A Rationale for Diagnosis and Treatment*. Ed 2, Quintessence Publishing Company, Chicago, 2011.

171. Nicoucar R, Giger GP, Harrison T, et al. Management of congenital fourth branchial arch anomalies: a review an analysis of published cases. *J Pediatr Surg*, 2009, 44: 1432–1434.

172. Soylu E, Orhan I, Yilmaz F, et al. Oropharyngeal branchial cyst in a young child. *J Craniofac Surg*, 2014, 25: e218–220.

Epidermoid Cyst

173. Davenport M. ABC of general surgery in children. Lumps and swellings of the head and neck. *Br Med J*, 1996, 312: 368–371.

174. Armon N, Sivan S, Maly A, et al. Occurrence and characteristics of head cysts in children. *Eplasty*, 2010, 10: e37.

175. Simirniotopoulos JG, Chicchi MV. Teratomas, dermoids and epidermoids of the head and neck. *Arch Radiographics*, 1995, 15: 1437–1455.

176. Yap EY, Hohberger GG, Bartley GB. Pilomatrixoma of the eyelids and eyebrows in children and adolescents *Ophthal Plast Reconstr Surg*, 1999, 15: 185–189.

177. DePonte FS, Brunelli A, Marchetti E, et al. Sublingual epidermoid cyst. *J Craniofac Surg*, 2002, 13: 308–310.

178. Oginni FO, Oladejo T, Braimah RO, et al. Sublingual epidermoid cyst in a neonate. *Ann Maxillofac Surg*, 2014, 4: 96–98.

Dermoid Cyst

179. Pryor S, Lewis JE, Weaver AL, et al. Pediatric dermoid cysts of the head and neck. *Otolaryngal Head and Neck Surgery*, 2005, 132: 938–942.

180. Armon N, Sivan S, Maly A, et al. Occurrence and charateristics of head cysts in children. *Eplasty*, 2010, 10: e37.

181. Marx RE, Stern D. *Oral and Maxillofacial Pathology: A Rationale for Diagnosis and Treatment*. Ed 2, Quintessence Publishing Company, Chicago, 2012, 660.

182. McAvoy JM, Zuckerbrown L. Dermoid cysts of the head and neck in children. *Arch Otolaryngol*, 1976, 102: 529–531.

183. Taylor BW, Erich JB, Dockerty MB. Dermoids of the head and neck. *Minn Med*, 1966, 49: 1535–1540.

184. Goins MR, Beasley MS. Pediatric neck masses. *Oral Maxillofac Surg Clin North Am*, 2012, 24: 457–468.

185. Cambiaghi S. Nasal dermoids sinus cyst. *Pediat Dermatol* 2007, 24: 646–650.

186. Blake WE. Nasal dermoids sinus cysts: a retrospective review and discussion of investigation and management. *Ann Plast Surg* 2006, 57: 535–540.

187. Ortlip T, Ambro BT, Pereira KD. Midline approach to pediatric nasofrontal dermoid cysts. *JAMA Otolaryngol Head Neck Surg*, 2015, 141: 174–177.

Teratoma (Teratoid Cyst)

188. Kadlub N, Touma J, Leboulanger N, et al. Head and neck teratoma: from diagnosis to treatment. *J Craniomaxillofac Surg*, 2014, 42: 1598–1603.

189. Smirniotopoulos JG, Chiechi MV. Teratomas, dermoids, and epidermoids of the head and neck. *Arch Radiographics*, 1995, 15: 1437–1455.

190. Tapper D, Lack EE. Teratomas in infancy and childhood. *Ann Surg* 1984, 198: 398–409.

191. Bale PM, Painter DM, Cohen D. Teratomas in childhood. *Pathology*, 1975, 7: 209–218.

192. Hassan S. Massive lingual teratoma in a neonate. *Singapore Med J*, 2007, 48: 212–214.

193. Grosfeld JL, Ballantine TVN, Lowe D, et al. Benign and malignant teratomas in children: analysis of 85 patients. *Surgery*, 1976, 80: 297–305.

194. Chakravarti A, Shashidhar TB, Naglot S, et al. Head and neck teratomas in children. A case study. *Indian J Otolaryngol Head Neck Surg*, 2011, 63: 193–197.

195. Wakhlu A, Wakhlu A. Head and neck teratomas in children. *Pediatr Surg Int*, 2000, 16: 333–337.

196. Chang AE, Ambro BT, Strome SE, et al. Immature teratoma of the maxillary sinus: a rare pediatric tumor. *JAMA Otolaryngol Head Neck Surg*, 2014, 140: 870–872.

Heterotopic Oral Gastrointestinal Cyst

197. Said-Al-Naief N, Fantasia JE, Sciubba JJ, et al. Heterotopic oral gastrointestinal cyst: report of 2 cases and review of the literature. *Oral Surg Oral Med Oral Pathol Oral Radiol Endod*, 1999, 88: 80–86.

198. Gruskin P, Landolfe FR. Heterotopic gastric mucosa of the tongue. *Arch Pathol*, 1972, 44: 184–186.

199. Takato T, Itoh M, Yonehara Y. Heterotopic gastrointestinal cyst of the oral cavity. *Annal Plast Surg*, 1990, 25: 146.

200. Mirchandi R, Sciubba J, Gloster ES. Congenital oral cyst with heterotopic gastrointestinal and respiratory mucosa. *Arch Pathol Lab Med*, 1989, 113: 1301.

201. Morgan WE, Jones JK, Flaitz CM, et al. Congenital heterotopic gastrointestinal cyst of the oral cavity in a neonate: case report and review of the literature. *Int J Pediatric Otorhinolaryngol*, 1996, 36: 69–77.

202. Srinivas T, Shetty KP, Sinivas H. Mixed heterotopic gastrointestinal cyst and glial tissue of the oral cavity with cleft palate. *Afr J Pediatr Surg*, 2011, 8: 237–240.

203. Chou L, Hansen LS, Daniels TE. Choriostomas of the oral cavity: a review. *Oral Surg Oral Med Oral Pathol*, 1991, 72: 584–593.

204. Coric M, Seiwerth S, Bumber Z. Congenital oral gastrointestinal cyst: an immunohistochemical analysis. *Eur Arch Otorhinolaryngol*, 2000, 257: 459–461.

Odontogenic Tumors

Robert O. Greer and Robert E. Marx

Classification of Odontogenic Tumors

Odontogenic tumors represent a unique set of neoplasms and aberrant attempts at tooth formation that in many instances are more properly classified as hamartomas. Convention, however, in both adults and children favors describing this group of lesions as neoplasms, and they will be classified as such here. The vast majority of odontogenic tumors are benign; however, malignant variants do occur. The World Health Organization (WHO) has established a classification schema for this group of lesions according to ectomesenchymal interactions.[1] The WHO classification of tumors is outlined in Box 8.1.

The WHO classification schema although quite complete, has proven to be cumbersome for both pathologists and clinicians when used as a practical tool. Thus, odontogenic tumors are most often regarded by the practicing pathologists, and surgeons who are called upon to diagnose and treat them, as neoplasms that are either: (1) ectodermally derived, (2) mesodermally derived or (3) of mixed ectodermal and mesodermal derivation (Box 8.2). This practical classification is to some extent simplistic in that it negates true epidermal/mesodermal interactions on a biologic level. However, we believe that it better serves to facilitate accurate and rapid communication between pathologists and clinicians, and more appropriately can be used to guide patient management than the WHO classification.

The discussion of odontogenic tumors in children that ensues will therefore center on this practical application, as has long been used by two of this book's authors (ROG, REM) and others, including Kumamoto,[2] who has used a similar classification scheme to codify those gene products and associated molecules, and infectious agents that have been found to be associated with odontogenic tumorigenesis and progression. Boxes 8.3 and 8.4 outline the various gene products and molecular aberrations that can be seen in odontogenic tumors according to Kumamoto.[2]

Odontogenisis and the Tooth Germ Apparatus

An appreciation of tooth development is mandatory to an understanding of the pathobiology of odontogenic tumors.

The developing tooth germ originates as an invagination of a tubular epithelial extension of basal cells from primitive stomodeal tissue that overlies what will become the alveolar ridges of the maxilla and the mandible. The tooth, including the crown, the root and the periodontal ligament will ultimately differentiate from these cells, which are ectomesodermal derivatives of the neural crest (Figure 8.1). These derivatives will differentiate to form both hard and soft tissue components of the tooth.

As development proceeds through the cap and bell stages of tooth development, remnants of these neural crest derived progenitor cells will remain entrapped within the jaws. These remnants represent the principal sources of odontogenic oncogenic change, and include (1) remnants of the dental lamina residing in mature adult gingiva, known as *rests of Serres*, (2) remnants of the radicular epithelial projections of the tooth germ (Hertwig's epithelial root sheath), that are present in the periodontal ligament, and are known as *rests of Malassez*, (3) remnants of the ameloblastic layer overlying the crowns of teeth and the outer enamel epithelium, known as *reduced enamel epithelium* and (4) *dental papilla remnants*. Odontogenic tumors and odontogenic cysts can develop from any of these odontogenic residuum.

Odontogenic Tumors in Children

Most odontogenic tumors that affect children and adolescents are benign and aside from the odontogenic keratocyst (OKC), which only a minority of investigators, worldwide, consider to be a true neoplasm, odontogenic tumors as a whole are rare in children.[3,4,5,6,7,8,9,10,11,12,13] Some investigators report that odontogenic tumors in children account for only 1 percent of all oral lesions in childhood, while others suggest that odontogenic tumors can account for as high as 28 percent of all oral lesions in children.[2,3] It is important to recognize that the reported frequency or infrequency of odontogenic tumors in patients in the pediatric age group may likely be related to ethnic or geographic considerations of the population studied.

Guerrisi,[3] in a series of 431 retrospectively reviewed odontogenic tumors in children and adolescents, found that the

Box 8.1 WHO histological classification of odontogenic tTumors*

- Odontogenic sarcomas
- Ameloblastoma fibrosarcoma
- Ameloblastic fibrodentintino and fibro-odontosarcoma

Benign Tumors

- Tumors of Odontogenic epithelium with mature, fibrous stroma without odontogenic ectomesenchyme
- Ameloblastoma, solid/multicystic type
- Ameloblastoma, extraosseous/peripheral type
- Ameloblastoma, desmoplastic type
- Ameloblastoma, unicystic type
- Squamous odontogenic tumor
- Calcifying epithelial odontogenic tumor
- Adenomatoid odontogenic tumor
- Keratocystic odontogenic tumor
- Tumors of Odontogenic epithelium with odontogenic ectomesenchyme, with or without hard tissue formation
- Ameloblastic fibroma
- Ameloblastic fibrodentinoma
- Ameloblastic fibro-odontoma
- Odontoma
- Odontoma, complex type
- Odontoma, compound type
- Odontoameloblastoma
- Calcifying cystic odontogenic tumor
- Dentinogenic ghost cell tumor
- Tumors of Mesenchyme and/or odontogenic ectomesenchyme with or without odontogenic epithelium
- Odontogenic fibroma
- Odontogenic myxoma/myxofibroma
- Cementoblastoma

Malignant Tumors

- Odontogenic carcinomas
- Metastasizing (malignant) ameloblastoma
- Ameloblastic carcinoma – primary type
- Ameloblastic carcinoma – secondary type (dedifferentiated), intraosseous
- Ameloblastic carcinoma – secondary type (dedifferentiated), peripheral
- Primary intraosseous squamous cell carcinoma – solid type
- Primary intraosseous squamous cell carcinoma derived from keratocystic odontogenic tumor
- Primary intraosseous squamous cell carcinoma derived from odontogenic cysts
- Clear cell odontogenic carcinoma
- Ghost cell odontogenic carcinoma

*From Barnes L, Everson JW, Richart P, Sidransky D. (eds), *World Health Organization Classification of Tumors. Pathology and Genetics of Head and Neck Tumors*. The International Agency for Research on Cancer (IARC) Press. 2005.[1]

Box 8.2 A practical classification of the most common odontogenic tumors*

Benign "Epithelial" Tumors

- Ameloblastoma and its variants
- Calcifying epithelial odontogenic tumor
- Adenomatoid odontogenic tumor (cyst)
- Squamous odontogenic tumor

Benign "Mesenchymal" Tumors

- Odontogenic fibroma and its central osseous and soft tissue variants
- Odontogenic myxoma
- Cementoblastoma

Benign "Dual/Mixed" Epithelial and Mesenchymal Tumors

- Ameloblastic fibroma
- Ameloblastic fibro-odontoma
- Odontoameloblastoma
- Odontoma and its variants

Malignant Odontogenic Tumors of Epithelial and Mesenchymal Origin

- Odontogenic carcinoma
- Malignant ameloblastoma
- Ameloblastic carcinoma
- Primary intraosseous squamous cell carcinoma
- Clear cell odontogenic carcinoma
- Odontogenic sarcoma
- Ameloblastic fibrosarcoma

*The odontogenic keratocyst and the calcifying odontogenic cyst are not considered to be neoplasms in this classification

Box 8.3 Odontogenic tumorigenesis: associated molecules

Molecules Possibly Associated with Tumorigenesis and/or Tumor Cell Differentiation

Oncogenes	*Fas, Myc, Ras*
Growth factors	FGF-1, -2< TGV-a,β. HGF
Regulators of cell cycle	Cyclin D1, p27,^{Kip1} p21 $^{WAFI/Cip1}$, p16^{INK4a}
Hard tissue related proteins	Enamelin, Amelogenin, Enamelysin, BSP, Ameloblastin, Osteonectin, BMP, Osteopontin, Osteocalcin
Oncoviruses	EBV, HPV, HSV
Tooth development regulators	Wnt pathway, SHH pathway
Tumor suppressor genes	APC, p53

Modified from Kumamoto H,[2] Molecular pathology of odontogenic tumors. *J Oral Pathol Med*, 2006, 35: 65–74.

odontoma represented the most commonly identified neoplasm. Table 8.1 documents the histologic types, relative incidence and distribution of tumors identified in the Guerrisi study according to age, gender and jaw location. Throughout the world there is little question that the odontoma is the most common of all odontogenic neoplasms, followed by the adenomatoid odontogenic tumor (AOT) or cyst and ameloblastoma of the so-called unicystic type. The mean age for all odontogenic tumors seen in children, when large reported series are accessed, is just under 13 years of age, with the lowest and highest mean ages reported to be 11 and 17.7 years respectively.[3,4,5,6,7,8,9,10,11,12,13]

General Management Principles for Odontogenic Tumors

The recommended curative treatment for each of the various types of odontogenic tumors will vary based upon their biologic behaviors as harmartomas, benign neoplasms or malignant neoplasms, as well as their individual size, location and duration. In general, lesions that fall into the hamartomatous category are usually cured with enucleation if they arise in bone and local excision if they arise in soft tissue. Biologically aggressive but benign odontogenic neoplasms are usually treated with resections encompassing 1 cm margins and more rarely excision of overlying soft tissue. Malignant odontogenic neoplasms are usually treated with resections encompassing 1.5 cm to 2 cm margins, with overlying soft tissue as required and adjunctive radiation therapy or chemotherapy in selected cases. A more complete and detailed discussion of the surgical management of odontogenic tumors along with reconstruction procedures can be found under a separate heading in this chapter.

Epithelial Odontogenic Tumors

Tumors of Odontogenic Epithelium with Mature, Fibrous Stroma without Odontogenic Ectomesenchyme, (WHO)

Ameloblastoma
Clinical Findings

Ameloblastoma is an uncommon odontogenic tumor in individuals in the pediatric age group. The tumor is generally considered to account for no more than 1 percent of all tumors and cysts of the jaw, although it has been reported to account for anywhere from 4.9 to 53.8 percent of all odontogenic tumors in children.[3,4,5,6,7,8,9,10,11,12,13] Zhang et al.[14] reviewed a series of 37 patients with ameloblastoma, in patients aged 18 years and younger, and reviewed the literature on the subject from 1970 to 2009. Of the 37 cases reviewed, 23 patients were male and 14 were female. The mean age for all patients was 14.8 years. Of all tumors reviewed by these investigators, 96.6 percent were in the mandible, and the tumors consisted of both solid and unicystic ameloblastoma subtypes. The posterior mandible and ramus were far more common sites of presentation than the mid mandible and anterior portion of the bone. Radiologically, the most common presentation for all tumors was that of a multilocular radiolucency, (Figure 8.2), with 56 percent of ameloblastomas in the study being multilocular.

The gender distribution of ameloblastoma among children and adolescents worldwide tends to be nearly equal, with males accounting for 53.6 percent of tumors and females 46.4 percent of tumors.[20] Painless swelling is the most common early symptom encountered. Radiographic differential diagnostic considerations may include central giant cell tumor (granuloma), odontogenic myxoma, OKC, ameloblastic fibroma (AF), dentigerous cyst or other lesions that can result in a unilocular or multilocular jaw radiolucency.

Classification of Ameloblastomas

The terminology used to define the clinical and histopathologic subclassification of ameloblastoma can be quite confusing. However, an understanding of that terminology is mandatory, since ameloblastomas in children have unique clinicopathologic and behavioral patterns. Zhang,[14] suggests that ameloblastomas in children should be classified into three clinical types; 1) solid or multicystic lesions, 2) unicystic lesions and 3) extraosseous or peripheral lesions.

Marx,[15] however, has noted that the use of such terms can be problematic and suggests that jaw lesions that arise de novo as solid or multicystic lesions within bone should be classified as central osseous invasive ameloblastomas of the jaws, whether in an adult or a child; whereas those lesions that arise in association with cysts should be classified as: *ameloblastoma in situ*, *microinvasive ameloblastoma* or *invasive* ameloblastoma, depending on whether they extend into and invade surrounding bone. *Microinvasive* ameloblastoma that is cyst associated would thus by definition represent a lesion that is confined to the connective tissue wall of a cyst, whereas *invasive ameloblastoma*, just as with its central osseous non-cystic

Table 8.1 Histologic types of odontogenic tumors. Incidence and distribution according to gender, age and tumor localization

Tumor Type	Cases		Gender M:F	Age (years)		Prevalent Localization
	N	%		0–10	11–20	
Odontoma	78	50.9	1:1.2	15	63	Maxilla, AS
Ameloblastoma	28	18.3	2:1	3	25	Mandible, PS
Myxoma	13	8.5	1:1.4	1	12	Mandible, PS
Adenomatoid odontogenic tumor	8	5.2	1:1	0	8	Maxilla, AS
Ameloblastic fibro-odontoma	7	4.6	6:1	3	4	Mandible, PS
Calcifying cystic odontogenic tumor	6	3.9	1.5:1	1	5	Maxilla, PS
Odontogenic fibroma	5	3.2	4:1	0	5	Mandible-maxilla
Cementoblastoma	3	1.9	2:1	0	3	Mandible, PS
Ameloblastic fibroma	3	1.9	1:2	0	3	Mandible, PS
Calcifying epithelial odontogenic tumor	2	0.13	1:1	0	2	Mandible, PS
TOTAL	153	100		23	130	

*AS: Anterior sector
*PS: Posterior sector
From: Guerrisi M, Piloni MJ, Keszler A. Odontogenic tumors in children and adolescents. A 15-year retrospective study in Argentina. *Med Oral Pathol Cir Buccal*, 2007, 12: 180–185.

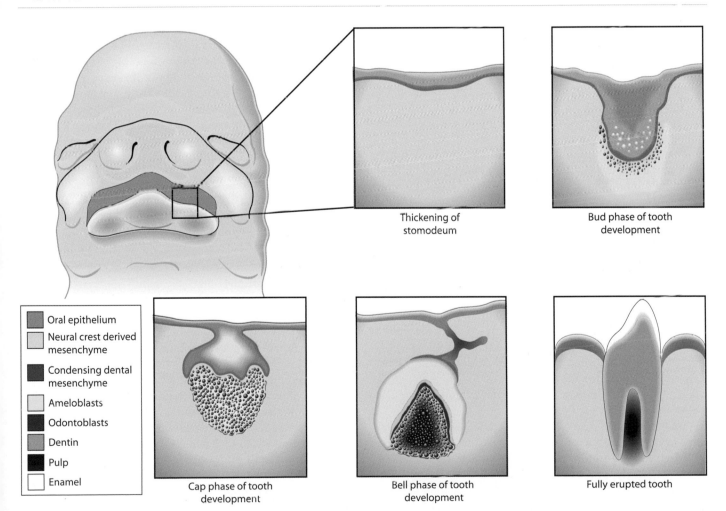

Thickening of stomodeum

Bud phase of tooth development

- Oral epithelium
- Neural crest derived mesenchyme
- Condensing dental mesenchyme
- Ameloblasts
- Odontoblasts
- Dentin
- Pulp
- Enamel

Cap phase of tooth development

Bell phase of tooth development

Fully erupted tooth

Figure 8.1 Initiation of tooth development from primitive neural crest cells to a fully formed tooth.

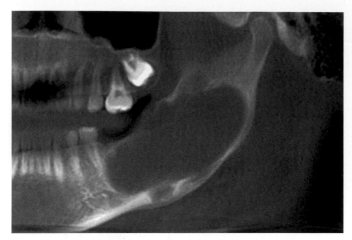

Figure 8.2 Ameloblastoma presenting as a multilocular radiolucency in the posterior mandible.

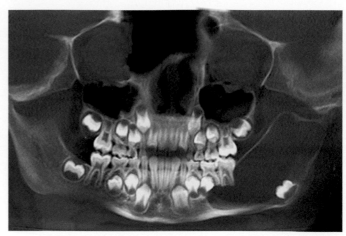

Figure 8.3 This unilocular radiolucency of the mandible demonstrates the classic radiographic pattern of the so-called unicystic or cystogenic ameloblastoma in a child, that of a large radiolucency associated with an impacted molar tooth. When examined microscopically, the lesion was further classified, according to the criterion of Marx, as an "intraluminal" lesion.

associated counterpart would represent a tumor that invades bone. Marx[15] further classifies microinvasive cystic associated lesions, (those that are confined to the connective tissue wall of the cyst in which they arise), into tumors that are *intramural*, tumors that are *transmural* and those lesions that are confined to the cyst lumen, or so-called *intraluminal* lesions.

The terminology suggested by Eversole and Leider[16] perhaps represents the most appropriate and useful umbrella term to describe ameloblastomas that arise from odontogenic cysts. These authors prefer the term *cystogenic ameloblastoma* to describe all ameloblastomas that arise from odontogenic cysts. Marx's further subclassification of these so-called cystogenic ameloblastomas into various subtypes would therefore seem quite appropriate.

Therefore in the subclassification of ameloblastomas employed in this text, we prefer using the combined and streamlined terminology suggested by Marx,[15] and Eversole and Leider[16] and favor classifying "cystogenic" ameloblastomas that arise in the walls of cysts in children in a broad sense as either 1) ameloblastoma in situ, 2) microinvasive ameloblastoma or 3) invasive ameloblastomas. We prefer not to use the confusing term "unicystic ameloblastoma." It remains important nonetheless, to discuss the often used term "unicystic ameloblastoma" from a historical perspective, especially since that form of ameloblastoma does indeed have a unique set of clinicopathologic features, and such lesions occur almost exclusively in children. In fact, half of the cases of so-called unicystic ameloblastoma reported in the literature have occurred in patients in the second decade of life.[14] A typical cytogenic ameloblastoma associated with an impacted molar tooth can be seen in Figure 8.3.

Ameloblastomas that arise in association with a cyst will often have nodular excrescences arising from the cyst lining epithelium, which will project into cyst lumen. It is therefore important for the surgical pathologist to carefully examine any cystic appearing tissue sample that is submitted, and inspect it

thoroughly to make certain that there is not an incipient ameloblastoma arising in the cyst wall.

The cyst lining epithelium of all "cystogenic ameloblastomas,"[16] regardless of how they are further subclassified, tends to be plexiform in character in 80 percent of cases. The proliferation index of tumor cells can be exceedingly high as the cyst lining epithelium ramifies throughout its supporting collagenous wall in a fashion that resembles the lining of an inflamed radicular or periapical cyst. Care must therefore always be taken to histologically separate a "cystogenic ameloblastoma" from a simple inflammatory cyst of dental origin that has a highly reactive epithelial lining.

Pathologic Features

On gross inspection, ameloblastomas that are *"cystogenic"* (the most common type of ameloblastoma to arise in children), tend to have the saccular appearance of a cyst, often with discernible invagination of the tumor into the cyst wall, whereas ameloblastomas that are *"solid"* non-cyst associated central osseous tumors to begin with, tend to be homogeneous, hemorrhagic, rubbery masses that on cut section, frequently appear honeycombed. The epithelial lining of an ameloblastoma that is arising in association with a cyst can extend into or fill the cyst lumen as a nexus-like (intraluminal) accumulation of hyperplastic plexiforme appearing strands (Figures 8.5) or extend into the supporting connective tissue wall as thin "transmural" strands and cords of interlacing cystic epithelium (Figures 8.6 & 8.7).[14] Cystogenic lesions can also arise as in situ growths in which the epithelial proliferation is confined to the cyst lining epithelium (Figure 8.8).

Ameloblastomas do not produce a calcified product and thus any microscopically identified hard tissue structures that

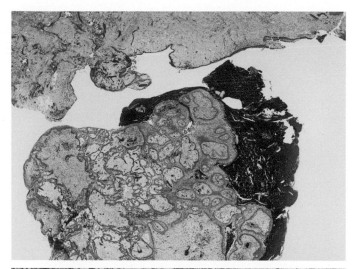

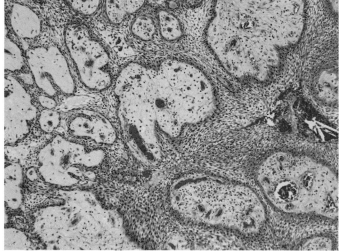

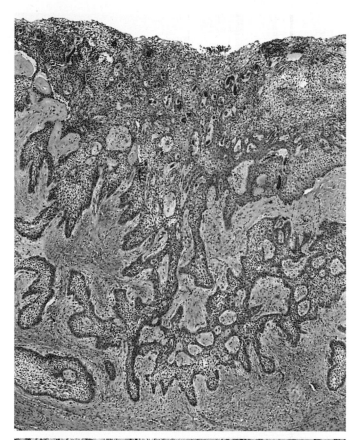

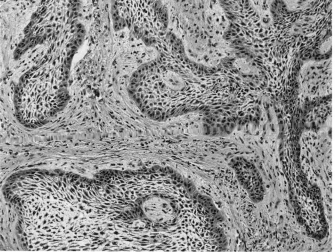

Figures 8.4 (top) & 8.5 (bottom) Low (Figure 8.4) and high power (Figure 8.5) photomicrographs of an "intraluminal ameloblastoma" in which anastomosing plexiforme tumor strands are confined entirely to the cystic lumen.

Figures 8.6 (top) & 8.7 (bottom) Low and high power photomicrographs of a "cystogenic ameloblastoma" confined to the connective tissue wall of the associated cyst as a "transmural" and microinvasive lesion. The ameloblastoma does not extend to the deep connective tissue excision margin, and thus the lesion can be classified as "transmural" but not invasive of the underlying bone.

are derived from the odontogenic apparatus, such as dentin and enamel, negate a diagnosis of ameloblastoma.

All of the histologic variants of ameloblastoma that have been reported in adults have also been documented in children. Those common histologic subtypes generally assigned to solid central osseous tumors include the *follicular, plexiform, desmoplastic, granular cell, acanthomatous* and *basal cell* forms of the tumor. Zhang et al.[14] in their study of childhood ameloblastomas, found that among solid central osseous ameloblastomas that were not otherwise classified as "unicystic," the follicular histologic pattern was identified in 48.7 percent of cases. The plexiform histologic pattern was observed in 10.8 percent of cases, and the remaining cases represented an admix of the various ameloblastoma histologic patterns.

Histologically, *follicular ameloblastoma* will be composed of sheets, islands and cords of odontogenically derived

epithelium. Tumor islands will be set in a matrix of collagen, and individual tumor islands will be marginated by tall columnar cells or palisaded pre-ameloblasts that surround an inner zone of fibroblast-like or triangular shaped cells that resemble

189

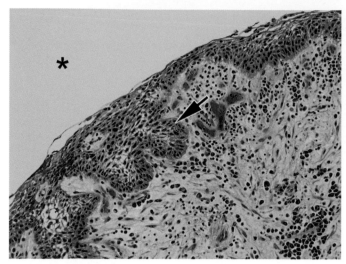

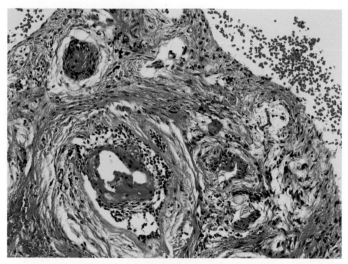

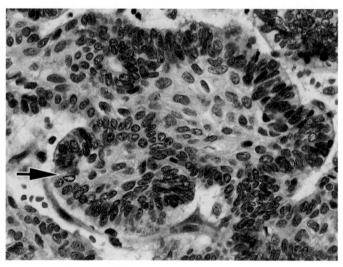

Figure 8.8 Unicystic ameloblastoma in which cyst lining epithelial cells show basal layer hyperplasia and loss of cellular polarity (arrow), consistent with in situ change. *Represents the cyst lumen.

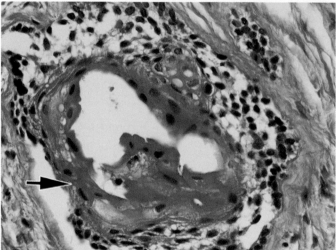

Figures 8.10 (top) & 8.11 (bottom) Low and high power photomicrographs of an acanthomatous ameloblastoma showing tumor islands with zones of central squamous metaplasia (Figure 8.11 arrow).

Figure 8.9 Follicular ameloblastoma demonstrating tumor islands marginated by tall columnar pre-ameloblasts (arrow).

the stellate reticulum of the tooth germ in its bell phase. (Figure 8.9). On occasion, the follicular ameloblastoma can undergo central cystic degeneration and microcysts can be observed histologically. Follicular ameloblastomas often undergo acanthomatous or squamous differentiation, to become *acanthomatous* ameloblastomas or combined follicular and acanthomatous ameloblastomas. (Figures 8.10 & 8.11) Some tumors undergo central tumor island *granular cell change*, in which case the tumor cells making up tumor islands will take on a central island granular cell and often eosinophilic appearance (Figures 8.12 & 8.13). On rare occasions, *basal cell ameloblastomas*, which resemble basal cell carcinoma histologically, have been reported in children. The *plexiform ameloblastoma* (Figure 8.14), the second most common pattern seen in children, will be composed of strands and cords of tumor cells that often appear rope-like, chain-like or streaming as they penetrate their supporting collagenous tumor matrix.

The peripheral columnar cells that surround ameloblastoma tumor islands, regardless of tumor subtype, will resemble pre-ameloblasts with cell nuclei that demonstrate reverse polarization. Cystic formation within a plexiform ameloblastoma is rare and tends to be seen more often in tumors of the follicular subtype.

The *desmoplastic ameloblastoma*, a rare histologic subtype of ameloblastoma, has infrequently been reported in children. The tumor, which most often involves the maxilla rather than the mandible, will be composed of widely dispersed cords and islands of tumor cells that are often composed of spindle shaped cells (Figure 8.15). The tumor islands of the desmoplastic ameloblastoma lack the peripheral palisading of pre-ameloblasts that are common to the follicular and plexiform subtypes of ameloblastoma. (Figure 8.16) The stroma of the desmoplastic ameloblastoma is also generally quite schirrous and hypocellular when

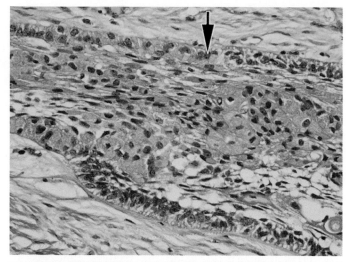

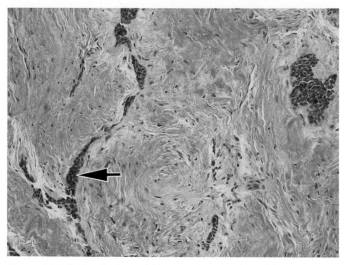

Figure 8.15 Desmoplastic ameloblastoma. Note thin basophilic crescent shaped tumor islands (arrow) set in a matrix of dense collagen.

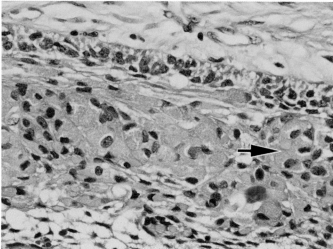

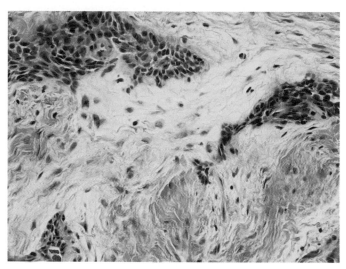

Figures 8.12 (top) & 8.13 (bottom) Granular cell ameloblastoma. The histologic pattern is otherwise follicular (arrow), (Figure 8.12) but the central stellate zones of tumor islands are filled with large eosinophilic granular cells (Figure 8.13)

Figure 8.16 High power photomicrograph demonstrating desmoplastic tumor islands that lack palisading pre-ameloblasts.

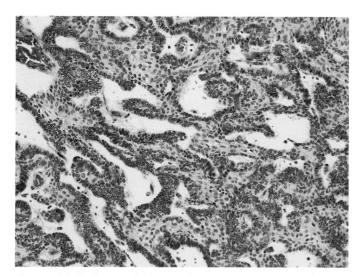

Figure 8.14 Plexiform ameloblastoma demonstrating an anastomosing braid-like network of tumor islands.

compared to other ameloblastoma histologic subtypes. Desmoplastic ameloblastomas were not reported in the large series of childhood ameloblastomas studied by Zhang et al.[14] however, they have rarely been documented in children.[15]

The *peripheral or extraosseous ameloblastoma* is a variant of ameloblastoma that accounts for no more than 1 percent of all ameloblastomas. It is exceedingly rare in children and the tumor accounts for no more than 1 percent of all ameloblastomas in both children and adults.[15]

Differential Diagnosis

Several lesions can closely resemble ameloblastoma microscopically. From a histologic differential diagnostic standpoint, *AOT, calcifying odontogenic cyst* (COC), *OKC (keratocystic odontogenic tumor)*, and *AF* can have similar histologies. The

191

AOT will demonstrate cells that surround tumor islands, and very much resemble the pre-ameloblasts seen in ameloblastoma tumor islands. However, these marginating cells will surround duct-like spaces rather than true solid tumor islands. These peripheral cells also will not demonstrate reverse polarization of their nuclei as seen in tumor islands of an ameloblastoma. The COC or *calcifying cystic odontogenic tumor* (CCOT), can also demonstrate cystic lining cells and epithelial nests that are rimmed by tall columnar basaloid ameloblastoma-like epithelial cells. The COC will however, typically contain an accumulation of ghost-like eosinophilic cells and focal psammomatoid appearing calcifications. These histologic findings are not typical of an ameloblastoma. The OKC (keratocystic odontogenic tumor), can sometimes be confused with ameloblastoma histologically, especially if the cyst lining epithelium is hyperplastic. However, the OKC will be lined by basal layer epithelial cells that will not exhibit reverse polarization of cell nuclei as is typical of ameloblastoma. The basal layer of the epithelium lining an OKC can, however, appear quite hyperchromatic and bud out in a pattern that is similar to ameloblastoma.

Finally, ameloblastoma can very easily be confused with *AF* histologically, since both lesions demonstrate islands and cords of odontogenic epithelium with marginating pre-ameloblasts at the periphery of tumor islands. However, AF is a neoplasm in which both the epithelial and mesenchymal components of the tumor are considered to be truly neoplastic. Thus the key and characteristic histologic feature of AF that is not seen in ameloblastoma, relates to a microscopically recognizable stromal difference between the two. The supporting stroma of an AF will be markedly cellular and composed of a loosely arranged rich proliferation of primitive stellate fibroblasts. The stroma of an ameloblastoma on the other hand, will classically be composed of mature and far less cellular collagen.

AF is also a tumor that occurs in a younger age group than ameloblastoma, with the exception of cystogenic ameloblastoma. The average age of patients with AF is 15.5 years.[15] AF is thus a more common tumor of childhood and adolescence than the standard central osseous solid or non-cystogenic ameloblastoma.

On a molecular level, ameloblastoma has been shown to be associated with mutations in the PTCH1 gene,[17] and Hye-Jung et al.[18] have shown that the tumor's rare malignant counterpart, ameloblastic carcinoma, will demonstrate expression of CK18, parenchymal MMP-2, stromal MMP-9 and Ki 67; IHC markers, all of which may be useful in differentiating this exceedingly rare tumor from the conventional benign ameloblastoma.

Clear cell ontogenic carcinoma[19] is a rare malignant odontogenic tumor that can resemble ameloblastoma. This tumor, which tends to be cystic in appearance clinically and radiographically, will show central acanthomatous and clear cell zones that are marginated by columnar cells that resemble ameloblasts. The tumor has only rarely been reported in children.

Treatment and Prognosis

The central osseous solid ameloblastoma should be treated by resection, observing a 1 cm medullary bony margin and one intact anatomic barrier (cortex or periosteum, or a cuff of muscle or mucosa at the periphery).[14] This treatment should be curative. Annual follow-up examinations are recommended. So-called Unicystic or cystogenic ameloblastomas may be limited to their cystic linings or to their respective connective tissue walls, or they may histologically extend well beyond radiographically evident margins of the tumor. Therefore, resection may be the only predictable cure for such lesions. Treating "cystogenic" ameloblastomas with enucleation results in a high probability of recurrence, and recurrences may not be clinically or radiographically evident for 10 to 15 years following initial surgery. It is therefore incumbent on pathologists to guide the treating clinicians by informing them as to whether a so-called cystogenic ameloblastoma shows intraluminal, transmural or bony invasion. This is best achieved when the entire surgical specimen can be examined.

Marx[15] suggests the palliative therapy for ameloblastomas, including all forms of "cystogenic" ameloblastoma, in which enucleation or curettage are employed, is indicated only in individuals who prefer and request palliation over curative resection, or for those individuals in which esthetic and surgical risks are too great to overcome a curative surgical approach.

The recurrence rates for ameloblastoma, regardless of any form of subclassification, using enucleation and curettage is in the 70 to 85 percent range and it often takes five years before palliative therapy can be identified as unsuccessful.[15] Ameloblastomas treated by resection, however, seldom recur and the cure rate for tumors treated by resection is around 98 percent.[15] One must consider, however, when dealing with children, that cosmesis can be of overwhelming concern to parents and thus conservative approaches to therapy, although not always warranted, do remain a treatment option.

Non-Jawbone Variants of Ameloblastoma

Craniopharyngioma is a non-glial intracranial tumor of the sella or parasella third ventricle region. The tumor is derived from oncogenically altered residual malformations of embryonic remnants of the obliterated craniopharyngeal duct of Rathke's pouch.[21] The craniopharyngioma, which is histologically similar to ameloblastoma, has an incidence of 0.5 to 2.0 cases per million persons per year.[21,22] Approximately 30 to 50 percent of all cases of craniopharyngioma are diagnosed during childhood or adolescence. The tumor represents 1.2 to 4.0 percent of all childhood intracranial tumors, and nearly 70 percent of all craniopharyngiomas harbor a mutation of the B-catenin gene, and will show associated inactivated Wnt signaling.[23] The vast majority of patients with a craniopharyngioma are diagnosed before the age of 18, with a median age at the time of diagnosis of 8.6 years. Craniopharyngiomas tend to cause non-specific symptoms associated with increased

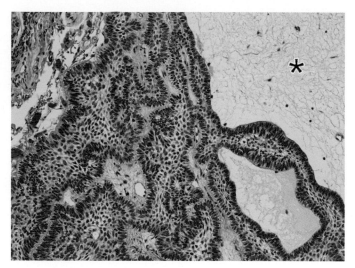

Figure 8.17 Craniopharyngioma demonstrating a plexiform ameloblastoma-like arrangement of tumor cell nests. Brain tissue (*).

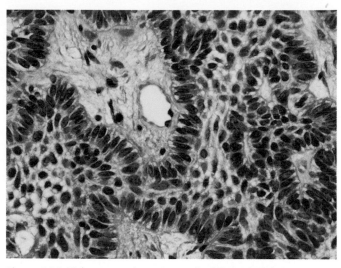

Figure 8.18 Higher power photomicrograph of Figure 8.17 showing peripheral palisading cells at the margins of tumor islands.

intracranial pressure. Early symptoms often include headache and nausea. Visual impairment and decreased growth rate as well as polydipsia and polyuria are also common symptoms.

Imaging studies typically demonstrate a mass localized to the supra-sella. A small percentage of craniopharyngiomas contain calcifications, which may show up radiographically. CT scans are mandatory for the detection of such calcifications and CTs are required imaging studies, if craniopharyngioma is considered to be a possible diagnosis in a child.[24,25,26]

Pathologic Features

On gross inspection, craniopharyngiomas typically present as a rubber or gelatinous mass at the inferior edge of the mid brain. Tumors are histologically similar to ameloblastoma and craniopharyngeomas are sometimes improperly referred to as *pituitary ameloblastoma*. The origin of the two neoplasms is to some extent similar, since Rathke's pouch does originate embryologically by invagination of oral epithelium, and the craniopharyngioma is composed histologically of a follicular or plexiform accumulation of epithelial cells that can mimic the pre-ameloblasts seen in an ameloblastoma. It is also possible that craniopharyngiomas occur as a result of the entrapment of oncogenically affected epithelial odontogenic rests, either rests of Malassez or rests of Serres that have become entrapped in an atypical anatomic location. However, most authorities continue to favor Rathke's pouch derived cells as the true tumor source.

Craniopharyngiomas demonstrate two distinctive histologic patterns. A *cystic pattern*, in which the tumor will demonstrate cystic or pseudocystic formations with associated keratinization, epithelial lobulation and the accumulation of eosinophilic, "ghost cells" and calcified material similar to what can be seen in a COC. A second *adamantinomatous* pattern can closely resemble either a follicular or plexiform ameloblastoma histologically, and individual epithelial islands tend to resemble plexiform ameloblastoma islands (Figure 8.17). These islands

can show peripheral palisading of cells at their margins in association with a central tumor island zone that resembles stellate reticulum of the tooth germ (Figure 8.18). The tumor, regardless of subtype, is usually slow growing without definitive encapsulation, and keratin formation is common.

Differential Diagnosis

Common differential diagnoses to consider, when confronted with a possible clinical diagnosis of craniopharyngioma in a child, include Langerhans cell histiocytosis, pituitary adenoma and hydrocephalus. Patients with craniopharyngioma will, unlike the aforementioned disorders, commonly have a history of obesity, hypothyroidism, delay in development of secondary sexual characteristics and occasional precocious puberty.

Treatment and Prognosis

Craniopharyngioma is a difficult tumor to manage surgically. Although it is slow growing in the manner of an ameloblastoma, with a similar locally invasive infiltrative pattern, recurrence after initial treatment is around 40 percent and the most notable adverse effect associated with management is severe hypothalamic obesity. The greatest challenge in managing patients with a craniopharyngioma is in identifying those candidates who are the most suitable patients for either appropriate radical or conservative surgery.[26,27,28] Recent studies have shown that complete or subtotal resection of the tumor, followed by radiation therapy, appear to be the most effective therapy. Even with such combined therapy, recurrence within three to four years of initial therapy occurs in approximately two-thirds of all patients. Recurrences are most often managed by either additional surgery or gamma knife radiosurgery.[26] Tumors that have a high degree of calcification within them, a feature that may be related to the ability of tumor cells to aggregate and adhere to brain tissue, tend to have a higher incidence of recurrence. Approximately 15 percent of patients diagnosed with craniopharyngioma will die from their tumor or from complications of therapy.[22]

Malignant Ameloblastoma, Ameloblastic Carcinoma and Clear Cell Odontogenic Carcinoma

Malignant ameloblastoma is exceedingly rare in children, with only 70 cases reported in the English-speaking literature between the years 1984 and 2011.[29] The term *malignant ameloblastoma* should be reserved for those tumors that show benign histologic features of classic ameloblastoma in both the primary neoplastic disease site and at any site of metastases. Cellular cytologic atypia need not be present to classify a tumor as a malignant ameloblastoma.

Ameloblastic carcinoma is a tumor that demonstrates the classic histomorphology of ameloblastoma with true cytologic atypia of tumor cells, regardless of whether or not there is associated tumor metastasis.[29,30] The WHO subclassifies ameloblastic carcinoma into primary, secondary, peripheral, osseous and solid subtypes. Too few tumors have been reported in children to determine if the subclassifications are truly meaningful in pediatric age group patients.

Both *malignant ameloblastoma* and *ameloblastic carcinoma* tend to present clinically as a multilocular radiolucencies of the jaw with bony expansion. Almost all cases of either malignant ameloblastoma or ameloblastic carcinoma have been reported to occur in the mandible, and most patients will ultimately have metastatic disease involving the lungs. Clinical signs that favor malignancy include ulceration, bleeding, fistulization, pain and tooth mobility and numbness at the tumor site. Malignant ameloblastoma may not show the same radiographically destructive pattern early on in its course as ameloblastic carcinoma.

From a differential diagnostic standpoint, a jaw tumor that shows rapid destruction of bone in a child could easily also represent metastasis from a viseral neoplasm, invasion of bone by an adjacent soft tissue malignancy, such as rhabdomyosarcoma, juvenile Hodgkin's disease, non-Hodgkin lymphoma or even a benign or malignant central osseous tumor, such as ossifying fibroma, chondrosarcoma and osteosarcoma. Ewing sarcoma, leukemia, neuroblastoma and Langerhans cell histiocytosis may also be included in the clinical differential diagnosis, for a rapidly growing bony destructive neoplasm.

Rare *clear cell odontogenic carcinomas* (CCOC) have been reported in children, but less than 80 cases in all age groups are known worldwide.[35] Histologically, CCOC can display three distinct patterns that have been designated monophasic, biphasic and ameloblastomatous. Most tumors are biphasic and will be made up of nests of clear cells along with islands of polygonal cells that are hyperchromatic with eosinophilic cytoplasm (Figures 8.18.1 and 8.18.2). Monophasic tumors will be made up of islands of clear cells alone, and ameloblastomatous

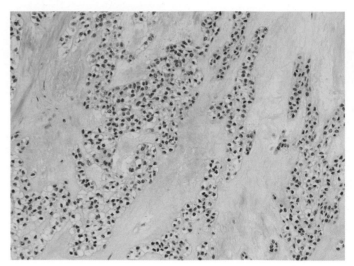

Figure 8.18.1 Low power photomicrograph of CCOC showing aggregates of clear cells in a collagenous stroma.

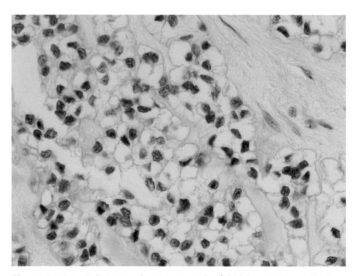

Figure 8.18.2 High power photomicrograph of CCOC. Note the cytologic atypia and minimal nuclear palisading at the periphery of tumor islands.

patterned tumors, which are rare, will have clear cells within an ameloblastomatous follicular tumor island network.

Pathologic Features

The histopathology of an *ameloblastic carcinoma* will be characterized by an accumulation of nests and cords of tumor cells with the distinctive features of an ameloblastoma, including the marginating of tumor islands by tall columnar or cuboidal preameloblastic basaloid cells, central tumor island cellular discohesiveness with a stellate reticulum-like pattern and focal cystic degeneration of island clusters. Identification of central tumor island cytologic atypia is mandatory in order to render a diagnosis of ameloblastic carcinoma and cells should demonstrate cytologic features of malignancy that will most often include loss of cellular polarity, hypercellularity, hyperchromatism and

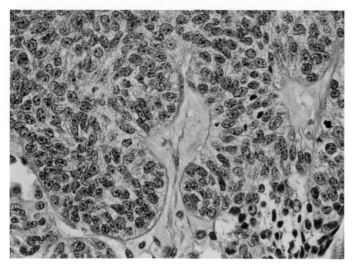

Figure 8.19 High power photomicrograph of ameloblastic carcinoma. Cells within tumor islands demonstrate hypercellularity and cytologic atypia with several atypical mitoses.

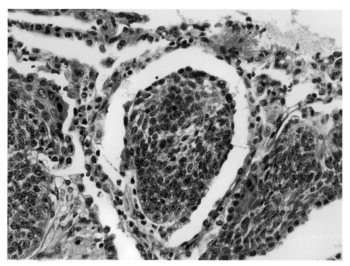

Figure 8.20 Ameloblastoma carcinoma metastatic to lung. Several ameloblastoma islands can be seen filling a lung alveolus.

atypical mitoses (Figure 8.19). Lung is a common metastatic site for this tumor (Figure 8.20).

Malignant ameloblastoma in contrast to ameloblastic carcinoma will demonstrate the classic benign histopathology of a common central osseous ameloblastoma without evidence of significant cytologic atypia. Metastasis of the jaw tumor to another anatomic site is the only feature that will establish the tumor's malignancy. Slootweg and Muller[31] reviewed a series of 26 cases of malignant ameloblastoma and found that patients had metastatic lung involvement in 20 instances. The second most common metastatic site was the lymph nodes.

Treatment

The treatment for *ameloblastic carcinoma, malignant ameloblastoma* and *CCOC* is wide surgical excision with lymph node dissection in those cases where there is lymph node involvement. Radiation therapy and chemo therapy are of limited value, although they may be helpful in managing locally advanced or metastatic disease. Osteonecrosis and secondary sarcomas may arise following radiation therapy. There is limited follow-up on the small number of cases of ameloblastic carcinoma and malignant ameloblastoma that have been reported. The median survival time after metastasis for malignant ameloblastoma in all age groups is approximately two years.[32] Once tumor spread has been documented for ameloblastic carcinoma, survival is equally as short.[33] Yazici et al. have reported a case of maxillary ameloblastic carcinoma in a child successfully treated with surgery and chemo therapy.[34] The chemotherapeutic agents of choice are Cisplatin, Adriamycin, Cyclophosphamide, Paclitaxel and Carboplatin.[29]

Calcifying Epithelial Odontogenic Tumor
Clinical Findings

The calcifying epithelial odontogenic tumor (CEOT), also known as the Pindborg tumor, was first described in 1958.[36] The lesion has a reported incidence of between 0.7 and 1.8 percent among all tumors of odontogenic origin. Franklin and Pindborg documented only one CEOT in a ten-year-old child among 113 cases they reviewed.[37] Ungari et al.[38] reported a CEOT in a nine-year-old child in a study of CEOTs in children, and Guerrisi et al.[39] in a review of cases from the archives of the Laboratory of Surgical Pathology of the School of Dentistry, University of Buenos Aires, found that 1.3 percent of the 156 odontogenic tumors they studied were CEOTs.

The premolar/molar region of the maxilla is the most common site for the CEOT in children,[38,39] and most lesions will present as an expansile mass or swelling that is painless. Extraosseous soft tissue variants of the CEOT, although reported in adults, appear to be undocumented in children.

The growth potential and biologic behavior of the CEOT in adults and children is considered to be similar to that of ameloblastoma, with the tumor demonstrating local invasiveness and a high recurrence potential. In children, however, the tumor does not seem to have the same propensity for developing in association with an impacted tooth, as it does in adults.[38]

The CEOT, which is thought to originate from a complex system of dental lamina remnants, will typically present as a well delineated radiolucent expansile unilocular or multilocular lesion. Approximately one-half of all CEOTs reported in adults have been described as containing radiopaque "calcified" zones radiographically, (Figure 8.21) leading to a differential radiographic diagnosis of COC, odontoma, odontoameloblastoma or ossifying fibroma. So few cases have been reported in children, that it is difficult to determine whether or not such a radiographic finding is also typical of childhood CEOTs. Ungari[38] has suggested that some CEOTs in children may in fact present as lesions that are totally radiolucent.

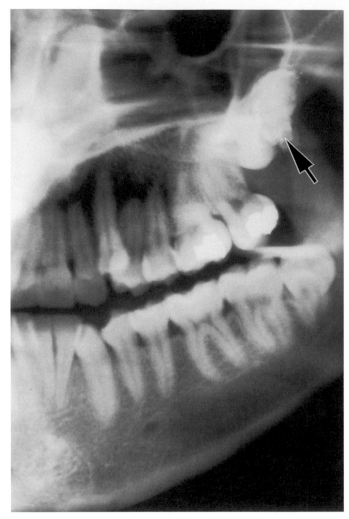

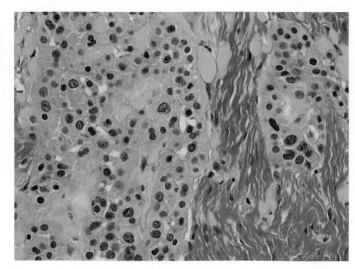

Figure 8.22 CEOT displaying characteristic islands of eosinophilic tumor cells set in a matrix of collagen.

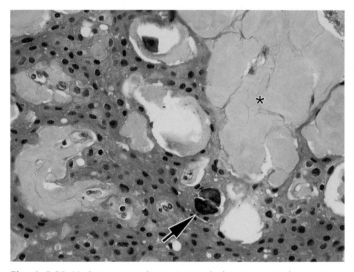

Figure 8.21 CEOT of the posterior maxilla in an 18-year-old boy. The densely radiopaque lesion is surrounded by a radiolucent zone and associated with an impacted tooth (arrow). (Reproduced with the permission of Cambridge University Press).

Pathologic Features

Grossly, the CEOT will most often be a homogenous tumor mass that may or may not contain a calcified product. Some semblance of a tumor capsule may be identified or the tumor may appear to extend beyond any limiting border and into marginating bone at the time of gross inspection.

The CEOT has a unique histology. Sheets, nests and cords of polyhedryl epithelial cells that stain deeply eosinophilic will be seen ramifying throughout a well vascularized collagenous stroma (Figure 8.22). Individual cells within tumor islands will demonstrate a significant degree of nuclear pleomorphism, and cellular hyperchromatism, which can be misinterpreted as malignant cytologic atypia. Round, calcified and ring-like aggregates are common to the tumor's histology. These calcified basophilic aggregates known as Liesegang ring calcifications are often coalescent. Pools of eosinophilic homogenous amyloid-like material will generally be seen admixed with tumor cells or within tumor islands (Figure 8.23). This

Figure 8.23 Medium power photomicrograph showing atypical appearing CEOT tumor cells. These "benign," but sometimes cytologically atypical appearing cells can display nuclear hyperchromatism, altered nuclear/cytoplasmic ratios and binucleation. Eosinophilic amyloid product (*), and Liesegang ring calcifications (arrow) are prominent.

material will stain positively for amyloid using thioflavin T staining, and congo-red stains will demonstrate the material to show an "apple green" birefringence when polarized. Most investigators agree that the amyloid-like substance which arises from destruction of lamina dense material is of epithelial origin.[42,43] The amyloid-like product has also been shown to be composed of N-terminal fragments of odontogenic ameloblast associated protein (ODAM).[40,41] The PTCH1 gene is believed to play a role in the genesis of the CEOT[44,45] and immunohistochemical reactivity for amelogenin in the neoplastic cells of the CEOT and in the tumor's associated amyloid-like product, has been documented.[41,44,45] Uncommon examples of CEOTs composed predominantly of clear cells have been reported.[46,47]

Differential Diagnoses

Squamous odontogenic tumor (SOT), COC, (CCOT) odontogenic fibroma (WHO type) and squamous cell carcinoma, can all resemble the CEOT histologically. The so-called ghost cells of the COC will stain negatively for amyloid product, however, allowing for a clear distinction between the CEOT and COC. The odontogenic fibroma, WHO type, will lack the Liesegang ring-like calcifications of the CEOT. Squamous cell carcinomas characteristically display the cytologic atypia of a malignant epithelial neoplasm whereas the CEOT will not. The "clear cell variant" of the CEOT[46] can resemble a clear cell salivary gland neoplasm, metastatic renal cell carcinoma, glycogen rich adenocarcinoma or CCOC, and although these neoplasms might be considered in the differential diagnoses of a clear cell CEOT in an adult, the clear cell CEOT is a distinct rarity in children.

Treatment and Prognosis

The CEOT is treated by a 1 to 1.5 cm marginal resection of bone and one uninvolved anatomic barrier margin, in a manner similar to ameloblastoma, although the CEOT will show intramedullary spread less often than ameloblastoma. Recurrence rates for the CEOT vary but recurrences are most often documented to be around 15 percent. Marx reports that CEOTs treated with enucleation and curettage will show a recurrence rate ranging from 15 to 30 percent after four years.[48] Close, long-term follow-up is recommended for pediatric patients diagnosed with a CEOT. The lesion has no malignant potential; however, clear cell variants of the CEOT have been reported to have a somewhat increased biological aggressiveness when compared with that of a conventional CEOT.[49]

Adenomatoid Odontogenic Tumor (Adenomatoid Odontogenic Cyst)

Clinical Findings

The AOT or cyst is much more common in pediatric age group patients than either ameloblastoma or CEOT, accounting for 3 to 7 percent of all odontogenic tumors.[50] Once known by the misleading term adenoameloblastoma, the AOT occurs most often between the ages of 10 and 20, with a mean occurrence age of 18.[51] Current theory suggests that the AOT is derived from the enamel organ or remnants of Hertwigs epithelial root sheath. Interestingly, Adebayo found the AOT to be the third most common tumor of children after ameloblastoma and myxoma in a study of Nigerian children.[52] However, more comprehensive worldwide statistics differ.

Marx[51] favors the term adenomatoid odontogenic cyst for this lesion because of its typical encapsulation, both clinically and grossly, and the almost invariable presence of a lumen. Females are affected much more commonly than males (2:1), and the most common clinical finding is that of a painless, slowly expansile swelling due to the underlying involvement of bone.[52,53,54] The AOT is usually identified in the maxillary

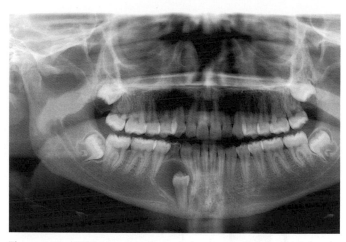

Figure 8.24 AOT. Panoramic radiograph showing a well-defined radiolucency surrounding a mandibular canine tooth.

canine, premolar or incisor region, although cases have been reported in the mandible. Seventy-five percent of reported cases have been associated with an unerupted or impacted tooth, the most common tooth being the maxillary cuspid.[53] Instances of extraosseous AOTs have been documented, but in children, such lesions are exceedingly rare.[52] Some investigators divide AOTs into follicular, extrafollicular and peripheral subtypes. Nearly all tumors in children are follicular in nature and arise in the maxillary canine region.[55]

Radiologically, the AOT will most often present as a unilocular solitary cyst-like growth associated with an impacted tooth (Figure 8.24). As a clinical differential diagnosis, dentigerous cyst, OKC and inflammatory cyst of dental origin (radicular cyst) should be considered. When an AOT is associated with an impacted tooth, the tumor will classically include a good portion of the root surface of that tooth within it. This feature helps to distinguish an AOT from a dentigerous cyst, a lesion which will generally encase only the crown of a tooth radiographically. Displacement of adjacent teeth is a common feature associated with the AOT. Calcifications can frequently be seen within the tumor or cystic mass, producing detectable radiopaque flecks or a ring of calcification near the cystic margin. The AOT will rarely grow to a size that results in penetration of the cortical plates, and if perforation of the cortex occurs, the clinical differential diagnosis should include a more aggressive odontogenic neoplasm.

From an embryological standpoint, there seems to be a distinct morphologic similarity between the cells that line the duct-like structures that can be seen in an AOT, and the cells of the inner enamel epithelium of the tooth germ. These duct-like structures may, in fact represent nothing more than an abortive attempt at formation.

Pathologic Features

Most AOTs will be small encapsulated growths measuring 1–3 cm in diameter. On cut section, the AOT tends to be yellow to white, with either a firm or a cystic cut surface. Multiple

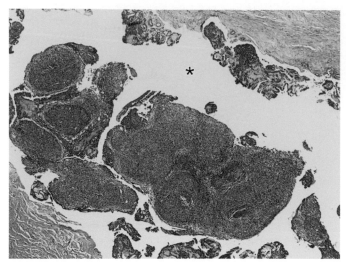

Figure 8.25 AOT showing a cavitation or cyst-like lumen (*) that is filled with nodular aggregates of basophilic spindle-like epithelial cells.

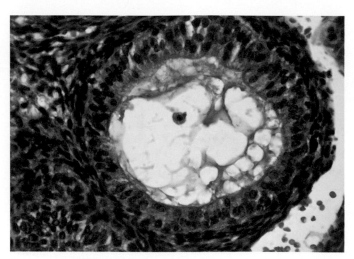

Figure 8.27 AOT tumor island showing columnar cells with their nuclei polarized away from the lumen and toward the basement membrane of the cell. Note characteristic aggregates of eosinophilic calcified material at the superior margins of spindle cell or cartwheel clusters.

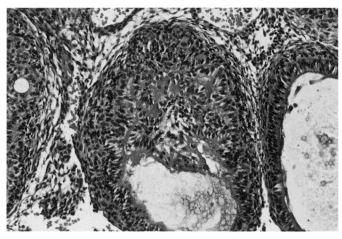

Figure 8.26 High power photomicrograph of AOT showing epithelial islands that contain duct-like spaces.

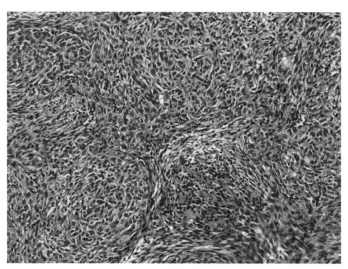

Figure 8.28 High power photomicrograph of AOT demonstrating swirling spindle shaped tumor cells.

sections through the gross specimen will nearly always reveal a cystic lumen. Any luminal area may contain gelatinous material, or a calcified "driven snow-like" product that will correlate with radiographic findings of radiopaque flecks.

Histologically, the AOT may appear cavitated or cystic, with a central luminal tumor mass (Figure 8.25). The AOT will be composed of a proliferation of sheets, nests and cords of neoplastic epithelial cells that differentiate along columnar lines to resemble ameloblasts (Figure 8.26). These tumor cell aggregates will form "ducts," "tubules" or "adenomatoid zones" with central lumena that will be surrounded by cuboidal or columnar cells. The cells lining the "duct-like" spaces stain deeply basophilic, and their nuclei will be polarized away from the lumen and toward the basement membrane in a manner opposite of that seen in an ameloblastoma (Figure 8.27). In addition to the tubular and ductal structures seen in the AOT, bands, sheets and clusters of tumor cells

arranged in a swirling spindle-like pattern can be identified (Figure 8.28). These cells tend to take on a cartwheel or cribriform pattern. Tumor nests, whether duct-like or swirling in their arrangement will be supported by a scant connective tissue stroma, in which eosinophilic dystrophic calcified material may be seen, These calcifications, which tend to develop primarily at junctions between aggregates of epithelial cells that form the tumor and the adjacent vascularized stromal tissues, have been shown to resemble enamel, pre-enamel or dentin morphologically.[53,54,55,56]

Poulson and Greer[56] reviewed the electron microscopic features of the AOT and identified two distinctly different cell types; polygonal cells and spindle cells. Polygonal to columnar cells tended to surround the tumor's duct-like structures, to form small nodules. These cells also tended to share common features with pre-ameloblasts and ultrastructurally resembled them, demonstrating an abundance of free ribosomes and a paucity of endoplasmic reticulum. Spindle-shaped cells appeared similar to cells of the stratum intermedium and stellate reticulum of the tooth germ. These cells demonstrated ovoid nuclei and appeared perpendicular to luminal cells. Ultrastructurally, the spindle cell type indeed to have a dense cytoplasm filled with numerous filaments and ribosomes.

Immunohistochemical attempts to identify the nature and source of the eosinophilic material that is often observed in the AOT suggest that the material is amyloid-like.[53] AOTs have also been shown to express a host of cytokeratins, and vimentin. The Ki-67 index fraction for the tumor is quite low.[57]

Differential Diagnosis

The duct-like structures found in the AOT, can histologically resemble ducts that can be seen in a salivary gland neoplasm. The AOT, with its polarizing tall columnar cells, can also resemble an ameloblastoma. Ameloblastoma, however, will demonstrate columnar cells at the periphery of tumor islands, which will have their nuclei polarized away from the basement membrane, whereas in the AOT, the nuclei of similar columnar cells that line "duct-like" spaces will be polarized toward the basement membrane. AOTs are also typically encapsulated growths whereas ameloblastomas are not.

Behavior and Management

The AOT grows slowly and generally will enucleate readily from the surrounding bone. The tumor shows little tendency toward recurrence,[50] and conservative surgical enucleation remains the treatment of choice.[58] It should be pointed out that some investigators[51] believe the AOT to be a hamartoma and not a true odontogenic neoplasm.

It is exceedingly important for the surgical pathologist to be able to separate the AOT from ameloblastoma because the biologic behavior of the two tumors is dramatically different. Although there can be a close histomorphologic resemblance between the cells of the AOT and the ameloblastoma, proper microscopic classification is mandatory.

Squamous Odontogenic Tumor

Clinical Findings

First characterized and reported in 1975, the SOT is a rare tumor of odontogenic origin that is thought to arise from residual rests of Malassez that remain in the periodontal ligament after tooth development, or from residual oral mucosal basal layer epithelium following tooth development.[59] The SOT remains an exceedingly rare odontogenic neoplasm with fewer than 200 cases reported worldwide.[60,61]

Most SOTs have been reported to occur in the third decade of life, although there are reports of the tumors occurring over a wide age-range, including documentation in children.[59,60,61,62,63,64] The SOT is characterized by a slight male

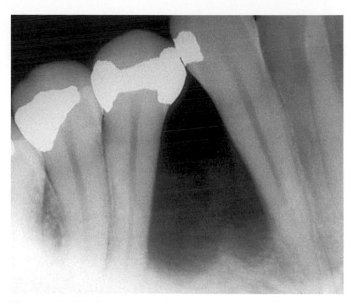

Figure 8.29 SOT demonstrating a large triangular shaped radiolucency.

predominance and the maxilla is affected more often than the mandible. Most SOTs will arise as a soft tissue mass within the premolar/canine region of the maxilla. The molar region of the mandible is the next most frequently affected site. The SOT will often present radiographically as a destructive triangular shaped lesion that occurs between the roots of adjacent teeth (Figure 8.29). SOTs can be multifocal and thus the tumor's clinical appearance may mimic that of generalized periodontal disease.[65,66] Parmar et al.[61] have recently documented the occurrence of SOT-like proliferations in the walls of radicular cysts.

A third of patients with SOT have no symptoms. When symptoms do occur, they most often fall into the category of a focal swelling and occasional pain. Although most reports describe the SOT as a hamartomatous-like central osseous like growth, extraosseous, and biologically aggressive central osseous cases have been reported.[66]

Pathologic Features

The SOT will be composed of bulbous islands of well differentiated acanthotic appearing and cytologically bland squamous epithelium (Figure 8.30). Tumor islands will lack marginating peripheral columnar cells. Individual tumor islands may contain areas of dystrophic calcification (Figure 8.31), globular bodies of keratin, clear cells or glassy lake-like eosinophilic pools of osteoid matrix. Tumor islands will typically be set in a collagenous matrix that may or may not be chronically inflamed.

Differential Diagnosis

Histologically, the SOT can resemble squamous cell carcinoma, the acanthomatous, or desmoplastic ameloblastoma, metastatic carcinoma or high grade mucoepidermoid carcinoma. SOT

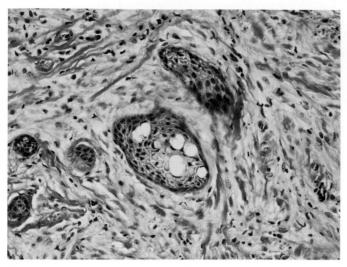

Figure 8.30 SOT showing aggregates of bland squamous epithelium set in a matrix of collagen.

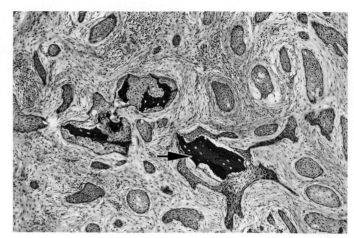

Figure 8.31 Zones of osseous metaplasia are common to tumor islands in the SOT (arrow).

tumor islands tend to be large, bulbous and round, whereas the individual tumor islands seen in desmoplastic ameloblastoma are more often thin and thread-like. Acanthomatous ameloblastoma tumor islands will tend to exhibit irregular shapes, and hyperchromatic columnar pre-ameloblastic appearing cells will marginate tumor islands, features that are not common and SOT. The cytologic atypia that is characteristic of squamous cell carcinoma or high grade mucoepidermoid carcinoma will not be seen in the SOT. The organ of Chievitz, a discrete aggregation of epithelial cells that are squamous in their appearance can also appear histologically similar to the SOT.

Behavior and Management

Treatment of SOT includes curettage or conservative surgical excision. New lesions can arise in a different location as frequently as 20 percent of the time; thus, close follow-up of the patient is mandatory. Peripheral, purely soft tissue SOTs can arise. Such soft tissue lesions are best managed by excision with a margin of normal tissue.[67]

Mesenchymal Odontogenic Tumors

Tumors of mesenchyme and/or odontogenic mesenchyme, with or without odontogenic epithelium (WHO)

Odontogenic Myxoma

Odontogenic myxoma is a rare odontogenic tumor that shows a wide age distribution. Servato et al. in a review of 431 childhood odontogenic tumors, found that odontogenic myxoma represented 5 percent of the total number of odontogenic tumors that were studied.[68] Guerrisi et al. report a somewhat higher incidence for odontogenic myxomas in the pediatric age group than Servato, with myxoma accounting for 8.5 percent of the 153 odontogenic tumors that were studied.[69]

There has been considerable debate in the literature as to whether or not myxomas of the maxillofacial skeleton are odontogenic in origin or of central osseous mesenchymal origin. Current thinking favors the premise that myxomas that arise in the jaws most likely originate from primitive odontogenic mesenchymal or embryonic connective tissue derivatives, while tumors that involve the sinonasal tract more than likely have an osseous rather than an odontogenic derivation.[70] Regardless of the tumor's source, the biologic behavior of all myxomas remains the same, and the vast majority of myxomas that have been studied ultrastructurally have been confirmed to arise from fibroblasts.[70,71]

Odontogenic myxomas of the jaws tend to show a peak incidence in the second and third decades of life. In children and adolescents, myxomas tend to occur slightly more often in boys than girls, with the mandible being slightly favored. Jaw expansion is the common presenting symptom.[72] Tumors in extragnathic sites are rare and primarily involve the maxillary sinuses with secondary extension into the nasal cavity. Soft tissue myxomas which are extremely rare in children have been reported in the pharynx, larynx, parotid gland and ear.[73]

Radiographically, the odontogenic myxoma will typically present as a painless multilocular radiolucency of the jaw that will cause a localized swelling and expansion of the bony cortex. (Figure 8.32) The clinical differential diagnosis for a suspected odontogenic myxoma, in a child with a multilocular or unilocular jaw radiolucency, should include AF, ameloblastoma, central giant cell granuloma (tumor) and OKC (keratocystic odontogenic tumor). The borders of a myxoma can be either poorly or well delineated radiographically, and the tumor frequently shows radiolucent scalloping between the teeth. Myxomas have been documented to occur in association with congenitally missing teeth and unerupted teeth as well as in the fully developed dentition. Displacement of nerves and root resorption are common radiographic findings associated with myxomas of the jaws. CT scans can be valuable in demonstrating expansion, medullary extension and perforation of the cortex by the tumor.

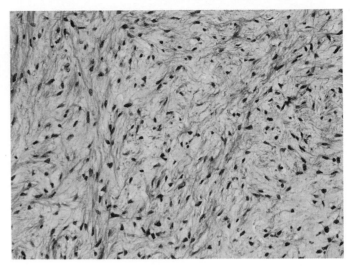

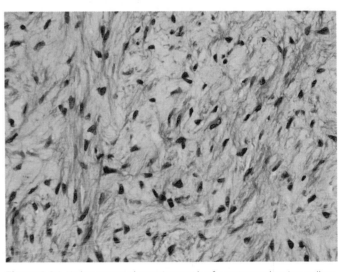

Figure 8.33 Odontogenic myxoma showing sparsely arranged fibroblasts set in a primitive collagen matrix with abundant ground substance.

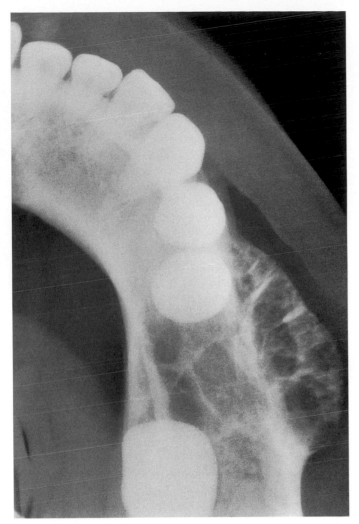

Figure 8.32 Odontogenic myxoma presenting as an expansile multilocular radiolucency. (Reprinted with the permission of Cambridge University Press).

Figure 8.34 Higher power photomicrograph of a myxoma showing stellate fibroblasts and primitive streaming bands of collagen.

Pathologic Features

Odontogenic myxomas will tend to have one of two common presentations on gross inspection. Tumors will present either as a mucoid gelatinous growth or as a gray/white to yellow solid mass. In either instance, the tumor will have a poorly defined unencapsulated peripheral margin. Tumors that are solid tend to be multinodular and bone will be frequently found within cut sections of the tumor.

Histopathologically, myxomas will be composed of a haphazard arrangement of stellate or spindle shaped cells that tend to have clear to eosinophilic cytoplasm and small hyperchromatic nuclei (Figure 8.33). These cells typically ramify throughout a loose myxoid or mucinous stroma (Figure 8.34). The degree of collagenization of that stroma will vary. Islands of odontogenic epithelium can be either prominent or quite sparse within the tumor, and it is not known if such epithelial rests and islands are simply a fetal remnant of odontogenesis or if they are mandatory for the genesis of the tumor.

Farman et al.[75] in an attempt to determine whether or not any specific histologic pattern is associated with odontogenic myxoma might be predictive of that tumor's biologic aggressiveness, found no microscopically predictive pattern. It has been shown, however, that maxillary myxomas tend to spread more rapidly than mandibular lesions, and that maxillary lesions present a more difficult management problem than those involving the mandible.

Zaho et al.[76] have shown that chondroitin 6-sulfate (CS-6) proteoglycans and hyaluronic acid (HA) are common to odontogenic myxomas. This finding tends to be helpful in separating odontogenic myxoma from fibrous histocytoma, which will stain negatively for both products.

Perdigao et al.[77] have suggested that odontogenic myxomas are linked developmentally to mutations in the PRKAR1 1A gene, which codes for the regulatory subunit of the protein kinase A. Goldblatt[78] has described two specific cell types in odontogenic myxomas: a non-secretory type I cell and a secretory type II cell. Both cells are thought to arise from a connective tissue source, and are most likely of periodontal ligament origin. The presence of these cells, which have been shown to have microfilament systems that allow them to function as myofibroblasts, supports the premise that a myofibroblast associated contractile mechanism, affords the odontogenic myxoma's tumor cells a degree of motility that enhances the bony destruction associated with the tumor.[76,77,78,79]

Differential Diagnosis

Odontogenic myxoma can resemble a host of neoplasms microscopically, including myxoid neurofibroma, chondromyxoid fibroma and myxoid chondrosarcoma. S100 protein staining should allow one to distinguish odontogenic myxoma from myxoid neurofibroma, in that the neurofibroma will stain positively for S100 protein. Cartilaginous or chondroid differentiation is common to the chondromyxoid fibroma and myxoid chondrosarcoma, a feature that tends to separate these two tumors from odontogenic myxoma, where cartilage formation is rare.

Cranial fasciitis in the child can also have a prominent myxoid background when viewed microscopically. However, this tumor will express smooth muscle actin, a feature that is not seen with odontogenic myxoma.

Odontogenic fibroma as well as the rare myxoid variant of desmoplastic fibroma can resemble odontogenic myxoma histologically. These two lesions, however, will most often demonstrate a dense interlacing collagenous tumor matrix whereas odontogenic myxomas will tend to be rich in ground substance and rarely demonstrate an interlacing mature collagenous pattern. Overexpression of matrix metalloproteinases is common to odontogenic myxoma, whereas desmoplastic fibroma and odontogenic fibroma will not show such over expression.

The surgical pathologist must always take care to distinguish odontogenic myxoma from a simple primitive tooth follicle, since the two processes can have similar microscopic appearances. Communication between the clinician or surgeon, and the pathologist, along with the appropriate evaluation of radiographs and CT scans is often necessary in order to prevent misinterpretation of a tissue sample from a hyperplastic tooth follicle as a myxoma.

Treatment and Prognosis

The treatment of choice for odontogenic myxoma is marginal surgical resection with a 1.0 to 1.5 cm bony margin and one non-involved anatomic barrier. Some investigators favor curettage for small myxomas, however, such conservative therapy is rarely adequate. The recurrence rate for odontogenic myxoma is typically in the 20 to 25 percent range. This high recurrence rate is thought to be largely due to undertreatment of the tumor using either enucleation or curettage. Although so-called malignant myxomas[80] have been reported in adults,

no appropriately documented cases have been reported in pediatric age group patients.

Central (Osseous) Odontogenic Fibroma

Central (osseous) odontogenic fibroma is an exceedingly rare tumor in pediatric age patients. Guerrisi et al. in an extensive 15-year study of odontogenic tumors in childhood and adolescents, found only 5 instances of central osseous odontogenic fibroma among 153 odontogenic tumors that were studied. The tumor, considered by most investigators to be of periodontal ligament origin, usually occurs posterior to the first mandibular molar in adults, where the tumor has a female predilection, (3:1).

Servato et al.[82] in a review of 431 cases of odontogenic tumors in children, found only 0.9 percent of the tumors evaluated to be odontogenic fibromas. Male and female involvement with the tumor was equal in the Servato study. Most pediatric age patients diagnosed with central odontogenic fibroma are between the ages of 11 and 20; unlike in their adult counterparts, the tumor shows neither a mandibular or maxillary predilection.

Peripheral odontogenic fibroma, the oral soft tissue counterpart of the central osseous form of the tumor, is rare in children, but slightly more common than the central osseous form of the tumor.

The diagnostic criterion established for central odontogenic fibroma were originally outlined by Gardner,[83] who subclassified the tumor into two histologic subtypes: tumors that contained epithelial odontogenic rests, and tumors that lack such rests. Handlers et al.[84] have suggested, however, that such subclassification is confusing, unnecessary and of little clinical significance, since such classification is not predictive of tumor behavior. The WHO, nonetheless continues to separate the tumor into two histological subtypes, which they define as; 1) epithelial poor or 2) epithelial rich.[85] Again, neither designation can be correlated with the biologic behavior of the tumor.

Clinical Findings

Central odontogenic fibromas inpatients in the pediatric age group, can present as either an asymptomatic or symptomatic swelling. When symptomatic, such swellings can be associated with loose teeth, pain, drainage, root resorption and even paresthesia. Tumors are most often radiolucent and unilocular (Figure 8.35) but they can also be multilocular in their presentation. Wesley et al.[86] found that 7 of 11 central odontogenic fibromas they studied were in close association with a crown of an impacted tooth. These investigators also reported that areas of calcification or opacity could often be identified radiographically within the lesional mass.

Pathologic Features

On gross inspection, the central osseous odontogenic fibroma will most often be a partially encapsulated neoplastic mass with a homogenous, firm glistening white to yellow cut surface.

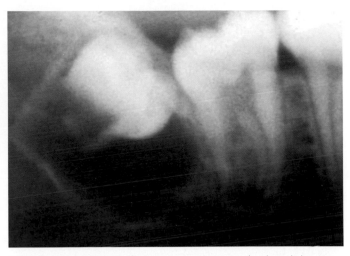

Figure 8.35 Odontogenic fibroma presenting as a unilocular radiolucency.

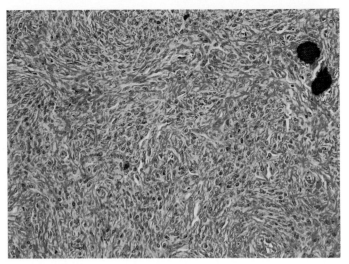

Figure 8.37 Central odontogenic fibroma showing dense eosinophilic collagen bands and an associated fibro-myxoid stroma. Calcifications are present within the tumor stroma.

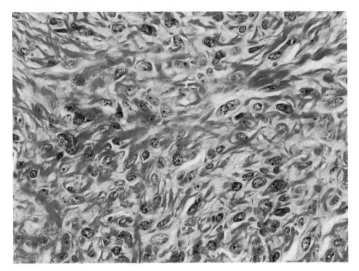

Figure 8.36 Central odontogenic fibroma demonstrating mature collagen and associated tumor cells, often with clear cytoplasm.

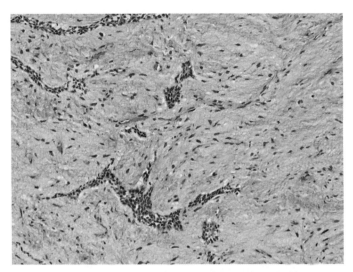

Figure 8.38 Central odontogenic fibroma. Odontogenic epithelial rests in a central odontogenic fibroma. Note both mature eosinophilic collagen bands and a myxoid stroma that resembles that of an odontogenic myxoma.

Histologically, the neoplasm will be composed of a moderately dense and relatively cellular proliferation of interlacing collagen fascicles (Figure 8.36). The distribution of fibroblasts throughout the tumor's largely collagenous architecture is usually uniform. On occasion, cementum or dentin-like calcifications may be identified within the neoplasm (Figure 8.37). The tumor may or may not contain odontogenic epithelium. When present, that epithelium will closely resemble epithelial odontogenic rests of Malassez (Figure 8.38). Portions of the tumor may appear histologically similar to odontogenic myxoma. However, myxoma will tend to be composed more often of scant amounts of mature collagen and an abundance of ground substance, giving that tumor a prominent myxoid appearance, rather than the more mature fibrotic appearance of odontogenic fibroma microscopically. When a suspected odontogenic fibroma tissue sample is viewed microscopically, a whirled pattern of the fibroblasts making up the tumor will tend to favor a diagnosis of odontogenic fibroma. Odontogenic epithelial rests tend to be more common to the central osseous odontogenic fibroma than odontogenic myxoma.

Central granular cell odontogenic fibroma, as described by Vincent et al.[87] is a rare variant of odontogenic fibroma. The tumor, which is almost exclusively seen in adults, shows a female predilection. Microscopically, the tumor will be composed of an abundance of not only fibroblasts and mature collagen, but it will also contain a prominence of polygonal cells with eosinophilic granular cytoplasm.

Odontogenic fibromas that show a high Ki67 index may be more biologically aggressive than those that do not; however, tumors that are rich in epithelium (odontogenic rests) and that show significant cytokeratin expression do not appear to have a more aggressive biologic behavior than those that do not.

Differential Diagnosis

Several tumors can closely resemble central odontogenic fibroma microscopically, included among those tumors are desmoplastic fibroma, CEOT and ameloblastoma. The desmoplastic fibroma tends to demonstrate interlacing fascicles of mature collagen more frequently than the central odontogenic fibroma. Desmoplastic fibroma will also lack odontogenic epithelial rests as part of its histopathology. The CEOT, unlike odontogenic fibroma will typically be composed of prominent eosinophilic polygonal cells and in contrast to odontogenic fibroma, the CEOT will contain amyloid in over 60 percent of cases. Ameloblastoma can possibly be confused with central odontogenic fibroma histologically. However, the epithelial tumor islands that are part of the ameloblastoma's histopathology will demonstrate tall columnar pre-ameloblastic cells at their periphery, a feature that will not be seen in the smaller immature odontogenic rest seen in odontogenic fibroma.

Ossifying fibroma also can resemble odontogenic fibroma microscopically, especially if one is dealing with a tumor that lacks a significant calcified component. However, the stroma of an ossifying fibroma is usually well vascularized, and granulomatous even, and the ossifying fibroma will be composed of less mature collagen than the central odontogenic fibroma. Fibrosarcoma may resemble central odontogenic fibroma histologically, however, fibrosarcoma will tend to have a fascicular pattern microscopically and the tumor will usually demonstrate significant cytologic atypia.

Peripheral odontogenic fibroma is a lesion that most often presents as a soft tissue nodule involving the gingiva (Figure 8.39). The mandibular arch is favored as a presentation site over the maxillary arch and the tumor will be histologically identical to its central osseous counterpart. Peripheral odontogenic fibroma must be distinguished histopathologically from the much more common childhood neoplasm, peripheral ossifying fibroma (peripheral fibroma with ossification). Peripheral ossifying fibroma will typically have reactive bone as a significant part of its histopathology (Figures 8.40 & 8.41); a

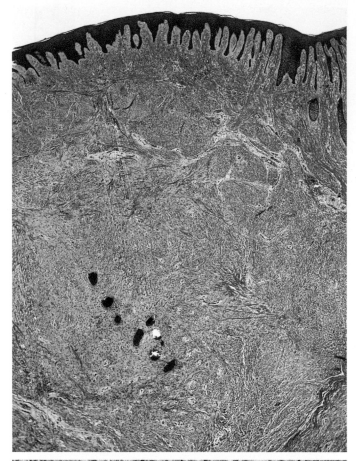

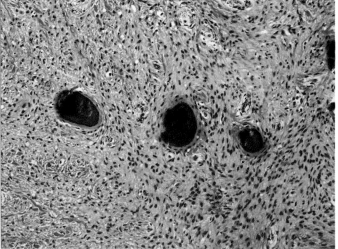

Figures 8.40 (top) & 8.41 (bottom) Peripheral ossifying fibroma at lower and intermediate magnification, showing calcifications.

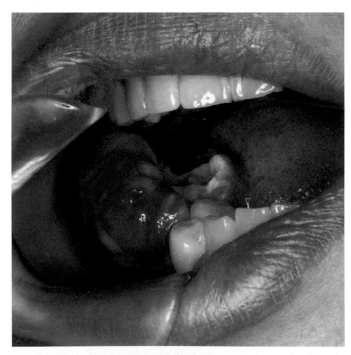

Figure 8.39 Nodular appearing peripheral odontogenic fibroma involving the mandibular gingiva of a child.

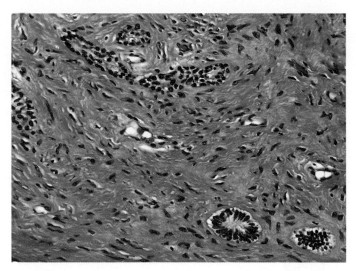

Figure 8.42 Peripheral odontogenic will generally lack such calcifications and more frequently display epithelial odontogenic rests, as a component of its histopathology.

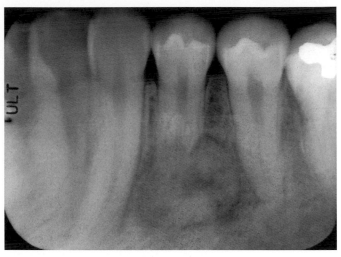

Figure 8.43 Cementoblastoma involving the root of a first bicuspid tooth. (Note that the tumor arises from the apical half of the root).

feature that is not classically part of the histopathology of a peripheral odontogenic fibroma. Both tumors can have epithelial odontogenic rests entrapped within their stroma, with the peripheral odontogenic fibroma more often demonstrating this rest entrapment phenomenon (Figure 8.42).

Treatment and Prognosis

Central (osseous) odontogenic fibroma is treated by local surgical enucleation and curettage. In children, the tumor is reported to have a recurrence rate of around 14 percent.[88] No instances of malignant transformation of odontogenic fibroma in children have been reported. The soft tissue or *peripheral odontogenic fibroma* is treated by complete excision of the tumor mass with a margin of normal tissue.

Cementoblastoma

Cementoblastoma, first described by Norberg[89] in 1930, has long been classified as an odontogenic neoplasm. The tumor is characterized by an apical proliferation of cementoblasts resulting in the encasement of the root apex or apices of the involved tooth by cementum. Both Servato et al.[90] and Guerrisi[91] in two extensive surveys of odontogenic tumors in children and adolescents report that cementoblastoma represented less than 2 percent of the tumors they reviewed. The tumor, which has a male predominance of approximately 2:1 is most often identified in patients between the ages of 10 and 20. Corio et al.[92] reviewed the clinicopathologic characteristics of cementoblastoma in all age groups, and found the mandibular premolar/molar region to be the most common anatomic site of predilection.

Clinical Findings

Cementoblastoma, which is always intimately associated with the apical half of the root or roots of a tooth, most often affects the mandibular permanent first molar tooth. An involved tooth will usually retain its vitality, even as the cementoblastoma occupies medullary bone and expands cortical bone. The tumor mass grows in such a fashion that there is often a thin radiolucent zone surrounding an area of dense apical calcification.[93] (See Figure 8.43.) Although cementoblastomas can be either radiolucent or radiopaque, they most often present as a radiopaque mass. In rare instances, the tumor can show invasion into the root canal of the associated tooth. Over time the tumor will result in bony expansion, tooth displacement or resorption and obliteration of the periodontal ligament space. Perforation of the bony cortex is rare; however, pain is a frequent symptom associated with cementoblastoma and some authorities consider cementoblastoma and osteoblastoma, which can also be quite painful, to be variants of the same neoplasm.[94]

Pathologic Features

The cementoblastoma will present grossly as a hard white to yellow or gray tumor mass that will be fused to the apex or apices of the involved tooth. The globular tumor mass can resemble hypercementosis. A thin margin of capsular connective tissue may be identified between the tumor and any surrounding bone.

Cementoblastoma is characterized microscopically by the proliferation of plump pleomorphic appearing cementoblastic cells that will typically marginate a concentric mineralized product that is consistent with cementum. The tumor will be attached directly to a tooth root or roots. The plump cementoblasts will have basophilic staining nuclei and globular to streaming eosinophilic cytoplasm. The nuclei of the cementoblasts can be markedly hyperchromatic and they will tend to be stacked on top of one another in a layer or lattice-like pattern. Tumor cells typically surround islands of cementum,

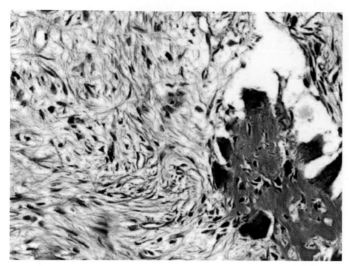

Figure 8.44 Plump proliferating cementoblasts marginating cementum characterize this cementoblastoma.

cementum-like product or osteoid-like material that ramifies throughout a thin fibrous stroma. (Figure 8.44) Rare foreign body giant cells may also be seen. Prominent basophilic reversal lines are common to the cementum or cementoid product. An associated fine microscopic birefringence, typical of true cementum, has been reported by Giansanti.[95]

Differential Diagnosis

Cementoblastoma can resemble osteosarcoma, osteoblastoma and osteoid osteoma microscopically. All four neoplasms can demonstrate prominent mitotic activity and cellular pleomorphism. However, osteoblastoma and osteoid osteoma will not be attached to the root or roots of teeth. Osteosarcoma will tend to show rapid growth, bony invasion and the production of malignant osteoid, in which nuclear pleomorphism and increased mitotic activity are common.[96] Human cementoblastoma derived protein (HCDP) has been identified in cementoblastoma, and the marker from this protein, CEMP1, may well prove to be helpful in distinguishing cementoblastoma from osteoblastoma and osteosarcoma in the future.[97]

Treatment and Prognosis

Although cementoblastoma can appear clinically and radiographically alarming because of its tendency to grow rapidly, expand bone, resorb root surfaces and cause pain, the tumor has a relatively limited growth potential. Extraction of the involved tooth along with the associated tumor mass along with curettage and peripheral ostectomy is the treatment of choice. In most cases, the tumor can easily be enucleated from the adjacent bone by sectioning of the tooth. Consideration may be given to immediate grafting of the socket to restore full height and width of the alveolus for future dental restorative purposes. Recurrence of cementoblastoma is rare.

Mixed Epithelial and Mesenchymal Odontogenic Tumors

Tumors with odontogenic epithelium, with ectomesenchyme, with or without hard tissue formation, (WHO)

Ameloblastic Fibroma
Clinical Findings

AF is a rare odontogenic tumor that accounts for between 1 and 2 percent of all odontogenic tumors seen in children and adolescents. The tumor, which has a slight male predilection,[98] occurs most frequently in the posterior mandible. AF occurs most often in the first and second decades of life and will generally present as an expansile, radiolucency of the jaw.[99] Ide et al.[100] have suggested that two types AFs occur: 1) a pericoronal hamartomatous form of the neoplasm that is most often associated with an impacted molar tooth and generally presents as an asymptomatic unilocular expansile lesion; and 2) a true neoplastic multilocular expansile radiolucent form of the tumor (Figures 8.45 & 8.46). The multilocular form of AF is reported to have a much higher recurrence rate than its pericoronal counterpart. The overall recurrence rate for AF is reported to be around 13 percent.[101,102]

Pathologic Features

AFs are solid fibrous tumors which may or may not be grossly encapsulated. Lesions tend to be tan to gray-white and are often translucent on gross inspection. Mineralized product may be identified on cross sectioning of the tumor.

Histologically AF is typically composed of sheets, cords and nests of epithelial tumor cells that ramify throughout an embryonal appearing primitive stellate reticulum-like connective tissue stroma (Figure 8.47). This frequently myxoid connective tissue matrix resembles the dental papilla of the tooth germ. The epithelial cells that marginate tumor islands are usually cuboidal or low columnar cells that resemble preameloblasts. These cells tend to be quite basaloid in appearance. Individual tumor islands can be arranged in a linear chain-like pattern or assembled as follicular islands of cells that are similar to the epithelial islands seen in an ameloblastoma. The central stellate areas within tumor islands sometimes undergo cystic degeneration.

Richardson et al.[103] report finding pigment in AF that is similar to the type of pigment that has been described in the CEOT. *MIB1* can be identified immunohistochemically in both the epithelial and mesenchymal components of AF, and some investigators suggest that high *MIB1* labeling indices are predictive of a more biologically aggressive neoplasm.[104] Since in rare instances, AF has been reported to show transition to ameloblastic fibrosarcoma, *MIB1* indices may prove to be of some significance in predicting which AFs have increased potential for such malignant transformation.[105]

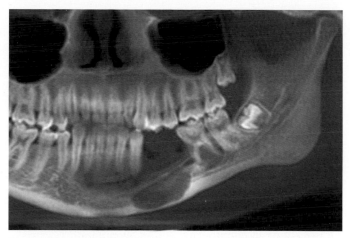

Figure 8.45 Large multilocular AF presenting as a well-demarcated expansile radiolucency of the mandible.

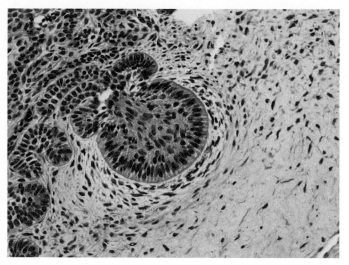

Figure 8.47 High power photomicrograph of an AF demonstrating ameloblastic islands, set in a loosely arranged fibro-myxoid matrix that is reminiscent of the dental papilla. Peripheral palisaded columnar cells demonstrating reverse nuclear polarity marginate the epithelial islands.

in the AF. Columnar pre-ameloblasts will marginate tumor islands in AF, a feature not seen in CEOTs. Finally, the CEOT will demonstrate a mature collagenous stroma rather than the primitive mesenchymal, dental papilla-like stroma that typifies AF. AOT will demonstrable duct-like spaces rimmed by tall columnar or cuboidal cells, and zones of epithelial organoid rosettes, features that is not part of the histologic pattern of AF. Odontomas are composed histologically of an admixture of calcified products (i.e., enamel, dentin, cementum). AF will not contain such calcifications, except in rare instances when a primitive dentinoid product may be seen.

Treatment and Prognosis

The treatment of choice for AF in a child or adolescent is enucleation and curettage.[106] In rare instances, large expansile neoplasms may require marginal resection. Chen et al. accessed 123 cases of AF over tumor progression periods that ranged from 4 months to 40 months and found that the tumors had an overall recurrence rate of 33.3 percent.[106] Ninety-three of the patients in the Chen et al. study were less than 22 years of age, and malignant transformation of AF to ameloblastic fibrosarcoma was reported in 14 cases (11.4 percent). The five year and ten year malignant transformation rates for AF in patients under and over 22 years of age were 10.2 percent and 22.2 percent respectively for patients in the study.

AF is one of the few odontogenic tumors that has been documented to undergo malignant transformation; thus close long-term follow-up of patients diagnosed with AF is mandatory. Fifty percent of AFs that undergo malignant transformation will transition to fibrosarcoma and the epithelial component of the tumor will have disappeared completely by the time a diagnosis of fibrosarcoma is rendered.[106]

AgNOR, PCNA and Ki67 labeling indices will tend to be higher in AF than in odontogenic myxoma, ameloblastic

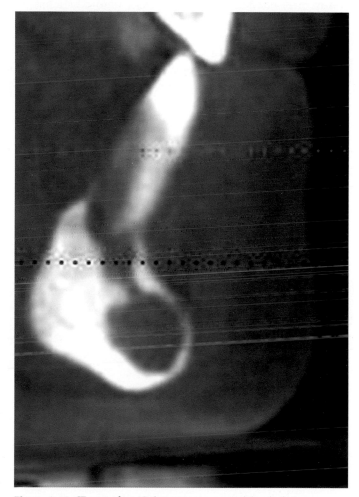

Figure 8.46 CT scan of an AF that presents as a multilocular lesion.

Differential Diagnosis

Histologically, AF can resemble CEOT, AOT or odontoma. CEOT is composed of tumor cells that have markedly hyperchromatic nuclei and eosinophilic cytoplasm, a feature not seen fibro-odontoma or the AOT.[107] These indices may therefore prove helpful in the follow-up and management of the child with AF.

Ameloblastic Fibro-Odontoma

Clinical Findings

The ameloblastic fibro-odontoma is a slow growing and exceedingly uncommon tumor of odontogenic origin that most often manifests as a clinically expansile lesion of bone. The tumor, which is normally encapsulated, represents the histological intermingling of an AF and an odontoma. The ameloblastic fibro-odontoma will usually present as painless swelling of the posterior mandible or maxilla. Slightly more than 50 percent of reported cases have occurred in the mandible. Although the tumor will most often manifest radiographically as a well defined radiolucency, focal areas of radiopacity will be distributed throughout the tumor approximately 50 percent of the time (Figure 8.48).

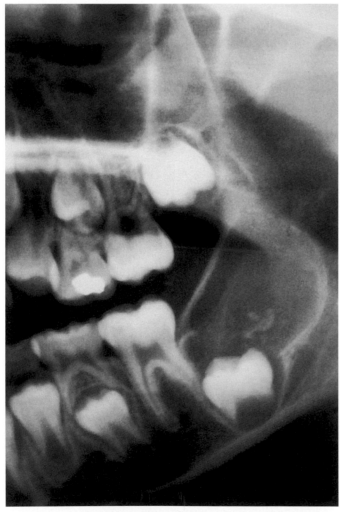

Figure 8.48 A well-defined, predominantly radiolucent ameloblastic fibro-odontoma can be seen associated with an unerupted molar. A small centrally located radiopacity is present within the larger radiolucency.

The WHO[108] recognizes ameloblastic fibro-odontoma as a distinct odontogenic tumor, although some investigators suggest that the lesion is in reality no more than a hamartomatous transitional phase in the developmental progression of a odontoma. Histologic resemblance of ameloblastic fibro-odontoma to both AF and a developing odontoma necessitates that clinicians appreciate the clinical and radiographic nuisances of the tumor, since all three tumors, which are common to childhood, have remarkably different biologic behaviors.

Small lesions that directly abut the occlusal surfaces of erupting teeth are very likely to be no more than developing odontomas and not true ameloblastic fibro-odontomas. The studies of Servato et al.[109] and Guerrisi et al.[110] have shown that ameloblastic fibro-odontoma represents between 1.6 and 4.6 percent of all odontogenic tumors in children. Tsagaris[111] reviewed a large series of ameloblastic fibro-odontomas and found the median age of patients in the study to be 13 years. Nearly three quarters of all ameloblastic fibro-odontomas in the Tsagaris study occurred in individuals younger than 20 years of age. Servato et al. have documented similar findings, reporting that half of the ameloblastic fibro-odontomas they reviewed in a series of 431 cases, occurred in children under ten years of age. The remainder of the tumors occurred in patients between the ages of 11 and 20.

The ameloblastic fibro-odontoma does not show a gender predilection[112] and nearly half of all tumors diagnosed are reported to arise as a swelling that is associated with an unerupted tooth. Clinical differential diagnoses for ameloblastic fibro-odontoma can include several lesions that can also present as mixed radiolucent or radiopaque lesions of the jaws of children, including CEOT, COC, AOT, ossifying fibroma and the rare odontoameloblastoma.

Pathologic Features

Ameloblastic fibro-odontoma will be composed of both odontogenic hard and soft tissue elements, such that on gross inspection, the tumor may appear denticle or tooth like, granular or gritty, myxoid or collagenous. Ameloblastic fibro-odontoma demonstrate three histologic components microscopically (Figures 8.49, 8.50 & 8.51): 1) an epithelial component, characterized by islands of epithelium with of palisading columnar or cuboidal pre-ameloblastic appearing cells that will marginate loosely arranged stellate cells, 2) a cell rich primitive immature collagenous stroma that resembles the developing dental pulp or the dental papilla of the tooth germ and 3) a mineralized component composed of recognizable immature or mature tooth structure that can resemble cementum, enamel or dentin.[111] *Ameloblastic fibrodentinoma* is a rare, poorly understood odontogenic tumor that can resemble ameloblastic fibro-odontoma. Although this tumor is recognized as a distinctive entity by the WHO,[108] it is regarded by the vast majority of practicing surgical pathologists to be simply an ameloblastic fibro-odontoma, in which dentin is the only mineralized product present within the tumor. Such a finding in

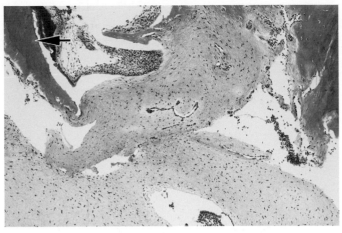

Figure 8.49 Ameloblastic fibro-odontoma. Note a solitary ameloblastic epithelial island abutting osteodentin (arrow) and the associated primitive supporting mesenchymal matrix.

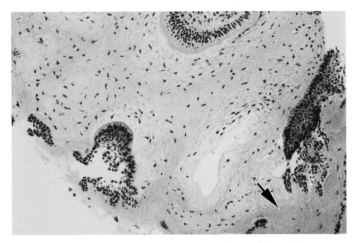

Figure 8.50 Medium power photomicrograph of ameloblastic fibro-odontoma showing ameloblastic islands, immature mineralized eosinophilic matrix (arrow) and myxoid stroma.

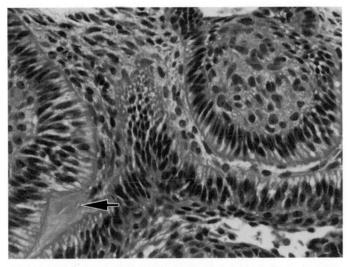

Figure 8.51 High power photomicrograph of ameloblastic-fibro-odontoma demonstrating classic ameloblastic epithelial islands with a focus of an induced (eosinophilic), dentin-like product (arrow).

the judgment of the authors (ROG, RM), although unusual, does not warrant assigning the lesion a separate name, especially since the biologic behavior of the tumor has not been documented to be any different from that of a more histologically typical ameloblastic fibro-odontoma.

Differential Diagnosis

The ameloblastic fibro-odontoma can be clinically difficult to distinguish from an odontoma. The fact that the ameloblastic fibro-odontoma will generally cause expansion of surrounding bone and undergo slow to rapid growth can serve to distinguish it from an odontoma clinically. Growth of a lesion that might be thought to be an odontoma, on the basis of radiographic findings alone, should cause one to consider the possibility that the lesion may in fact actually represent an ameloblastic fibro-odontoma. The presence of ameloblastoma appearing epithelial islands in an ameloblastic fibro-odontoma, can make the separation of that tumor from ameloblastoma and odontoameloblastoma difficult. However, the stromal elements of an ameloblastic fibro-odontoma will always appear mesenchymally primitive histologically, resembling the dental papilla, or the pulpal tissue of a tooth, whereas the stroma of both ameloblastoma and odontoameloblastoma will always consist of mature connective tissue.

Odontoameloblastoma

Odontoameloblastoma is a rare odontogenic tumor in which both epithelial and mesenchymally (ectomesenchymal) derived odontogenic components proliferate. Mosqueda-Taylor et al.[114] reviewed the world's literature related to odontoameloblastoma and found less than 50 cases of odontoameloblastoma documented in the English, speaking dental literature. These authors added 14 cases of their own to that total, but to date fewer than 150 lesions have been appropriately documented in the world literature. The Mosqueda-Taylor et al. study reported that males outnumber females with the tumor and that the average age of their patients was 20.2 years. The sample size of the study does not lend itself, however, to a clear identification of any gender or age predilection, other than to suggest a childhood predilection for the tumor, which is supported by the studies of Thompson et al.[115] who reported an average age of 12 in their studies of odontoameloblastomas. Servato et al.[116] in their study of 431 odontogenic tumors in children and adolescents, recorded no examples of odontoameloblastoma, nor did Guerrisi et al.[117] in a 15-year retrospective study of 153 odontogenic tumors in children and adolescents.

The pathogenesis of the odontoameloblastoma is unknown, although some investigators suggest that the mineralized dental tissues that are seen in the neoplasm histologically form as hamartomatous proliferations in response to inductive stimuli produced by the proliferation of epithelium within mesenchymal tissue.[114] Dive et al.[118] reported a case of odontoameloblastoma and reviewed the literature related to odontoameloblastoma in a 2011 investigation. The Dive study found odontoameloblastomas

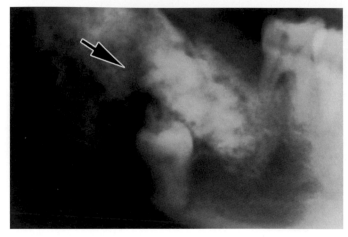

Figure 8.52 Odontoameloblastoma of the mandible. Note the expanding mixed radiopaque and radiolucent lesion (arrow). A large globular zone of calcification can be seen superior to an impacted molar tooth.

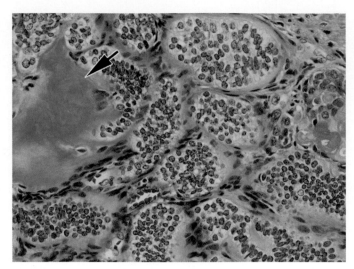

Figure 8.53 Poorly aggregated ameloblastic islands, marginated by columnar cells with clear cytoplasm, can be seen at the periphery of tumor islands in this odontoameloblastoma. Tumor cell nuclei are polarized toward the center of tumor islands. A large eosinophilic zone of osteodentin (arrow) that is surrounded by tumor islands can also be seen.

to be a tumor that is rarely identified in the anterior mandible, and is most often a lesion of the posterior mandible.

Clinical Findings

Radiographically, most odontoameloblastomas have been reported to be either a unilocular or multilocular radiolucency that contains variable amounts of mineralized dental product, causing the lesion to, most often, have a mixed radiolucent/radiopaque radiographic appearance (Figure 8.52). The tumor is typically well margined and the tumor will often cause displacement of surrounding erupted teeth rather than produce root resorption.[115] The odontoameloblastoma is generally a slow growing, painless mass that causes expansion of the alveolus and bony cortex. The tumor may cause permanent teeth not to erupt, but pain has not been documented as a common initial clinical symptom. From a radiographic and clinical differential diagnostic standpoint, the odontoameloblastoma can mimic a developing odontoma, a COC or an ameloblastic fibro-odontoma. A developing odontoma will not result in bony expansion or bone invasion, however, and ameloblastic fibro-odontoma can easily be histologically separated from odontoameloblastoma, on the basis that ameloblastic fibro-odontoma will characteristically demonstrate a primitive pulp-like or dental papilla type of tumor stroma, rather than a stroma made up of mature connective tissue.

Pathologic Features

The odontoameloblastoma will be composed of an admixture of ameloblastoma islands and mesenchymally derived dental tissues that range from primitive odontogenic mesenchyme to hard tissue structures that can include dentin, cementum, a cementum-like product and enamel (Figure 8.53). These calcified structures will demonstrate a variable degree of maturity. On occasion, pigmented, melanin positive cells that are dendritic in appearance can also be seen in the supporting stromal collagen. The ameloblastoma component of the tumor will be made up of ameloblastic islands, sheets, nests and cords of tumor cells that are marginated by pre-ameloblasts. Stellate cells, granular cells or acanthomatous zones will fill the center of tumor islands. The odontoma portion of the neoplasm may be composed of rudimentary tooth-like aggregates, or a minimal amount of osteodentin, or the histologic process may be dominated by classic ameloblastoma and very little calcified product may be evident.

Yamamoto et al.[119] evaluated a series of mixed odontogenic tumors and found that all of the tumors, including odontoameloblastoma, stained positively for cytokeratin as detected by the antibody KL-1. These investigators also found that tenascin stained the cells positively in only the immature dental papilla-like mesenchymal tissue in the tumors studied, including odontoameloblastoma. Vimentin staining in the tumors studied was limited to areas in the immature dental papilla-like areas, and in the basement membrane of the odontogenic epithelial component of the ameloblastomas that were studied. This investigation suggests that the tumor cells in mixed odontogenic tumors, including odontoameloblastoma, may possess certain proteins that are associated with tumor proliferation.

Treatment and Prognosis

Odontoameloblastoma is considered to have a behavior pattern similar to that of ameloblastoma; thus, marginal resection using a 1.0 to 1.5 cm bony excision margin, with one uninvolved anatomic barrier margin is the treatment of choice.[120] Recurrence of this tumor is quite high when curettage or enucleation are employed, but occasionally when pallative therapy is appropriate, enucleation and curettage can be beneficial.

Odontoma

Clinical Findings

Odontoma, recognized as the most common of all odontogenic tumors is, in reality, no more than a hamartomatous growth of odontogenic epithelial and ectomesenchymal elements, interacting in an abortive attempt at tooth formation. Servato et al.[121] found that of a total of 431 odontogenic tumors they studied in children and adolescents, odontomas were divided almost equally between males and females. The ages of subjects in their study ranged from 1 to 18, and most odontomas were identified in the anterior mandible. Guerrisi, et al.[122] in a study of 153 odontogenic tumors in children, found that odontomas represented 50.9 percent of the total number of cases reviewed. The majority of odontomas in the Guerrisi study were identified in the anterior maxilla, and the average age of subjects in the study was 15.

Odontomas have traditionally been classified into two subtypes; 1) *compound* and 2) *complex*. Compound odontomas most often appear radiographically as asymptomatic, tooth-like aggregates (Figure 8.54); whereas complex odontomas tend to present radiographically as sclerotic radiopaque masses that are well demarcated from the surrounding bone (Figure 8.55). Budnick et al.[123] in a review 149 odontomas, found that 76, or 51 percent, of the lesions studied were histologically complex, and were composed of a mass of haphazardly arranged dentin enamel, cementum and connective tissue. The tumors showed little resemblance to normal tooth morphology. The remainder of the cases in the Budnick study were of the compound variety, and were composed of tooth-like or denticle-like structures arranged in a morphologic pattern that resembled a tooth or teeth.

In children, as a rule, complex odontomas tend to be more common in the posterior jaws whereas compound odontomas typically present in the anterior jaws.[124,125] Odontomas are usually asymptomatic but, on occasion, they can cause bony expansion and intraoral swelling. Odontomas can arise over impacted teeth, and cause tooth eruption problems. Tumors in children rarely exceed 2.5 cm in diameter, and they usually do not exceed the size of a normal tooth. The majority of odontomas are asymptomatic, and the tumors rarely cause pain, swelling or bony expansion. Rare extra osseous odontomas have been reported.[126]

Pathologic Features

Grossly, odontomas will be composed of an aggregate of denticle-like structures or an aborted mass of calcified tissue that may resemble a tooth (Figure 8.56). Odontomas will be composed, histologically, of an accumulation of ectomesenchymally derived or epithelially derived dental products including enamel, enamel matrix, dentin, periodontal ligament, cementum and pulpal tissue (Figure 8.57). Tumor components can be arranged in a haphazard pattern, as is the case with most complex odontomas, or in a pattern resembling

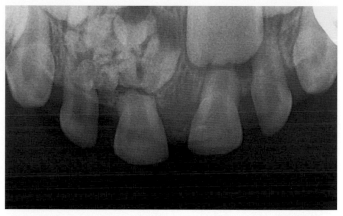

Figure 8.54 Compound odontoma composed of radiopaque denticle-like aggregates. (Courtesy of Dr. Thomas Borris).

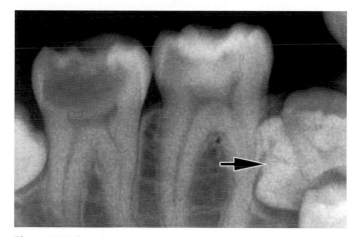

Figure 8.55 Complex odontoma demonstrating characteristic radiodense sclerotic mass.

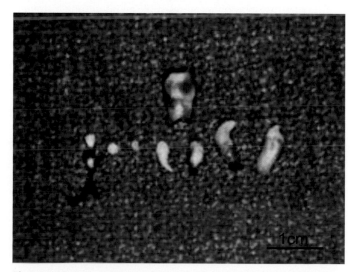

Figure 8.56 Gross inspection of the compound odontoma will be reveal aggregates of small tooth or denticle-like hard tissue structures.

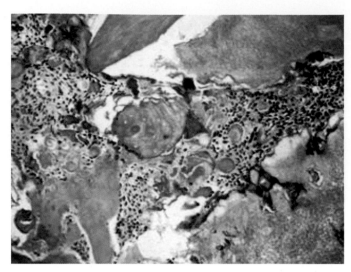

Figure 8.57 Complex odontoma composed of a haphazard accumulation of dentin, poorly decalcified enamel and reduced enamel epithelium.

normal tooth structure, which is most common with compound odontomas. Epithelial "ghost cells" can be identified within the tumor in some instances, similar to cells that can be seen in the COC.[127]

Differential Diagnosis

It may be difficult to distinguish an ameloblastic fibro-odontoma from an early developing complex odontoma, and in fact, the distinction between the two may be of minimal clinical significance. As a rule, ameloblastic fibro-odontomas are neoplasms that cause jaw expansion and growth, a feature that would be quite uncommon for an odontoma. AFs will be histologically composed of ameloblastic islands, nests, and cords that will be set in a primitive mesenchymal matrix. Hard tissue (calcified) odontogenic derivatives such as dentin, enamel and cementum will be absent.

Odontoameloblastoma can resemble an odontoma histologically, but the odontoameloblastoma will contain true ameloblastic islands and the lesion will show destructive growth radiographically. Supernumerary teeth and residual root tips resulting from incomplete tooth extraction can also resemble an odontoma.

Treatment and Prognosis

Odontomas are tumors that have a limited growth potential and rarely do they enlarge. Most odontomas are treated by surgical excision or enucleation and curettage. Since the odontoma can have multiple hard and soft tissue components, it is important that radiographs be taken interoperatively to make certain that the entire neoplastic component has been removed. In most instances the bony defect following surgery will fill in within one year.

Ameloblastic Fibrosarcoma

Ameloblastic fibrosarcoma represents the only malignant tumor of mesenchymal origin that has been reported with any

frequency in childhood or adolescence.[128,129,130] Chen et al.[130] report a 11.4 percent transduction rate of AF to ameloblastic fibrosarcoma, with five and ten year transition rates of 10.2 percent and 22.2 percent respectively in patients under the age of 22. See AF for a more complete discussion of this tumor.

Pediatric Benign Odontogenic Tumors and Reconstructive Surgery

In the subset of benign odontogenic tumors, most actually represent disturbed attempts at tooth formation and represent hamartomas instead of neoplasia e.g. odontomas, ameloblastic fibro-odontomas, AFs etc. These are treated for cure with an enucleation procedure. Those benign odontogenic tumors that possess a true neoplastic biology are treated with resection. These include the ameloblastoma, odontogenic, myxoma, odontogenic fibroma, the calcified epithelial odontogenic tumor, which occurs only very rarely in children and the odontoameloblastoma, which occurs only very rarely in anyone. In younger children (12 and under) who have not received either previous surgery or radiation, spontaneous bone regeneration often occurs, making bone grafting of the surgical defect unnecessary (Figures 8.58 & 8.59). In children who have had previous surgery or radiation – which reduces the ability of resident osteoprogenitor cells and stem cells to independently regenerate bone in the defect – and in late teenagers, some bone grafting is usually necessary.

The Enucleation Procedure: Enucleation is defined as removing a lesion from bone and separating it from the native bone via a capsule or a natural cleavage plane. If curettage is added to the procedure, adopting the often used term "enucleation and curettage," this adds to definition, the removal of 1 to 2 mm of the bony wall.

For these non-neoplastic odontogenic hamartomas a mid-crestal or neck of tooth incision is best (Figure 8.60). A broad based full thickness mucoperiosteal flap will provide the best access to the lesion. The buccal cortex may be expanded and thinned allowing the surgeon to remove it by flicking off the thinned cortex with a periosteal elevator. Otherwise the author uses an acrylic burr to thin down and remove the cortex. This can be facilitated by inserting a periosteal elevator under the cortex in the initial area where the cortex has been completely removed and safely removing bone over the instrument protecting the lesion. When a sufficient uncovering of the lesion is gained, it is separated from its bony crypt using the back end of a #4 molt curette or similar instrument to deliver the specimen (Figure 8.61). Once the lesion is removed, it is advised to inspect the bony crypt to confirm that the entire lesion was removed.

In most cases in children, bone regeneration can be anticipated obviating the need for grafting. In the unusual case where a graft is required, the author (REM) prefers a composite graft of crushed cancellous allogeneic bone, platelet rich plasma and recombinant human bone morphogenetic protein, which avoids

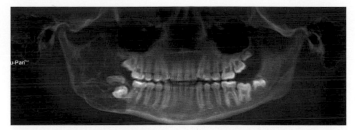

Figure 8.58 Benign tumor of the mandible in a 12-year-old. (Reprinted from Marx R, Stern D. *Oral and Maxillofacial Pathology: A Rationale for Diagnosis and Treatment* with permission from Quintessence Publishing Company).

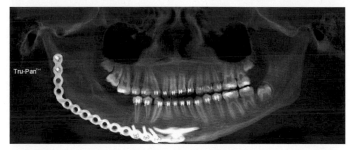

Figure 8.59 Complete native bone regeneration seen at six months after resection. (Reprinted from Marx R, Stern D. *Oral and Maxillofacial Pathology: A Rationale for Diagnosis and Treatment* with permission from Quintessence Publishing Company).

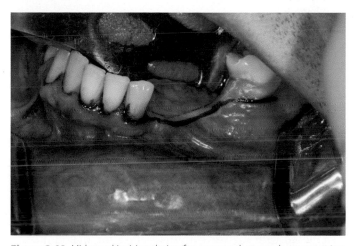

Figure 8.60 Midcrestal incision design for a transoral approach. (Reprinted from Marx R, Stern D. *Oral and Maxillofacial Pathology: A Rationale for Diagnosis and Treatment* with permission from Quintessence Publishing Company).

the donor site morbidity inherent in harvesting autogenous bone, while predictably regenerating bone throughout the defect. However, autogenous bone may also be used if it is preferred by the patient, the patient's parents or the surgeon with the acceptance of a donor site. If a dental implant is planned to be placed into the area of the defect, a six-month bone maturation time should be anticipated with all bone regeneration schemes. It should also be noted that regenerated bone, whether by native bone regeneration or grafted bone regeneration, will grow normally along with the native mandible. Therefore, placing dental implants into the regenerate bone in patients aged 16 years or under should be done with caution due to the potential for the implants to become submerged.

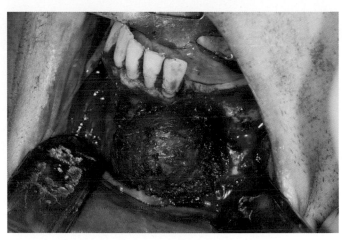

Figure 8.61 Odontogenic hamartoma exposed for enucleation. (Reprinted from Marx R, Stern D. *Oral and Maxillofacial Pathology: A Rationale for Diagnosis and Treatment* with permission from Quintessence Publishing Company).

Resection of Odontogenic Tumors: Resections for cure of true odontogenic neoplasms in the mandible require 1.0 to 1.5 cm bony margins and one tumor-free anatomic barrier. Therefore, most will require an extraoral approach. To minimize and conceal the resultant scar, it is advised to place it within a natural skin fold in the neck. (Figure 8.62) Since many children have not as yet developed such skin folds, the incision is best concealed by making it curvilinear, following the contours of the mandible about 2 cm to 3 cm inferior to it. It is also advised to avoid lip split techniques, which are unnecessary, and vertical trajectories of the incision that are sometimes used near the midline. Each of these goes against resting skin tension lines and will result in an unnecessarily wide scar.

The inferior border of the mandible is approached in a plane deep to the facial vein so as to avoid injury to the marginal mandibular branch of the facial nerve. If the CT scan has shown an intact cortex, a subperiosteal dissection is pursued as the cortex itself will serve as the anatomic barrier for the en-bloc resection (Figure 8.63). If the CT scan has shown a perforation of the cortex or one is observed during the dissection, the periosteum becomes the intact anatomic barrier and a supraperiosteal dissection pursued. Figure 8.64 In the rare event that the tumor has breached the periosteum in a local area, a supraperiosteal dissection is pursued up to that area, and a cuff of adjacent tissue excised and examined with a frozen section to confirm a clear margin.

Based upon radiographs and scans, the appropriate tumor resection margins are outlined in the cortex and any tooth in the line of the planned resection cut is removed (Figure 8.65). If the lateral expansion of the tumor is negligible, it is ideal to adapt a rigid 2.4 mm or 2.9mm titanium reconstruction plate to the intact mandible and fixate it with four tapped and measured bicortical locking screws (Figure 8.66). This will index the correct occlusion and maintain the condyle in its proper position in the temporal fossa once the resection is completed. The titanium plate is then removed and each screw is dedicated so as to be replaced in the same position after the

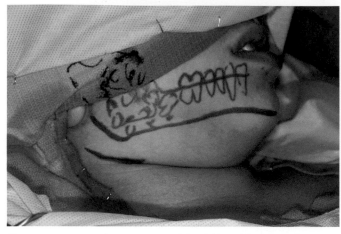

Figure 8.62 Incision design in a natural skin fold used for extraoral approaches. (Reprinted from Marx R, Stern D. *Oral and Maxillofacial Pathology: A Rationale for Diagnosis and Treatment* with permission from Quintessence Publishing Company).

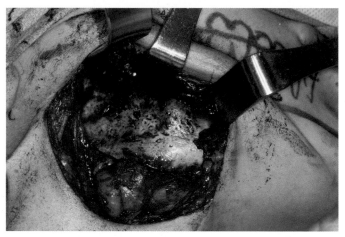

Figure 8.63 Subperiosteal reflection is used to access the mandible in cases where the cortex is intact. (Reprinted from Marx R, Stern D. *Oral and Maxillofacial Pathology: A Rationale for Diagnosis and Treatment* with permission from Quintessence Publishing Company).

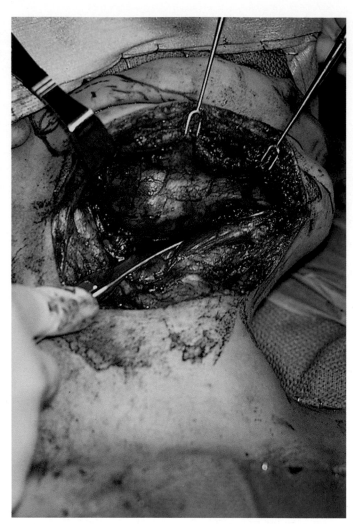

Figure 8.64 Supraperiosteal reflection is used for tumors that have broken through the cortex. (Reprinted from Marx R, Stern D. *Oral and Maxillofacial Pathology: A Rationale for Diagnosis and Treatment* with permission from Quintessence Publishing Company).

resection. (Figure 8.67) Tapping each screw hole is highly recommended as compared to self-tapping screws. This will ensure retaining full axial compression strength when the screw is fixated to the plate after the resection.

It is best to accomplish the anterior resection margin first. This is associated with less bleeding during the resection, and will allow the surgeon to lateralize the mandible so as to gain direct visual access to the lingual area. The posterior or proximal resection cut is accomplished next. Since it is often through the inferior alveolar neurovascular bundle, more bleeding is encountered during this resection. Therefore, separating the stable proximal segment and the resection specimen quickly will allow clamping or cautery of the bleeding point, and reduce the overall blood loss.

Once the specimen has been freed of all its soft tissue attachments, the author (REM) recommends that a specimen radiograph be taken so as to check the adequacy of the bony margins. (Figure 8.68) Any soft tissue oral opening is then closed with mattress sutures before the titanium plate is re-fixated to the mandible. At this juncture, the neck incision may be closed and the bony reconstruction deferred for a later time or an immediate bony reconstruction performed.

Alternative Resection Techniques to Preserve the Inferior Alveolar Nerve

Transecting and removing a section of the inferior alveolar nerve along with the odontogenic tumor represents a time honored and accepted outcome. However, the following are two surgical methods which can preserve part or all of the nerve sensation to the ipsilateral lip and chin without reducing the curative ability of the resection:

The Nerve Pull Out Technique: This surgery transects the inferior alveolar neurovascular bundle at the anterior resection

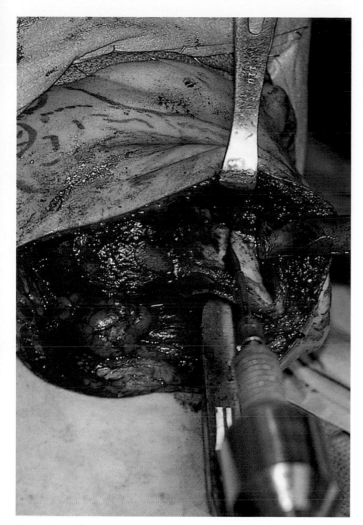

Figure 8.65 The anterior resection for a continuity resection is accomplished first. (Reprinted from Marx R, Stern D. *Oral and Maxillofacial Pathology. A Rationale for Diagnosis and Treatment* with permission from Quintessence Publishing Company).

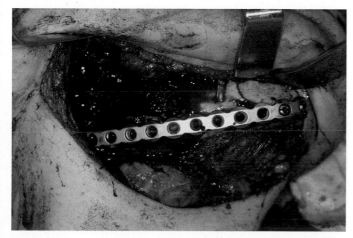

Figure 8.66 Titanium reconstruction plate fixated to the intact mandible. (Reprinted from Marx R, Stern D. *Oral and Maxillofacial Pathology: A Rationale for Diagnosis and Treatment* with permission from Quintessence Publishing Company).

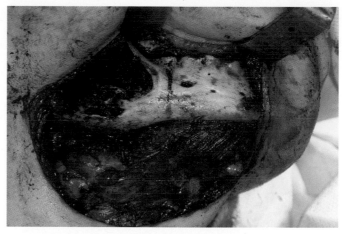

Figure 8.67 Removed titanium plate with resection margin outlined. (Reprinted from Marx R, Stern D. *Oral and Maxillofacial Pathology: A Rationale for Diagnosis and Treatment* with permission from Quintessence Publishing Company).

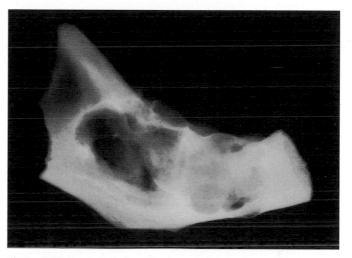

Figure 8.68 Specimen radiograph of resected tumor. (Reprinted from Marx R, Stern D. *Oral and Maxillofacial Pathology: A Rationale for Diagnosis and Treatment* with permission from Quintessence Publishing Company).

margin or just after emerging from the mental foramen before it branches. If the posterior resection margin is anterior to the lingula of the ramus, the immediate area is decorticated laterally. The neurovascular bundle is then pulled back to this area from the anterior resection margin so that the bony resection can be accomplished (Figure 8.69). If the resection is in the mid area of the ramus just posterior to the lingula, this resection is accomplished and the specimen turned laterally to expose the neurovascular bundle entering the lingual foramen (Figure 8.70). In either situation, the neurovascular bundle is gently tractioned to break the fibers entering the teeth apices and pulled back through the bony mandibular canal as the specimen is delivered. The nerve strand is separate from the artery and the vein at the anterior resection edge. Each blood vessel is either clipped with a small vascular metal clip or coagulated with bipolar cautery. The nerve is then immediately re-anastamosed with 7-0 or 8-0 nylon sutures at the epineurial level using either 3.5 x or greater loops or the operating

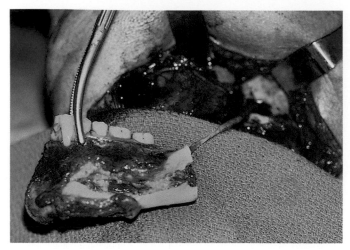

Figure 8.69 Neurovascular bundle pulled back out of the mandibular canal. (Reprinted from Marx R, Stern D. *Oral and Maxillofacial Pathology: A Rationale for Diagnosis and Treatment* with permission from Quintessence Publishing Company).

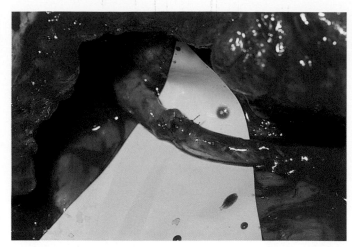

Figure 8.71 Microanastamosis of the entire neurovascular bundle. (Reprinted from Marx R, Stern D. *Oral and Maxillofacial Pathology: A Rationale for Diagnosis and Treatment* with permission from Quintessence Publishing Company).

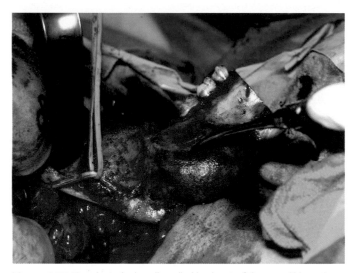

Figure 8.70 Neurovascular bundle pulled back out of the mandible at the lingual foramen.

microscope (Figure 8.71). After the nerve is re-anastamosed, the titanium reconstruction plate can be placed and either an immediate bone graft is accomplished or a closure of the wound for a staged bone graft later. Return of sensation, in the author's (REM) experience, with this technique in patients of all ages as compared to a sural nerve graft is excellent. In children and teenagers, the return of sensation is over 90 percent between six and nine months, due to their youth supporting a greater nerve regeneration through the epineurial sheath following Wallerian degeneration of the distal nerve segment. It should be noted that this technique is only indicated for surgeries removing benign tumors which displace but do not invade the neurovascular sheath.

The Double En-Bloc Resection Technique

Based on the same fact that benign tumors do not invade the neurovascular sheath, this approach first accomplishes a wide

decortication of the lateral cortex over the tumor as well as anterior and posterior to the tumor. This is usually accomplished by placing bur holes through the lateral cortex in a wide rectangular design using a 702 burr and then connecting the bur holes. In this manner the lateral decortication can be accomplished in a single en-bloc segment in this double en-bloc technique (Figure 8.72). The neurovascular bundle is then identified and separated from any cancellous bone or tumor adjacent to it (Figure 8.73). Both the anterior and posterior resections can then be made while protecting the neurovascular bundle. At this time, the surgeon will find the cable of the intact neurovascular bundle to lay lateral to the resected specimen. The adherent soft tissue on the lingual side is then separated from the specimen. The specimen can then be delivered by pushing the specimen lingually and rotating it underneath the cable of the neurovascular bundle as it is lifted superiorly with nerve hooks (Figure 8.74).

In this technique, the neurovascular bundle is never violated and the nerve is never transected. The nerve remains 100 percent intact as does the sensation to the ipsilateral lip and chin.

It should be noted that neither of these two techniques applies to resections of benign tumors in the maxilla. All such resections are inferior to the infraorbital nerve and its course through the orbital floor. It should also be noted that neither of these two techniques apply to resections for malignant tumors as they often invade the neurovascular sheath.

Bony Reconstruction of Mandibular Continuity Defects in Children

Immediate Versus Staged Grafting

Due to an uncompromised and usually non-radiated tissue bed, benign tumor related defects lend themselves to immediate reconstruction. However, it remains the surgeon's decision. If the opening in the oral mucosa is large or cannot be closed

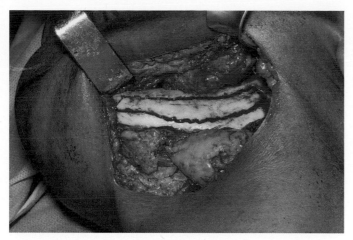

Figure 8.72 Lateral decortication outline of the double en-bloc technique. (Reprinted from Marx R, Stern D. *Oral and Maxillofacial Pathology: A Rationale for Diagnosis and Treatment* with permission from Quintessence Publishing Company).

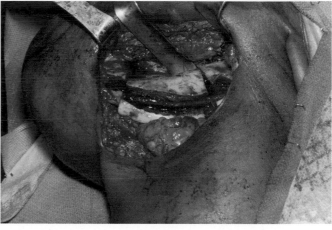

Figure 8.74 Tumor resection specimen delivered showing empty mandibular canal. (Reprinted from Marx R, Stern D. *Oral and Maxillofacial Pathology: A Rationale for Diagnosis and Treatment* with permission from Quintessence Publishing Company).

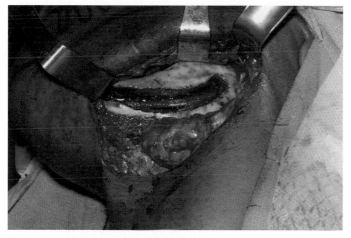

Figure 8.73 Exposed neurovascular bundle that will be transposed to avoid its unnecessary removal during tumor extirpation. (Reprinted from Marx R, Stern D. *Oral and Maxillofacial Pathology: A Rationale for Diagnosis and Treatment* with permission from Quintessence Publishing Company).

completely, then a staged reconstruction is preferred. Similarly, if the tumor expansion orally has resulted in biting trauma to the mucosa, or the teeth within or adjacent to the tumor have accumulated significant plaque or calculus, or have chronic abscesses, the risk of a graft infection increases and may prompt a decision to stage the bone graft.

Bony Reconstruction with Autogenous Cancellous Bone and Cellular Marrow (ACBCM)

ACBCM grafts are a time honored standard and may be used for immediate or staged reconstructions. To limit the time between bone harvest and placement, the donor site is most often harvested simultaneously by a second surgical team or after the recipient bed has been prepared. Due to the presence of the tibial epiphysical growth plate in children, harvesting bone in this area, as is often accomplished in adults, is

discouraged. Therefore, the anterior or posterior ilium is the preferred donor sites in children. In both adults and children, the available bone that can be harvested from the anterior ilium will be that amount limited to a four centimeter mandibular defect. In larger defects, the posterior ilium is preferred due to its 2.0 to 2.5 times greater bone availability. If the anterior ilium is used, the medial approach is preferred. This is due to the fact that the reflection of the iliacus muscle that is attached to the medial aspect of the ilium is not active during normal walking motions and therefore has less pain. The lateral anterior ilium approach reflects the tensor fascia latta muscle which traverses the hip joint and the knee joint. Therefore it is active in every bend of either the knee or hip producing postoperative pain. While the downsides of the anterior ilium is greater postoperative discomfort with either the medial or lateral approach and the limited bone availability, its advantage is that the patient does not need to be moved on the operating room table. In this manner, one team of surgeons can be harvesting the graft while another team is resecting the tumor or preparing the recipient site. This of course saves operating room time and resources.

If the posterior ilium is the surgeon's choice, the patient will be required to be turned onto a prone position after the tumor resection or the recipient site preparation, and turned back to the supine position once the donor site is closed. This also requires a temporary closure of the recipient site before the initial turn to the prone position. In the posterior ilium harvest, the best site of entry and harvest is the area of the attachment of the gluteus maximus muscle. This area contains the greatest reservoir of cancellous marrow, and the gluteus maximum is not inherently activated in normal walking or bending of the hip joint. The advantages of the posterior ilium harvest are the greater amount of graftable bone available and a reduced blood loss of harvesting. This latter advantage is gained by placing a support roll under the anterior thighs, a

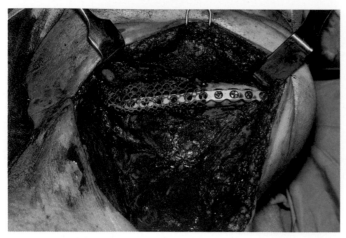

Figure 8.75 Titanium plate and mesh positioned to contain the bone graft. (Reprinted from Marx R, Stern D. *Oral and Maxillofacial Pathology: A Rationale for Diagnosis and Treatment* with permission from Quintessence Publishing Company).

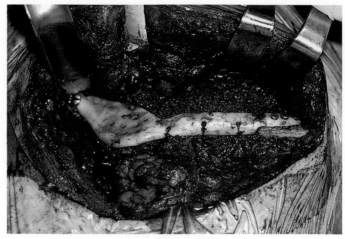

Figure 8.77 Allogeneic mandible crib containing the bone graft. (Reprinted from Marx R, Stern D. *Oral and Maxillofacial Pathology: A Rationale for Diagnosis and Treatment* with permission from Quintessence Publishing Company).

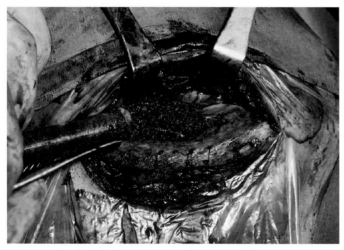

Figure 8.76 Allogeneic iliac crest is used here to contain the bone graft. (Reprinted from Marx R, Stern D. *Oral and Maxillofacial Pathology: A Rationale for Diagnosis and Treatment* with permission from Quintessence Publishing Company).

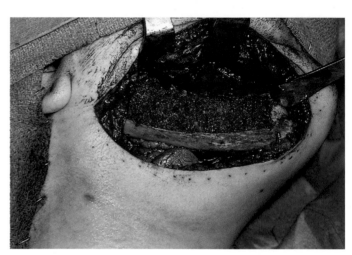

Figure 8.78 Allogeneic split rib segment replaces the inferior border and allows the graft to be compacted on top of it. (Reprinted from Marx R, Stern D. *Oral and Maxillofacial Pathology: A Rationale for Diagnosis and Treatment* with permission from Quintessence Publishing Company).

roll in each axilla and positioning the operating table in a reverse flex position of about 210 degrees.

It should be noted that a cartilage cap is usually present over both the anterior and posterior iliac crests in children 13 years and under. This cartilage represents an ossification area, not a growth plate. Therefore, growth disturbances are not seen when a graft is harvested from the ilium. However, to avoid a contour irregularity of the iliac crest, the entry point of the harvest should ideally be placed below this cartilage cap. Marx and Stevens have described in detail the techniques used to harvest bone from all sites for jaw reconstruction, including the anterior and posterior ilium.[128]

Once the ACBCM has been harvested, it is best to temporarily store it in a small amount of saline, platelet rich plasma, bone marrow aspirate or bone marrow aspirate concentrate. Hypotonic solutions, particularly distilled water or D5W and warmed solution are to be avoided. Hypotonic solutions will burst the osteoprogenitor and stem cells in the graft and solutions above body temperature will coagulate the membranes of these cells. Once harvested the graft material is placed within the recipient bed and contained using either a titanium reconstruction plate with a "U" shaped configuration for the inferior border (Figure 8.75) as can be obtained from an allogeneic ilium specimen, Figure 8.76 or an allogeneic mandible hollowed out to receive the graft (Figure 8.77). Additionally, allogeneic split ribs used at the inferior border or as a buccal-lingual containment also contain the graft well (Figure 8.78). For the best outcome it is best to compress the graft material into the containment crib so as to gain the maximum cellular density.

Bony Reconstruction Using In situ Tissue Engineering

Due to a greater number of resident osteoprogenitor and stem cells at the resection edges as well as those circulating from the bone marrow, children and teenagers have an excellent track record of regenerating large segments of resected bone by using in situ tissue engineering. This requires completing the classic tissue engineering triangle of cells, signal and matrix in constructing a composite graft. This is done by relying on the native resident stem cells and by using platelet rich plasma (PRP) along with its natural and circulating host stem cells (the cells) together with recombinant human bone morphogenetic protein/acellular collagen sponge (rhBMP-2/ACS) (the signal), and cancellous allogeneic bone (the matrix) (Figure 8.79). It should also be realized that the cell adhesion molecules in PRP (fibrin, fibronectin and vitronectin) are also part of the matrix, which together with the cancellous allogeneic bone forms an ideal scaffold for bone formation.

The author (REM) uses sufficient cancellous allogeneic bone to fill the defect, 10 ml of PRP derived from 60 ml of autologous whole blood validated to contain at least 1 million platelets per ml and 1 mg of rhBMP-2/ACS per 1 cm of continuity defect in either jaw.

This in situ tissue engineering graft will regenerate viable functional bone equal to a 100 percent autogenous graft in six months. The graft will grow along with the native mandible as does a 100 percent autogenous graft. By six months, type II or III bone is seen capable of gaining primary stability if dental implants are placed. By six months all of the cancellous allogeneic bone will be resorbed and replaced by viable native bone (Figures 8.80 & 8.81).

The obvious advantages to in situ tissue engineering is the avoidance of donor site morbidity, a reduced blood loss, a shorter operative time, a shorter hospital stay and a faster return to family and school activities. The main disadvantage of this approach is the postoperative edema, which will be twice that of an autogenous graft and last somewhat longer. This is apparently due to the very nature of the rhBMP-2/ACS, i.e., it is chemoattractive to circulating stem cells, and proliferates resident stem cells that increase the cellular mass of the graft. The rhBMP-2/ACS is also a hypertonic solution which draws water into the area thereby increasing the clinical edema. Because of this mechanism, preoperative or intraoperative steroids do not significantly prevent this edema. Nevertheless this increased edema has not resulted in an airway compromise when used in jaw reconstruction and does subside completely.

Fixation for All Types of Grafts Used to Reconstruct Mandibular Continuity Defects

Whether an autogenous graft or an in situ tissue engineered graft is used to provide stability to support vascular in-growth, cellular proliferation and cellular differentiation is crucial. If a rigid titanium plate is used, maxillomandibular fixation need only be there so as to stabilize the graft during this period of revascularization and cellular activity. Beyond three weeks, the rigid titanium plate will support the strength characteristics required as the graft matures. However, if an allogeneic crib or a titanium mesh is used without the internal stability offered by a rigid titanium plate, the maxillomandibular fixation time needs to be extended to six weeks.

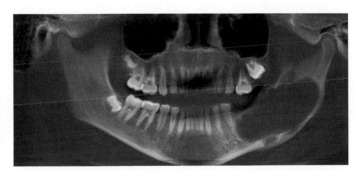

Figure 8.79 In situ tissue engineered graft consisting of Platelet Rich Plasma, recombinant human bone morphogenetic protein and freeze dried allogeneic bone. (Reprinted from Marx R, Stern D. *Oral and Maxillofacial Pathology: A Rationale for Diagnosis and Treatment* with permission from Quintessence Publishing Company).

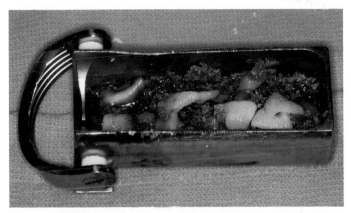

Figure 8.80 Ameloblastoma of mandible. (Reprinted from Marx R, Stern D. *Oral and Maxillofacial Pathology: A Rationale for Diagnosis and Treatment* with permission from Quintessence Publishing Company).

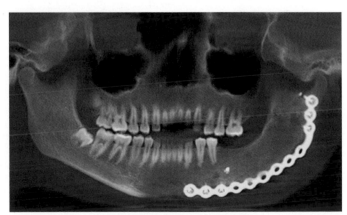

Figure 8.81 Defect in Figure 8.80 with complete bone regeneration from in situ tissue engineering. (Reprinted from Marx R, Stern D. *Oral and Maxillofacial Pathology: A Rationale for Diagnosis and Treatment* with permission from Quintessence Publishing Company).

Special Considerations in Reconstructing Maxillary Defects

Reconstructing maxillary defects in children and teenagers may be accomplished using the same principles as those discussed for mandibular reconstruction with some notable differences. Due to the fact that the maxilla is a stable non-moving bone, the placement of a titanium plate at the time of resection or reconstruction, or the use of maxillomandibular fixation for the reconstruction is unnecessary. If the tumor removal is limited to the alveolar bone and does not communicate with a maxillary sinus or the nasal cavity, an immediate reconstruction using either of the graft concepts already discussed will be predictable (Figure 8.82). However, if the resection creates an opening into the maxillary sinus or the oral cavity, the author (REM) recommends a closure and plans for a staged reconstruction four to six months later. It is also advised to avoid placing a spacer in such defects as the rate of infection about a foreign body in this situation is very high.

By four to six months, sufficient soft tissue has formed in the resected area as to allow the surgeon to develop a recipient bed than spans the bony resection edges without entering the nasal or sinus cavities. A tissue pocket is formed between the anterior resection margin and the zygomatic maxillary buttress (Figure 8.83). The graft of either autogenous bone or the in situ tissue engineered graft is placed into this pocket which is contained within a titanium mesh crib or allogeneic bone crib (Figure 8.84). The crib is firmly fixated with monocortical screws, and the lateral soft tissue thoroughly undermined to achieve a tension free primary closure. It is advised to avoid temporary appliances that might compress the graft during the entire healing period. This can be accomplished by avoiding such appliances for the entire six-month maturation period, or by using a tooth supported appliance that does not contact the

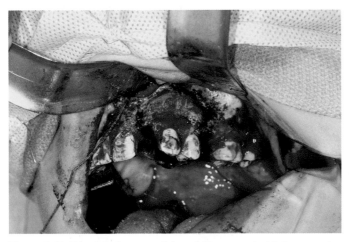

Figure 8.82 Odontogenic tumor of the maxilla removed with 1 cm margins. (Reprinted from Marx R, Stern D. *Oral and Maxillofacial Pathology: A Rationale for Diagnosis and Treatment* with permission from Quintessence Publishing Company).

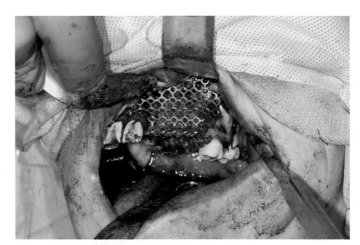

Figure 8.84 Titanium mesh used to contain in situ tissue engineered graft. (Reprinted from Marx R, Stern D. *Oral and Maxillofacial Pathology: A Rationale for Diagnosis and Treatment* with permission from Quintessence Publishing Company).

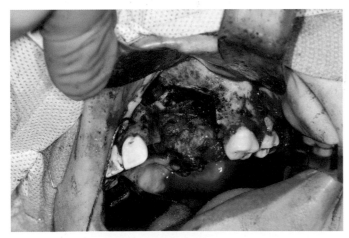

Figure 8.83 Maxillary defect after tumor removal. (Reprinted from Marx R, Stern D. *Oral and Maxillofacial Pathology: A Rationale for Diagnosis and Treatment* with permission from Quintessence Publishing Company).

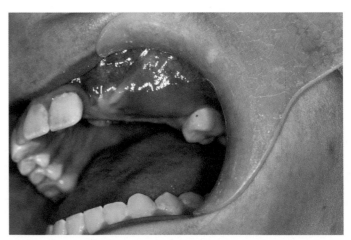

Figure 8.85 Final bony ridge after tumor removal and graft placement. (Reprinted from Marx R, Stern D. *Oral and Maxillofacial Pathology: A Rationale for Diagnosis and Treatment* with permission from Quintessence Publishing Company).

graft such as an Essex appliance. This is especially important during the first three weeks after graft placement because this is the time of vascular ingrowth and cellular migration to and within the graft. The graft will mature over six months and allow for the placement of dental implants that can replace any lost teeth (Figure 8.85).

References

Odontogenic Tumors, Introduction

1. Barnes L, Everson JW, Richart P, Sidransky D. (eds) *World Health Organization Classification of Tumors Pathology and Genetics of Head and Neck Tumors*. IARC Press, Lyon, 2005.

2. Kumamoto H. Molecular pathology of odontogenic tumors. *J Oral Pathol Med*, 2006, 35: 65–74.

3. Guerrisi M, Piloni MJ, Keszler A. Odontogenic tumors in children and adolescents. A 15-year retrospective study in Argentina. *Med Oral Pathol Cir Buccal*, 2007, 12: 180–185.

4. Ulmansky M, Lustmann J, Balkin N. Tumors and tumor-like lesions of the oral cavity and related structures in Israeli children. *Int J Oral Maxillofac Surg*, 1999, 28: 291–294.

5. Tanrikulu R, Erol B, Haspolat K. Tumors of the maxillofacial region in children: retrospective analysis and long-term follow-up outcomes of 90 patients. *Turk J Pediatr*, 2004, 46: 60–66.

6. Ajayi OF, Ladeinde AL, Adeyemo WL, Ogunlewe MO. Odontogenic tumors in Nigerian children and adolescents – a retrospective study of 92 cases. *World J Surg Oncol*, 2004, 2: 39.

7. Al-Khateeb T, Al-Hadi Hamasha A, Almasri NM. Oral and maxillofacial tumours in North Jordanian children and adolescents: a retrospective analysis over 10 years. *Int J Oral Maxillofac Surg*, 2003, 32: 78–83.

8. Adebayo ET, Ajike SO, Adeyeke EO. Odontogenic tumors in children and adolescents: a study of 78 Nigerian cases. *J Cranio Maxillofac Surg*, 2002, 30: 267–272.

9. Tanaka N, Murata A, Yamaguchi A, Kohama G. Clinical features and management of oral maxillofacial tumors in children. *Oral Surg Oral Med Oral Pathol Oral Radiol Endod*, 1999, 88: 11–15.

10. Ulmansky M, Lustmann J, Balkin N. Tumors and tumor like lesions of the oral cavity and related structures in Israeli children. *Int J Oral Maxillofac Surg*, 1999, 28: 291–294.

11. Chen YK, Lin LM, Huang HC, et al. A retrospective study of oral and maxillofacial biopsy lesions in a pediatric population from southern Taiwan. *Pediatr Dent*, 1998, 20: 404–410.

12. Sato M, Tanaka N, Sato T, et al. Oral and maxillofacial tumours in children: a review. *Br J Oral Maxillofac Surg*, 1997, 35: 92–95.

13. Jones AV, Franklin CD. An analysis of oral and maxillofacial pathology found in children over a 30-year period. *Int J Paediatr Dent*, 2006, 16: 19–30.

Ameloblastoma and its Variants

14. Zhang J, Zexu G, Jiang L, et al. Ameloblastoma in children and adolescents. *Br J Oral Maxillofac Surg*, 2010, 48: 549–554.

15. Marx RE, Stern D. *Oral and Maxillofacial Pathology: A Rationale for Diagnosis and Treatment*. Ed2, Quintessence Publishing Company, Chicago, 2012, 674–680.

16. Eversole RE, Leider A. Radiographic characteristics of cystogenic ameloblastoma. *Oral Surg Oral Med Oral Pathol*, 1984, 57: 572–577

17. Ponti G, Pollio A, Mignogna MD. Unicystic ameloblastoma associated with novel K729M PTCH1 mutation in a patient with nevoid basal cell carcinoma (Gorlin) syndrome. *Cancer Genet*, 2012, 205: 177–181.

18. Hye-Jung Y, Byoung-Chan J, Wui-Jung S, et al. Comparative immune-histochemical study of ameloblastoma and ameloblastic carcinoma. *Oral Surg Oral Med Oral Pathol Oral Radiol Endod*, 2011, 112: 767–771.

19. Yamamoto H, Inui M, Mori A, et al. Clear cell odontogenic carcinoma. A case report and literature review of odontogenic tumors with clear cells. *Oral Surg Oral Med Oral Pathol Oral Radiol Endod*, 1998, 86: 86–89.

20. Oliaitan AA, Adekeye E. Clinical features and management of ameloblastoma of the mandible in children and adolescents. *B J Oral Maxillofac Surg*, 1996, 34: 248–251.

Craniopharyngioma

21. Bunin GR, Surawicz TS, Witman PAZX, et al. The descriptive epidemiology of craniopharyngioma. *J Neuro Surg*, 1998, 90: 547–551.

22. Muller HL. Consequences of craniopharyngioma in children. *J Clin Endocrine and Metabolism*, 2011, 96: 1981–1991.

23. Hoisken A, Buchfielder M, Fahlbusch R, et al. Tumor cell migration in adamantinomatous craniopharyngioma is promoted by inactivated Wnt-signaling ACTA. *Neuropathol*, 2010, 119: 631–639.

24. Byrne MN, Sessions DG. Nasopharyngeal craniopharyngioma: case report and literature review. *Ann Otol Rhinol Laryngol*, 1999, 99: 633–639.

25. Ahsan F, Rashid H, Chapman A, et al. Infrasellar craniopharyngioma presenting as epistaxis, excised via Denker's medial maxillectomy approach. *J Laryngol Otol*, 2004, 110: 895–898.

26. Muller HL, Kaatsch P, Warmuth-Metz M, et al. Childhood craniopharyngioma – current concepts on diagnosis and therapy. *Monatsschr Kinderheilkd*, 2003, 151: 1056–1063.

27. Puget S, Garnet M, Wray A, et al. Pediatric craniopharyngiomas: classification and treatment according to the degree of hypothalamic involvement. *J Neuropath*, 2007, 106: 3–12.

28. Poretti A, Grotzer MA, Ribi K, et al. Outcome of craniopharyngioma in children: long-term complications and quality of life. *Der Med Child Neurol*, 2004, 46: 220–229.

Malignant Ameloblastoma, Ameloblastic Carcinoma, and Clear Cell Odontogenic Carcinoma

29. Horvath A, Horvath E, Popsor S. Mandibular ameloblastic carcinomas in a young child. *Romanian J Morph and Embryology*, 2011, 53: 179–183.

30. Ramesh M, Sekar B, Murali S, et al. Ameloblastic carcinoma – review and histopathology of five cases. *Oral Maxillofac Pathol*, 2011, 2: 154–160.

31. Slootweg PJ, Muller H. Malignant ameloblastoma or ameloblastic carcinoma. *Oral Surg, Oral Med, Oral Pathol*, 1984, 57: 168–176.

32. Laughlin EH. Metastasizing ameloblastoma. *Cancer*, 1989, 64: 776–780.

33. Dhin K, Sciubba J, Tufano RP. Ameloblastic carcinoma of the maxilla. *Oral Oncol*, 2003, 39: 736–741.

34. Yazici N, Karagoz B, Varan A, et al. Maxillary ameloblastic carcinoma in a child. *Pediat Blood Cancer*, 2008, 50: 175–176.

35. Swain N, Dhariwal R, Gopal Ray J. Clear cell odontogenic carcinoma of the maxilla: a case report and mini review. *J Oral Maxillofac Pathol*, 2013, 17: 89–94.

Calcifying Epithelial Odontogenic Tumor

36. Pindborg JJ. A calcifying epithelial odontogenic tumor. *Cancer*, 1958, 98: 206–211.

37. Franklin CD, Pindborg JJ. The calcifying epithelial odontogenic tumor. A review and analysis of 113 cases. *Oral Pathology*, 1976 42: 753–762.

38. Ungari C, Poladas G, Giovannetti F, et al. Pindborg tumors in children. *J Craniofacial Surg*, 2006, 17: 365–369.

39. Guerrisi M, Piloni MJ, Kesler A. Odontogenic tumors in children and adolescents. A 15-year retrospective study in Argentina. *Med Oral Path Oral Cir Bucal*, 2007, 12: 180–185.

40. Anderson HC, Kim B, Minkowitz S. Calcifying epithelial odontogenic tumor of Pindborg: an electron microscopic study. *Cancer*, 1969, 24: 585–596.

41. Kestler DP, Foster JS, Macy SD. Expression of odontogenic ameloblast-associated protein (ODAM) in dental and other epithelial neoplasms. *Mol Med*, 2008, 14: 318–326.

42. Liu AR, Liu Z, Shao J. Calcifying epithelial odontogenic tumors: a clinico-pathologic study of nine cases. *J Oral Pathol*, 1982, 11: 399–406.

43. Abrams AM, Howell FV. Calcifying epithelial odontogenic tumor: report of four cases. *J Am Dent Assoc*, 1967, 74: 1231–1240.

44. Zachary S, Peacock DC, Schmidt BL. Involvement of PTCH1 mutations in the calcifying epithelial odontogenic tumor. *Oral Oncology*, 2010, 46: 387–392.

45. Kumamoto H. Molecular pathology of odontogenic tumors. *J Oral Pathol Med*, 2006, 35: 65–74.

46. Krolls JO, Pindborg JJ. Calcifying epithelial odontogenic tumor. A survey of 23 cases and discussions of histomorphologic variations. *Arch Pathol*, 1974, 98: 206–211.

47. Greer RO, Richardson JF. Clear-cell calcifying odontogenic tumor viewed relative to the Pindborg tumor. *Oral Surg Oral Med Oral Pathol*, 1976, 42: 775–779.

48. Marx RE, Stern D. *Oral and Maxillofacial Pathology: A Rationale for Diagnosis and Treatment*. Ed 2, Quintessence Publishing Company, Chicago, 2012, 696.

49. Hicks MJ, Flaitz CM, Wong MEK, et al. Clear cell variant of calcifying epithelial odontogenic tumor. Case report and review of the literature. *Head and Neck*, 1994, 16: 272–277.

Adenomatoid Odontogenic Tumor

50. Philipsen HP. Adenomatoid odontogenic tumor: biologic profile on 499 cases. *J Oral Pathol Med*, 1991, 20: 149–158.

51. Marx RE, Stern D. *Oral and Maxillofacial Pathology: A Rationale for Diagnosis and Treatment*. Ed 2, Quintessence Publishing Company, Chicago, 2012.

52. Adebayo ET, Ajike SD, Adekeye EO. Odontogenic tumors in children and adolescents. A study of 78 Nigerian cases. *J Craniofac Surg*, 2002, 30: 267–272.

53. Courtney RM, Kerr DA. The odontogenic adenomatoid tumor. A comprehensive study of twenty new cases. *Oral Surg Oral Med Oral Pathol* 1975, 39: 424–435.

54. Giansanti JS, Someren A, Waldron CA. Odontogenic adenomatoid tumor (adenoameloblastoma). Survey of 111 cases. *Oral Surg Oral Med Oral Pathol*, 1970, 30: 69–88.

55. Lee SK, Kim YS. Current concepts and occurrence of epithelial odontogenic tumors. I: ameloblastoma and adenomatoid odontogenic tumor. *Korean J Pathol*, 2013, 47: 191–202.

56. Poulson TC, Greer RO. Adenomatoid odontogenic tumor: clinicopathologic and ultrastructural concepts. *J Oral Surg*, 1983, 41: 818–824.

57. Leon JE, Mata GM, Fregnani ER, et al. Clinicopathological and immunohistochemical study of 39 cases of adenomatoid odontogenic tumor: a multicentric study. *Oral Oncology*, 2005, 41: 835–842.

58. Bhullar A, Bhullar RPK, Kler S. Adenomatoid odontogenic tumor involving the maxillary sinus in a child. *Indian J Dent*, 2012, 3: 25–28.

Squamous Odontogenic Tumor

59. Adebayo ET, Ajike SO, Adekeye EO. Odontogenic tumors in children and adolescents: a study of 78 Nigerian cases. *J Craniomaxillofac Surg*, 2002, 30: 267–272.

60. Philipsen HP, Reichart PA. Squamous odontogenic tumor (SOT): a benign neoplasm of the peridontium: a review of 36 reported cases. *J Clin Periodontol*, 1996, 23: 922–926.

61. Pamar RM, Brannon RB, Fowler CB. Squamous odontogenic tumor-like proliferations in radicular cysts: a clinicopathologic study of forty-two cases. *J Endod*, 2011, 37: 623–626.

62. Ruhin B, Raould F, Kolb O, et al. Aggressive maxillary squamous odontogenic tumor in a child: his dilemma and adaptive surgical behavior. *Int J Oral Maxillofax Slurg*, 2007, 36: 868–866.

63. Goldblatt LI, Brannon RB, Ellis GL. Squamous odontogenic tumor: report of five cases and review of the literature. *Oral Surg Oral Med Oral Pathol*, 1982, 54: 187–196.

64. Schwartz-Arad D, Lustman J, Ulmansky M. Squamous odontogenic tumor: review of the literature and case report. *Int J Oral Maxillofac Surg*, 1990, 19: 327–330.

65. Jones BE, Sarathy AP, Ramos MB, et al. Squamous odontogenic tumor. *Head and neck*, 2011, 5: 17–19.

66. Hopper TL, Sadeghi EM, Pricco DF. Squamous odontogenic tumor: report of a case with multiple lesions. *Oral Surg Oral Med Oral Pathol*, 1980, 50: 404–410.

67. Baden E, Doyle J, Mesa M, et al. Squamous odontogenic tumor: report of three cases including the first extra osseous case. *Oral Surg Oral Med Oral Pathol Oral Radiol Endod*, 1993, 75: 733–738.

Odontogenic Myxoma

68. Servanto PS, deSouza PE, Hortu M, et al. Odontogenic tumors in children and adolescents: a collaborative study of 431 cases. *Int J Oral Maxillofac Surg*, 2012, 41: 768–773.

69. Guerrisi M, Piloni MJ, Keszler A. Odontogenic tumors in children and

adolescents. A 15 year retrospective study in Argentina. *Med Oral Pathol Oral Cir Bucal*, 2007, 12: 180–185.

70. White DK, Chess SY, Mohnac AM, et al. Odontogenic myxoma. A clinical and ultrastructural study. *Oral Surg*, 1975, 39: 901–917.

71. Hasleton PS, Simpson W, Craig RDP. Myxoma of the mandible – a fibroblastic tumor. *Oral Surg*, 1978, 46: 396–406.

72. Keszler A, Dominguez FV, Giannuzio G. Myxoma in childhood. An analysis of 10 cases. *J Oral Maxillofac Surg*, 1995, 53: 518–521.

73. Andrews T, Kountakis SE, Millard AA. Myxoma of the head and neck. *Am J Otolaryngol*, 2000, 21: 184–189.

74. Rios D, Valles V, Torres-Vera AM, et al. Periocular myxoma in a child. *Case Rep Ophthalmol Med*, 2012, doi. 10.1155/2012/739094.

75. Farman AG, Nortje CJ, Groteposs FW, et al. Myxofibroma of the jaws. *Br J Oral Surg*, 1977; 15: 3–18.

76. Zaho M, Lu Y, Takata T, et al. Immunohistochemical and histochemical characterization of the muco-sustance of odontogenic myxoma: histogenesis and differential diagnosis. *Path Res Pract*, 1999, 195: 391–395.

77. Perdigao PF, Stergiopoulos SG, DeMarco L, et al. Molecular and immunohistochemical investigation of protein kinase a regulatory subunit type 1A (PRKAR1A) in odontogenic myxomas. *Genes Chromosomes Cancer*, 2005, 44: 204–211.

78. Goldblatt LI. Ultrastructural study of an odontogenic myxoma. *Oral Surg Oral Med Oral Pathol*, 1976, 42: 206–220.

79. Marx RE, Stern D. *Oral and Maxillofacial Pathology: A Rationale for Diagnosis and Treatment*. Ed 2, Quintessence Publishing Company, Chicago, 2012.

80. Pahl S, Henn W, Binger T, et al. Malignant odontogenic myxoma of the maxilla: case with cytogenetic confirmation. *J Otolaryngol Otol*, 2000, 114: 533–535.

Central (Osseous) Odontogenic Fibroma

81. Guerrisi M, Piloni MJ, Keszler A. Odontogenic tumors in children and adolescents. A 15 year retrospective study in Argentina. *Med Oral Pathol Oral Cir Buccal*, 2007, 12: 180–185.

82. Servato JPS, deSouza PEA, Horta DC, et al. Odontogenic tumors in children and adolescents: a collaborative study of 431 cases. *Int J Oral Maxillofac Surg*, 2012, 41: 768–773.

83. Gardner DG. The central odontogenic fibroma, an attempt at clarification. *Oral Surg Oral Med Oral Pathol*, 1980, 50: 425–432.

84. Handlers JP, Abrams A, Melrose RJ. Central odontogenic fibroma: clinicopathologic features of 19 cases and a review of the literature. *J Oral Maxillofac Surg*, 1991, 47: 46–54.

85. Barnes L, Everson JW, Richart P, Sidransky D. (eds) *World Health Organization Classification of Tumors. Pathology and Genetics of Head and Neck Tumors*. IARC Press, Lyon, 2005.

86. Wesley RD, Wysachi GP, Mintz SM. The central odontogenic fibroma. Clinical and morphologic studies. *Oral Surg Oral Med Oral Pathol*, 1975, 40: 235–245.

87. Vincent SD, Hammond HI, Ellis GI, et al. Central granular cell odontogenic fibroma. *Oral Surg Oral Med Oral Pathol*, 1987, 63: 715–721.

88. Taylor-Mosqueda A, Martinez-Mata G, Carlos-Bregi R, et al. Central odontogenic fibroma: new findings and a report of a multicentric collaborative study. *Oral Surg Oral Med Oral Pathol Oral Radiol Endod*, 2011, 112: 349–358.

Cementoblasatoma

89. Norberg O. Zur Kenntis der dysontogenetischen Geschwulste der Zieferknochen. *Vierteljahrsschrift Zahnh*, 1930, 46: 321.

90. Servato JPS, deSouza PEA, Horta DC, et al. Odontogenic tumors in children and adolescents: a collaborative study of 431 cases. *Int J Oral Maxillofac Surg*, 2012, 41: 768–773.

91. Guerrisi M, Piloni MJ, Keszler A. Odontogenic tumors in children and adolescents. A 15 year retrospective study in Argentina. *Med Oral Pathol Oral Cir Bucal*, 2007, 12: 180–185.

92. Corio RL, Crawford BE, Schaberg SJ. Benign cementoblastoma. *Oral Surg Oral Med Oral Pathol*, 1976, 41: 524–530.

93. Cherrick HM, King OH Jr, Lucatorto FM, et al. Benign cementoblastoma. *Oral Surg Oral Med Oral Pathol*, 1974, 37: 54–63.

94. Abrams AM, Kirby JW, Melrose RJ. Cementoblastoma. *Oral Surg Oral Med Oral Pathol*, 1974, 38: 394–403.

95. Giansanti JS. The pattern and width of collagen bundles in bone and cementum. *Oral Surg Oral Med Oral Pathol*, 1970, 30: 508–514.

96. Bilodeau E, Collins B, Costello B, et al. Case report: a pediatric case of cementoblastoma with histologic and radiographic features of osteoblastoma and osteosarcoma. *Head and Neck Pathol*, 2010, 4: 324–328.

97. Komaki M, Iwasaki K, Arzate H, et al. Cementum protein 1 (CEPM1) induces a cementoblastic phenotype and reduces osteoblastic differentiation in periodontal ligament cells. *J Cell Physiol*, 2012, 227: 649–657.

Ameloblastic Fibroma

98. Guerrisi M, Piloni MJ, Keszler A. Odontogenic tumors in children and adolescents. A 15-year retrospective study in Argentina. *Med Oral Pathol Oral Cir Bucal*, 2007, 12: 180–185.

99. Servato JPS, deSouza PEA, Horta DC, et al. Odontogenic tumors in children and adolescents: a collaborative study of 431 cases. *Int J Oral Maxillofac Surg*, 2012, 41: 768–773.

100. Ide F, Kitada M, Tanaka A, et al. Ameloblastic fibroma: a critical review of reported cases provides evidence of two types. *Oral Mcd and Pathol*, 2002, 7: 55–59.

101. Chaudry AP, Stickel FR, Gorlin RJ, et al. An unusual odontogenic tumor. Report of a case. *Oral Surg Oral Med Oral Pathol*, 1962, 15: 86–88.

102. Trodahl JN. Ameloblastic fibroma. A survey of cases from the Armed Forces Institute of Pathology. *Oral Surg Oral Med Oral Pathol*, 1972, 33: 547–558.

103. Richardson JF, Balogh K, Merk F, et al. Pigmented odontogenic tumors of jawbone. A previously undescribed expression of neoplastic potential. *Cancer*, 1974, 34: 1244–1251.

104. Sano K, Yoshida S, Ninomiya H, et al. Assessment of growth potential by M1B1 immunohistochemistry in ameloblastic fibroma and related lesions of the jaws compared with ameloblastic fibrosarcoma. *J Oral Pathol Med* 1998; 27: 59–63.

105. Kobayashi K, Murakami R, Fujii T. Malignant transformation of ameloblastic fibroma to ameloblastic fibrosarcoma: case report and review of the literature. *J Cranio-Maxillofac Surg*, 2005, 33: 352–355.

106. Chen Y, Jing MW, Tie JL. Ameloblastic fibroma: a review of published studies with special reference to its nature and biologic behavior. *Oral Oncology*, 2007, 43: 960–969.

107. Martins C, Carvalho YR, doCarmo MA. Argyrophilic nucleolar organizer regions (AgNORs) in odontogenic myxoma (OM) and ameloblastic fibroma (AF). *J Oral Path Med*, 2001, 30: 389–493.

Ameloblastic Fibro-Odontoma

108. Barnes L, Everson JW, Richart P, Sidransky D. (eds) *World Health Organization Classification of Tumors. Pathology and Genetics of Head and Neck Tumors*. IARC Press, Lyon, 2005.

109. Servato JPS, deSouza PEA, Horta DC, et al. Odontogenic tumors in children and adolescents: a collaborative study of 431 cases. *Int J Oral Maxillofac Surg*, 2012, 41: 768–773.

110. Guerrisi M, Piloni MJ, Keszler A. Odontogenic tumors in children and adolescents. A 15-year retrospective study in Argentina. *Med Oral Pathol Oral Cir Bucal*, 2007, 12: 180–185.

111. Tsagaris GT. *A Review of Ameloblastic Fibro-Odontoma. Thesis.* Geroge Washington University, Washington DC, 1972.

112. DeRui G, Meloni S, Contini M, et al. Ameloblastic fibro-odontoma. Case report and review of the literature. *J Cranio-Maxillofac Surg*, 2010, 38: 141–144.

113. Pontes HAR, Pontes FSC, Rodrigo AGL. Report of four cases of ameloblastic fibro-odontoma in mandible and discussion of the literature about the treatment. *J Cranio-Maxillofac Surg*, 2012, 40: 59–63.

Odontoameloblastoma

114. Mosqueda-Taylor A, Carlos-Bregni R, Ramirez-Amador V, et al. Odontoameloblastoma. Clinico-pathologic study of three cases and critical literature review. *Oral Oncol*, 2002, 38: 800–805.

115. Thompson IO, Phillips VM, Ferrevia R, et al. Odontoameloblastoma. A case report. *Br J Oral Maxillofac Surg*, 1990, 28: 347–349.

116. Servato JPS, deSouza PEA, Horta DC, et al. Odontogenic tumors in children and adolescents: a collaborative study of 431 cases. *Int J Oral Maxillofac Surg*, 2012, 41: 768–773.

117. Guerrisi M, Piloni MJ, Keszler A. Odontogenic tumors in children and adolescents. A 15-year retrospective study in Argentina. *Med Oral Pathol Oral Cir Bucal*, 2007, 12: 180–185.

118. Dive A, Khandekar S, Bodhade A. Odontoameloblastoma. *J Oral Maxillofac Pathol*, 2011, 15: 60–64.

119. Yamamoto K, Yoneda K, Yamamoto T, et al. An immunohistochemical study of odontogenic mixed tumours. *Eur J Cancer*, 1995, 31: 122–128.

120. Marx RE, Stern D. *Oral and Maxillofacial Pathology: A Rationale for Diagnosis and Treatment*. Quintessence Publishing Company, Chicago, 2012.

Odontoma

121. Servato JPS, deSouza PEA, Horta DC, et al. Odontogenic tumors in children and adolescents: a collaborative study of 431 cases. *lnt J Oral Maxillofac Surg*, 2012, 41: 768–773.

122. Guerrisi M, Piloni MJ, Keszler A. Odontogenic tumors in children and adolescents. A 15-year retrospective study in Argentina. *Med Oral Pathol Oral Cir Bucal*, 2007, 12: 180–185.

123. Budnick SO. Compound and complex odontomas. *Oral Surg Oral Med Oral Pathol*, 1976, 42: 501–506.

124. Patil S, Rahman F, Tipu SR. Odontomas: review of the literature and report of a case. *J Oral and Maxillofac Pathol*, 2012, 3: 224–227.

125. deOliveria BH, Carepos V, Marcae S. Compound odontoma - diagnosis and treatment: three case reports. *Pediatr Dent*, 2001, 23: 151–157.

126. Gomel M, Seckin T. An erupted odontoma case report. *J Oral Maxillofac Surg*, 1989, 47: 999–1000.

127. Hong SP, Ellis GL, Hartman KS. Calcifying odontogenic cyst. A review of ninety-two cases with re-evaluation of their nature as cysts or neoplasms, the nature of ghost cells and sub-classification. *Oral Surg Oral Med Oral Pathol*, 1991; 72: 56–64.

Ameloblastic Fibrosarcoma

128. Sano K, Yoshida S, Ninomiya H, et al. Assessment of growth potential by M1B1 immunohistochemistry in ameloblastic fibroma and related lesions of the jaws compared with ameloblastic fibrosarcoma. *J Oral Pathol Med*, 1998, 27: 59–63.

129. Kobayashi K, Murakami R, Fujii T. Malignant transformation of ameloblastic fibroma to ameloblastic fibrosarcoma: case report and review of the literature. *J Cranio-Maxillofac Slurg*, 2005, 33: 352–355.

130. Chen Y, Jing M-W, Tie JL. Ameloblastic fibroma: a review of published studies with special reference to its nature and biologic behavior. *Oral Oncology*, 2007, 43: 960–969.

Odontogenic Tumor Reconstructive Surgery

131. Marx RE, Stevens MR. *Atlas of Oral and Extraoral Bone Harvesting*. Quintessence Publishing Company, Chicago, 2010.

Non-Neoplastic Diseases of Salivary Glands

Sherif Said, Robert O. Greer and Robert E. Marx

Non-Neoplastic Diseases of Salivary Glands

Introduction

The production and secretion of human saliva is an important physiologic function that is accomplished by three pairs of major salivary glands (Tubulo-acinar exocrine type glands); the parotid glands with acini that produce purely serous secretions; the submandibular gland with acini that produce mixed serous and mucinous secretions and the sublingual gland with acini that produce purely mucinous secretions. Additionally, hundreds of minor seromucinous salivary glands are scattered throughout the nasopharyngeal, oral and oropharyngeal submucosa, the larynx and tracheobronchial tree.

The ductal system of the salivary glands originates as small, cuboidal cell lined "intercalated ducts" arising from the acini. These ducts intersect larger tall columnar cell lined ducts with basal infolding known as "striated ducts," which are particularly rich in mitochondria. The striated ducts join larger pseudostratified columnar epithelially lined "interlobular ducts" that ultimately terminate as "excretory" ducts. Contractile "myoepithelial cells" surround the salivary gland acini and their contraction helps in evacuating and maintaining a stream of salivary secretions (Figure 9.1). A host of developmental anomalies, as well as benign and malignant neoplasms can arise from the salivary glands in infants and adolescents.

Developmental Abnormalities

Agenesis of Salivary Glands

Genesis of the major salivary glands occurs between the fourth and eighth weeks of embryonic life with an oral ectodermal growth into the underlying mesenchymal tissue.[1] The parotid gland is the first gland to develop followed by the submandibular and sublingual glands. Agenesis of salivary glands is[2] rare and may occur alone or in combination with other first branchial arch anomalies.[3,4,5] Most reported cases of salivary gland agenesis are sporadic, without an established family history, however, familial instances of salivary gland agenesis has been reported.[6,7,8,9,10,11]

Depending on the degree and extent of gland agenesis, patients can present without symptoms, or they may suffer a considerable decrease in saliva production with consequential dry mouth, caries, periodontal disease, oropharyngeal infections and difficulty in chewing and swallowing. Most pediatric age group instances of salivary gland agenesis will result in minimal symptoms. The diagnosis can be usually confirmed

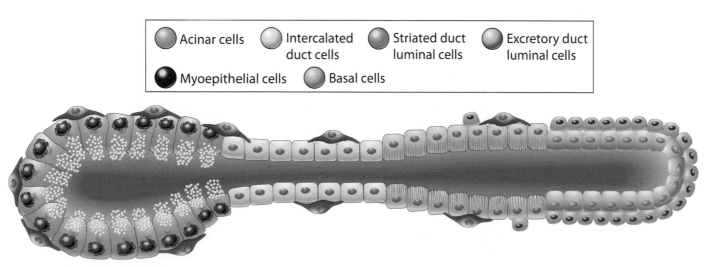

Figure 9.1 Structure of the salivary gland unit consisting of the salivary gland acinus and the attached ducts.

by scintigraphy, which will show "99mTcO4" uptake to be lacking in the affected sites.

Treatment of salivary agenesis is largely symptomatic and includes the need for strict oral hygiene and appropriate dietary and dental management. Regular oral hydration should be the rule and saliva substitutes may be necessary. *Hypoplasia* of salivary gland is usually asymptomatic. However, hypoplasia can result in compensatory enlargement of the major salivary glands in children. *Congenital atresia* of major salivary gland ducts has also been reported in children.[12]

Polycystic (Dysgenetic) Salivary Gland Disease

Mihalyaka[13,14] provided the first clinical description of polycystic salivary gland disease, a disorder that is characterized by the formation of multiple cysts of variable sizes, which replace the salivary gland parenchyma, while at the same time preserving the lobular architecture of the gland. The associated cysts, which give the gland a spongy consistency, arise from the intercalated duct segment of the gland. Although most reported cases occur in adults, the condition will start in childhood, with most children complaining of recurrent painless salivary gland swelling and lack of saliva flow.[13] Ultrasound, MRI or CT scans are all effective ways of demonstrating the cystic nature of the lesion and a biopsy is generally confirmatory.

Pathologic Findings

Histologically, the cysts identified in polycystic salivary gland disease will contain altered salivary secretions, which are diastase resistant/periodic acid Schiff positive.[15] Incomplete septae will extend into the cyst lumen and an hour glass cyst narrowing of cystic spaces will characterize many of the cyst formations seen in this disease.[16,17] The cysts ultimately replace the salivary gland parenchyma, producing a honeycomb appearance microscopically (Figure 9.2).

The exact etiology of the disorder remains unknown, although developmental malformations of the salivary gland duct system have been suggested as the cause.[18,19] Parotidectomy has been employed to manage the condition, largely for cosmetic reasons.

Salivary Gland Heterotopia (Choristoma)

Salivary gland heterotopia (SGH) represents the occurrence of salivary gland tissue outside of the major or minor salivary glands. SGH can be encountered as either ductal or acinar inclusions within the *parotid lymph nodes* (Neisse Nicholson rests) (Figure 9.3). These inclusions have been linked etiologically to the origin of Warthin's tumors and benign lymphoepithelial lesions in the parotid gland. Such inclusions can also be less frequently encountered in the middle ear,[20] the gingiva,[21] the external auditory canal,[22] the lower neck,[23] the thyroglossal duct cyst,[24] the thyroid and parathyroid,[25,26] the mandible,[27,28] the pituitary gland[29] and the cerebellopontine angle,[30] and other craniofacial sites in children.[31,32,33,34,35,36,37,38]

The *clinical consequences* of a salivary gland heterotopic are variable. Patients can present with a draining sinus, or an asymptomatic or symptomatic nodule at the point that surgery is required.

Heterotopic salivary gland of the middle ear, first reported by Taylor and Martin in 1961,[39] can occur in the pediatric population.[40] Patients usually present with conductive hearing loss that may be associated with cholesteatomas or other ear anomalies.[24]

Lesions involving the ear have been linked to first and second branchial arch anomalies that occur prior to the fourth month of intrauterine development.[41,42] Rare pleomorphic adenomas have also been reported to arise from the middle ear in association with these rare choristomas.[43] The lesions consist histologically of an admix of neoplastic seromucinous glands and adipose tissue in a normal acinar arrangement.

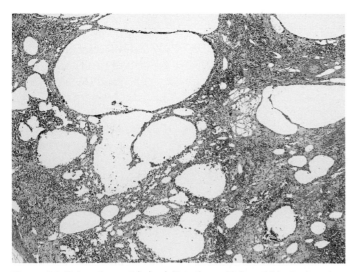

Figure 9.2 Polycystic parotid gland. Note the multiple variable sized cystic spaces and the chronically inflamed intervening parenchyma.

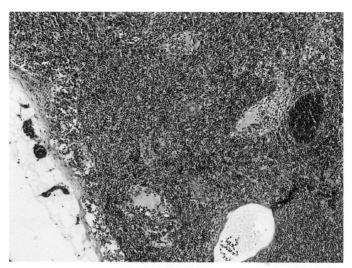

Figure 9.3 A periparotid lymph node showing ductal inclusions within the substance of the lymph node. Notice the subcapsular sinus with histiocytes confirming lymph node formation.

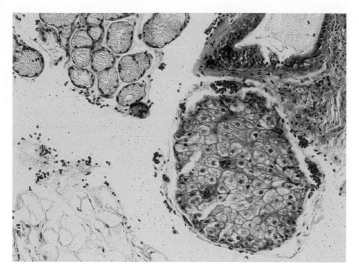

Figure 9.4 Sebaceous cell aggregates adjacent to the wall of the salivary gland intralobular duct.

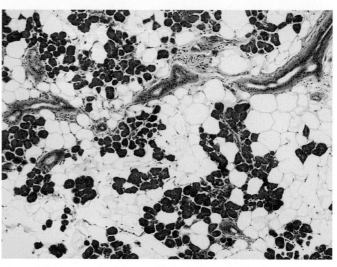

Figure 9.5 Lipomatosis of the parotid gland. Notice the distribution of mature fat cells among normal appearing acini and ducts within a salivary gland lobule.

Ducts may or may not be identified. *Heterotopic salivary glands of the lower neck* are usually identified near the sterno-clavicular joint in the lower neck and are most often noticed shortly after birth as a painless unilateral growth.[44,45] HSGT, whether symptomatic or asymptomatic, ends up being excised.

Mucoviscidosis (Cystic Fibrosis)

Mucoviscidosis, an autosomal recessive condition that primarily affects the lungs, is in fact a disease of exocrine gland function, including the salivary glands. Salivary gland component of the disease is characterized by secretion of abnormally viscid thick glandular secretions that can result in duct obstruction and glandular atrophy. The etiology of the disorder is related to defects in both copies of the cystic fibrosis gene that codes for a protein transmembrane conductance regulator (CFTR). CFTR is an ABC transporter-class ion channel that codes for a protein that conducts chlorine and thiocyanate across epithelial cell membranes.[46] Histologically, the affected gland will show dilated obstructed ducts with thick eosinophilic secretions, and acinar atrophy with fibrosis and chronic inflammation.[47,48]

Ectopic Sebaceous Gland Differentiation

Sebaceous differentiation is common within the major salivary glands, particularly the parotid gland [49]. It usually shows bimodal peaks with the first peak occurring in the pediatric age group (10 to 20 years old) and the second peak in the adult population over [50] 70 years of age (Figure 9.4).

Conditions resulting in tissue type or metaplastic changes, and infiltrations in salivary glands:

Fat Replacement (Lipomatosis)

Lipomatosis is a poorly defined entity that is considered to be a non-neoplastic deposition of adipose tissue throughout salivary gland tissue with resulting glandular enlargement over time. The disorder will primarily affect the major salivary glands, particularly the parotid, although it has been reported in minor salivary glands.[51] In adults, fat content increase in salivary glands is most often associated with alcoholism, liver cirrhosis, diabetes, chronic sialoadenitis, Sjögren syndrome (SS) and increasing age. The disorder is quite rare in the pediatric age group, and Krolls et al.[52] found only three cases of lipomatosis among 430 salivary gland lesions in children (up to 15 years) that were studied at the Armed Forces Institute of Pathology (AFIP). Other similar studies report no instances of lipomatosis in children.[53] Some investigators have suggested that the coxsackie B virus may be involved in the etiology of the disorder.[54] Preoperative diagnosis of lipomatosis can be difficult. CT imaging is considered to provide the best diagnostic results, when a diagnosis of lipomatosis in a child is a consideration.[55]

Pathologic Findings

Grossly, the gland involved by lipomatosis will show enlargement, usually in a multinodular fashion. Microscopically, uniloculated mature fat cells will be distributed totally or partially in an interstitial fashion throughout the gland (Figure 9.5).

Treatment and Prognosis

Treatment of symptomatic lipomatosis usually involves a superficial or total parotidectomy with facial nerve preservation.

Iron Deposition in Salivary Glands

Iron deposition in salivary glands in the pediatric age group can be encountered in neonatal hemochromatosis,[56] Thalassemia major[57] and in instances where there have been repeated blood transfusions for various hematologic disorders.[58] Chronic and persistent iron deposition in major and minor salivary glands can eventually lead to glandular functional changes due to chronic inflammation, acinar atrophy and fibrosis.

Pathologic Findings

Labial lip biopsy of minor salivary glands has been employed to diagnose neonatal hemochromatosis. Microscopically, the histologic changes that are seen include chronic inflammation, atrophy of acinar elements, fibrosis and hemosiderin deposition within the acini. These findings, however, can be quite minimal and non-diagnostic.

Amyloidosis

Amyloidosis involving salivary glands is quite rare.[59,60] In children, the most frequent forms of amyloidosis include the reactive AA amyloidoses that are associated with the hereditary periodic fever group of syndromes: familial Mediterranean fever, periodic fever syndrome and juvenile idiopathic arthritis.[61]

Pathologic Findings

Labial minor salivary gland biopsy can be used to detect amyloidosis in a large majority of cases involving children.[62,63] The associated amyloid deposition will occur in the form of a homogenous eosinophilic, proteinaceous and acellular product that is predominantly periductal and periacinar. Congo-red and Sirius-red stains can be used to highlight amyloid deposits, which will demonstrate an apple green/orange birefringence under polarized light. Thioflavin T stains for amyloid are considered to be equally or more diagnostic.

Non-Developmental Salivary Gland Cysts

Mucocele

Mucoceles of the extravasation, retention and superficial subtypes are the most commonly encountered cystic lesions of salivary glands in children.[64,65] The lesions most often occur due to trauma, with the lower lip being the most common site of occurrence.[65,66,67] (Figure 9.6) Lesions can involve any oral site and there is a slightly higher incidence in girls than boys. Most mucoceles present as bluish dome like swellings that are usually less than 1 cm in diameter. Mucoceles that involve the floor of mouth are classified as *ranulas* and they can be much larger than mucoceles (Figure 9.7). Ranulas tend to originate in the sublingual glands, either in the body or duct systems, or in the submandibular gland or Wharton duct.[68] Ranulas that herniate through the mylohyoid muscle into the neck to present as a submental or submandibular neck mass are defined as *plunging ranulas* (Figure 9.8), and they will histologically consist of a dilated mucin-filled channel that will be surrounded by granulation tissue and chronic inflammatory cells (Figure 9.9).

Pathologic Findings

The so-called extravasation type of mucocele will consist of a cavity rimmed by granulation tissue. The cavity will frequently be lined by flattened fibroblasts. The cavity may or may not contain mucin. The extravasated mucin, if significant can incite a chronic inflammatory response with numerous histiocytes (mucinophages) (Figure 9.10). The *retention mucocele* also known as a mucous retention cyst will demonstrate a cystic channel or cavity that is lined by a thin layer of attenuated cuboidal or columnar epithelium. On occasion, retention mucoceles may be lined by metaplastic squamous or oncocytic epithelium.[69] Superficial *mucoceles*, or mucous retention phenomena will present as a raised surface blister that usually involves the immediate subepithelial connective tissue, such that mucin is retained just beneath the overlying squamous epithelium[70] (Figure 9.11). These lesions are usually seen in children in the region of the palatoglossal fold.

Treatment and Prognosis

Mucoceles are typically treated by complete excision or marsupialization.[71] Recurrence in children can range as high as 12 percent.

Lymphoepithelial Cyst

Lymphoepithelial cysts are primarily seen in the parotid gland in both children and adults. Less commonly they can involve

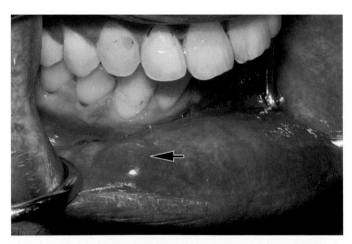

Figure 9.6 Mucocele of the lower lip in a teenager with a history of chronic lip biting. (Reprinted from Marx R, Stern D. *Oral and Maxillofacial Pathology: A Rationale for Diagnosis and Treatment* with permission from Quintessence Publishing Company).

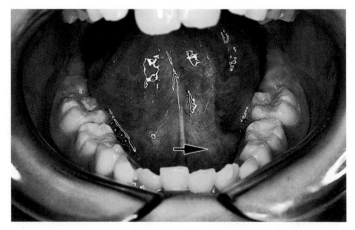

Figure 9.7 Ranula involving the floor of the mouth in a child. (Reprinted from Marx R, Stern D. *Oral and Maxillofacial Pathology: A Rationale for Diagnosis and Treatment* with permission from Quintessence Publishing Company).

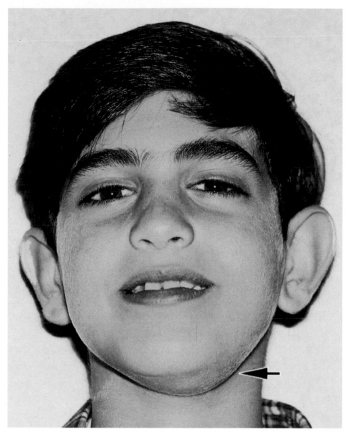

Figure 9.8 Plunging ranula that has herniated through the mylohyoid muscle in the neck. (Reprinted from Marx R, Stern D. *Oral and Maxillofacial Pathology: A Rationale for Diagnosis and Treatment* with permission from Quintessence Publishing Company).

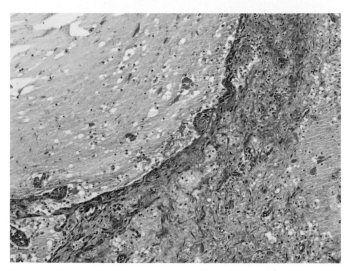

Figure 9.10 Mucous extravasation phenomenon demonstrating a mucin filled cavity that is marginated by flattened fibroblasts and granulation tissue.

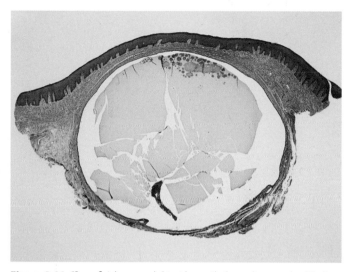

Figure 9.11 "Superficial mucocele" just beneath the oral mucosal epithelium. Note the thin attenuated epithelial lining of the mucin filled channel.

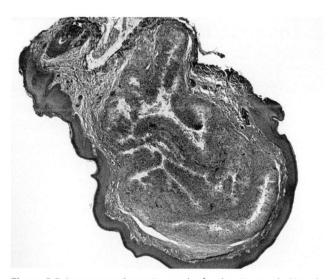

Figure 9.9 Low power photomicrograph of a plunging ranula. Note the dilated central channel surrounded by chronic inflammatory cells and granulation tissue.

the posterior-lateral tongue and floor of the mouth.[72,73,74] Originally, these cysts were thought to arise from embryonic remnants of the branchial arch system. More recent theories suggest that lymphoepithelial cysts originate from Neisse

Nicholson rests within lymph nodes or from the formation of a dense periductal lymphocytic infiltrates within the parotid gland.[75] Most patients will present with a mass in the preauricular area or infra-auricular region. The vast majority of lesions will be mobile and non-tender.

Bilateral parotid lymphoepithelial cystic lesions (BLELs) have been linked to Sjögren's syndrome or an HIV-positive status (see benign HIV associated lymphoepithelial cysts in this chapter). [76]

Pathologic Findings

The benign HIV associated lymphoepithelial cystic lesions (BLEC) are usually lined by squamous, cuboidal or respiratory type epithelium that may show sebaceous or mucous metaplasia (Figure 9.12). The connective tissue wall of the cyst will be rich with lymphoid tissue that may contain germinal centers.

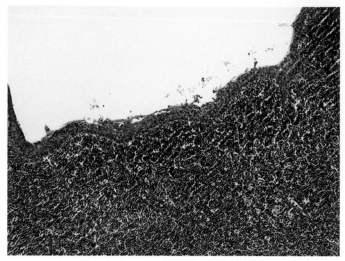

Figure 9.12 Lymphoepithelial cyst with a lining of squamous epithelium.

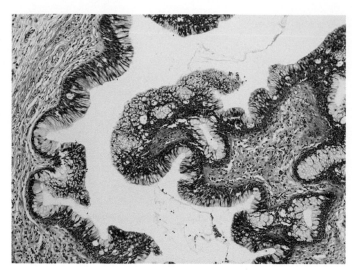

Figure 9.14 Salivary duct cyst within Stensen's duct. Note the surrounding fibrous tissue and chronic inflammation and extensive mucinous metaplasia of the duct's normal stratified columnar epithelium.

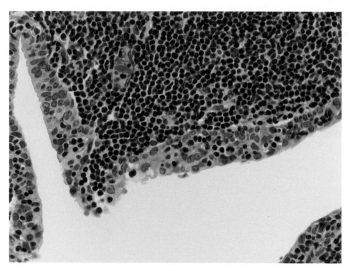

Figure 9.13 A dense lymphocytic infiltrate present in the cyst wall.

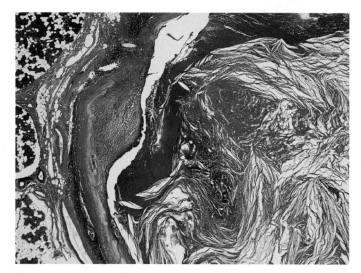

Figure 9.15 Intraparotid salivary duct cyst. Note the cystic dilation of the duct and the surrounding fibrosis.

(Figure 9.13) Lymphoepithelial cysts in children can arise in association with other lymphoproliferative disorders including Castleman's disease.

Treatment and Prognosis

Superficial partial parotidectomy is the treatment of choice for parotid lesions. Minor salivary gland lesions should be completely excised.

Salivary Duct Cyst (Sialocyst)

The salivary duct cyst is a rare cyst that generally arises in association with the parotid gland duct and only rarely in minor salivary glands, as a painless swelling that is usually no more than 3 cm in diameter. Duct obstruction by a mucous plug with consequential cystic dilatation of the duct and swelling are common presenting symptoms. The affected duct will be lined by cuboidal or columnar epithelium with occasional oncocytic metaplastic or mucous changes (Figure 9.15 & 9.16) Children are only rarely affected, and surgical excision of the cyst is curative.[77,78]

Sialadenitis

Sialadenitis, or inflammation of major or minor salivary glands is common to the pediatric population and encompasses a variety of lesional sub types, some of which appear similar clinically, while others have specified well defined patterns as well as etiologic factors. Clinicopathologic correlation is therefore required in many instances in order to determine the exact nature of the disease process.

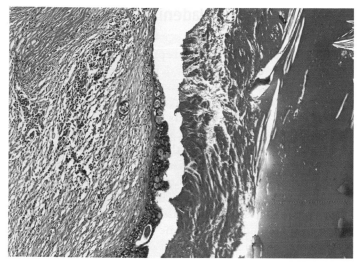

Figure 9.16 The duct contains proteinaceous thickened eosinophilic material and there is focal mucinous metaplasia of the cyst lining epithelium.

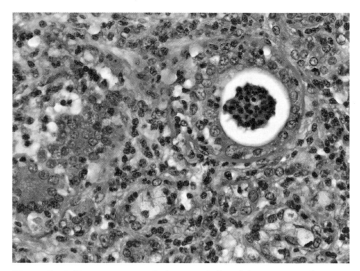

Figure 9.18 Extensive acute sialadenitis with ductal destruction and microabscess formation are evident.

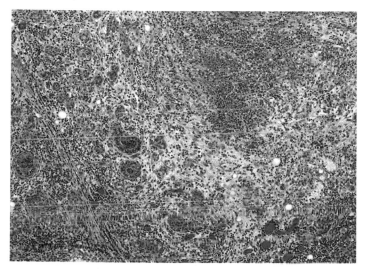

Figure 9.17 Acute suppurative sialadenitis demonstrating polymorph nuclear leukocyte infiltrate and inflammation with residual ductal epithelium and acinar elements.

Acute Suppurative Sialadenitis

Acute suppurative sialadenitis is a common form of pediatric sialadenitis that most often affects the parotid gland.[79] The etiology of the disorder can be viral or bacterial.[79,80,81] Newborn preterm infants with a propensity for dehydration tend to be quite susceptible to such infections. Children with an underlying systemic illness such as glomerulonephritis, immunosuppressive disorders such as an immunoglobulin deficiency, or acute lymphocytic leukemia are also more prone to the causally associated bacterial and viral infections. The mean age of onset for pediatric acute suppurative sialadenitis has been reported to be 4.4 years of age.[80]

Clinically, most affected children will present with a tender indurated swelling of the involved gland. Intraoral inspection may demonstrate an edematous erythematous Stensen's papillae with or without a purulent discharge from Stensen's duct.

Retrograde infection precipitated by bacterial microorganisms, most often *Staphylococcus aureus* tends to be the most common trigger for the disorder. *Streptococcus pneumonia, Streptococcus pyogenes, Streptococcus viridans, Haemophilus influenzae, Klebsiella pneumonia, E. coli and Pseudomonas aeruginosa* have also been implicated as potential bacterial sources for the disorder. Mumps parotitis (parotitis epidemica) is the most common viral cause of the disorder.[82]

Submandibular gland suppurative sialadenitis in children is a rare disorder that is usually associated with obstructive causes, most often salivary stone formation.[83,84]

Sialolithiasis of the parotid gland, common in adults, is rarely observed in pediatric age group patients.[85] The disorder may be accompanied by bouts of acute suppurative sialadenitis that eventuates to *chronic obstructive sialadenitis.*

Pathologic Findings

Histologically, acute suppurative sialadenitis will be characterized by edema, interstitial vascular prominence and periductal and interstitial neutrophilic infiltrates (Figure 9.17). Acinar and ductal destruction of the gland with microabscess formation is common (Figure 9.18).

Treatment and Prognosis

Treatment is usually conservative and will typically involve antibiotic therapy, oral hygiene instruction, gland message and adequate hydration. Incision and drainage of the gland may be required if abscess formation develops. In cases of salivary gland stone formation, an intraoral sialolithectomy may be necessary

Juvenile Recurrent Parotitis

Juvenile recurrent parotitis (JRP) is a typically self-limiting, non-obstructive and non-suppurative form of recurrent or

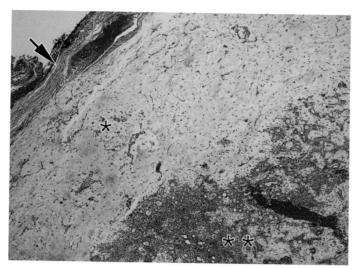

Figure 10.16 Pleomorphic adenoma. Note the exceedingly thin connective tissue capsule surrounding the tumor (arrow). The tumor is both stromal(*) and tumor cell(**) rich.

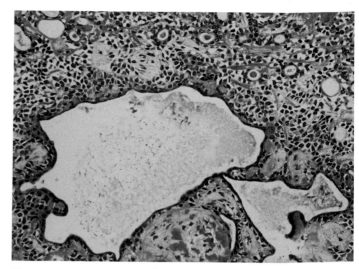

Figure 10.18 Pleomorphic adenoma demonstrating cystic areas that are not an unusual occurrence in pediatric age group pleomorphic adenomas.

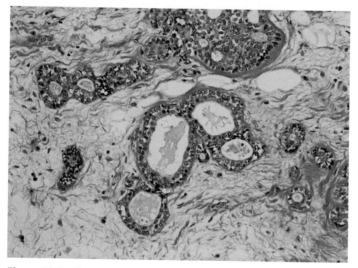

Figure 10.17 Pleomorphic adenoma displaying ductal and tubular formations that are surrounded by one or more layers of myoepithelial cells. These classic myoepithelial cells blend in with modified myoepithelial cells to form the tumor stroma.

in a stroma derived from by modified myoepithelial cells. The proportion of the stoma to the tumor's epithelial/myoepithelial components can be quite variable, and in so-called cellular pleomorphic adenomas, the epithelial/myoepithelial component of the tumor can be so significant that the stromal component of the tumor may appear to be absent.

Pleomorphic adenomas of major salivary glands are typically marginated by fibrous connective tissue of variable thickness. (Figure10.16)[110,111] In minor salivary glands a marginating capsule tends to be less apparent or deficient than in major salivary gland neoplasms. Microscopic satellite tumor nodules, tumor pseudopodia and foci of capsular penetration may be seen external to the tumor capsule. These excrescences, which are largely the reason for the recurrence

of pleomorphic adenomas, can be left behind at the time of surgical excision because they may not be easily appreciated by the naked eye.[110,111]

The epithelial component of the tumor will consist of epithelial and myoepithelial nests islands, and cords of cells with divergent growth patterns that can include a trabecular or tubular, papillary, cystic or solid architectures. Tumor cells that exhibit myoepithelial features[112,113] can be quite common or tumor cells may have a plasmacytoid, epithelioid, spindle, oncocytic or clear cell morphology. The epithelial component of the tumor will not demonstrate significant cytologic atypia.

The ducts and tubules that are seen in pleomorphic adenomas will be lined by an inner cuboidal or columnar cellular layer (Figure 10.17). These cells will have eosinophilic cytoplasm and will be marginated by an outer myoepithelial cell layer of one or more cell rows.[89,90,94,114] The outer myoepithelial layer will tend to merge into the surrounding stroma where cells will be dispersed or grouped as modified myoepithelial cells. Tumor-associated ducts may contain eosinophilic secretory material and, on occasion, they may become distended and form multiple microcysts or even larger cysts (Figure 10.18).

The modified myoepithelial cells of the tumor produce a richly variable stromal component which may appear mucoid, myxoid, hyaline-like, chondroid, myxochondroid or osseous (Figures 10.19, 10.20, 10.21 & 10.22).[89,90,115,116] Some investigators have suggested that a prominent hyalinized stroma can be correlated with tumors that may have a propensity for malignant change.[117,118] The proportion of tumor parenchymal elements to stromal elements can be variable, and thus tumors are often subdesignated as either epithelial cell-rich, or myoepithelial cell-rich.

Pleomorphic adenomas in children can occasionally exhibit unusual epithelial and stroma components that can include sebaceous cell nests, fibroadipose rich stromal elements and crystal formations that can include tyrosine or oxalate crystals (Figure 10.23).[119,120,121,122]

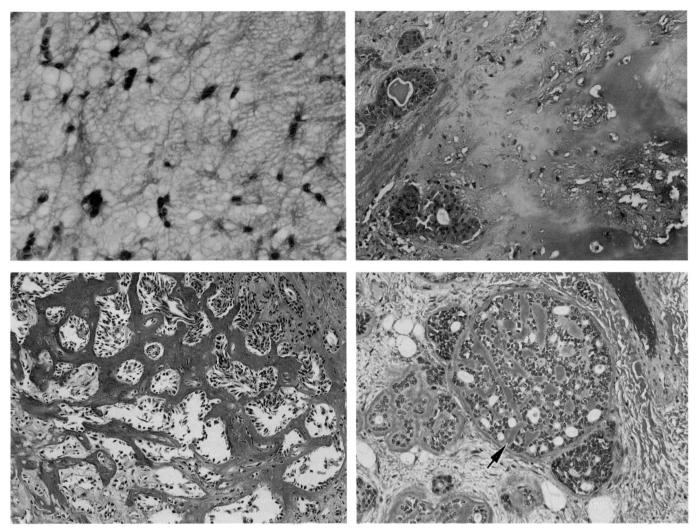

Figures 10.19 (top left), 10.20 (top right), 10.21 (bottom left) & 10.22 (bottom right) Pleomorphic adenoma demonstrating myxoid, chondroid, hyalinized and reduplicated basement membrane (arrow) stromal elements respectively.

Necrosis or increased mitosis are not commonly encountered in pleomorphic adenoma, and pleomorphism of tumor cells or extracapsular extension, should not necessarily be interpreted as harbingers of malignant change in the absence of additional corroborating evidence. The occasional presence of benign tumor fragments within vascular spaces in pleomorphic adenomas, or within the immediate peritumoral vasculature is thought to result from perioperative manipulation of the tumor during surgical resection and should not be interpreted as evidence of vascular invasion.[89,90,116]

Differential Diagnosis

Focal stromal hyalinization, with cribriform and cylindromatous differentiation of the epithelial component of a pleomorphic adenoma, can mimic the histolomorphology of adenoid cystic carcinoma and polymorphous low grade adenocarcinoma. However, the presence of more typical areas of

pleomorphic adenoma and the absence of malignant features, particularly the perineural invasion common to the aforementioned tumors, should help to distinguish pleomorphic adenoma from these two malignant neoplasms.

Myoepithelioma, best defined as a cellular mixed tumor, and discussed separately in this text, will show no glandular differentiation, and the tumor will lack a hyalinized or myxochondroid matrix. Basal cell Adenoma (BCA), with which a mixed tumor can be confused, will also fail to demonstrate the myxochondroid stroma of a mixed tumor. Additionally, BCA will also be composed of relatively uniform basaloid cells that tend to be surrounded by a prominent basal lamina. *Carcinoma ex-pleomorphic adenoma*, unlike a benign mixed tumor, will demonstrate cellular cytologic atypia, necrosis, perineural invasion, vascular invasion and infiltration of the tumor beyond its capsular margins. (Figure 10.24)

In most instances, the diagnosis of pleomorphic adenoma is made via recognition of the characteristic histomorphology

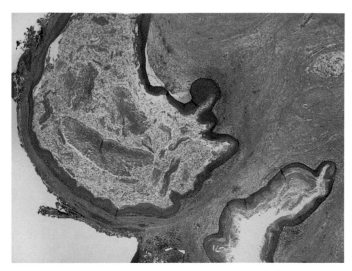

Figure 10.35 Keratocystoma. Low power photomicrograph showing multicystic, benign, squamous, epithelially lined cysts containing lamellated keratin and intervening fibrous tissue.

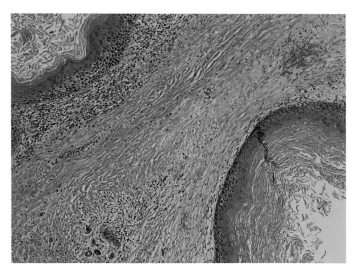

Figure 10.36 Higher magnification of the squamous lining of keratocystoma cysts. The epithelial lining lacks a granular cell layer.

Microscopically, the neoplasm will be composed of cysts of variable size. The cysts will be lined by stratified keratinizing squamous epithelium that lacks a granular cell layer (Figure 10.35). The cyst lumena will contain lamellar keratin. (Figure 10.36). Cystic spaces will be randomly, rather than lobularly, arranged and solid, well-defined stromal squamous islands can be observed penetrating an inflamed fibrous connective tissue stroma. Rupture of any of the cysts can be accompanied by a foreign body giant cell reaction.

Differential Diagnoses

Differential diagnoses for the keratocystoma include primary or metastatic squamous cell carcinoma, mucoepidermoid carcinoma, metaplastic Warthin tumor and tumor associated squamous metaplasia of the type that can occur in other salivary gland tumors, especially pleomorphic adenoma.

Necrotizing sialometaplasia is probably the lesion that most resembles the keratocystoma histologically. Keratocystomas will, however, lack a normal lobular glandular configuration of necrotizing sialometaplasia; fail to show simultaneous metaplasia of acini and other ductal epithelium and lack a prominence of granulation tissue that is typical of necrotizing sialometaplasia.

Epidermoid cysts and odontogenic keratocysts (OKC) can resemble a keratocystoma. Epidermoid cysts are usually unicystic, however, and they will demonstrate a granular cell layer in their epithelial lining. Soft tissue OKCs will have a nearly identical histology to the keratocystoma except for the fact that the cyst lining epithelium in the OKC will typically be parakeratinized. Still, clinicopathologic correlation will be necessary to separate the two entities.

Immunohistochemically, the squamous epithelium lining the cystic space of a keratocystoma will stain positively for AE1/AE3 and CK5/6 and will be focally positive for CK7. P63 will be strongly positive and P53 weakly positive.

Treatment and Prognosis

The treatment of choice for the keratocystoma is surgical excision, usually by superficial parotidectomy. No recurrences have to date been reported for the tumor.

Basal Cell Adenoma
Clinical Features

BCAs are benign salivary gland neoplasms[224,225] that generally affect adults. The tumor accounts for 2 to 3 percent of all salivary gland neoplasms, and only in rare instances has this tumor been reported in children, occasionally as a congenital lesion.[226,227,228,229] BCA in the pediatric age group can involve the parotid gland, the submandibular gland and oral and lacrimal minor salivary glands.[226,227,228] Most tumors will involve the parotid gland, and while in adults, females are favored, no gender predilection has been documented in children. BCAs will present clinically as a firm, mobile, painless, well defined nodular swelling or mass (Figure 10.37) that on occasion may have a cystic consistency.[224,229,230] At one time, BCA, along with canalicular adenoma were classified broadly as *monomorphic adenomas*. These tumors are now, however, regarded as distinct and unique entities.

Pathologic Findings

Grossly, the BCA will tend to appear as grey to brown, firm, 1 to 3 cm, well circumscribed nodule with a homogenous cut surface that at times may be cystic. Microscopically, the tumor will consist of small round to ovoid basaloid cells.[224,225,231] The tumor tends to be well encapsulated when occurring in the major salivary glands and non-encapsulated when occurring in a minor salivary gland.[228] Tumor cells will be set in a sparse barely evident connective tissue stroma. Four histologic subtypes are reorganized: solid, trabecular, tubular and membranous.

The solid histologic variant of the tumor will be composed of basaloid epithelial cells arranged in sheets, nests and cords

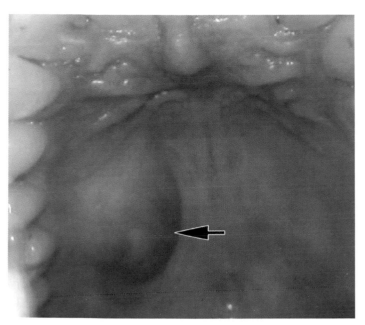

Figure 10.37 BCA of the palate presenting as a nodular swelling.

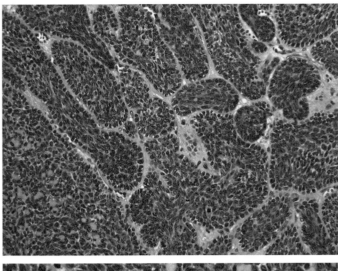

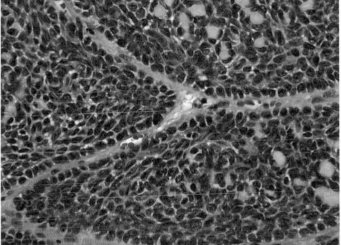

Figure 10.38 (top) & 10.39 (bottom) Low and high power photomicrographs of the solid variant of BCA respectively. Note the peripheral palisading of tumor island marginating cells in the high power view.

(Figure 10.38). Peripheral palisading columnar or cuboidal basaloid cells will marginate tumor cell nests (Figure 10.39).

The trabecular histologic variant of the tumor will consist of narrow anastomosing trabeculae of basaloid cells separated by thin well vascularized stromal tissue that may contain modified myoepithelial cells.[232] (See Figure 10.40.) On occasion, ductal lumina are present among the basaloid cells, resulting in a tubulo-trabecular pattern. The tubular histologic variant of the tumor will show a predominance of small ductal type formations (Figure 10.41). Tubules will be lined by cuboidal cells with eosinophilic cytoplasm. The lumina of the tubules will often contain eosinophilic colloid like material.

The membranous histologic variant, sometimes known as the *dermal analogue tumor* will demonstrate islands and nests of basaloid cells that are encased or surrounded by an eosinophilic hyaline product (Figure 10.42). Tumor cell nests are often integrated into a mosaic pattern. The membranous variant of the tumor is the variant most often associated with multinodular growth.

Differential Diagnosis

Adenoid cystic carcinoma and basal cell adenocarcinoma can mimic BCA histologically, however, tumor necrosis, the presence of angiolymphatic and/or perineural invasion and cytologic atypia will tend to distinguish these malignant neoplasms from BCA.

Although extraosseous ameloblastoma can resemble BCA, the peripheral palisading cells of ameloblastoma tumor islands will show reverse cellular polarity of the tumor cell nuclei, a feature not seen in BCA.

Immunohistochemistry

Immunohistochemically, the epithelial cells of BCA will show variable reactivity with cytokeratin stains. Inner luminal cells

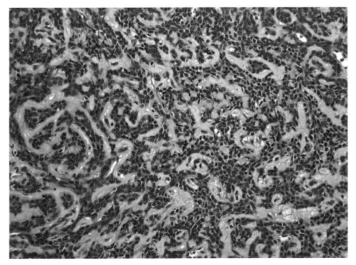

Figure 10.40 Trabecular BCA displaying anastomosing cords of basaloid cells that are separated by thin septa of collagen.

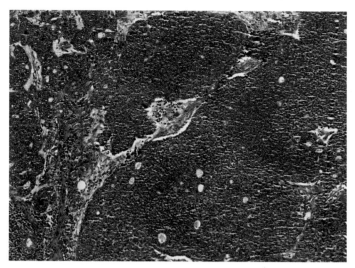

Figure 11.21 ACC. Solid variant. Note the distinctive solid nesting of tumor cells and the marked basophilia.

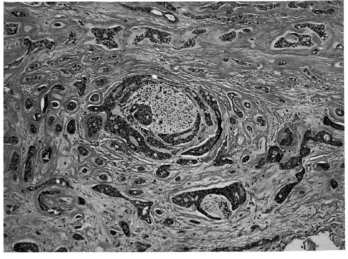

Figure 11.22 ACC demonstrating extensive perineural invasion by tumor cells.

This form of ACC predominantly affects minor salivary glands and has not been reported in the pediatric population.

When accessed immunohistochemically, the cells lining true lumina in ACC will be immunoreactive and stain for CEA, EMA, Pancytokeratins, CK6, CK14, CK17 and CK19, and S100 protein. BFAP may be focally positive.[80]Duct luminal cells will express 1-ACT. ACC will also express C-Kit (CD117), B-Catenin, E-cadherin, and demonstrate high expression levels of P53 and Bcl-2, and low KI-67 expression.[67,80]

Tumor pseudocysts will contain diastase resistant periodic acid Schiff (PAS) positive and mucicarmine positive material. Although ACC will stain positively for CD117 (C-kit) on an immunohistochemical level, C-kit mutations may not be seen in ACC on a molecular level.[81] EGFR over expression has been reported in the tumor's myoepithelial layer of cells.[82,83]

Translocation between chromosomes 6 and 9 leading to MYB and NFIB gene fusion and loss of the MYB3 target gene and ultimate loss of cell cycle control has been reported in ACC.[84] Additionally, isolated genomic allelic loss of heterozygosity can be seen at 6q 23–25, and chromosomal losses at 12q, 1p and 9p can be identified in ACC.[85,86,87]

Differential Diagnosis

Common differential diagnoses include pleomorphic adenoma, basal cell adenoma, polymorphous low grade adenocarcinoma (PLGA), sialoblastoma and carcinoma ex mixed tumor. Pleomorphic adenoma, unlike ACC, will not display a malignant infiltrative pattern and will lack evidence of perineural invasion, as will basal cell adenoma.

PLGA will demonstrate a targetoid perineural pattern of growth or feature columns of tumor cells arranged in a single file. PLGA will also show little pleomorphism, tumor cells will not display angular nuclei, and atypical mitoses, unlike what can be seen in ACC, will be rare. Sialoblastoma, a tumor seen

almost exclusively in children will be rich in basaloid cells and show peripheral palisading of nuclei, features that are not common to ACC.

Carcinoma ex mixed tumor will be associated with a previously existing pleomorphic adenoma, histologic features of a benign mixed tumor will be present and cytologically atypical features of malignancy will readily be evident. It must be noted, however, that the malignancy in a malignant mixed tumor can in fact be an ACC.

Treatment and Prognosis

The management modality of choice for ACC in children and adolescents includes wide and sometimes radical surgical excision, generally with margins that are 3 cm around the tumor mass.[88,89] Adjuvant radiation therapy is often employed; however, its effectiveness is still debated.[89,90]

Chemotherapy plays a limited role in the management of ACC.[91] Recent studies have shown a tumor response to Imatinib mesylate, a potent inhibitor of KIT tyrosine kinase, an enzyme involved in the pathogenesis of the ACC.[92] Recurrence rates for ACC are high, with metastatic foci within the lungs commonly showing up decades after removal of the primary tumor. Although the short term prognosis for ACC in a child or adolescent is generally good, the long term prognosis is poor, with 15-year survival rates ranging between 29 and 55 percent.[89,90]

Polymorphous Low Grade Adenocarcinoma (PLGA)

PLGA, originally described using the term lobular carcinoma, is largely a tumor of palatal minor salivary glands.[93,94,95] PLGA occurs only rarely in major salivary glands, and even then, primarily as a component of carcinoma ex pleomorphic adenoma. PLGA is considered to originate from the intercalated terminal ducts of the salivary gland duct system. Presentation

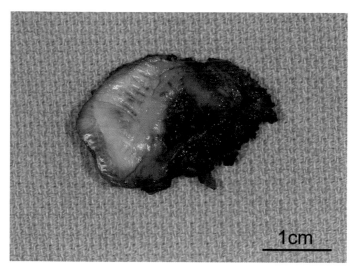

Figure 11.23 PLGA gross specimen, indicating the volume tumor of tissue needed to obtain tumor free margins. (Reprinted from Marx R, Stern D. *Oral and Maxillofacial Pathology: A Rationale for Diagnosis and Treatment* with permission from Quintessence Publishing Company).

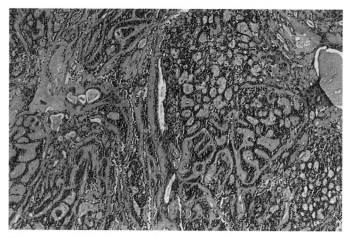

Figure 11.25 PLGA demonstrating Various architectural patterns, ductal aggregates and single file columns of tumor cells.

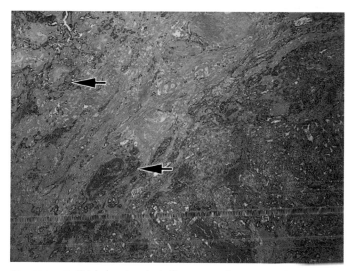

Figure 11.26 PLGA showing single file pattern of tumor growth (arrows) within a dense fibrous stroma.

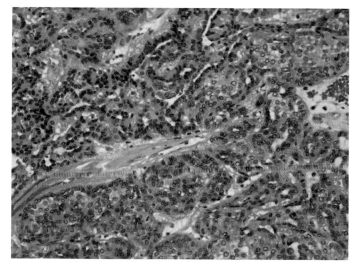

Figure 11.24 PLGA. Note the isomorphic uniform bland appearing tumor cells arranged in a streaming pattern.

outside the minor salivary glands of the oral cavity is quite rare,[96] and the tumor, when encountered in the pediatric age group, is almost uniformly seen in adolescents in the 12 to 18 year age group.[97,98,99,100]

Clinical Findings

Although tumors have been reported in the lacrimal glands, the nasopharynx and the sinonasal tract, the vast majority of tumors will present in the palate[98,99,100] as a firm, painless, slow growing submucosal mass that will occasionally ulcerate. PLGAs average 2 cm in diameter in most cases, and they are usually well circumscribed. Rarely do tumors show marginal infiltration of surrounding tissues, but bone invasion can occur.

Pathologic Findings

On gross inspection, PLGA will be an unencapsulated or but typically well circumscribed nodular mass (Figure 11.23). Histologically, PLGA will show an infiltrative growth pattern that will feature bland ovoid aggregates of streaming tumor cells with uniform isomorphic nuclei and only rare atypical cytologic features (Figure 11.24). Tumor cell aggregates can be arranged in various architectural patterns including *solid, trabecular, papillary, fascicular, cribriform and tubular patterns*. Individual tumor cells tend to be cuboidal and form small duct like structures or cribriform aggregates (Figure 11.25). Tumor cells may also be arranged in a whorled/targetoid, pattern, particularly when they are associated with nerves and blood vessels. In some instances, tumor cells will be arranged in a single-file pattern (Figure 11.26) as they penetrate a dense collagenous or muco-collagenous stroma. This pattern will particularly be seen at the peripheral margins of the tumor.

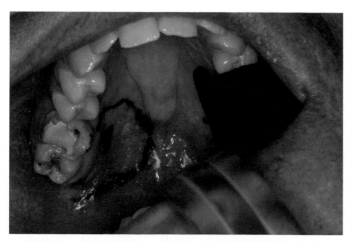

Figure 11.50 Palatectomy demonstrating the outline of the excision margins. (Reprinted from Marx R, Stern D. *Oral and Maxillofacial Pathology: A Rationale for Diagnosis and Treatment* with permission from Quintessence Publishing Company).

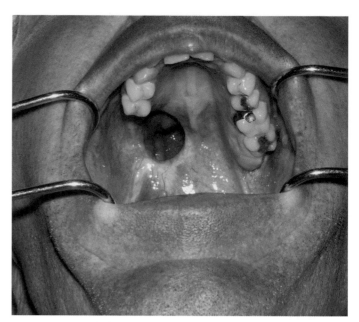

Figure 11.52 Healed palatectomy defect in an adult patient. (Reprinted from Marx R, Stern D. *Oral and Maxillofacial Pathology: A Rationale for Diagnosis and Treatment* with permission from Quintessence Publishing Company).

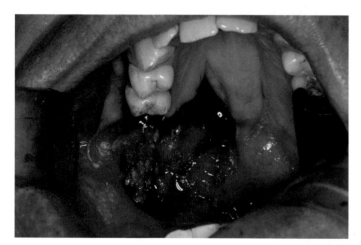

Figure 11.51 Initial wound after palatectomy. (Reprinted from Marx R, Stern D. *Oral and Maxillofacial Pathology: A Rationale for Diagnosis and Treatment* with permission from Quintessence Publishing Company).

The resultant defect is best managed with the use of a premade denture like palatal acrylic splint lined with a soft tissue liner, which is left in place for approximately ten days. The exposed palatal bone and any exposed soft palate musculature readily granulates to fibrous repair and wound completion in six weeks or less.

Palatectomy: A palatectomy is indicated in low grade salivary gland malignancies that have evidence of invasion into the bony palate and intermediate grade malignancies. This primarily encompasses intermediate grade MECs and some PLGAs.

The surgical excision should begin with a circumscribing incision over the anterior portion of the tumor from the 9 o'clock position to the 3 o'clock position similar to that employed for a soft tissue palatal tumor excision. However, with a palatectomy, periosteum is not reflected and the soft tissue component of the excision continues around the entire lesion. If the tumor extends posterior to the soft palate, the excision must extend through the thickness of the soft palate

into the nasal vault. A reciprocating saw is then inserted into the soft tissue incision so as to osteomize the palate in the same circumscribed fashion as the soft tissue incision (Figure 11.50). The tumor en-bloc within the palate can then be delivered with a resultant oral-antral-nasal communication (Figure 11.51). Because the alveolar ridge and any teeth within the alveolus will remain, an immediate surgical obturator only needs to cover the palate. As with a soft tissue palatal excision, the surgical obturator is best lined with a soft tissue liner and held in place by wiring it to several teeth or via a palatal screw if sufficient bony palate remains. This surgical obturator will need to be re-fitted over the first six months it is in place, because the surgical wound will diminish in size as soft tissue partially fills in the surgical defect and matures. Between six months and nine months the surgical wound becomes dimensionally stable and a permanent palatal obturator can be constructed with teeth if teeth are missing, in a fashion similar to a conventional denture as seen in examples in an adult patient (Figures 11.52 & 11.53).

Hemimaxillectomy: A formal hemimaxillectomy is indicated in children and adolescents most commonly for sarcomas such as osteosarcoma, fibrosarcoma, chondrosarcoma and rhabdomyosarcoma. However, the procedure may also be required for high grade MECs and the rare ACC in children. Most hemimaxillectomies are accomplished via a transoral approach. However, a Weber–Ferguson access is preferred if the tumor extends into the orbit, ethmoids, through the posterior wall of the maxilla into the retromaxillary space.

Transoral Hemimaxillectomy: A transoral hemimaxillectomy begins with a soft tissue excision circumscribing the clinical tumor and incudes both the labial and palatal extent of the

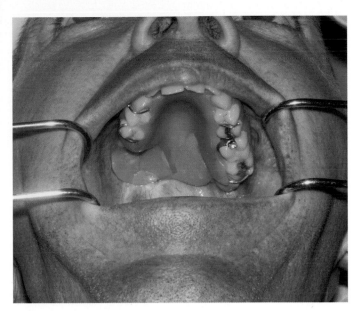

Figure 11.53 Partial denture like obturator for a palatectomy defect in an adult patient. (Reprinted from Marx R, Stern D. *Oral and Maxillofacial Pathology: A Rationale for Diagnosis and Treatment* with permission from Quintessence Publishing Company).

tumor thereby excising the alveolar ridge and the teeth contained therein. The osteotomy follows a 2.0 cm margin in bone. It is advisable to avoid a midline osteotomy between the central incisors because the nasal septum will deflect the saw cut and the remaining central incisor will be lost due to rotation into the defect. Therefore, it is best to accomplish most hemimaxillectomies through maxillary lateral incisor area, thereby leaving or removing both central incisors. The resultant defect is best obturated with an immediate acrylic surgical obturator splint fixated to remaining teeth via direct wiring, a palatal screw if sufficient palatal bone remains, clasping to remaining teeth or a fixation plate to the zygomatic-maxillary buttress.

Weber–Ferguson Approach Hemimaxillectomy: A Weber–Ferguson approach to a hemimaxillectomy is a lip split procedure which provides enhanced direct access for tumor removal. The inherent scar and potential for upper lip retraction, which can result in a postsurgical snarling appearance, can be minimized by the specifics of the incision design. The best cosmetic outcome is achieved using a midlid incision which dissects to the maxilla without incising through the orbicularis oculi. This is accomplished by retracting the muscle's inferior edge superiorly as the incision is deepened to the infraorbital rim. The skin incision moves to curve around the medial angle of the eye at the level of the lower eye lid and progresses around the nose. It is important to stay 1 to 1.5 mm away from the alar and subnasal creases. Placing the incision within these creases will cause the alar flare to roll inward, distorting the contour of the nose and affecting nasal breathing through that nostril. Additionally, the vertical lip split is best placed at the height of the philtrum ridge rather than the absolute midline between the two philtrum ridges.

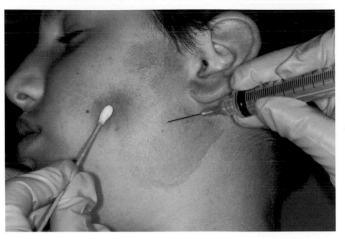

Figure 11.54 FNA biopsy. (Reprinted from Marx R, Stern D. *Oral and Maxillofacial Pathology: A Rationale for Diagnosis and Treatment* with permission from Quintessence Publishing Company).

The incision at the height of the ipsilateral philtrum ridge will end at the height of Cupid's bow of the upper lip. At this point the incision is carried along the vermillion–skin junction to the midline, where the lip split is completed through the vermillion. The right angle turns at the subnasal–philtrum junction and the philtrum–vermillion junction will act as "Z" plasty to prevent an upward retraction of the lip upon healing.

The oral component of the Weber–Ferguson incision encompasses the labial extent of the tumor from the midline to the tuberosity area, reflecting periosteum. Combined with the lip split and skin incisions the entire maxilla will come into view including the infraorbital rim, zygoma and pterygoid plates. The tumor can then be removed with the appropriate osteomies under direct vision. The resultant defect is manage with a surgical obturator splint fixated with wires or plates to the best available remaining bone, which is most often the zygoma. The Weber–Ferguson flap is then draped over the surgical obturator and closed in a layered fashion for the skin incisions, and as a single layer for the mucosa.

Parotid Surgeries

Fine Needle Aspirate (FNA): FNA is useful to assess masses in the parotid and to distinguish between inflammatory and neoplastic disease, or to distinguish between benign and malignant neoplasms, if neoplastic cells are observed.

The technique requires a 10 cc syringe, a 22 to 26 gauge needle, a dry glass microscopic slide and a fixative. The skin over the mass is anesthetized with local anesthetic and prepared with an antiseptic solution. The surgeon should stabilize the mass between his/her index and middle finger with one hand and hold the syringe-needle complex as one would hold a dart so as to gain maximum tactile sense. (Figure 11.54) The surgeon will note resistance entering the epidermis, followed by little resistance once that needle is in the subcutaneous layer or native parotid, followed by a second resistance indicating entry into the mass. The surgeon can confirm the needles location in the mass by toggling the mass between the middle

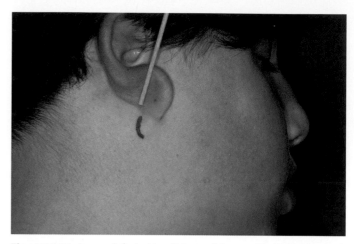

Figure 11.56 Approach for incisional biopsy of the parotid with incision made under the lobule of the ear. (Reprinted from Marx R, Stern D. *Oral and Maxillofacial Pathology: A Rationale for Diagnosis and Treatment* with permission from Quintessence Publishing Company).

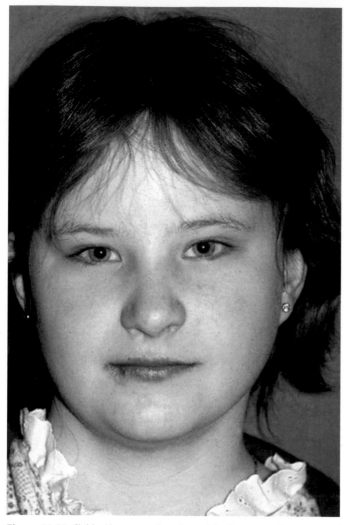

Figure 11.55 Child with xerostomia and parotid enlargement due to a mixed connective tissue autoimmune disease. (Reprinted from Marx R, Stern D. *Oral and Maxillofacial Pathology: A Rationale for Diagnosis and Treatment* with permission from Quintessence Publishing Company).

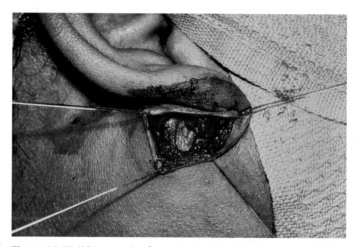

Figure 11.57 White capsule of parotid gland identifies the location of the incisional parotid biopsy. (Reprinted from Marx R, Stern D. *Oral and Maxillofacial Pathology: A Rationale for Diagnosis and Treatment* with permission from Quintessence Publishing Company).

and index finger. If the syringe moves with the mass it confirms the location of the needle in the mass. At that time, the surgeon should draw back forcibly on the plunger and withdraw the needle maintaining some negative pressure. The contents of the needle-syringe may not be seen by the naked eye as it represents only a few cells. The contents should be forcibly ejected onto the dry glass slide and smeared as thin as possible to create a monolayer, then quickly placed into the fixative or sprayed with a fixative spray to avoid drying and crenation of the cells.

Incisional Parotid Biopsy: An incisional parotid biopsy is only indicated as a diagnostic procedure in children for that rare instance in which a systemic disease enlarges the parotid gland or when there is suspicion of a disease such as sarcoidosis, Sjögren's disease or mixed connective tissue disease or the like. (Figure 11.55) If the lesion in question is a solid mass or a known parotid neoplasm, an incisional biopsy of the parotid is contraindicated.

The incisional biopsy is accomplished under local anesthesia with or without sedation. An incision is made under the lobule of the ear so as to access the tail of the parotid (Figure 11.56). In this location, the facial nerve is 3.2 cm deep to the skin and is therefore not at risk. The incision needs only to be 1.0 cm to 1.5 cm in length. It is deepened to the glistening white parotid capsule (Figure 11.57). A 1 cm wedge of parotid, including the capsule is excised from the tail of the parotid and submitted for a histopathologic examination (Figure 11.58). The capsule and skin are then closed in two layers. This excision of a superficial aspect of the parotid avoids any major ducts thereby avoiding the development of sialoceles.

The diagnostic yield of an incisional parotid sample is far superior to minor salivary gland biopsies even if the parotid is of normal size. The incisional biopsy will identify systemic disease sooner, and document a more advanced form of most

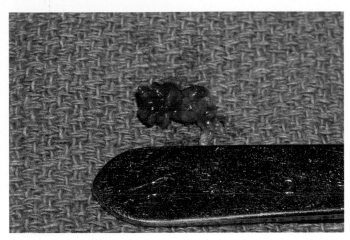

Figure 11.58 Diagnostic tissue obtained from the incisional parotid biopsy. (Reprinted from Marx R, Stern D. *Oral and Maxillofacial Pathology: A Rationale for Diagnosis and Treatment* with permission from Quintessence Publishing Company).

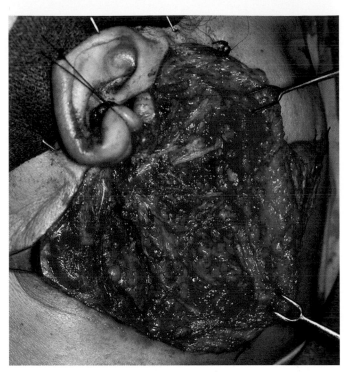

Figure 11.60 Identification of the facial nerve during a superficial parotidectomy. (Reprinted from Marx R, Stern D. *Oral and Maxillofacial Pathology: A Rationale for Diagnosis and Treatment* with permission from Quintessence Publishing Company).

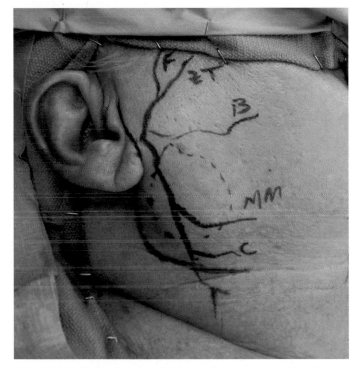

Figure 11.59 Outline for a superficial parotidectomy. (Reprinted from Marx R, Stern D. *Oral and Maxillofacial Pathology: A Rationale for Diagnosis and Treatment* with permission from Quintessence Publishing Company).

diseases, especially connective tissue disease, than minor salivary gland biopsies. It is therefore the preferred diagnostic procedure for suspected systemic diseases.

Superficial Parotidectomy: The superficial parotidectomy is the most common therapeutic surgical procedure performed on the parotid gland. The procedure is safe, avoids facial nerve encounters, and is accurate. This is due both to the fact that 80 percent of parotid masses are benign and that 80 percent of the gland volume is the superficial lobe leaving only 20 percent as the deep lobe through which the facial nerve

passes. The procedure is indicated for solitary masses in the superficial lobe that have a benign or low grade malignant suggestion by CT or MRI scans or a FNA demonstrating benign cells.

The Classic Central Superficial Parotidectomy: This approach has been a long time standard one in which the superficial lobe is initially dissected through in order to identify the trunk of the facial nerve after it exits the stylomastoid foramen. The incision is termed the "Blair" incision and incorporates a preauricular incision with a Risdon incision inferior to the inferior border of the mandible. These two incisions are connected by a curvilinear incision around the tail of the parotid (Figure 11.59). This completed incision allows the creation of an anterior based skin flap which can be sutured forward to expose the parotid gland.

The trunk of the facial nerve is found between four classic anatomic landmarks: the posterior border of the mandibular ramus, the cartilage meatus of the ear, the mastoid tip and the transverse process of the Atlas (C-1). The substance of the parotid is dissected through anterior to the anterior border of the sternocleidomastoid muscle, testing for nerve activation with an appropriate nerve tester. The trunk of the facial nerve is also located posterior to and at the same depth as the retromandibular vein.

Once the trunk of the facial nerve is identified and confirmed by stimulation, a hemostat is placed on the nerve with the beaks pointed upward and any parotid tissue swept off the hemostat. This process is followed anteriorly to the bifurcation

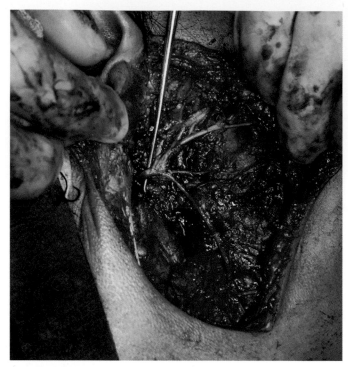

Figure 11.61 Completely skeletonizing the facial nerve risks a paresis due to disrupting the blood supply to the nerve. (Reprinted from Marx R, Stern D. *Oral and Maxillofacial Pathology: A Rationale for Diagnosis and Treatment* with permission from Quintessence Publishing Company).

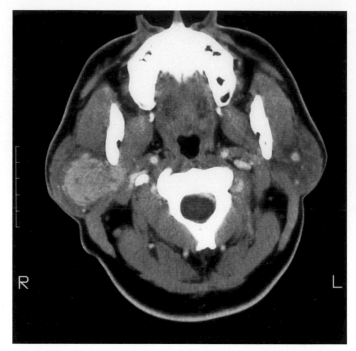

Figure 11.62 CT scan of a tumor extending into the deep lobe of the parotid referred to as a "dumbbell" shaped tumor. (Reprinted from Marx R, Stern D. *Oral and Maxillofacial Pathology: A Rationale for Diagnosis and Treatment* with permission from Quintessence Publishing Company).

of the inferior and superior nerve divisions. (Figure 11.60) As each division is followed, branching into the five classic branches, the tumor mass contained within parotid parenchyma follows. This composite continues to be swept anteriorly using a bipolar cautery to coagulate the small blood vessels that run along the nerve until the superficial lobe ends over the masseter muscle and the specimen is delivered. At this point, all branches of the facial nerve should be visible, with parotid parenchyma surrounding each branch to some degree. It is neither wise nor necessary to skeletonize the facial nerve or its branches. (Figure 11.61) Such disruption of the blood supply to the epineurium may result in as much as a 10 percent loss of facial nerve conduction.

The resultant defect is largely closed primarily with the return of the skin flap. The hollow concavity that results is usually well tolerated by individuals of thin or normal build. However, in those patients with a chubby or abundant cheek appearance of the type that often exists in teens, placement of a dermal fat graft, supported with platelet rich plasma, can be employed to reconstruct facial symmetry.

The Peripheral Superficial Parotidectomy Approach: This surgical approach achieves the same total removal of the superficial lobe of the parotid as the classic approach, but approaches the trunk of the facial nerve from outside the parotid. Its advantages are that it is more straightforward in locating the facial nerve and can more directly accomplish a

subtotal superficial parotidectomy in those cases where the tumor is limited to the tail of the parotid.

This peripheral approach begins with the same Blair incision previously outlined and the development of an anterior based skin flap. However, instead of a somewhat tedious dissection through 3 cm of parotid substance in order to locate the facial nerve trunk, the cervical branch is more easily located outside of the parotid gland and followed into the gland. Therefore, this approach starts in the neck and identifies the external jugular vein just deep to the platysma muscle. The cervical branch of the facial nerve always courses along the vein. The surgeon then dissects along the superficial surface of this branch into the parotid, identifying the cervico-facial division and the marginal mandibular branch, and sweeping the parotid parenchyma off these branches. The cervico-facial division is followed to the trunk of the facial nerve where the buccal branch and zygomatic-temporal division are identified. The tumor within the parenchyma of the gland's superficial lobe is then swept off these branches as well, ending anteriorly as the gland becomes extinguished as in the central approach.

For those tumors limited to the tail of the parotid this approach can end at the level of the buccal branch of the facial nerve without exposing or dissecting along the zygomatic-temporal branches.

Total Parotidectomy with Nerve Preservation: This surgical procedure is a variation of the superficial parotidectomy surgery. It is indicated for the uncommon finding of a tumor in

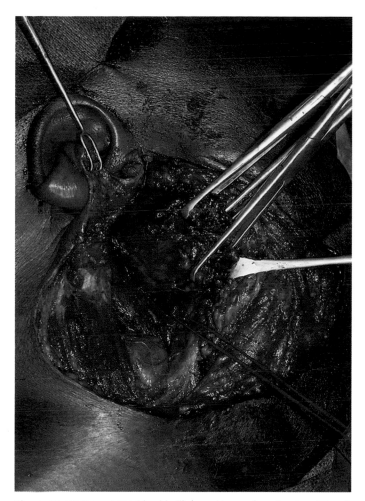

Figure 11.63 Removing a "dumbbell" shaped tumor from the deep lobe of the parotid in an adult. (Reprinted from Marx R, Stern D. *Oral and Maxillofacial Pathology: A Rationale for Diagnosis and Treatment* with permission from Quintessence Publishing Company).

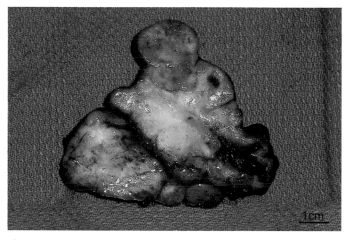

Figure 11.64 Large specimen removed via the "Attia" approach. (Reprinted from Marx R, Stern D. *Oral and Maxillofacial Pathology: A Rationale for Diagnosis and Treatment* with permission from Quintessence Publishing Company).

the superficial parotid lobe that extends into the deep lobe between the upper and lower divisions of the facial nerve in so-called dumb-bell tumor fashion (Figure 11.62).

The incision and dissection approaches are the same as that of either of the two previously outlined approaches to the superficial parotidectomy. However, when the zygomatic-temporal division and the cervico-facial nerve divisions are identified, each division is retracted. That is, the zygomatic-temporal division is retracted superiorly and the cervico-facial division retracted inferiorly. Depending on the origin of the buccal branch of nerve, this branch may be retracted with either of the other two divisions to allow direct access to the deep lobe while keeping all nerve branches intact (Figure 11.63).

Total Parotidectomy with Nerve Transection and Nerve Grafting: This is a lesser used surgical procedure today than in the past, due to the more common use of the nerve preservation approach just discussed. This approach is also a variation of either of the superficial parotidectomy approaches. Once the facial nerve and all its branches are exposed, each branch that blocks the access to the deep lobe (usually the zygomatic, temporal and buccal branches) are transected and tagged. The access to the deep lobe that is gained is used to remove the tumor, after which the nerve branches are re-anastamosed under magnification, or nerve grafts from the greater auricular nerve branches are performed. Due to the retraction of the transected nerve branches and the swelling in the surgical field, direct anastamosis of the facial nerve branches is often under tension making the use of nerve grafting more likely.

Deep Lobe of the Parotid Excision via Mandibular Osteotomy: This surgical approach offers direct access to any tumor within the deep lobe of the parotid or within the lateral or retropharyngeal space without risking injury to the facial nerve.

It is an approach that requires an extended submandibular retromandibular incision to gain direct access to the mandible. Once the mandible is exposed with reflection of its lateral soft tissue attachments, rigid 2.0 to 2.8 mm titanium plates are placed on the intact mandible anticipating osteotomies between the first and second bicuspid teeth or a tooth socket and a horizontal osteotomy above the lingula on the ramus. After fixating the plates using tapped screw holes and bicortical looking screws, the plate is removed and the anticipated osteomies accomplished. The mandibular segment between the two osteotomies is retracted superiorly creating direct access to the deep lobe of the parotid and lateral pharyngeal space. The osteotomized segment of the mandible becomes a vascularized bone flap by virtue of an intact inferior alveolar neurovascular bundle. The tumor and deep lobe (Figure 11.64) are subsequently removed and the viable mandibular segment replaced and fixated by reattaching the original plates. Known as the "Attia procedure," this approach is the preferred approach to the deep lobe of the parotid and the parapharyngeal spaces.

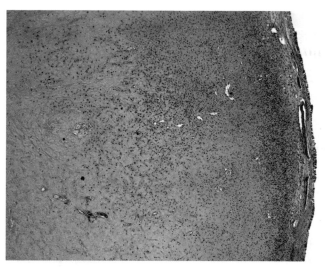

Figure 12.7 Low power photomicrograph of nasal chondro-mesenchymal hamartoma demonstrating proliferating fibroblasts and cartilage.

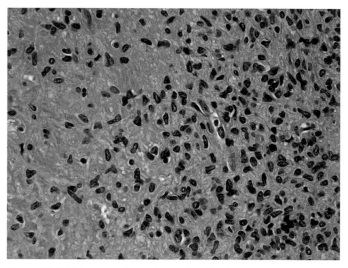

Figure 12.8 High power photomicrograph of the lesion seen in Figure 12.7 showing an admix of fibroblasts and myofibroblasts with areas of immature cartilage and a myxoid stromal component.

more often seen in older children (Figure 12.8). Blood-filled spaces lined by osteoclast like giant cells can sometimes be present. Nuclear atypia, necrosis or atypical mitosis will not be seen.

A unique *immunohistochemical* staining pattern has been reported for NCMH, which includes weak staining of stromal cells for CD68; moderate to strong staining of the lesion's stromal component for SMA; strong S100 protein staining of the cytoplasm and nuclei of the cartilaginous component of the lesion and focal weak S100 protein staining in both the stromal and the cartilaginous component of the lesion.

Complete surgical excision is the *treatment* of choice for NCMH. Treatment can be challenging due to the anatomic complexity of the nasal and paranasal sinus anatomic architecture. Recurrence, however, is uncommon.

Non-Neoplastic Diseases and Infections of the Nasal Cavity, Paranasal Sinuses and Nasopharynx

Sinonasal Polyps (SNP)

SNPs occur, albeit rarely, throughout the pediatric age-range without gender preference. However, SNPs are seldom seen in children under five years except in cases of cystic fibrosis (CF) where polyps are encountered in the late first decade and the second decades. The incidence of SNPs in patients with CF ranges from 6 to 48 percent.[47] In pediatric patients, asthma and nasal polyps can also occur successively and concurrently although the incidence is lower than in CF, ranging from 5.6 to 16 percent.[47,48]

SNPs are simply defined as a "non-neoplastic inflammatory swelling of the sinonasal mucosa." Their etiology is not well defined, but linked polyps have causally infection, allergy, CF, diabetes mellitus and aspirin hypersensitivity.[46]

The use of specific terms to define a nasal polyp include "allergic" or "inflammatory polyp" can be misleading as the etiology of any particular case may not be necessarily related to an established allergic, infectious or inflammatory condition.

Clinical Features

Pediatric age group patients will usually present with variable degrees of nasal obstruction, sneezing and rhinorrhea. Headaches are common as well. *Samtar's triad* is a term that has been used to describe children presenting with a combined history of asthma, aspirin intolerance and nasal polyposis. Nasal polyps can be single or multiple, unilateral or bilateral and the vast majority of nasal polyps arise along the lateral nasal wall and ethmoidal recess.

Radiographically, nasal polyps will present as mucosal thickening or density of soft tissue. Only rarely will polyps be destructive of bone; however, lesions can be large and dense enough to result in nasal sinus and paranasal sinus opacification.

Spontaneous lesional regression is rare although regression has been reported to be as high as 30 percent in children with CF.[49] Endoscopically, nasal polyps will demonstrate a so-called mulberry pattern in which the nasal turbinate becomes swollen and edematous.

Pathologic Findings

On gross inspection, the typical polyp appears soft, edematous with glistening surface and a delicate fine surface vascularity; older polyps tend to become more opaque and firm in consistency due to increased fibrosis. The size of a nasal polyp can vary from a few millimeters to many centimeters in largest dimension.

On microscopic examination, the mucosal surface is usually covered by respiratory type epithelium (Figure 12.9), unless continuous friction and surface irritation or ulceration results in squamous metaplasia (Figure 12.10). The lesional

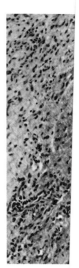

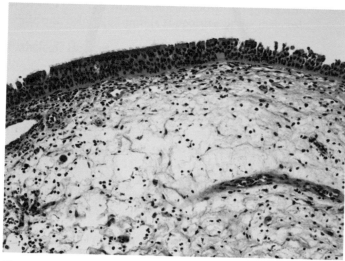

Figure 12.9 Nasal polyp covered by respiratory type epithelium. A prominent underlying myxoid/edematous stroma that contains a scattered chronic inflammatory cellular infiltrate is evident.

Figure 12.17 of lymphocyte

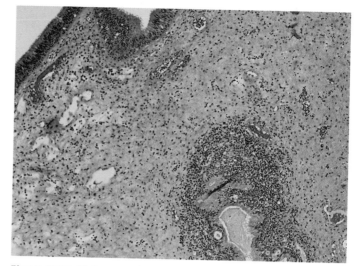

Figure 12.11 High power photomicrograph of a nasal polyp showing a fibrotic stroma with a chronic lymphoplasmacytic infiltrate and occasional eosinophils.

Rhinosinι

Rhinosinus
virus initia
affects the
Exceedingl·
can be acuι
to months.

The etiι
is multifac
ing most o
cations, pε
mucosa aι
dysfunctio
disease.[91,9]

In add
have been

Sympt
include na
and heada
lent disch

The cl
prompted
classificat

Imagi
rhinosinu
clinical e:
sal thicke
complica
rule out
or mass.

Pathologi

Rhinosin
features
respirato

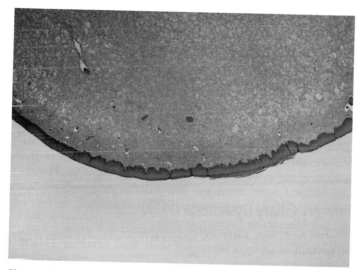

Figure 12.10 Nasal polyp showing squamous metaplasia of the epithelial surface and a dense underlying fibrotic stroma.

stroma is typically loose, edematous and may contain mucous glands and a chronic lymphoplasmacytic inflammatory infiltrate with eosinophils (Figure 12.11). Polyps that are left untreated start to show structural changes including increased surface ulceration, parenchymal increased vascularity and fibrosis, and glandular hyperplasia. The deposition of an amyloid like substance within the tumor stroma and cartilaginous and osseous metaplasia may be seen. Foci of granuloma formation may also be seen either as a spontaneous reaction to injury, or secondary to the use of intranasal medications. Mucous retention cysts can also be seen in association with nasal polyps. These cysts can rupture and create a significant inflammatory tissue reaction.[50,52]

Atypical stromal cells can become quite prominent in some SNPs, so much so that they can simulate malignant cells. These cells in fact represent a cellular reactive response to injury and likely represent myofibroblastic differentiation.[53]

The differential diagnosis for nasal polyps can be quite extensive and can include schneiderian papillomas, nasopharyngeal angiofibromas, REAH, infections (e.g. tuberculosis and sarcoidosis), heterotopic glial tissue and encephaloceles, Wegner's granulomatosis (WG) and malignant tumors, including rhabdomyosarcoma. Papillomas will have a multilayer corrugated epithelial surface. REAH will feature a prominent glandular component. Nasopharyngeal angiofibroma will be characterized by vascular spaces that do not have a smooth muscle wall. Glial tissue and encephaloceles with be IHC positive for GFAP. WG will be rich in eosinophils and giant cells, and rhabdomyosarcoma will be IHC positive for myogenic markers.

Antrochoanal polyps[54,55,56] represent a form of SNP that originates from the maxillary sinus ostium, or from a stalk that extends through the sinus ostium into the nasal cavity, where it can continue to grow, often extending into the nasopharynx. Tumors are usually single and unilateral and they are histologically similar to SNP except for the presence of fewer mucous cells and eosinophils in the tumor stroma. The presence of a long stalk in these types of polyps predisposes them to infarction. The polyp may show extensive vascularization almost simulating a vascular tumor. (Figure 12.12) Rarely, sphenochoanal polyps arising in the sphenoid sinus can present simultaneously with antrochoanal polyps.[58]

The antrochoanal polyp can resemble nasopharyngeal angiofibroma, or a vascular neoplasm microscopically.

Treatment and Prognosis

Nasal polypectomy is the treatment of choice. A caldwell luc sinus entry procedure can be used to treat antrochoanal polyps, as can functional endoscopic sinus surgery, which has decreased patient morbidity considerably. Approximately one-half of patients will experience a recurrence.

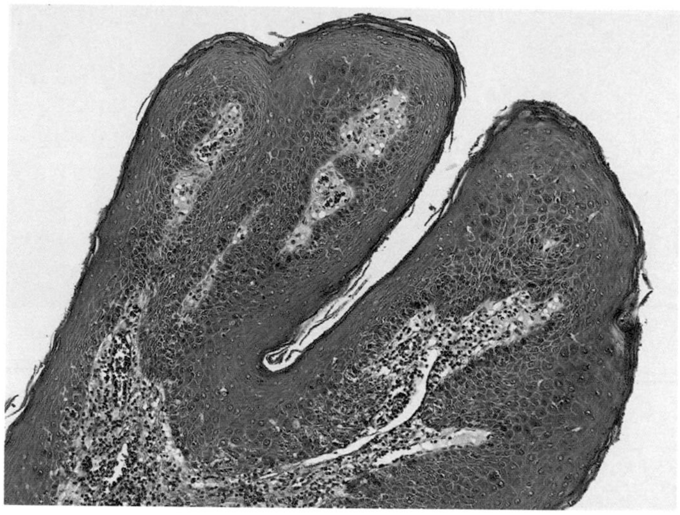

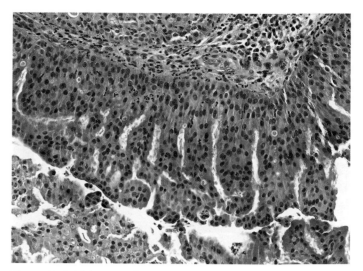

Figure 13.6 Exophytic (septal) papilloma showing squamous epithelial fronds covered by a thin layer of keratin and parakeratin.

Figure 13.8 High power photomicrograph of a Schneiderian oncocytic papilloma showing oncocytic change in the tumor's multilayered epithelium.

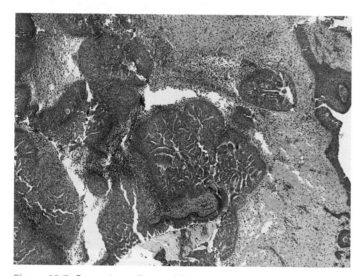

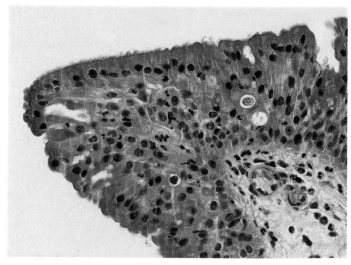

Figure 13.7 Oncocytic papilloma exhibiting an endophytic growth pattern.

Figure 13.9 Schneiderian oncocytic papilloma demonstrating the formation of round isolated intraepithelial mucin cysts.

failed to confirm any acceptable cases in the pediatric age group. Most tumors will occur in patients over 50 years of age. However, a lack of reports of such cases does not exclude their presence in children.[16]

On gross inspection, the oncocytic papilloma will be a brown to red corrugated/polypoid firm to friable nodule or mass. On microscopic examination, the lesion will be composed of both exophytic and endophytic epithelial components that will consist of proliferating, multilayered epithelial fronds 5 to 10 cells in thickness (Figure 13.7). Columnar tumor cells, which display granular eosinophilic cytoplasm, vesicular nuclei with prominent nucleoli and occasional cilia can be seen (Figure 13.8). Ultrastructurally, tumor cells can be confirmed to be oncocytes rich in mitochondria.[16] Intraepithelial mucous cysts (Figure 13.9), or microabscesses containing neutrophils may be present, and the intervening and supporting tumor

stroma is generally myxoid to fibrous. Dysplasia and malignant transformation occurs in between 4 and 17 percent of cases in adults.[17] Transition in children is exceedingly rare. The tumor must be differentiated from rhinosporidiosis and low grade papillary oncocytic carcinoma of the nasal cavity and paranasal sinuses. Rhinosporidiosis will display submucosal as well as intraepithelial cysts that will be filled with microorganisms, unlike the oncocytic papilloma. Oncocytic carcinomas will appear cytologically malignant.

Treatment and Prognosis of Schneiderian Papillomas

Functional endoscopic sinus surgery with complete surgical excision is the treatment of choice for the entire group of benign Schneiderian neoplasms of the nasal and paranasal sinuses. Incomplete resection will most often result in a recurrence. Unfortunately, there are no reliable features that enable one to predict the propensity for this polypoid group of tumors to undergo malignant transformation.[18] However, the presence of focal dysplasia should alert the pathologist to perform a thorough search of all submitted tissue for any evidence of malignancy. Treatment for rare malignancies reported in adults will include surgery and radiation therapy. Malignant transition of tumors in the pediatric age group is, however, unreported.

Vascular Tumors

Juvenile Nasopharyngeal Angiofibroma (JNA)

JNA is a rare highly vascular, hormonally influenced tumor that was first documented by Chauveau in 1906, and later, further characterized by Friedberg in 1940.[19,20,21] The tumor is typically seen in adolescent males. JNA is thought to be testosterone dependent, and has been shown to contain androgen receptors. JNA accounts for only 0.1 percent of all head and neck neoplasms.[21,22] However, the reported incidence of JNA is 3.7 cases per million when considering the population at risk,[22] adolescents to young men less than 20 years of age. JNA originates in the nasopharynx and although the tumor is benign, it is locally aggressive and destructive, and thus problematic in terms of its initial management, and recurrence.

Clinical Features

Most individuals with JNA will present with frequently recurrent, and sometimes severe, epistaxis, obstructive nasal symptoms, anosmia and cranial nerve deficits. Facial swelling, proptosis, diplopia and otitis media may also be manifest. The tumor most commonly occurs in the posterolateral portion of the roof of the nasal cavity. If left untreated, it can extend beyond the nasal cavity, and into the pterygopalatine fossa or into the intracranial cavity and base of the skull.[23] A familial predisposition to JNA can be seen familial adenomatous polyposis

(FAP) patients who have been shown to have an increased incidence of JNA in age matched groups[24].

CT scans and MRI scans will tend to demonstrate bone and soft tissue destruction by the tumor, and an anterior bowing of the posterior wall of the maxillary sinus on CT, with displacement of the pterygoid plates posteriorly, is highly supportive of a JNA diagnosis. Angiography is important in identifying tumor feeder vessels, and tumor embolization prior to surgery is often employed in order to reduce blood loss from the tumor, which can be quite significant.[25] Consumptive coagulopathy has been reported in some patients with JNA and although classification systems have been devised to categorize the various forms of JNA in terms of tumor extension, no general consensus on a standard classification schema has been adopted.[26]

Pathologic Findings

On gross inspection, tumors can be either a red, tan or grey, sessile or pedunculated nodular to multi-nodular mass with a rubbery consistency. On microscopic examination, JNA will consist of a fibrocollagenous neoplastic growth that is admixed with variably sized small to large thin walled vessels that may have a staghorn appearance (Figure 13.10) and vessels will be lined by a flat or plump single layer of endothelial cells (Figure 13.11). A smooth muscle layer of variable thickness and continuity may be seen surrounding these vessels. No elastic fibers will be seen. Tumor stromal cells will be spindle to stellate with plump nuclei, and tumor cells will radiate around the vessels (Figures 13.12, 13.13 & 13.14). Mast cells may be seen. Tumor cell nuclear pleomorphism is usually mild if present. Tumors may show evidence of embolization within blood vessels when treated (Figure 13.15).

On immunohistochemical assessment of the neoplasm, CD31 and CD34 stains will highlight the endothelial cell component. Smooth muscle immunohistochemical (IHC) markers, including smooth muscle actin (SMA) and calponin will be

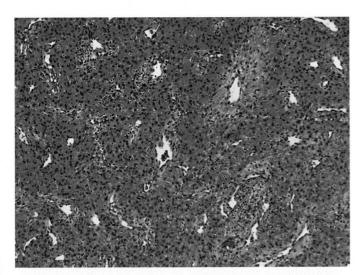

Figure 13.10 JNA. Low power photomicrograph exhibiting the major histomorphologic components of the lesion: a fibrous stroma, and thin walled vessels with a dilated staghorn or slit-like appearance.

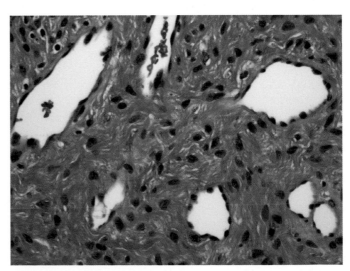

Figure 13.11 High power photomicrograph of JNA demonstrating vessels lined by plump endothelial cells.

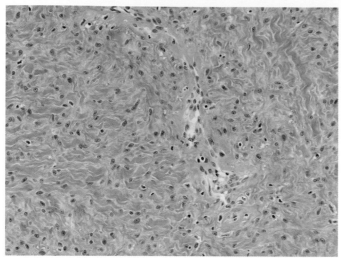

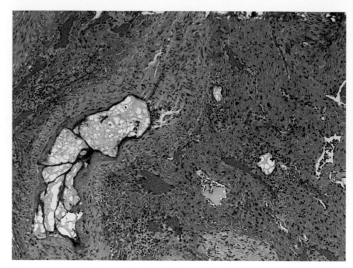

Figure 13.15 JNA demonstrating a blood vessel containing embolization material within the lumen.

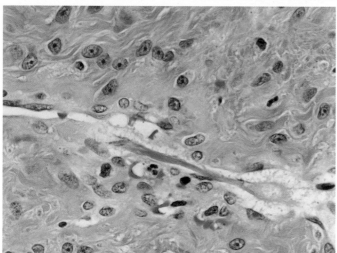

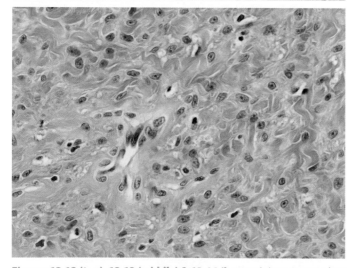

Figures 13.12 (top), 13.13 (middle) & 13.14 (bottom) Low, intermediate and high power photomicrographs of a JNA showing endothelially lined blood vessels set in a stroma composed of spindle cells and stellate cells radiating around vessels.

strongly positive in the muscle of vessel walls. Stromal stellate cells will be vimentin positive, and stromal and endothelial cells will be androgen receptor positive.

Differential diagnoses include antrochoanal polyp, inflammatory angiomatous polyp, lobular capillary hemangioma (LCH) and nerve sheath tumor. Antrochoanal polyps will lack the vascularity of a JNA, as will inflammatory angiomatous polyps. The LCH (pyogenic granuloma) will be rich in granulation tissue and richly chronically inflamed, unlike HNA.

Treatment and Prognosis

The approaches to treatment of JNA are not uniformly agreed upon. Open surgical resection, pure endoscopic resection or endoscopic assisted surgery has most often been employed.[21] Data from a number of studies suggest surgery that is purely endoscopic and open surgical approaches are equally as effective without a significant difference in recurrence rate identified between the two. Recurrence rates for the tumor vary between 6 and 24 percent. Embolization angiography and radiation therapy have also been employed successfully as treatments. Malignant transformation is quite uncommon, and when it occurs, the transformation been linked to previous radiation therapy.[27]

Sinonasal-type Hemangiopericytoma (Glomangiopericytoma) (SNHPC)

Hemangiopericytoma, first described by Stout and Murray in 1942,[1] is considered to be an uncommon benign vascular tumor with indolent behavior, although some investigators consider the tumor to have borderline/low-grade malignant potential. Fifteen to twenty-five percent of all hemangiopericytomas occur in the head and neck region.[2] The tumor is encountered more commonly in adults than children, with approximately 5 to 10 percent of cases occurring in children. Pediatric SNHPCs tend to behave in a more benign manner than those of adults.

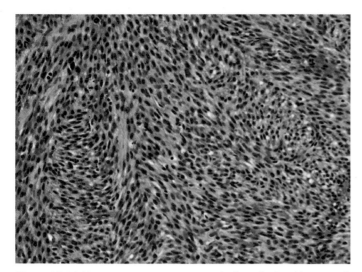

Figure 13.16 Hemangiopericytoma composed of spindle shaped tumor cells with ovoid to spindle shaped nuclei with blunted ends. Note the tumor's fascicular growth pattern.

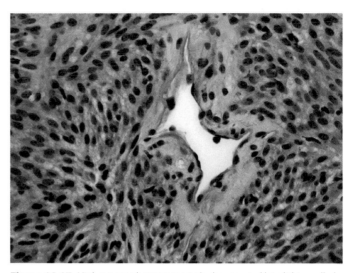

Figure 13.17 High power photomicrograph showing a dilated thin walled staghorn type vessel in a hemangiopericytoma with associated perivascular hyalinization.

HNTHPC is derived from perivascular modified smooth muscle cells, the so-called myloid/pericytic cells.[3] No definitive etiology for the tumor has been documented.

Thompson et al.[4] in a study of 104 sinonasal hemangiopericytomas including tumors in pediatric age group patients, concluded that the SNHPC, with its characteristic glomus-like differentiation has a distinctly different lesion, histopathologically, from soft tissue hemangiopericytomas.[4] Tumors present over a wide age-range with the seventh decade representing the mean; however, tumors have been reported to have an age-range of 5 to 86 years.[4] There is no significant gender predilection and the age at which tumors present has little bearing on the ultimate outcome.

Clinical Features

Patients with HNTHPC will commonly present with a unilateral nasal mass causing obstructive symptoms and epistaxis. Other non-specific symptoms including sinusitis, headaches, pain, difficulty breathing, changes in the sense of smell and discharge have been reported.[3,4] Radiologic findings including CT imaging will depend upon the size and location of the tumor mass and may show a multitude of findings including sinus opacification, bone erosion by the tumor, bone expansion or sclerosis.[4] The cribriform plates are normally spared and angiograms may be characterized by a so-called tumor blush. Tumors in females tend to be slightly larger than those in males, averaging 3 cm in diameter, while tumors in males average 2.5 cm in diameter.

Pathologic Features

On gross inspection, tumors will be pink to red, firm and polypoid.[2,4,5] On microscopic examination,[2,4,5] the tumor will be covered by respiratory epithelium with a subjacent proliferation of spindle to ovoid tumor cells. Tumor cell nuclei will have blunted ends and hyperchromatic chromatin. A wide variety of growth patterns can be seen, including a whorled, storiform, fascicular, palisaded or reticular pattern of tumor cell growth. Tumor cells will have indistinct borders and clear to eosinophilic cytoplasm without significant pleomorphism or mitosis as they proliferate syncytially (Figure 13.16). The tumor can exhibit zones of marginally hyalinized vascular spaces, or dilated thin wall vascular channels that display an irregular Staghorn appearance (Figure 13.17). Extravasated red blood cells and inflammatory cells are usually seen scattered throughout the tumor stroma. Foci of keloid-like collagen deposition similar to that seen in the solitary fibrous tumor (SFT) may be seen.

Reticulin stains will highlight individual tumor cells outlined by a distinct cell membrane. Vimentin, muscle specific actin (MSA), SMA and factor XIII/a IHC stains will be positive in nearly all cases with factor VIIIA stains showing the most frequent negative immunoreactivity among the three. Variable target cell reactivity for CD34, S100 protein and epithelial membrane antigen (EMA) can be seen as in (Figure 13.18), but these stains are more often negative than positive. The tumor will stain negatively for pancytokeratin, Factor VIII, CD99, CD68, Neurone specific enolase (NSE) and CD117.

Differential diagnoses microscopically can include LCH, nasopharyngeal angiofibroma, glomus tumor, solitary fibrous tumor (SFT), fibrosarcoma, synovial sarcoma and mesenchymal chondrosarcoma. The SFT will, unlike HNTHPC, display dense collagen deposition that is often scar-like. Fibrosarcoma will be only vimentin positive, cytologically atypical, largely, and be composed of elongated spindle cells. Nasopharyngeal angiofibroma will demonstrate a more marked hyalinization of its tumor stroma than HNTHPC, and sarcomas, be they mesenchymal or synovial, will display significant tumor cell cytologic atypia.

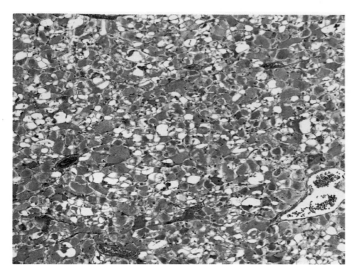

Figure 13.23 Nasal rhabdomyoma showing closely packed polygonal skeletal muscle cells.

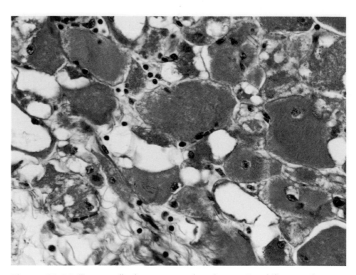

Figure 13.24 Tumor cells demonstrate abundant eosinophilic granular cytoplasm, often with peripheral vacuoles and cross striations.

Smooth muscle tumors of uncertain potential (SMTUMP)[47,48] represent neoplasms which are histopathology characterized by increased cellularity, moderate nuclear pleomorphism and no more than 4 mitosis/10 high power field. These tumors are primarily encountered in uterine leiomyomas, but have also occasionally been described in the nasal cavity in children.[46,49]

Treatment and Prognosis

Complete surgical excision of the nasal leiomyoma is curative.

Nasal Rhabdomyoma

Rhabdomyoma is a rare benign neoplasm of rhabdomyoblasts that can be seen in both children and adults. The tumor shows a predilection for the head and neck region, with *nasal fetal rhabdomyoma* representing the most common presentation in the pediatric age group.[50,51,52,53]

On microscopic examination, the tumor will show aggregates of rhabdomyoblasts in various stages of differentiation including strap cells and atypical appearing spindle cells. In spite of its primitive histologic appearance, the lesion is usually well defined and marginated clinically and it will not show evidence of invasion, necrosis or the typical cytologic features associated with rhabdomyosarcoma. More differentiated adult type rhabdomyomas, which rarely can occur in pediatric age group patients[54] will demonstrate sheets of large, well differentiated skeletal muscle cells. Most adult type cases have occurred in the tongue, however, and Veziroglu et al. report in an extensive literature review that only 160 total cases of adult rhabdomyoma have been documented in the entire head and neck region in children.[54] Tumor cells are round or polygonal with abundant eosinophilic fibrillar or granular cytoplasm that shows frequent cross striations or intracytoplasmic rod-like inclusions (Figures 13.23 & 13.24). Tumor cell nuclei are small, round and vesicular, and may have prominent nucleoli.

Osseous, Fibro-osseous, Cartilaginous and Fibro/Myxoid Tumors

Sinonasal Osteoma

Osteomas are benign slow growing osteogenic tumors that are composed of mature, compact or cancellous bone. They are the most common non-epithelial tumors of the facial region,[55] seen most frequently in the mandible (particularly the angle) and far less frequently in the nasal sinuses. The frontal sinus will be involved in 96 percent of cases, the ethmoid sinus in 2 percent of cases and the maxillary sinuses in 2 percent of cases. The sphenoid sinus is rarely involved.[56,57] Osteomas have a peak incidence in the fourth and sixth decades of life, but can be also seen in the pediatric age group.[55,58,59]

Many sinonasal osteomas are asymptomatic and are only discovered incidentally during radiologic examination for other reasons such as minor trauma to the involved region. However, paranasal sinus tumors can be associated with pain, headache, facial distortion proptosis and sinusitis. Imaging studies will show a radiodense compact mass with focal radiolucencies. Most patients are conservatively followed up without surgical intervention.[60] However, tumors that cause symptomology may require resection.

Pathologic Features

Grossly, osteomas can be sessile or polypoid. They generally will have a smooth or Bosselated surface and cut sections can show so-called ivory bone, trabecular bone or both. Histologically, tumors will be composed of dense mature lamellar bone, with associated interosseous spaces that may contain adipose tissue and bone marrow elements (Figures 13.25 & 13.26). Nasal osteomas as well as and other craniofacial sinus osteomas do not have the potential for malignant transformation and some investigators suggest that they may indeed not represent a true neoplasm, but are rather an end-stage reactive, or fibro-osseous proliferation.[61,62]

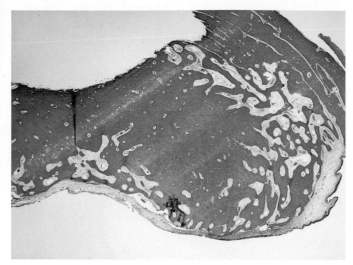

Figure 13.25 Sinonasal osteoma of the frontal sinus made up of dense compact bone.

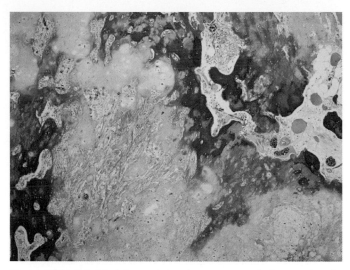

Figure 13.27 Lobulated sinonasal chondroma composed of aggregates of cytologically bland chondrocytes and marginated by bony trabecula.

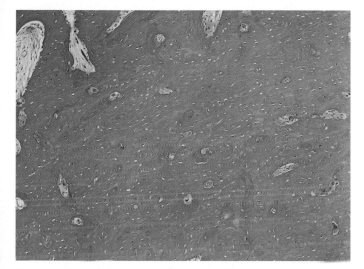

Figure 13.26 Sinonasal osteoma showing lamellar bone trabeculae and a peripheral focus of fibrovascular stroma.

Treatment and Prognosis

Surgical excision is curative. The type of the surgical procedure employed will depend on the size of the tumor. Small tumors can be endoscopically removed, while larger lesions may require an external surgical approach.

Fibro-Osseous Lesions

The most commonly encountered fibro-osseous lesions that present in the sinonasal tract include ossifying fibroma, psammomatoid ossifying fibroma, cemento-ossifying fibroma and fibrous dysplasia. All of these lesions can be seen in pediatric age group patients, particularly fibrous dysplasia and psammomatoid ossifying fibroma, both of which tend to present most frequently in the first and second decades of life. Psammomatoid ossifying fibroma has a particular predilection for the ethmoid sinus and supraorbital frontal lesion. These disorders are discussed in detail in Chapter 16.

Sinonasal Chondroma

Chondromas arise only rarely in the sinonasal region,[63] and their presence in the head and neck region is most commonly in the larynx.[64,65] Those sinonasal chondromas that are seen in pediatric age group patients occur most often in the adolescents. The peak age of occurrence when all age groups are considered, is between 20 and 30 years of age. Tumors are thought to originate from embryonic remnants of cartilaginous cells that are not resorbed. [66]

Chondromas are slow growing tumors[63,65] that in the sinonasal tract will most frequently arise from the paranasal sinuses (particularly the sphenoid and ethmoid sinuses), the nasal bone and the nasal septum, primarily the posterior septum.

The location and size of the tumor will largely determine symptomatology, which can range from a lack of symptoms to obstruction and even disfigurement. Tumors are typically well defined on CT scans, presenting as a well-defined radiodense mass. On microscopic inspection, chondromas will be lobulated tumors that are usually surrounded by a fibrous capsule, and composed of mature hyaline cartilage with bland, cytologically normal appearing chondrocytes (Figures 13.27 & 13.28). Differential diagnoses can include well differentiated chondrosarcoma, however, the nuclear atypia, focal necrosis and abnormal mitosis, typical of that tumor, will not be evident microscopically in the chondroma.

Treatment and Prognosis

The treatment of choice for the sinonasal chondroma is surgical excision, and recurrences are infrequent.

Myxoma and Fibromyxoid Tumors

Nasal myxomas and fibromyxoid tumors are rare in the pediatric age group.[67,68,69,70,71,72] Most such neoplasms in

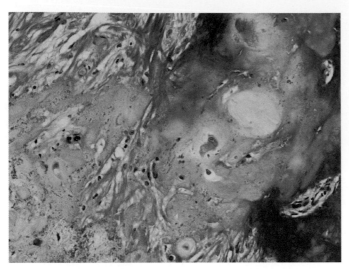

Figure 13.28 High power photomicrograph of sinonasal chondroma demonstrating bland, cytologically normal appearing chondrocytes.

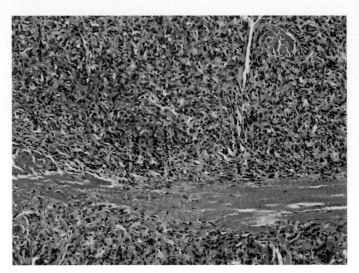

Figure 13.29 SFT demonstrating a spindle cell neoplasm that shows no specific cellular pattern of arrangement. Aggregates of collagen fibers (amianthoid fibers) and variable tumor vascularity is evident.

the head and neck region are of odontogenic origin and occur in the jaws.

Myxomas in the nasal sinuses can present as an asymptomatic mass or they can produce obstructive symptoms. Radiologically, tumors will be well circumscribed with a calcified rim and they may demonstrate zones of calcification. Most tumors in pediatric age group patients will occur in adolescents and while most tumors will involve bone, rare soft tissue myxomas can occur.[73]

Pathologic Features

On microscopic examination, myxomas tend to be lobular or multinodular with a surrounding shell of lamellar bone. The tumor will consist of spindle cells or ovoid cells with vesicular nuclei, eccentrically located nucleoli and eosinophilic cytoplasm. The tumor stroma can be fibromyxoid, hyalinized or collagenized, and cartilage formation and osteoid formation may be seen. Nasosinus tumors, unlike jaw tumors, are considered not to have an aggressive pathobiology.

Major differential diagnoses can include inflammatory sinonasal polyp peripheral nerve sheath tumor, chondroid syringoma, myxoid chondrosarcoma and epithelioid smooth muscle tumors.

Clonal chromosomal aberrations have been detected in myxomas in this site, including a 6p21 mutations, and balanced or unbalanced (6; 12)(p21; q24) translocations. Overexpression of EAAT4 and underexpression of PMP22 may also be seen, as well as a loss of INI-1 at 22q11.2. PHF1 gene rearrangement at 7q21 has also been identified in sinonasal myxomas.[74,75,76,77,78]

Treatment and Prognosis

Sinonasal myxomas can be treated by enucleation and curettage. However, the considerable recurrence rate, although not as high as in the jaws, has led some investigators to favor resection. An alternative approach can include peripheral

osteotomy to remove the peripheral margins. Recurrence of bone around the tumor can range as high as 25 percent.

Solitary Fibrous Tumor (SFT) of the Nasal Cavity

The SFT of the nasosinuses is quite rare in pediatric age patients.[80,81] Tumors which will be composed of spindle cell aggregates of tumors cells in a so-called patternless arrangement (Figure 13.29) are discussed in detail in Chapter 2.

Ectopic Pituitary Adenoma

Sinonasal ectopic pituitary adenomas are rare benign pituitary gland neoplasms that occur separate from, and without involvement of, the sella turcica. The anterior pituitary will be normal in patients with this tumor;[82,83,84] however, instances of sinonasal pituitary adenomas associated with an empty sella have been documented[84] in both adults and children.[82] Tumors, which are functional, are considered to be a derivative of remnants of the embryonic pituitary gland that are left behind during the gland's migration from Rathke's pouch.

Clinical Features

Pediatric age individuals with an ectopic pituitary adenoma may be asymptomatic or they may complain of chronic sinusitis, obstructive symptoms, headache and visual field defects. Females are more often affected than males. CT and MR imaging studies and CT scans are crucial to the discovery of ectopic pituitary adenoma,[85] and will classically show an isointense mass within the sphenoid sinus.

Pathologic Features

On microscopic inspection, the tumor will usually have a lobular, sheet-like infiltrative growth pattern. Tumor cells will be small, with round to ovoid shaped nuclei and the nuclear chromatin will display a neuroendocrine appearance with

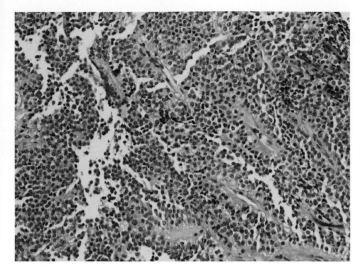

Figure 13.30 Ectopic pituitary adenoma composed of infiltrative groups of small neuroendocrine appearing cells.

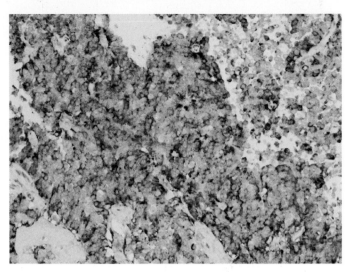

Figure 13.32 Ectopic pituitary adenoma. Immunohistochemical staining with the neuroendocrine marker chromogranin stains target tumor cells, confirming the neuroendocrine nature of the tumor.

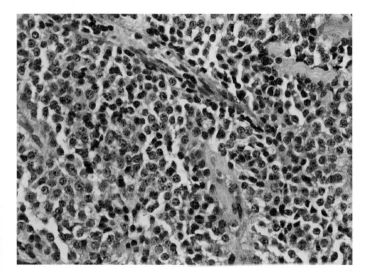

Figure 13.31 Round to oval tumor cell nuclei demonstrate a so-called salt and pepper appearance with clumping of nuclear chromatin in this ectopic pituitary adenoma.

so-called salt and pepper clumping (Figure 13.30). The tumor's growth pattern can be organoid, trabecular, glandular or insular, and the tumor's stroma will be fibrous and well collagenized. (Figure 13.31)

Tumor cells may have grooves, folds and intranuclear inclusions, and the cytoplasm of tumor cells can range from amphophilic, to eosinophilic, to granular, to clear. Rare psammoma bodies may be seen.

The neoplasm will display variable positive IHC staining for pancytokeratin and cam 5.2. Synaptophysin, CD56 and chromogranin[82] represent the most sensitive endocrine markers for the tumor (Figure 13.32).

Differential microscopic diagnoses will include olfactory neuroblastoma, melanoma, meningioma, paraganglioma, neuroendocrine carcinoma and Ewing/PNET sarcoma. Olfactory

neuroblastoma will stain negatively for chromogramin and keratin markers, as will Ewing sarcoma/PNET. Meningioma will have a whorled appearance rather than a lobular or sheet-like one, and will display intranuclear inclusions, while staining negatively for neuroendrocrine markers. Melanoma will tend to be made up of epithelioid or spindle cells and will stain positively for S100 protein, melan-A, HMB-45 and negatively for neuroendocrine markers.

Treatment and Prognosis

Surgical excision of the tumor is the treatment of choice for the ectopic pituitary adenoma. Radiotherapy has been employed for large tumors, although its risks, macular ischemia, vasculopathy and optic neuropathy, are significant. The use of Bromocriptine, a dopamine antagonist has been employed to control the tumor's associated hormonal effects. The prognosis for patients is excellent if the tumor is completely excised.

Sinonasal Meningiomas

Primary extracranial sinonasal meningiomas are quite rare in both adults and pediatric age group patients.[86,87,88,89] The average age for such tumors is 40 to 50 and females are slightly favored. Two types of sinonasal meningiomas occur: 1) Meningiomas that arise in the sinonasal tract from extracranial extension of an intracranial meningioma and 2) primary extracranial meningiomas that arise from ectopic arachnoid tissue in the nasal cavity, nasopharynx or sinuses.[90] Etiologically, extracranial sinonasal meningiomas of either type have several developmental sources:[91,92]

- The accumulation of arachnoid cells from sheaths of cranial and spinal nerves or vessels that migrate through the skull foramina and suture lines.

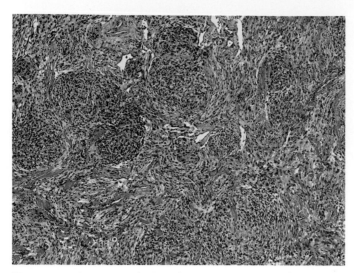

Figure 13.33 Meningioma showing characteristic small nests of tumor cells arranged in a whorled pattern.

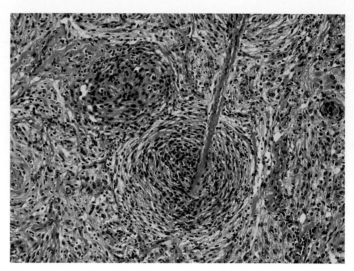

Figure 13.34 High power photomicrograph showing hyperchromatic tumor cells within tumor nests with no distinct borders.

- Displaced pachydermal body detachment during embryogenesis.
- Trauma or cerebral hypertension that displaces arachnoid islets.
- Undifferentiated multipotent mesenchymal cells.

Clinical Features

Patient symptomatology will vary in the pediatric age group patient with a sinonasal meningioma, and depending on the anatomic site of the tumor, symptoms may include obstructive symptomatology, sinusitis, headache, rhinitis, occasional epistaxis exopthalmous, periorbital edema and ptosis.[93]

Pathologic Features

Grossly, tumors will be gray to tan with an intact mucosal surface and a firm to gritty cut surface. Histopathologically, meningiomas can be classified as meningothelial, fibroblastic, syncytial or transitional neoplasms. The meningotheliomatous meningioma represents the most common histologic subtype. Microscopically, the tumor will show a lobular whorled growth pattern with an intervening fibrous tissue (Figure 13.33). Hyperchromatic tumor cells that have round, oval or spindle-shaped nuclei (Figure 13.34). The cytoplasm of tumor cells will be pale with indistinct borders. Intranuclear inclusions and psammoma bodies may be seen.

Immunohistochemically, tumors will be reactive to EMA but show no reactivity to neuroendocrine markers including chromogranin and synaptophysin.

Differential diagnoses include olfactory neuroblastoma, melanoma and paraganglioma. Olfactory neuroblastoma will demonstrate rosette and pseudo rosette formations of cells, unlike meningioma. Melanoma will show positive immunoreactivity to melanoma IHC markers and paraganglioma will be immunoreactive to S100 protein, unlike meningioma.

Treatment and Prognosis

Treatment includes complete surgical extirpation without the need for adjuvant therapy and the prognosis for pediatric age patients with an ectopic meningioma is excellent.[89]

Juvenile Fibromatosis of the Nose and Paranasal Sinuses (Desmoid Type Fibromatosis)

The juvenile fibromatoses are a group of non-metastasizing, well differentiated fibrous connective tissue proliferations that have a tendency to invade locally.[94,95,96,97] Head and neck fibromatoses account for 23 percent of all extra-abdominal desmoid fibromatoses that are seen in adults, and 33 percent of such lesions in children.[94,98,99] In the sinonasal and nasopharyngeal regions, the maxillary sinus is the most common site of involvement, but the nasal cavity, ethmoid sinuses and, to a lesser extent, the nasopharynx can be involved. No distinct causal factor has been identified for the disorder; however, trauma and the secretion of estrogen during pregnancy have been sighted as possible causes. Males are affected more often than females (2:1), and bilateral disease can be seen in a quarter of all cases.

Clinical Features

Symptoms vary according to the location of the lesion and can include chronic sinusitis, nasal obstruction, epistaxis, eye symptoms including exophthalmos and diplopia, facial swelling and tenderness. Tumors tend to range in size from 2 cm to up to 7 cm.

Pathologic Features

On macroscopic examination, the tumor mass will generally be firm, white to grey in color and will often demonstrate a whorled or trabeculated appearance on cut section.

Microscopically, juvenile fibromatosis will typically consist of a poorly circumscribed infiltrative growth made up

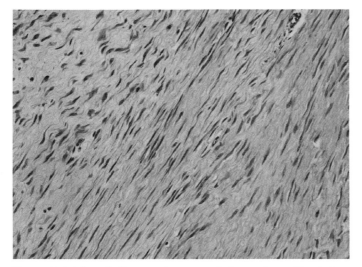

Figure 13.35 Juvenile fibromatosis composed of streaming and interlacing aggregates of fibroblasts without significant tumor cellular pleomorphism are set in a myxoid stroma.

of well demarcated bands of spindle shaped cells that will show mild nuclear pleomorphism. Tumor cell nuclei will be oval and the tumor matrix will range from myxoid to densely collagenous (Figure 13.35). Tumors will tend to be vimentin reactive on IHC. Tumor cells will stain negatively for melanocytic, myogenic, epithelial, neural and vascular markers.

Differential diagnoses include reactive fibrosis or scar, SFT, nerve sheath tumors, nodular fasciitis, myofibroblastic tumors and well differentiated fibrosarcoma. Scar tissue will show dense collagenation with scant or no vascularity. The SFT, unlike juvenile fibromatosis, will be CD34 and Bcl-2 immunoreactive. Myofibroblastic tumors will stain for vimentin, S100 protein and myoglobin. Fibrosarcoma will generally be cytologically atypical and infiltrative.

Treatment and Prognosis

The treatment for juvenile fibromatosis is wide surgical excision of the neoplasm and the overall prognosis is good. However, an infiltrating tumor margin in the nasosinuses may render the surgery difficult, and therefore significant morbidity and major loss of function can ensue. Radiotherapy and chemotherapy have been used to decrease tumor recurrences,[94,95,96,97,98,99] however, these modalities are usually reserved for surgical failures or for cases in which the tumor is not amenable to exploration.[94,95,96,97,98,99] Approximately 2 to 3 percent of all tumors display malignant transformation, although metastasis is rare.[100,101]

Neural Tumors

Tumors of nerve sheath origin, principally Schwannomas and neurofibromas have been described in the sinonasal tract and nasopharynx in the pediatric age group. These tumors are described in detail in Chapter 2.

References

Nasal Papillomas

1. Ward N. A mirror of the practice of medicine and surgery in the hospitals of London: London hospital. *Lancet* 1854; 2:480–482.

2. Hyams VJ. Papillomas of the nasal cavity and paranasal sinuses. *Ann Oto Rhinol Laryngal* 1971; 80: 192–206.

3. Ganzer D, Donath K, Schmelzle R, Geschwulste der inneren Nase, der Nasennebenhohlen, des ber- und unterkiefers. In: Naumann HH, Helms J, Herberhold C, Kastenbauer E, eds. *Oto-Rhino-Laryngologie in Klinik und Praxis Vol2*. Stuttgart New York: Thiem, 1992:312–359.

4. Eggers G, Muhling J, Hassfeld S. Inverted papillomas of the paranasal sinuses. *J Cranio Maxillofac Surg* 2007; 35:21–29.

5. Michaels L. Benign mucosal tumors of the nose and paranasal sinuses. *Semin Diagnost Pathol* 1996; 13:113–117.

6. Lampertico P, Russel WO, MacComb WS. Squamous papilloma of the upper respiratory tract. *Arch Pathol* 1963; 75:293–302.

7. Stanley RJ, Kelley JA, Matta II, Falkenberg J. Inverted papilloma in a 10 year old. *Arch Otolaryngol* 1984; 110.813–815.

8. Ravey ED. Inverted papilloma of the nose and paranasal sinuses in childhood and adolescence. *Laryngoscope* 1985; 95:17–23.

9. Ozcan C, Gorur K, Talas D. Recurrent inverted papilloma of a pediatric patient: clinico-radiological considerations. *Int J Pediatr Otorhinolaryngol* 2005; 69:861–864.

10. D' Angelo AJ, Marlowe A, Marlowe FI, McFarland M. Inverted papilloma of the nose and paranasal sinuses in children, *Ear Nose Throat J* 1992; 71:264–266.

11. Syrjanen KJ. HPV infections in benign and malignant sinonasal lesions. *J Clin Pathol* 2003; 56:174–181.

12. Gaffey MJ, Frierson HF, Weiss LM, et al. Human papillomavirus and Epstein-Barr virus in sinonasal Schneiderian papillomas. An in situ hybridization and polymerase chain reaction study. *Am J Clin Pathol* 1996 Oct; 106(4):475–482.

13. Macdonald MR, Le KT, Freeman J, et al. A majority of sinonasal inverted papillomas carries Epstein Barr virus genomes. *Cancer* 1995; 75(9):2307–2312.

14. Barnes L, Tse L, Hunt J. Schneiderian papillomas. In: Barnes L, Eveson J, Reichert P, Sidransky D, eds. *WHO Classification of Tumors, Pathology and Genetics of Head and Neck Tumors*. Lyon, France: IARC Press, 2005: 28–32.

15. Barnes L. Schneiderian papillomas and non salivary glandular neoplasms of the head and neck. *Mod Pathol* 2002; 15:279–297.

16. Barnes L, Benedetti C. Oncocytic schneiderian papilloma: a reappraisal of cylindrical cell papilloma of the sinonasal tract. *Hum Pathol* 1984; 15:344–351.

17. Vorasubin N, Vira D, Suh J, et al. Schneiderian papillomas: comparative review of exophytic, oncocytic and inverted types. *Am J Rhinol Allergy* 2013; 27:287–292.

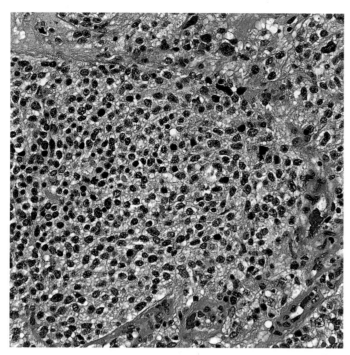

Figure 14.19 Grade II ONB demonstrating a moderate degree of nuclear pleomorphism including occasional mitosis, and a loss of tumor lobular architecture.

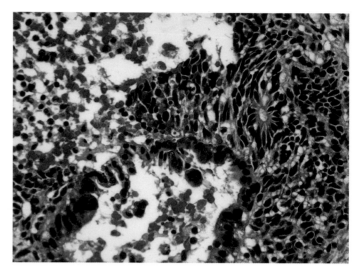

Figure 14.21 Grade IV neuroblastoma showing Flexner–Wintersteiner rosette formation (clusters of cuboidal or columnar tumor cells arranged around a central lumen). Note that tumor cell nuclei tend to be displaced away from lumen.

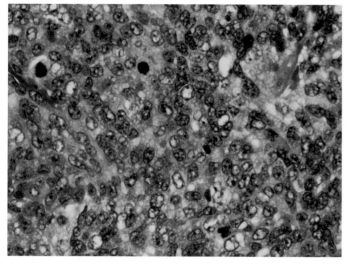

Figure 14.20 Grade IV ONB showing marked nuclear pleomophism and significant mitotic activity among tumor cells.

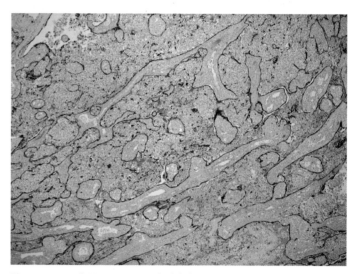

Figure 14.22 S100 protein stain highlighting sustentacular cells surrounding tumor lobules in this well differentiated ONB.

a gradual shift toward increased cellular pleomorphism, with a loss of the tumor's lobular architecture. (Figure 14.19) Increased mitoses, necrosis and appearance of the true Flexner–Wintersteiner rosettes characterize high grade tumors (Figures 14.20 & 14.21).

Tumor cells will be strongly reactive to neuroendocrine markers including; chromogranin, synaptophysin, CD56 and NSE. S100 protein stains will stain the sustentacular cells at the periphery of tumor lobules (Figure 14.22). Tumor cells are usually negative for immunohistochemical epithelial

markers, melanocytic markers, lymphoid markers, muscle markers and CD99.

Molecular and cytogenetic studies of ONB have shown overexpression of DNA chromosomal material on chromosome 19, partial gains on the long arm of chromosomes 8, 15, 22, deletion of the entire long arm of chromosome 4 and several gains and losses on chromosomes 3p, 6q, 9q, 10q, 13q and 17q.[10,11,12]

The differential diagnoses for ONB are lengthy and include: 1) sinonasal undifferentiated carcinoma (SNUC), 2) nasopharyngeal undifferentiated carcinoma, 3) small cell carcinoma, 4) sinonasal lymphoepithelial carcinoma, 5) malignant melanoma, 6) NK/T-cell lymphoma, 7) RMS and 8) PNET/EWS. Perhaps the most significant differential

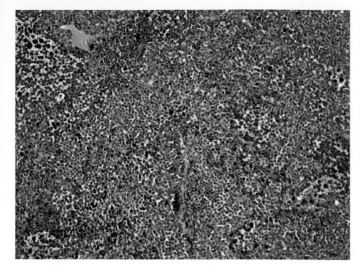

Figure 14.23 Sinonasal malignant melanoma showing solid sheets of malignant melanocytes with foci of pigmentation.

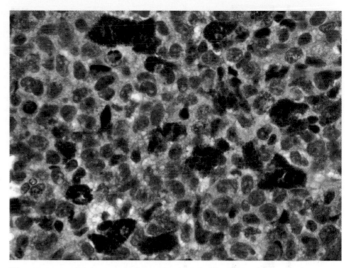

Figure 14.24 High power photomicrograph illustrating the marked pleomorphism of tumor cells and an abundance of melanin pigment in this mucosal malignant melanoma.

diagnostic consideration, PNET/EWS, can be excluded on the basis that ONB will show a t(11;22) (q24;q12) fusion transcript.

Treatment and Prognosis

Complete surgical resection with post-operative radiation is the treatment of choice for ONB. Endoscopic resection can be employed for small tumors. Chemotherapy has shown limited success; however, it can be employed as a palliative measure for unresectable or disseminated disease.

Low grade tumors in children have an 80 percent five-year survival rate, while high grade tumors show only a 40 percent survival after five years.

Sinonasal Mucosal Malignant Melanoma

Nasal mucosal malignant melanomas are of neuroectodermal origin and arise from neural crest derived melanocytes in the nasal mucosa. These tumors are extremely rare in the pediatric population.[14,15] Most patients will present with a mass in the nasal cavity or nasal sinus and accompanying non-specific symptoms, including nasal obstruction, recurrent epistaxis and epiphora.

Although formaldehyde exposure and smoking have been implicated in the etiology of melanoma in adults, it is not clear in the pediatric population that these agents play a role in tumor development.

Pathologic Features

Grossly, tumors will be polypoid, often pigmented and rarely larger than 2 cm in diameter. On microscopic examination, tumor cells will show a varied morphology that can include a proliferation of small round cells, spindle cells, plasmacytoid or epithelioid appearing cells. Fifty to seventy percent of cells will contain pigment (Figure 14.23). Tumor cells usually exhibit prominent eosinophilic nucleoli and a high nuclear cytoplasmic ratio, along with cellular pleomorphism, bizarre

shaped nuclei (Figure 14.24) and occasionally increased mitosis. Tumors will usually express S100 protein, HMB45, Tyrosinase and Melan A/MART1. CD4, CD8 and CD56 stains as well as stains for cytokeratins, smooth muscle markers and lymphoma will be negative.

Differential diagnoses can include many of the undifferentiated malignant neoplasms of the sinonasal region including RMS, ONB, PNET/EWS and SNUC. All of the aforementioned tumors, unlike melanoma, will be HMB45, melan A/MART1 and tyrosinase negative. Immunohistochemical staining patterns for significant malignant pediatric nasosinus tumors can be seen in Table 14.1.

Treatment and Prognosis

Although mucosal melanoma of the nasosinuses carries a grave prognosis in adults, the prognosis in the pediatric population is somewhat better. Treatment includes complete excision of the tumor, with adjuvant chemotherapy, radiation therapy and high dose immunotherapy.

Small Cell Undifferentiated Neuroendocrine Carcinoma (SCUNC)

Malignant neuroendocrine tumors include the carcinoid tumor (well differentiated neuroendocrine carcinoma, low grade), atypical carcinoid (well differentiated neuroendocrine carcinoma), intermediate grade(moderately differentiated neuroendocrine carcinoma), and high grade tumors (including SCUNC and large cell neuroendocrine carcinoma).[16]

Among this group of neoplasms, only extremely rare reports of SCUNC have been identified with any frequency in the sinonasal tract of pediatric age patients.[2] Most such tumors have occurred in the nasal cavity while the ethmoid are maxillary sinuses have been spared.

Clinical symptomatology can include epistaxis nasal obstruction, facial pain or exophthalmos.

Table 14.1 Immunohistochemical staining patterns in malignant pediatric nasosinus tumors

	S100	NSE	CG	SYN	CK	HMB	LCA	CD56	CD99	VIM	DES	Myf-4
Mucosal melanoma	+	–	–	–	–	+	–	–	–	+	–	–
T/NK lymphoma	–	–	–	–	–	–	(+ –)	+	–	(+ –)	–	–
ONB	+[a]	+	(+ –)	(+–)	–	–	–	–	–	–	–	–
SNUC	–	(+ –)	–	–	+	–	–	–	–	–	–	–
RMS	–	–	–	–	–	–	–	–	–	+	+	+
SCC	–	–	–	–	+	–	–	–	–	–	–	–
PNET/EWS	(+–)	(+–)	–	(+–)	–	–	–	–	+	+	–	–
SCUNC	+	+	+	+	+	–	–	–	–	–	–	–

NSE = Neuron-specific enolase
CG = Chromogranin
CK = Cytokeratin
DES = Desmin
HMB45 = Melanin marker
LCA = Leukocyte common antigen
S100 = S100 protein
CD56 = Neuroendocrine marker
VIM = Vimentin
CD99 = Ewing sarcoma/PNET marker
CG = Chromogranin
SYN = Snaptophysin
Myf-4 = Rhabdomyosarcoma markers
+ –= variable
ONB = Olfactory neuroblastoma
SNUC = Sinonasal undifferentiated carcinoma
RMS = Rhabdomyosarcoma
SCC = Squamous cell carcinoma
PNET/EWS = Primitive neuroectodermal tumor (Ewing sarcoma)
SCUNC = Small cell undifferentiated neuroectodermal carcinoma

Pathologic Features

On microscopic examination, SCUNC will be composed of hypercellular, hyperchromatic small blue cells or spindle shaped cells, typically growing in sheets, cords and ribbons.[17,18] The tumor may show increased mitotic activity as well as single cell and confluent necrosis with significant associated crush artifact. (Figure 14.25) Tumors show a propensity for lymphovascular invasion, perineural invasion and metastasis, and tumor cells may demonstrate a high degree of pleomorphism and hyperchromatism. SCUNC tumor cells will stain positively for CD56 and variably positive for synaptophysin (Figure 14.26), chromogranin and neurone specific enolase. Cytokeratin staining shows variable positivity and Cam 5.2 is usually positive.

Treatment and Prognosis

In the adult population, SCUNC is a highly malignant tumor that is associated with a guarded prognosis. The paucity of cases in the pediatric population does not allow for a definitive assessment of the tumor's behavior in that population. Most SCUNCs in pediatric age group patients have been treated with systemic chemotherapy and therapeutic radiation.

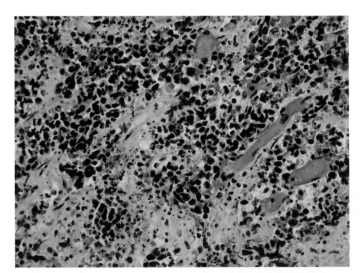

Figure 14.25 SCUNC showing infiltrating sheets of small, round, blue tumor cells that exhibit significant and characteristic crush artifact and necrosis.

Sinonasal Ewing Tumor Family (ETF); Ewing Sarcoma / Primitive Neuroectodermal Tumor (EWS/PNET)

EWS/PNET represents a malignant high grade primitive round cell neuroectodermal neoplasm that primarily affects

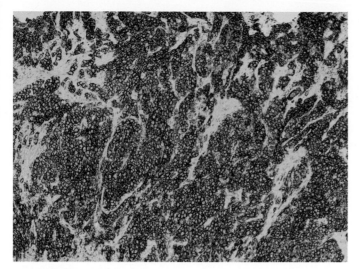

Figure 14.26 SCUNC demonstrating strong synaptophysin reactivity.

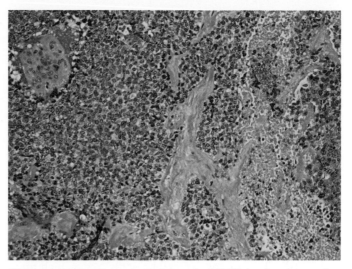

Figure 14.27 Low power photomicrograph of SNUC showing clusters of basophilic staining round to polygonal shaped cells.

pediatric age group and young adult patients.[19,20,21,22,23] Most individuals of EWS/PNET in the sinonasal region will present with nasal obstruction, pain and epistaxis. Extra-sinonasal extension into the orbit or brain has also been recorded. A complete discussion of the clinicopathology of EWS/PNET can be found in Chapter 16.

Epithelial Neoplasms

Sinonasal Undifferentiated Carcinoma (SNUC)

Most malignant neoplasms of the sinonasal tract will represent keratinizing or non-keratinizing squamous cell carcinomas. However, non-epithelial malignancies that are undifferentiated can also occur. SNUC is an aggressive malignancy for which the causation and histogenesis are unknown. The tumor was first described in 1986 by Frierson et al.[1] and radiation has been postulated as a possible etiologic factor, along with somatic mutation at the RB1 locus.[2] Epstein Barr virus (EBV) has also been implicated in the genesis of this tumor.[3] Only rare sporadic cases have been reported in the pediatric age group.[4,5]

Most SNUCs will be large nasal obstructive tumors which may extend intracranially on presentation.[1,2,3,4,5,6] Symptoms can include sinusitis, epistaxis, cranial nerve palsies, convulsions, drowsiness, severe headaches, orbital symptoms that include proptosis, visual disturbance and paresis.[5] Symptoms usually have a rapid onset of just a few weeks to a few months.

Pathologic Features

Grossly the tumor will consist of a rubbery fungating mass with poorly defined margins. Histologically SNUC will be composed of pleomorphic small to large, polygonal shaped cells with a high nuclear to cytoplasmic ratio and hyperchromatic round to oval nuclei (Figures 14.27 & 14.28). One or more prominent nucleoli may be seen. Multiple foci of apoptosis and confluent necrosis will be seen and the tumor's growth pattern can be sheet-like, trabecular, lobular or organoid.

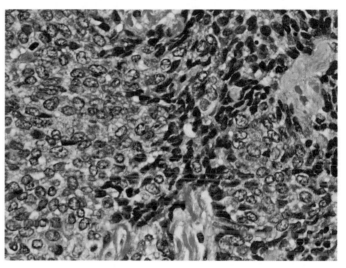

Figure 14.28 SNUC characterized by sheets of oval to spindle shaped cells admixed with lymphocytes.

SNUC, which shows a high propensity for angiolymphatic and perineural invasion, must be differentiated from similar poorly differentiated tumors occurring in the region including, RMS, ONB, SCUNC, nasopharyngeal undifferentiated carcinoma, poorly differentiated squamous carcinoma and NK/T Cell lymphoma. Immunohistochemical stains of SNUC tumor cells will show positive reactivity for keratins including pancytokeratin, cam 5.2 and occasionally for simple keratins (CK7, 8, 9).

The tumor will mark negatively for muscle markers, hematolymphoid markers, melanocytic markers and Ewing / PNET markers (CD99). Only rare sporadic staining for S100 protein, synaptophysin and chromogranin will be seen. Focal staining for NSE and CD56 may also be observed.

Genetic polymorphism has recently been reported within the promotor region of VEGF in SNUCs.[7]

Treatment and Prognosis

Following surgical tumor resection, multimodality therapy is usually employed in the treatment of SNUC, including neoadjuvant chemotherapy. Although the tumor's prognosis in pediatric age patients is difficult to determine due to the paucity of cases, adult patients have an overall poor survival rate with a high incidence of local recurrence and local and distant metastasis.

Sinonasal Adenocarcinoma

Extremely rare instances of sinonasal adenocarcinoma have been reported in the pediatric population.[1] Two main categories of tumor are encountered in the sinonasal region.[1] An intestinal type tumor that can appear papillary, colonic, solid, mucinous or mixed (Figures 14.29, 14.30 & 14.31); and a non-intestinal form of tumor that can be either low or high grade (Figure 14.32). All of the tumor variants are mucosal surface epithelially derived with adenomatous differentiation, and most will occur in the lateral nasal walls, causing nasal obstruction. EGFR alterations are common to intestinal type tumors, while KRAS and BRAF mutations are infrequent.[2] Complete surgical excision is curative.

Basaloid Squamous Cell Carcinoma (BSCC)

BSCC represents a high grade variant of squamous cell carcinoma. The tumor is rare in the nasosinus and generally affects adults, rather than pediatric age individuals. Laryngeal tumors and tumors of the hypopharynx far exceed the number of sinonasal tumors, and laryngeal tumors tend to be more biologically aggressive than sinonasal tumors, often presenting as multifocal growths. Symptoms depend on the anatomic site of presentation of the tumor and may include hoarseness, dysplasia, swelling of the neck or pain.

Microscopically BSCC will be composed of a predominance of basaloid cells with an associated squamous cell carcinoma component that will show a trabecular, cribriform, solid, glandular or cystic growth pattern.

Treatment and Prognosis

Tumors are treated by radical surgical excision and neck dissection and nasosinus tumors tend to have a better prognosis than BSCC in other head and neck sites.

Germ Cell Tumors (GCT)

Yolk Sac Tumor (YST) (Endodermal Sinus Tumor)

The vast majority of GCTs in children that develop in the head and neck area are benign.[1,2,3,4] Extragonadal YST, a malignant germ cell neoplasm is extremely uncommon in children[2,3] although it represents the leading non-seminomatous type of GCT to occur in the perinatal period and throughout childhood.[3] Even so, YST is extremely rare in the sinonasal tract.[4,5,6,7] Tumor related symptoms will vary and are rather non-specific. Nasal obstruction, epistaxis and sinusitis may be

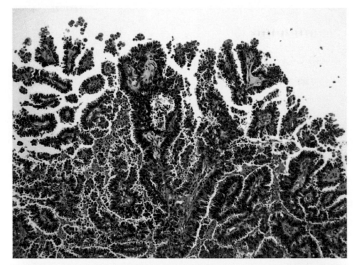
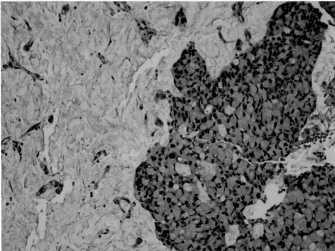
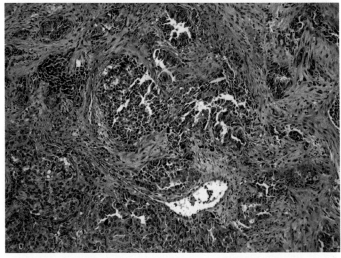

Figures 14.29 (top), 14.30 (middle) & 14.31 (bottom) Intestinal type sinonasal adenocarcinomas that are papillary, mucinous, and colonic respectively can be seen in these three photomicrographs. Note the classic glandular pattern of each tumor subtype.

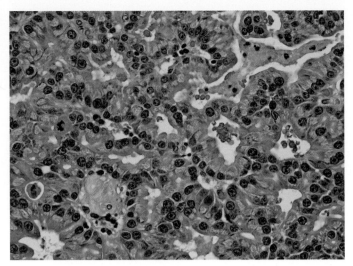

Figure 14.32 Non intestinal sinonasal type adenocarcinomas. This high power photomicrograph demonstrates a low grade oncocytoid (non-intestinal type) adenocarcinoma.

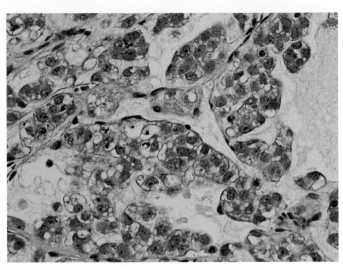

Figure 14.34 High power photomicrograph showing pleomorphic tumor cells that marginate a cystic spaces in a YST.

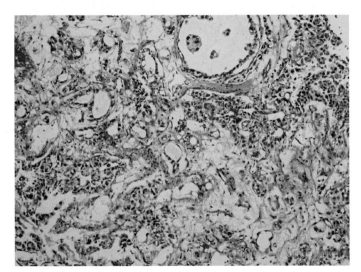

Figure 14.33 Low power photomicrograph of a YST showing microcystic, interconnected web-like collections of tumor cells.

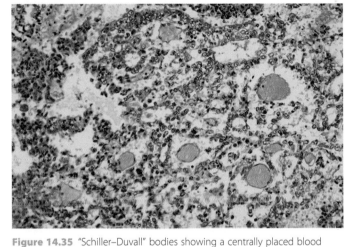

Figure 14.35 "Schiller–Duvall" bodies showing a centrally placed blood vessels surrounded by flattened malignant tumor cells that marginate a cystic space.

seen. The tumor produces alpha-fetoproteins, (AFP) a homologue of albumin, and thus AFP can be used as a diagnostic marker in follow-up of the patient during post treatment. Clinically tumors of the nasosinus in pediatric patients will be characterized by persistent nasal bleeding, and CT and MRI will tend to demonstrate a lobulated soft tissue mass in the sinus or paranasal sinus region.

Pathologic Features

Microscopically the YST will demonstrate pleomorphic cuboidal type cells arranged in a microcystic pattern that results in an interconnected web-like network (Figures 14.33 & 14.34). The tumor can also demonstrate an endodermal sinus pattern in which a central vessel will be surrounded by malignant cells that lie within a cystic space that will be lined by flattened tumor cells, or so called Schiller–Duvall bodies. (Figure 14.35)

Tumors can also appear solid, glandular, myxomatous, macrocystic, hepatoid, polyvesicular, festooned or parietal. The tumor will commonly contain hyaline globules (1–50u) that are periodic acid positive (PAS)/diastase resistant, as well as aggregates of an eosinophilic band-like protein product representing extracellular basement membrane material.

Tumor target cells will stain for AFP (Figure 14.36) and low molecular weight cytokeratin, AFP and occasionally for Placental alkaline phosphatase (PLAP) and Glypican 3.[8]

Microscopic differential diagnoses include RMS, adenocarcinoma, ONB, undifferentiated carcinoma and other GCT types (embryonal carcinoma, choriocarcinoma, dysgerminoma and teratoma). Molecular studies have demonstrated loss of the long arm of chromosome 6, the short arm of

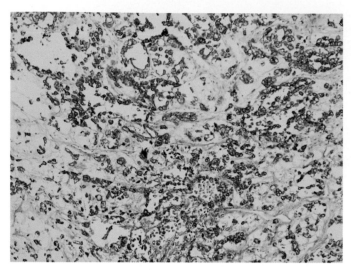

Figure 14.36 AFP positive immunohistochemical staining of YST cells.

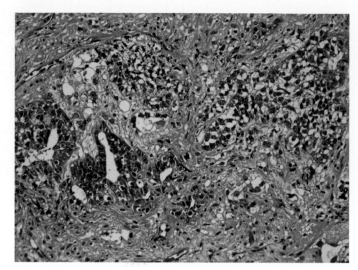

Figure 14.38 Malignant epithelial tumor component of a sinonasal teratocarcinosarcoma composed of pleomorphic poorly differentiated cells that show focal glandular formations.

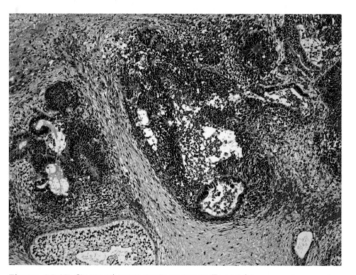

Figure 14.37 Sinonasal teratocarcinosarcoma. Teratoid tumor component composed of immature small round blue tumor cells set in a neurofibrillary matrix.

chromosome 1 or gains in the long arm of chromosomes 1 and 20 in YST.[9] These cytogenetic findings can be helpful in differentiating YST from the more common small round cell neoplasms that are seen in pediatric age patients.

Treatment and Prognosis

Surgical excision with combined chemotherapy and radiation therapy is the treatment of choice for YST. The most common chemotherapy employed is a combined carboplatin based JEB regimen.[6] Although the tumor is biologically aggressive, most cases reported in children have shown a good prognosis with survival rates ranging from 4 to 14 years. However, it should be noted that the number of cases assessed to date is too limited to make firm conclusions about the *prognosis* of YST in the sinonasal tract of children.

Sinonasal Teratocarcinosarcoma / Teratocarcinoma

Sinonasal teratocarcinosarcoma is an extremely rare highly malignant polymorphous paranasal sinus neoplasm that shows combined histologic features of both a teratoma and carcinosarcoma. With fewer than 100 reported cases in the literature, tumors in pediatric age patients are exceptionally rare.[10,11,12,13,14,15,16,17] Most reported tumors have involved the ethmoid sinus, maxillary sinus, sphenoid sinus and nasopharynx. Tumors are thought to arise from either primitive naso-sinus embryonic tissue or from a multipotential adult somatic stem cell with divergent pathway differentiation.[18]

Patients can present with a myriad of symptoms ranging from nasal obstruction and epistaxis to dizziness. Clinical examination will often reveal an ulcerated nasal mass. MRI and CT will commonly demonstrate a mass filling the affected sinus cavity.

Pathologic Features

Microscopically tumors will demonstrate a teratoid component and a carcinosarcoma component. The teratoid component can be composed of neuroepithelium and neuroectodermal/blastemal cells that will be small, round and blue and resemble neuroblastoma. Tumor cells are generally set in a neurofibrillary matrix (Figure 14.37).

The tumor's epithelial component will consist of benign appearing glandular or ductal structures, fetal type clear cell squamous epithelium and foci or aggregates of squamous carcinoma and/or adenocarcinoma (Figure 14.38).

The tumor's mesenchymal component can demonstrate an admix of benign or malignant fibroblasts, myofibroblasts, zones of RMStous tissue, foci of osteoid formation or osteosarcoma (Figure 14.39). Benign, mature and immature cartilage or foci of chondrosarcoma may also be seen.

Differential diagnoses can include ONB, EWS/PNET, RMS, craniopharyngioma, adenocarcinoma, poorly differentiated

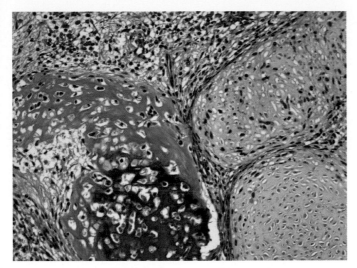

Figure 14.39 Sinonasal teratocarcinosarcoma demonstrating osteosarcoma in its mesenchymal component.

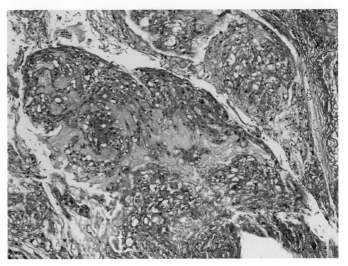

Figure 14.40 Low power photomicrograph of a chordoma showing large round (physaliphorous) tumor cells set in an abundant fibro-myxoid stroma.

squamous carcinoma, adenocarcinoma, SNUC and high grade sarcomas.

Treatment and Prognosis

The sinonasal teratocarcinoma is a highly malignant neoplasm that requires aggressive therapy in adults, including surgical resection, adjuvant chemotherapy and radiation therapy. In the adult population the average patient survival is less than two years. Follow-up of reported pediatric cases is too limited to draw any firm conclusions about long term prognosis. However, Agrawal et al. have reported a case in a 15-year-old male, in which the patient was treated with combined surgery and chemoradiation. The patient at the time of follow-up had no evidence of recurrence after 45 months.

Notocord Derived Tumor

Chordoma

Chordomas represent malignancies of low grade to intermediate grade potential that arise along the length of the neuraxis from embryonic notochordal remnants. Chordomas only rarely occur in extraaxial locations including the nasopharynx and the sinonasal tract.[1,2,3,4] They are more commonly present in a sacro-coccygeal or sphenooccipital location.[5] Most tumors will affect adults; however, tumors have been recorded in the pediatric age group. Tumors occur at the rate of less than 0.7 per 100,000 of the population on an annual basis, and they represent less than 0.2 percent of all tumors that involve the nasopharynx.[6] Males are more often affected than females.

Clinically lesions commonly present as a lobulated or expansile mucoid, friable nasosinus mass, accompanied by gradual nasal obstruction, headaches, diplopia, sensory motor compromise or pain.

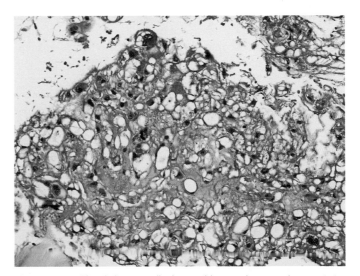

Figure 14.41 Physaliphorous cells show mild to moderate nuclear atypia in this medium power photomicrograph.

Pathologic Features

Histologically chordomas will be composed of sheets and cords of large round to epithelioid polygonal cells with vacuolated cytoplasm (Physaliphorous cells). (Figure 14.40) Tumor physaliphorous cells may show mild to moderate nuclear atypia (Figure 14.41). The tumor stroma will most often appear either myxoid or chondroid. Tumors displaying a chondroid stromal matrix are more common in pediatric age group patients and women.

Immunohistochemical staining of the tumor target cells will be positive for pancytokeratin, S100 protein and epithelial membrane antigens.

Genes showing increased expression in chordoma[7] are frequently located on chromosomes 2, 5, 1 and 7. Interphase cytogenetics studies have demonstrated gains of chromosomal material in chordoma, with gains being most prevalent on chromosome 7q.[7]

Differential diagnoses include chondrosarcoma, which will lack physaliphorous cells; chordoid meningioma, which will be S100 protein negative, liposarcoma, which will be keratin and EMA negative and chordoid glioma, which will stain positively for glial markers.

Treatment and Prognosis

Surgery remains the treatment of choice for chordomas, although adjuvant radiation therapy can be used in cases where there has been incomplete surgical resection. Traditional chemotherapy has not been shown to be effective; however, clinical trials have shown clinical efficacy of imatinib mesylate in the treatment of chordoma.[8]

Malignant Tumors of the Nasopharynx

Nasopharyngeal carcinoma (NPC) carcinoma is a form of squamous cell carcinoma that arises from nasopharyngeal mucosa. In order to be classified as such, a tumor must demonstrate light microscopic or ultrastructural evidence of squamous differentiation.

NPC can be classified histologically as: 1) keratinizing or 2) non-keratinizing. Non-keratinizing NPC can be further classified as differentiated or undifferentiated. A rare BSCC variant is also recognized.

In the pediatric age group the median age of occurrence for NPC is 13 years. The tumor is more common in males than females and occurs more frequently in the black population with a significant northern and central African demographic. NPC also accounts for nearly 20 percent of all cancers in China with the non-keratinizing type accounting for 60 percent of such cases. However, only 15 to 20 percent of NPC cases in China occur in the pediatric patient age group.[2,3] As a whole, NPC constitutes from 20 to 50 percent of all primary nasopharyngeal malignant tumors in children.[4,5]

NPC has a close causal association with EBV which has been found in the genome of NPC tumor cells, and the tumor is associated with a type of neoplastic latency in which EBNA1 nuclear protein, LMP1, LMP2 nuclear proteins and EBER proteins are ultimately expressed in a clonal fashion in tumor cells.[6] Antibody titers of IgG and IgA against early EBER antigen or viral capsid antigens are encountered in patients with NPC at high levels, and titer expression assessment is currently widely used for early screening of high risk groups.

Differences in the world-wide incidence of NPC are thought to be related to genetic and environmental factors. Individuals with a HLA.AW33 haplotype are reported to have a lesser risk for development while polymorphism of some metabolic enzymes including Glutathione-S-transferase and Cytochrome – P450 2E1 are related to an increased NPC incidence and risk.[7,8]

The undifferentiated NPC common to southern China and Hong Kong, Southeast Asia, the Mediterranean basin particularly northern Africa and Alaska has been related causally to the consumption of food stuffs that are rich in volatile nitrosamines, such as salted fish, the use of tobacco, exposure to chemical fumes and dust, formaldehyde and radiation exposure.[9]

NPC can be a symptomless lesion or it can present with nasal obstructive symptoms including, blood tinged nasal discharge, bleeding and blockage of the Eustachian tubes with consequential otitis media, earache and tinnitus. Many patients will present initially with a painless cervical neck mass that will represent metastatic NPC that is ultimately determined by clinical investigation to be of nasopharyngeal origin. As many as 25 percent of NPCs invade the skull base, causing cranial nerve deficits.[6]

MRI assessment is the method of choice for determining the extent of the tumor's soft tissue involvement and for assessing any intracranial extension, while CT scans are more helpful in determining evidence of bone erosion.[8,10,11] Detection of EBV using in situ hybridization or by employing PCR will demonstrate EBV in 80 to 90 percent of non-keratinizing NPC.

Cytogenetic abnormalities in the form of deletions in chromosome 3p, 9p, 11q, 13q and 14q have been found in patients with NPC, suggesting that tumor suppressive genes are deficient. Other significant genetic alterations include inactivation of P53, rearrangement of retinoblastoma tumor suppressor genes and genetic polymorphism of the CYP2E1 gene. Tumor associated chromosome 12 gene gains, and allelic loss on 11q, 13q and 16q have been linked to the neoplasms invasive potential.[6,12,13,14] Children with NPC have been shown to have significant T- lymphocyte suppression.[15]

Non-keratinizing NPC, which rarely occurs in patients under 40, has an affinity for the lateral nasal wall. Clinical symptoms are similar to the non-keratinizing form of the disease, however this form of the disease has not been linked to EBV.

Pathologic Features

NPC in the pediatric population will most frequently be of the non-keratinizing undifferentiated histologic subtype. Tumors will demonstrate a cellular syncytium of often highly basophilic, large, sometimes overlapping tumor cells (Figure 14.42). Tumor cell nuclei will be vesicular to round to ovoid with nuclei, prominent nucleoli and amphophilic cytoplasm (Figure 14.43).

Less frequent differentiated tumors, common to adults, will demonstrate a pattern reminiscent of what in the past has been referred to as transitional cell carcinoma, with cellular stratification and tumor cell pavementing.

The growth pattern of differentiate NPCs can be solid, plexiform or trabecular. Tumor cells will have well-defined cell margins and sometimes vague intercellular bridges, and there may be occasional keratinizing cells. Tumor cells will have

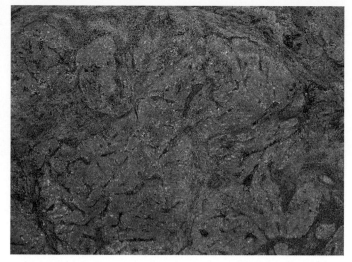

Figure 14.42 Low power photomicrograph of undifferentiated non-keratinizing NPC, demonstrating the tumor's considerable basophilia and lobularity.

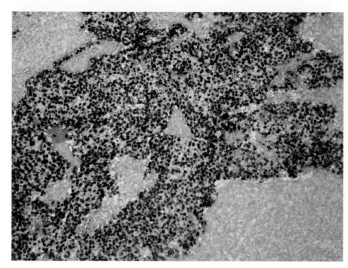

Figure 14.44 Positive in situ hybridization stain showing EBV (encoded for early RNA (EBER) in a non-keratinizing NPC.

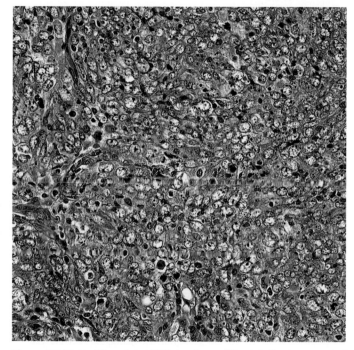

Figure 14.43 Undifferentiated NPC showing a diffusely infiltrative tumor cell syncytium made up of large cells with vesicular hyperchromatic oval nuclei. Tumor cells characteristically have indistinct cell margins.

high nuclear cytoplasmic ratios and the nuclei will be small and less prominent than in the undifferentiated form of the tumor. More differentiated tumors may show focal keratinization.

Lymphocytes and plasma cells have a great affinity for NPC and they will be seen in the stroma between tumor islands or infiltrating tumor islands. The tumor's lymphoid cells will represent a mixture of T and B cells in which T cells and polyclonal plasma cells predominate. Spindle cells, sometimes

arranged in a fascicle-like pattern, are more common to differentiated NPC than non-keratinizing undifferentiated forms of the tumor.[16]

EBV, which is associated with non-keratinizing NPC in nearly all cases, can be demonstrated by in situ hybridization for EBV, encoded for early RNA (EBER) (Figure 14.44).

Immunohistochemical staining of non-keratinizing forms of NPC will show strong staining for pancytokeratin, and high molecular weight keratins (CK5/6). Epithelial membrane antigen will be focal to absent, while low molecular weight keratins such as CK7 and 20 will be negative or weak.

Differential diagnoses for the more common undifferentiated NPC that affects pediatric age group patients can include melanoma, RMS, lymphoma, ONB, EWS/PNET, SNUC and primitive neuroectodermal tumors.

Immunohistochemical markers, including B cell markers for lymphoma, HMB-45, melan-A and tyrosinase for melanoma and myogenic markers including desmin for RMS should allow one to distinguish these tumors which can appear similar on routine H & E staining from one another.[17,18]

Treatment and Prognosis

The treatment of choice for NPC is super voltage radiotherapy.[17] Surgery is reserved for radioresistant and recurrent tumors. Direct tumor extension into the skull base, paranasal sinuses, orbit and basal foramina is common. NPC will demonstrate a high incidence of both hematogenous spread and lymph node metastasis at presentation, particularly, to the jugulo-digastric node and the posterior cervical chain. Chemotherapy is usually reserved for disseminated advanced stage disease and is generally given in concert with radiation therapy. If metastases develop, they usually occur within three years of the initial presentation of the neoplasm.

Pathologists should be aware that the radiation changes induced in fibroblasts can last for years in a NPC patient, and thus such changes should not be over interpreted to

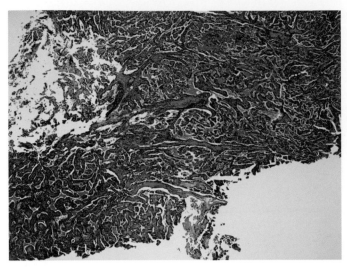

Figure 14.45 Low power photomicrograph of papillary nasopharyngeal adenocarcinoma demonstrating the tumors' characteristic papillary nature.

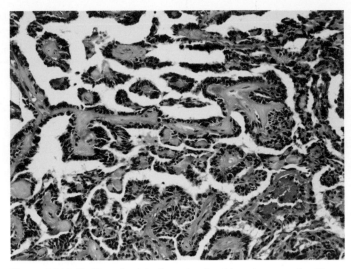

Figure 14.46 Papillary glandular formation, lined by columnar cells with bland, round to oval nuclei characterize this LGNPPA.

represent spindled carcinoma, in those instances where there is a re-biopsy or re-excision.

Pediatric NPC has a better prognosis than the adult form of the disease. The overall five-year survival rate for patients in all age groups ranges as high as 98 percent for stage I disease to as low as 73 percent for stage IV disease.

Low Grade Papillary Nasopharyngeal Adenocarcinoma (LGNPPA)

Glandular nasopharyngeal tumors have two sources of origin: minor salivary glands and surface mucosal epithelium. LGNPPAs arise from mucosal surface epithelium.[1] These tumors which are exceedingly rare in pediatric age patients[2,3] have a median occurrence age of 37, and can arise from the roof, lateral wall or posterior wall of the nasopharynx. Most patients will present with obstructive nasal symptoms including nasal fullness, blood tinged saliva and nasal discharge. Pediatric age patients will have increased otitis media symptomatology.

Pathologic Features

Histologically, LGNPPA will be composed of delicate papillary fronds and back to back, often cribriform glandular formations that are neoplastic (Figure 14.45). Glandular spaces will be lined by pseudostratified columnar or cuboidal epithelium with large round to oval often overlapping nuclei with small nucleoli (Figure 14.46). Psammoma bodies may be seen within the fibrovascular tumor stroma.[3]

Immunohistochemical staining will demonstrate target cells that will stain positively for CK7, CK19. Tumor cells will stain negatively for thyroglobulin, CK5/6 or CK20,[4] and tumors will be EMA and TTF-1 positive. Mucicarmine stains will be positive for intraluminal mucin.

Treatment and Prognosis

LGNPPA is an indolent, slow growing tumor that does not metastasize. Complete surgical excision is accompanied by cure and an excellent prognosis.

References

Introduction

1. Benoit M, Bhattacharya N, Faquin W, Cunningham W. Cancer of the nasal cavity in the pediatric population. *Pediatr* 2008; 121:e141–e145.

2. Yi JS, Cho GS, Shim MJ. Malignant tumors of the sinonasal tract in the pediatric population. *Acta Otolaryngol* 2012; 132 Suppl (1):S21–S26.

Rhabdomyosarcoma

3. Benoit M, Bhattacharya N, Faquin W, Cunningham W. Cancer of the nasal cavity in the pediatric population. *Pediatr* 2008; 121:e141–e145.

4. Fyrmpas G, Wurm J, Athanassiadou F, et al. Management of pediatric sinonasal rhabdomyosarcoma. *J Laryngol Otol* 2009; 123:990–996.

5. Wurm J, Constantinidis J, Grabenbauer G, Iro H. Rhabdomyosarcoma of the nose and paranasal sinus: treatment results in 15 cases. *Otolaryngol Head Neck Surg* 2005; 133:42–50.

6. Parham DM, Barr FG. Embryonal rhabdomyosarcoma. In: Fletcher C, Unni K, Mertens F, editors, *WHO Classification of Tumors. Pathology and Genetics of Tumors of Soft Tissue and Bone.* Lyon, France: IARC Press. 2002; 146–154.

7. Lawrence W, Anderson JR, Gehan EA, Maurer H. Pretreatment TNM staging of childhood rhabdomyosarcoma study group. *Cancer* 1997; 80: 1165–1170.

8. Newton WA, Gehan EA, Webber BL, et al. Classification of rhabdomyosarcoma and related sarcomas: pathologic aspects and proposal for a new classification – an intergroup rhabdomyosarcoma study. *Cancer* 1995; 76:1073–1085.

9. Parham DM, Webber B, Holt H, et al. Immunohistochemical study of childhood rhabdomyosarcomas and related neoplasms. Results of

an intergroup rhabdomyosarcoma study project. *Cancer* 1991; 67: 3072–3080.

10. Koufos A, Hansen MF, Copleland NG, et al. Loss of heterozygosity in three embryonal tumors suggest a common pathogenetic mechanism. *Nature* 1985; 316:330–334.

11. Koi M, Johnson LA, Kalikein LM, et al. Tumor cell growth arrest caused by subchromosomal transferable DNA fragments from chromosome 11. *Science* 1993; 260:361–364.

12. Wang Wuu S, Soukup S, Ballard E, et al. Chromosomal analysis of sixteen human rhabdomyosarcomas. *Cancer* 1988; 48:983–987.

13. Barr FG. Molecular genetics and pathogenesis of rhabdomyosarcoma. *J Pediatr Hematol Oncol* 1997; 19: 483–491.

14. Barr FG, Galili N, Holick J, et al. Rearrangement of PAX3 paired box gene in the pediatric solid tumor alveolar rhabdomyosarcoma. *Nat Genet* 1993; 3:113–117.

15. Davis RJ, Barr FG. Fusion genes resulting from alternative chromosomal translocations are overexpressed by gene specific mechanisms in alveolar rhabdomyosarcoma. *Proc Natl Acad Sci USA* 1997; 94:8047–8051.

16. Weiner ES. Head and neck rhabdomyosarcoma. *Semin Pediatr Surg* 1994; 3:203–206.

17. Rodeberg DA, Anderson JR, Arndt CA, Comparison of outcomes based on treatment algorithms for rhabdomyosarcoma of the bladder/prostate: combined results from the Children's Oncology Group, German Cooperative Soft Tissue Sarcoma Study, Italian Cooperative Group, and International Society of Pediatric Oncology Malignant Mesenchymal Tumors Committee. *Int J Cancer* 2011; 128:1232–1239.

Other Sarcomas

18. Ozzello L, Stout AP, Murray MR. Cultural characteristics of malignant histiocytomas and fibrous xanthomas. *Cancer* 1963; 16:331–344.

19. De Rosa J, Smith J. Myxoid malignant fibrous histiocytoma presenting as a midline nasal mass. *ENT J* 2012; 91: e3–e5.

20. Wang CP, Chang YL, Yang TL, et al. Malignant fibrous histiocytoma of the sinonasal tract. *Head & Neck* 2009; 31:85–93.

21. Weiss SW, Enzinger FM. Malignant fibrous histiocytoma: an analysis of 200 cases. *Cancer* 1978; 41:2250–2266.

22. Barnes L, Kanbour A. Malignant fibrous histiocytoma of the head and neck. A report of 12 cases. *Arch Otolaryngolo Head Neck Surg* 1988; 114:1149–1156.

23. Gadwaal SR, Gannon FH, Fanburg-Smith JC, et al. Primary osteosarcoma of the head and neck in pediatric patients. *Cancer* 2001; 91:598–605.

24. Singh J, Gluckman J, Kaufman R, et al. Osteosarcoma of the nasal bone in a child. *Head Neck*; 4:246–250.

25. Gadwal SR, Famburg-Smith JC, Gannon FH, Thompson L. Primary chondrosarcoma of the head and neck in pediatric patients. *Cancer* 2000; 88:2180–2188.

26. Krishnamurthy A, Shanmugasundaram G, Majhi U. Pediatric chondrosarcoma of the sinonasal region. *J Can Res Ther* 2013; 9:163–164.

27. Lacovara J, Patterson K, Reaman GH. Primary nasal chondrosarcoma. The pediatric experience. *Am J Pediatr Hematol Oncol* 1992; 14:158–162.

28. Shukla GK, Gupta KR, Dayal D. Angiosarcoma of the palate and nose. *Ind J Otol* 1973; 25:120–124

29. Kimura Y, Tanaka S, Mitsuru F. Angiosarcoma of the nasal cavity. *J Laryngol Otol* 1992; 106:368–369.

30. Sharma B, Nawalcha P. Angiosarcoma of the maxillary antrum: report of a case with brief review of the literature. *J Laryngol Otol* 1979; 79:181–186.

31. Palacios E, Lam E. Infantile fibrosarcoma of the maxillary sinus: significant response. *ENT J* 2012; 3: 98–99.

32. Kim KI, Yoo SL. Infantile fibrosarcoma in the nasal cavity. *Otolaryngol Head Neck Surg* 1996; 114: 98–102.

33. Swain RE, Sessions DG, Ogura JH. Fibrosarcoma of the head and neck in children. *Laryngoscope* 1976; 86: 113–116.

34. Steelman C, Katzenstein H, Parham D. et al. Unusual presentation of congenital infantile fibrosarcoma in seven infants with molecular genetic analysis. *Fetal Pediatr Pathol* 2011; 30:329–337.

35. Chung EB, Enzinger FM. Infantile fibrosarcoma. *Cancer* 1976; 38:729–739.

36. Goswami S, Kundu I, Majumdar P, et al. Neurofibrosaroma of the nasal cavity. *Ind J Otolaryngol Head Neck Surg* 2001; 53:129–132.

Neuroendocrine and Neuroectodermal Tumors

37. Broich G, Pagliari A, Ottaviani F. Esthesioneuroblastoma: a general review of the cases published since the discovery of the tumor in 1924. *Anticancer Res* 1997; 17:2683–2706.

38. Benoit M, Bhattacharya N, Faquin W, Cunningham W. Cancer of the nasal cavity in the pediatric population. *Pediatr* 2008; 121:e141–e145.

39. Bisogno G, Soloni P, Conte M, et al. Esthesioneuroblastoma in pediatric and adolescent age. A report from TREP project in cooperation with Italian neuroblastoma and soft tissue sarcoma committees. *Cancer* 2012; 12:117–121.

40. Eich HT, Hero B, Staar S, et al. Multimodality therapy including radiotherapy and chemotherapy improves event free survival in stage C esthesioneuroblastoma. *Strahlentheronkol* 2003; 179:233–240.

41. Kumar M, Fallon RJ, Hill JS, Davis MM. Esthesioneuroblastoma in children. *J Pediatr Hematol Oncol* 2002; 24:482–487.

42. Kupeli S, Yalcin B, Buyukpamukcu M. Olfactory neuroblastoma in children: results of multimodality treatment in 2 patients. *Pediatr Hematol Oncol* 2011; 28:56–59.

43. Kadish S, Goodman M, Wang CC. Olfactory neuroblastoma. A clinical analysis of 17 cases. *Cancer* 1976 Mar; 37(3):1571–1576.

44. Morita A, Ebersold MJ, Olsen KD, et al Esthesioneuroblastoma: prognosis and management. *Neurosurgery* 1993; 32:706–714.

45. Dias FL, Sa GM, Lima RA, et al. Patterns of failure and outcome in esthesioneuroblastoma. *Arch Otolaryngol Head Neck Surg* 2003; 129:1188–1192.

46. Hyams VJ. Olfactory neuroblastoma (case6). In: Batsakis JG, Hyams VJ, Morales AR, editors. *Special Tumors of the Head and Neck*. Chicago: ASCP Press. 1982; 24–29.

47. Wenig BM, Duluguerove P, Kapadia S, et al. Tumor of the nasal cavity and paranasal sinuses: neuroectodermal

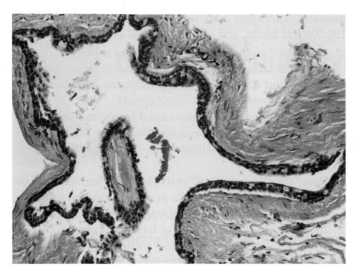

Figure 15.3 Laryngeal "saccular" cyst lined by respiratory epithelium.

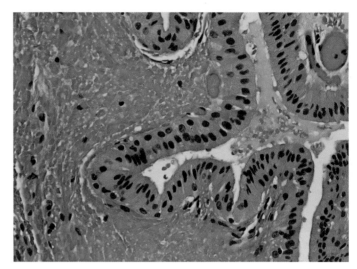

Figure 15.5 Higher power photomicrograph of (A) demonstrating a cyst lining made up of eosinophilic granular oncocytic cells.

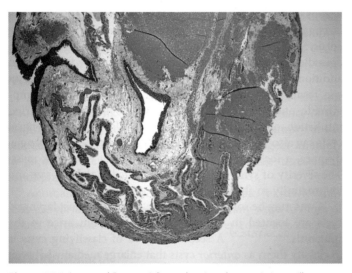

Figure 15.4 Laryngeal "oncocytic" cyst showing characteristic papillary invaginations.

chronically inflamed connective tissue wall (Figure 15.3). Tonsillar cysts will be lined by squamous epithelium. The lumen will typically be keratin filled and the connective tissue wall of the cyst will contain lymphoid tissue. Ductal cysts will be lined by a dual layer of often flattened or cuboidal epithelium. Oncocytic cysts will be lined by eosinophilic cells displaying granular cytoplasm (Figures 15.4 & 15.5).

Treatment and Prognosis

Endoscopic marsupialization or de-roofing of laryngeal cysts has been the most common mode of treatment employed. However, the risk of recurrence of the *saccular* type of cyst is quite high and obstruction and infection can occur. Complete endoscopic excision and external surgery have been treatment modalities as well. Multiple therapeutic procedures can eventually result in scarring and narrowing of the airway.

Laryngocele

While laryngeal cysts are defined primarily in terms of their pathogenesis and histopathology, true laryngoceles are formed in the laryngeal ventricle of Morgagni, a small blind ended recess between the true and false vocal cords, and represent abnormal saccular dilations that maintain communication with the laryngeal lumen.

Three types of laryngoceles have been described, (1) internal (within the laryngeal lumen), (2) external (in the neck) and (3) mixed (in both locations). Laryngoceles occur only rarely in the pediatric population where they can be further categorized as either congenital or acquired.[32,33,34]

Clinical Features

The clinical course associated with laryngoceles can be a lengthy one often requiring multiple endoscopic evaluations before a diagnosis is rendered.[33] Laryngoceles in children are most often clinically characterized by coughing, dyspnea/intermittent airway obstruction, dysphagia, hoarseness and if infected, pain and tenderness. External or combined external and internal laryngoceles can present as a soft anterolateral neck swelling (Figure 15.6). Many pediatric age patients will require tracheostomy, occasionally under emergency conditions,[33] and an MRI or computerized tomography to confirm the diagnosis of a laryngeal luminal lesion.

Pathologic Findings

In infants, the laryngocele will be lined by an epithelial mucous membrane, which will often show papillary formations, with associated prominent submucosal lymphoid aggregates. In adolescents and adults the laryngocele saccule is more often lined by respiratory type epithelium without associated submucosal lymphoid aggregates. Squamous metaplasia of the cyst lining epithelium may be seen as a sequel to infection, and oncocytic metaplasia may also be seen. Differential

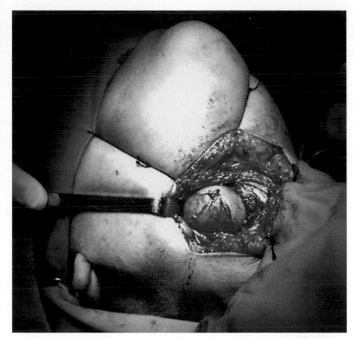

Figure 15.6 External laryngocele arising in the neck. Wikipedia.org/wiki/Laryngocele.

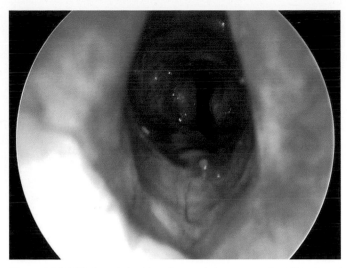

Figure 15.7 SGS characterized by a laryngeal airway narrowing. Wikipedia.org/wiki/Laryngotracheal stenosis.

microscopic diagnoses can include classic laryngeal cysts, oncocytic papillary cystadenoma and branchial cleft cyst.

Treatment and Prognosis

Laryngoceles in pediatric age patients are generally treated by excision using an endoscopic or external approach. As with laryngeal cysts, scarring and narrowing of the airway can result from multiple invasive procedures. A relationship between true laryngoceles and squamous cell carcinoma (SCC) is recognized and SCC occurs in up to 25 percent of adult laryngoceles. Such transformation is rare in pediatric patients however.

Subglottic Stenosis (SGS)

SGS can occur as a congenital or acquired airway narrowing disorder that develops in the anatomic region below the laryngeal glottis and above the first tracheal ring. (Figure 15.7) It is a common cause of stridor in neonates, infants and children.[35]

Acquired SGS is the most common acquired anomaly of the larynx in the pediatric age group, and the most common abnormality necessitating tracheostomy in children less than one year of age.[35,36] In the past, acquired SGS was usually related to an infection (syphilis, TB, diphtheria and typhoid) or caused by trauma.

Currently, however, long term intubation in neonates who require prolonged ventilation,[37] often results in SGS.[38,39] Other factors that play a role in acquired SGS include bacterial infections, gastroesophageal reflux (GERD), rare laryngeal tumors and factors that affect or alter wound healing in general.

Congenital SGS, first described by Holinger et al. in 1954, was originally thought to occur as a result of malformation of the cricoid cartilage.[40] However, incomplete recanalization of the laryngo-tracheal tube during the third month of gestation is more likely the true case. SGS can occur as a *membranous form* in which there is submucosal gland hypoplasia with excessive fibrosis or as a *cartilaginous form* in which there is an abnormality in cricoid cartilage.[41] The disorder improves as the larynx grows and in most cases SGS associated symptoms resolve within a few years of initiation.[42]

The clinical findings seen in SGS are variable and largely depend upon the degree of obstruction.[43] In neonates, obstructed breathing and stridor are the most common chief complaint, while in older children, SGS may only be induced by significant exercise. Children with marginal SGS can become symptomatic when they have an associated viral or bacterial infection that results in edema of the laryngeal lining mucosa. Hoarseness of voice may also occur in these children.

Direct laryngoscopy and bronchoscopy are the usual methods by which one evaluates a child for SGS. A plain anteroposterior and lateral neck radiograph will show the subglottis to have a thin narrow and peaked appearance or a so-called steeple sign. Fluoroscopy can also be used to evaluate a child for and identify SGS.

Pathologic Features

SGS usually begins immediately below the level of the true vocal with associated progressive laryngeal narrowing toward the cricoid cartilage. Maximum stenosis will be seen at the level of the cricoid cartilage and upper trachea.

Histopathologic findings can include fibrosis or granulomatous inflammation and fibrosis (Figure 15.8) that can be keloid-like. The respiratory lining epithelium overlying the area of fibrosis may be unchanged or it may demonstrate significant squamous metaplasia (Figure 15.9). Microscopic differential diagnoses include Wegener's granulomatosis, collagen vascular disease, infectious disease or neoplasia, all of which can be assessed and accurately diagnosed on the basis of routine histopathology, in-situ hybridization (ISH) and special stains.

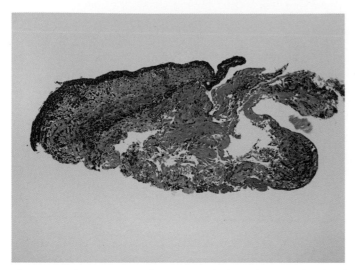

Figure 15.8 SGS. Low power photomicrograph of SGS showing subepithelial fibrous tissue.

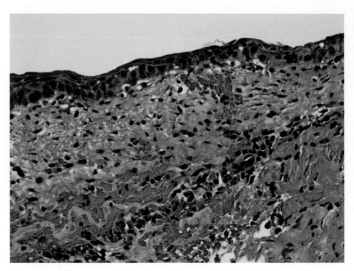

Figure 15.9 Squamous metaplasia of the surface epithelium with submucosal dense fibrosis are evident.

Treatment and Prognosis

Conservative supportive treatment alone may be sufficient to manage most cases of mild SGS. Moderate SGS will respond to endoscopic laser resection and dilation, or to open reconstructive surgery. Mitomycin can be employed postoperatively to reduce scar formation. In severe cases of SGS, laryngeal reconstructive surgery with crico-tracheal resection may be required.[35]

Wegener's Granulomatosis

Wegner's granulomatosis can on rare occasion affect the larynx, subglottic area and lungs of children. The pathobiology and histopathology of Wegener's granulomatosis are described in detail in Chapter 12.

Congenital Laryngeal Webs

Congenital laryngeal webs represent rare laryngeal abnormalities that occur due to incomplete recanalization of the laryngotracheal tube during the third month of gestation. Most laryngeal webs occur anteriorly at the glottis, at the true vocal fold level or at the posterior inter-arytenoid area. Laryngeal webs can also occur in the supraglottic or subglottic region. Web formation can be significant enough to cause airway compromise and even stridor.

Laryngeal webs may be associated with other anatomic anomalies. The association between anterior glottic area webs and velocardiofacial syndrome has been well reported in association with a (22q11.2) deletion. Other syndromes associated with laryngeal webs include Di–George syndrome and CATCH 22 syndromes.[44,45]

Patient evaluation usually involves the use of rigid laryngoscopy and bronchoscopy to assess the location and extent of the web. Radiologic evaluation may demonstrate a characteristic radiographic "sail sign" due to a persistence of tissue between the vocal cords and the subglottis.

Pathologic Features

Histologically, laryngeal webs will be made up of a core of hyperplastic fibrous tissue that is covered by benign laryngeal mucosa. Treatment of laryngeal webs will depend on the degree of airway compromise that is encountered. Asymptomatic lesions require no treatment. Surgical management of severe cases may include surgical division using laryngeal knives, laryngeal microscissors or galvanocautery. Therapy can also include radio-frequency current or laser therapy.[46,47,48]

Laryngeal Atresia
Clinical Features

Laryngeal atresia is an extremely rare congenital entity that results from failure of laryngeal canalization during embryogenesis.[49] The condition may accompany other anomalies including tracheoesophageal fistula, esophageal atresia, low set ears, limb defects and urinary tract anomalies.[49,50]

The condition can be avoided by careful prenatal ultrasound evaluation which usually shows evidence of "Congenital high airway obstruction syndrome" (hyperechogenic enlarged lungs, flattened or inverted diaphragm, fluid filled dilated airway distal to the obstruction, polyhydramnios and fetal hydrops).[49,51] If this is undiscovered, the baby will present with severe respiratory distress at birth, which requires immediate tracheostomy. Tracheolaryngeal reconstruction is typically performed at a later stage in infancy or childhood, and children can recover normally.[49,52]

Pediatric Vocal Fold Nodules or Polyps (Vocal Cord Nodules or Polyps, VFNPs or Singer's Nodule)
Clinical Features

Vocal fold nodules (VFNP) are the most common cause of dysphonia in children. VFNPs occur in 3 to 20 percent of

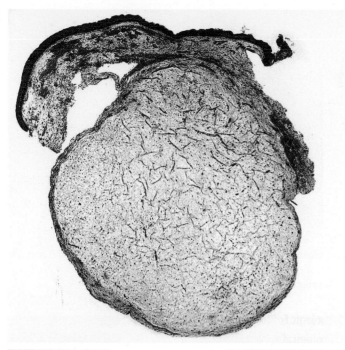

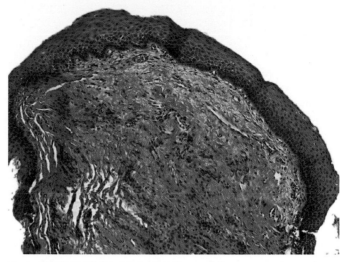

Figure 15.12 Epithelial acanthosis and stromal fibrosis are evident in this fibrous vocal cord nodule.

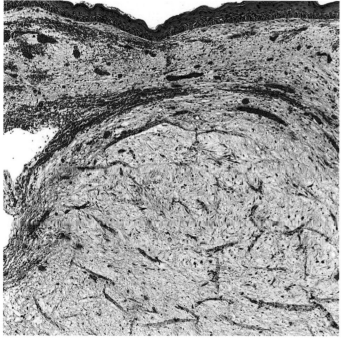

Figures 15.10 (top) & 15.11 (bottom) Low and intermediate power views of vocal cord nodule of the myxoid type demonstrating significant myxoid and edematous stromal change.

pediatric patients.[53,54,55] Classified as a non-neoplastic stromal reactive response, the lesions are related to repeated phonotraumatic or inflammatory insults which affect the true vocal folds of the larynx. VFNPs can be categorized as nodules (sessile lesions), or as polyps (pedunculated lesions). More than one million children in the United States are reported to have vocal cord nodules and slightly more than 2 percent of children worldwide have VFNPs.

VFNPs show a male predominance and peak between the ages of five and ten.[56,57,58] Polyps have been documented, however, in infants less than seven months of age.[58]

Nodules tend to be bilateral while polyps are most often unilateral. Nodules are most often identified anterior to the mid-portion of the true vocal cord. Polyps favor the aryepiglottic fold or the vocal fold.

VFNPs in children arise primarily due to vocal abuse or misuse that can include crying, yelling, singing or talking for prolonged periods. Allergic conditions, infections associated with excessive cough or throat clearing, gastric reflux and dehydration have also been implicated in the etiology of the disorder.[57] Endocrine dysfunction and a genetic predisposition toward polyp formation may be additional causal factors.[54,57,59]

Symptoms vary with the disorder, but commonly include hoarseness, reduced pitch, dysphonia, laryngeal hyperfunction and a breathy vocal quality.

Eating and sleeping habits, including mouth breathing, as well as smoking and alcohol abuse can also be contributory.[55,60,61] The single most important diagnostic procedure used to diagnose vocal cord nodules in children is flexible fiber optic laryngoscopy.[60,62,63] Lesions tend to occur most frequently as bilateral growths at the junction of the anterior third and posterior two-thirds of the true vocal folds. Ultra sonography can be employed as a diagnostic tool as well.

Pathologic Features

VFNPs present grossly as sessile or pedunculated rubbery nodules,[64] that are usually no greater than 0.5 cm in diameter. Five histologic variants of VFNPs can occur[65] and include an edematous *myxoid type* (Figures 15.10 & 15.11), a *fibrous type,* (Figure 15.12), a *hyaline type* (Figures 15.13 & 15.14), a

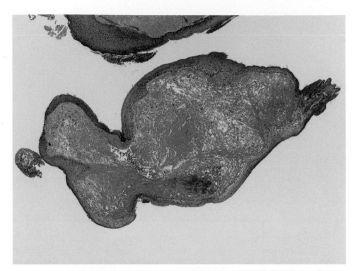

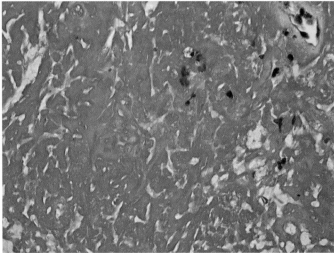

Figures 15.13 (top) & 15.14 (bottom) Low and high power photomicrographs showing stromal hyalinization in this hyaline type vocal cord polyp.

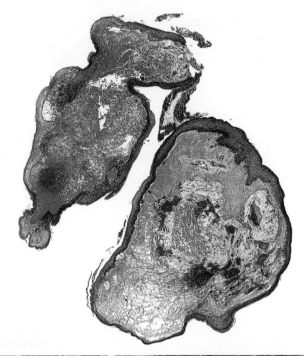

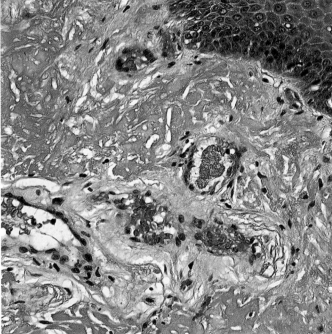

Figures 15.15 (top) & 15.16 (bottom) Considerable stromal vascularity can be seen in this vocal cord nodule.

vascular type (Figures 15.15 & 15.16) and *mixed lesions*. The latter two subtypes can contain any of the elements of the three more common subtypes.

The squamous epithelium overlying the hyperplastic nodule or polyp may show acanthosis, hyperkeratosis or parakeratosis, and may thus also be hyperplastic. Lesions can also appear atrophic, ulcerated and inflamed. On rare occasions the stroma of the lesion may show atypical appearing myofibroblasts similar to those seen in nasal polyps. This atypia is reactive in nature, rather than sarcomatous. Dysplasia of the overlying epithelium may also be seen. Although in-situ SCC and invasive carcinomas have been reported to arise from VFNPs in adults, no such changes have been reported in pediatric age group patients.

Differential microscopic diagnoses can include myxoma, fibroma, amyloidosis and hemangioma for one or more of the various histologic variants of the VFNPs. Immunohistochemical (IHC) assessment of tissue, including appropriate connective tissue and amyloid markers should allow appropriate classification of lesions.

Treatment and Prognosis

Treatment of VFNPs can include conservative management such as voice therapy, drug therapy or surgical excision of the

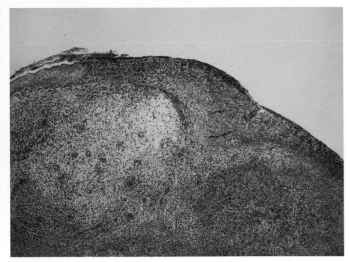

Figure 15.17 Laryngeal contact ulcer showing denuded epithelium and an ulcer base of inflamed granulation tissue.

lesions. Conservative management which always includes voice therapy first, focuses on managing the underlying causes of the disorder, prevention of reflux disease and corrective speech therapy.

Laryngeal Contact Ulcers (Contact Granulomas)

Contact ulcers of the laryngeal mucosa are rare in children. First described in 1928,[66,67] these lesions arise due to the mechanical effect of the arytenoid cartilages colliding and causing mucosal breakdown and ulcer formation. Lesions can be classified as specific and non-specific.[68]

Contact ulcers are also commonly related to mucosal irritation from intubation, particularly from prolonged endotracheal and nasogastric intubation. However, voice abuse and laryngeal/esophageal reflux are also causal factors. Contact ulcers most often involve the posterior vocal cord area where there is the greatest friction during the opening and the closing of the glottis. At this site the mucosa and mucoperichondrium are thin and there is only sparse supportive subepithelial connective tissue.[69] Hoarseness, sore throat, cough with difficulty breathing, occasional choking and throat pain are common to the disorder.

Pathologic Features

On microscopic examination, laryngeal contact ulcers will present as a polypoid ulcerated lesion similar to a pyogenic granuloma. Granulation tissue with acute and chronic inflammation is common to the ulcer base (Figure 15.17). Multinucleated giant cells may also be seen within the fibro-granulomatous complex. Differential diagnoses in children should include infectious diseases, and vascular tumors.

Treatment and Prognosis

The vast majority of laryngeal contact ulcers resolve on their own. Surgery is discouraged as the primary treatment modality for laryngeal contact ulcers, as it is associated with a high recurrence rate and the need for multiple additional surgeries. Voice rest and other treatment modalities including the emerging role of botulinum toxin type A in the treatment of ulcers can be a first line of treatment.[70] The use of topical anti-inflammatory agents such as mitomycin-C and flash lamp pulse dye laser therapy have also been investigated as possible additional therapies.

Laryngeal Amyloidosis (Amyloidoma)
Clinical Features

Laryngeal amyloidosis,[71,72] reported to account for 0.2 to 1.2 percent of all benign tumorous masses in the larynx is exceedingly rare in children.[73,74,75,76,77]

Amyloid is an extracellular insolvable or acellular fibrillar protein material with characteristic microscopic, histochemical and ultrastructural characteristics. Amyloidosis of the larynx can present as an isolated idiopathic solitary lesion, it can be a component of a systemic familial or hereditary disorder,[78] or it can occur secondary to an underlying disease or malignancy.[76,79] The aberrant subepithelial deposited amyloid can eventually lead to interference with laryngeal function. Most laryngeal cases of amyloidosis will contain light chain amyloid A immunoglobulin, and are thus subclassified as fibril in type.[76]

Symptoms will vary in children with laryngeal amyloidosis depending on the size of the formed amyloid mass. Progressive hoarseness is typically the most prominent symptom. Dysphagia may also develop, and although airway obstruction is a theoretical possibility, it has not been reported in children. On laryngoscopic examination, a localized laryngeal mass will be found.[73,74,75,76,77] MRI, the imaging technique of choice, to detect amyloidosis will show amyloid deposits characterized by an intermediate T1-weighted signal intensity and low T2-weighted signal intensity.

Pathologic Features

Histologic examination of laryngeal tissue involved by amyloidosis will demonstrate an extracellular eosinophilic, amorphous material deposited in the submucosa (Figure 15.18). Deposition will be prominent around blood vessels and in the walls of blood vessels. An associated chronic inflammatory infiltrate may be present and a foreign body giant cell reaction, prominently seen around the edges of the amyloid is common.

Thioflavin T staining of the amyloid product will be positive and Congo red stains will show a characteristic green birefringence when the amyloid product is viewed with polarized light. Foreign body giant cell reactivity may be seen. Electron microscopic examination of the amyloid product will classically show an accumulation of linear non-branching

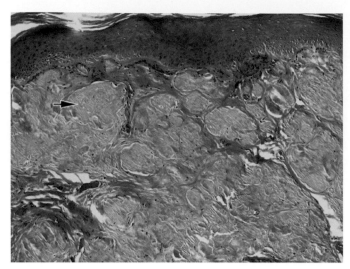

Figure 15.18 Laryngeal amyloidosis. Extracellular eosinophilic acellular amorphous matrix material deposited in the submucosa characteristic of amyloidosis (arrow).

fibrils with a B-pleated sheet-like configuration, varying in size from 50 to 150 Ångstrom in diameter, and 7.5 to 10 nm in width. Plasma cell light chain restriction may also be identified in IHC stained tissue sections. Vocal cord polyps and lipid proteinosis can simulate amyloidosis; however, vocal cord polyps will lack an inflammatory component and amyloid matrix. Amyloid stains will be non-reactive in the case of lipid proteinosis.

Treatment and Prognosis

Resection of the amyloid mass is the treatment of choice for laryngeal amyloidosis. The paucity of cases in children and the lack of long term assessment of such patients make the long term prognosis in children unclear, but persistent and recurrent cases have been reported in adults.

Laryngeal Melanosis

Benign pigmented lesions of the laryngeal mucosa that are histologically characterized by pigmentation of the basal keratinocyte layer, with a slight increase in melanocytes (Figure 15.19) occur primarily in smokers, and most previously reported cases in the literature have been in adults[80] and not in children, however, it is interesting to note that melanosis has been reported in the gingiva of children whose parents have been heavy smokers.[81]

Laryngopharyngeal Reflux Disease (LPRD)

Laryngopharyngeal reflux disease is a disorder in which there is a retrograde flow of gastric contents (acid/pepsin) to the upper aero-digestive tract including the larynx, oropharynx or nasopharynx.[82,83] It is estimated that one in five children suffer some degree of LPRD reflux.[82].

Infants with LPRD will present with failure to thrive, regurgitation, vomiting, dysphagia, recurrent croup, loss of appetite and chronic nasal congestion. School age children

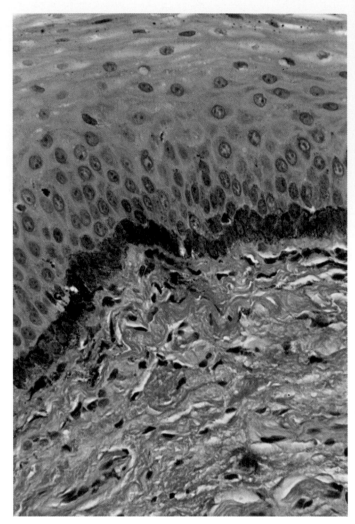

Figure 15.19 Laryngeal melanosis characterized by melanocytic hyperplasia within the basal epithelial layer and rare melanocytes in the superficial collagen.

typically complain of chronic cough, dysphonia, dyspnea, sore throat, globus sensation and halitosis. Older children usually complain of regurgitation, nausea and vomiting, heartburn and chronic respiratory issues.[82,83,84,85]

LPRD is believed to contribute to many pediatric laryngeal disorders, including recurrent respiratory papillomatosis (RRP), laryngomalacia, vocal cord nodules and SGS. Eustachian tube dysfunction, otitis media, chronic sinus disease, poor wound healing after laryngotracheal reconstruction, chronic cough, hoarseness and aspiration have also been reported as a component of the disease.[82,83,84]

The diagnosis of LPRD is generally established on the basis of patient symptomatology, pH probes, endoscopy and radiographic studies.[84]

Pathologic Features

Postcricoid mucosal biopsies from patients with LPRD will demonstrate basal cell hyperplasia of the epithelium, elongation of epithelial rete pegs and eosinophilia. It should be noted, however, that negative biopsies may be seen in symptomatic patients.

Treatment and Prognosis

Treatment of LPRD includes the use of histamine blockers, proton pump inhibitors and lifestyle modification, including patient avoidance of food types that precipitate reflux (spicy food, chocolate, mints and juices). Postural positioning particularly during sleep can be quite beneficial. Surgical treatment may be needed for children with severe disease. Nissan fundoplication is the surgical treatment of choice for such patients.[86]

Benign Neoplasms

Juvenile Onset Recurrent Respiratory Papillomatosis (JORRP)

RRP is the most common benign neoplasm of the larynx[87] in children. JORRP is caused by Human Papilloma Virus (HPV) genotypes 6 and 11 in 90 percent of all cases.[88,89] Other HPV genotypes, including types 16, 18, 31, 33, 35 and 39 are causally implicated. The mode of viral transmission is not clear although perinatal transmission during delivery through an infected maternal birth canal is one presumed method. Sexual transmission or reactivation of a perinatally acquired infection, represent additional causal factors. The incidence of JORRP is approximately 1.7 to 4.3 per 100.000 in children annually.[90]

The condition primarily affects the vocal cord area of the larynx, but can also involve the oral cavity, trachea, bronchi, lung parenchyma and esophagus, and will peak before five years of age or between the second and fourth decades of life. Males are more commonly affected than females at a rate of 3:2.

Although JORRP is a benign disorder, arising from viral replication in squamous mucosal cells, it is a problematic condition due to its unpredictable nature, its preferential ability to spread to other parts the respiratory tract, its malignant potential which is approximately 3 to 7 percent, and its operative risk. The disease also carries with it a social, monetary and psychological toll for affected children and families.[90,91]

The younger an individual's age at disease onset, the more likely the patient will have a more severe disease course. Children with HPV 11 associated disease appear to be at higher risk for recurrence and obstructive problems.[89,90,91,92] It is likely that the host humoral and cellular immune response in children with JORRP is compromised and that the degree of an individual's immune-competence will affect the clinical course of the disease.

Clinical Features

Hoarseness is the principle presenting symptom in JORPP, largely because the vocal cord is the predominant site of papilloma formation.[94] Stridor resulting from increased lesional tissue density is the second most common presenting symptom. Disease associated stridor will initially be inspiratory and later biphasic.[95] Additional symptoms can include chronic cough,

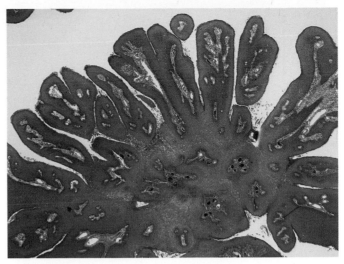

Figure 15.20 Laryngeal papilloma. Low power photomicrograph of a laryngeal papilloma showing characteristic papillary fronds.

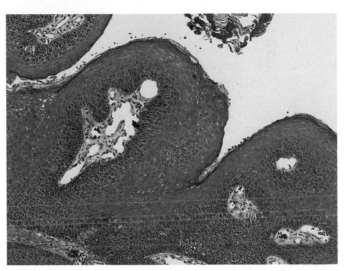

Figure 15.21 Higher power view of the tumor's exophytic fronds and fibrovascular cores

recurrent pneumonia, dyspnea, dysphagia and acute respiratory distress.[95] The biologic course of the disease is quite unpredictable and varies from spontaneous tumor regression, to persistent multifocal disease requiring periodic surgery.[96]

A number of clinical staging systems have been devised in an attempt to assess the severity of JORRP; however, no single universal staging system has gained wide acceptance.[97]

Pathologic Features

On gross inspection, JORRP papillomas appear as exophytic solitary or multiple wart-like, friable, tan to red rubbery growths of less than 1 cm in diameter. Histologically the lesions of JORRP will be composed of squamous epithelial papillary fronds that are supported by a well vascularized connective tissue stromal core (Figures 15.20 & 15.21). Koilocytes may be seen within the epithelium and some degree of

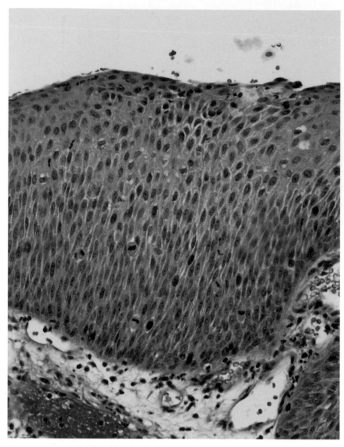

Figure 15.22 Papillary fronds displaying mild atypia that is characterized by increased mitoses and a loss of cellular polarity in this laryngeal papilloma.

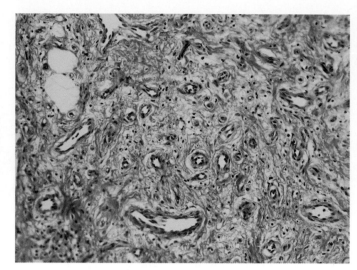

Figure 15.23 Subglottic capillary hemangioma composed of small capillary sized vessels lined by bland, cytologically normal appearing endothelial cells.

reactive nuclear atypia may also be present. P16 can be employed as a surrogate HPV marker, while PCR or ISH can be employed to detect HPV genotypes.

Differential diagnoses include laryngeal verruca vulgaris (reported in adults but not in children), verrucous carcinoma, papillary SCC and condyloma acuminatum. Rarely dysplastic changes can occur in the squamous mucosa of a papilloma (Figure 15.22) with subsequent cancer development. However, such changes are exceptionally rare in pediatric age patients.

Treatment and Prognosis

No single treatment modality has been found to be uniformly effective in managing JORRP. Management of the condition requires a skilled and cooperative team of clinicians. Neonatal JORRP will often require tracheostomy and carries with it a greater mortality risk. The mortality rate for the disease in children is less than 2 percent and is usually related to pulmonary disease, asphyxia or malignancy. Surgery that is most often laser based or performed as a micro-debridement endoscopic procedure is the most common form of treatment. Adjuvant therapy that includes antiviral modalities such as interferon, ribavirin, acyclovir and cidofovir can prove to be effective. Dietary supplements including Indole-3-Carbinol, cox2 inhibitors, retinoids and mumps vaccine injections into

lesions have also been employed with varying degrees of success. Emerging gene therapies may prove to be beneficial in the future. However, no single adjuvant therapeutic measure is wholly effective in curing JORRP.[95]

The recently introduced HPV vaccine has shown promise in decreasing the incidence of JORRP, and in providing protection against HPV6 and 11 associated laryngeal papillary lesions.[98,99]

Congenital Laryngeal Subglottic Hemangioma

Congenital laryngeal subglottic hemangiomas are rare, typically asymptomatic lesions that arise at birth. However, this unique form of hemangioma tends to grow rather rapidly, and within 2 to 12 months of birth, most affected individuals will be symptomatic with a chief complaint of progressive respiratory compromise. Rigid bronchoscopy is typically employed to establish the diagnosis in the subglottis.

PHACES syndrome, characterized by posterior fossa brain malformations, hemangiomas, cardiac anomalies, coarctation of the aorta and eye anomalies with or without sternal clefting should be excluded when one encounters a subglottic hemangioma in an infant or child.[100,101,102]

Pathologic Features

Grossly, the subglottic hemangioma will be a sessile and easily compressible hemorrhagic growth or mass. Microscopically, most lesions represent simple capillary hemangiomas. Less frequently, lesions can be cavernous or present as a mixed capillary/cavernous hemangioma. Histologically, tumors will be composed of endothelially lined vascular spaces that ramify throughout the supporting lamina propria (Figure 15.23), to often involve the perichondrium of the underlying cartilage, or extend between the tracheal rings.[101] Inflammation will be variably present in the stromal component of the neoplasm.

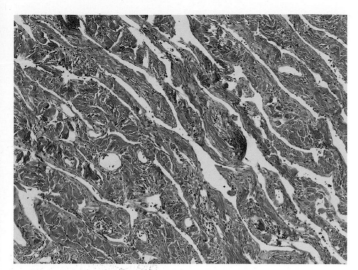

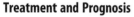

Figure 15.24 Laryngeal lymphangioma demonstrating variably sized lymphatic channels lined by attenuated endothelial cells. Pericytes and smooth muscle support are absent.

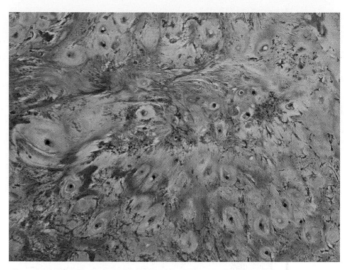

Figure 15.25 Laryngeal chondroma composed of hyaline cartilage with normal appearing bland chondrocytes within lacunae.

Treatment and Prognosis

Treatment of subglottic hemangiomas can vary. Periodic to long term observation for small lesions that do not cause significant obstruction may be sufficient. Tracheostomy may be required in patients until larger lesions regress, which usually occurs by the age of five. Small and medium sized lesions may respond to steroid injections and involute. Laser ablation therapy, cryosurgery, intralesional interferon injection, sclerosing agent injection, systemic steroids and more recently propranolol therapy have all been used to treat subglottic hemangiomas.[103,104,105] When these treatment modalities fail, surgery remains the treatment of choice.

Congenital Laryngeal Lymphangioma

Congenital lympangiomatous malformations of the larynx are rare. Fifty percent of all such lesions are recognized in the neonatal period of life, while approximately 75 percent are diagnosed by the age of one.[106,107,108] Symptoms are variable and depend largely on the size of the lesion. Voice changes, progressive dyspnea and even stridor can occur.[106,107,108,109,110]

Pathologic Features and Treatment

Microscopically, lymphangiomas are composed of variably sized lymphatic channels that are lined by attenuated endothelial cells (Figure 15.24). These channels lack pericytes and smooth muscle support.

Treatment and Prognosis

Various treatment options are available to manage congenital lymphangioma including surgical excision, laser debulking of the lesion, sclerotherapy and corticosteroid therapy.[111] Recurrence or persistence of disease after surgical excision is common and the overall incidence of permanent cranial nerve injury is 20 percent.

Chondroma

Laryngeal chondromas in pediatric age group patients are rare lesions that occur most frequently within the cricoid or thyroid cartilage as endochondral ossifications.[112,113,114,115,116] Chondromas can occur congenitally in which case the affected infant may present with stridor.[113] Most chondromas however, will present as a laryngeal mass that causes dysphonia, hoarseness or dyspnea. Radiologically, laryngeal chondromas will present as a well defined hypodense compartmentalized laryngeal mass that may exhibit calcific foci. Endoscopically, tumors will present as a laryngeal space projection.

Pathologic Features

Tumors rarely reach a size of 2 cm in greatest dimension. On microscopic examination, most tumors will appear as a submucosal lobulated or nodular growth that will be composed of normal appearing lacunae located chondrocytes without cellular pleomorphism or marked hyperchromatism (Figure 15.25). The overlying epithelium will be intact. Chondrometaplasia can resemble the chondroma histologically; however, it will present as an elastic cartilage nodule without cartilage unification.

Treatment and Prognosis

The treatment of choice for small chondromas of the larynx is surgical excision of the mass via an endolaryngeal approach. An extralaryngeal approach is typically required to manage larger lesions. Tumors must be evaluated by the pathologist using appropriate sampling since well differentiated chondrosarcoma can be a diagnostic consideration. Recurrence is in the 10 to 15 percent range and while chondrosarcoma develops in nearly 5 percent of cases, it only rarely occurs in children.

Lipoma

Lipomas of the larynx in pediatric age group patients are uncommon, with less than 100 cases reported in the literature.[117,118,119,120,121] Lipomas in this site are thought to originate from either a pluripotent primitive regional cell, or more likely from lipomatous tissue normally found below the false vocal cord, epiglottis and aryepiglottic fold. Most pediatric lipomas are slow growing neoplasms that will cause upper airway compromise, hoarseness and more rarely sleep apnea. CT scans usually will typically demonstrate a low attenuation non-enhanced mass.

Pathologic Features

Histologically, the laryngeal lipoma will be composed of encapsulated mature adipose tissue that is made up of adipocytes that are uniform in their size, shape and cytology. Tumors may have a prominent myxoid stroma. The primary differential microscopic diagnoses include well differentiated liposarcoma or myxoid liposarcoma, and myxoid vocal cord polyp. Liposarcomas will tend to display some degree of cytologic atypia, while myxoid vocal cord polyps will be made up of cells that are more loosely arranged and myxoid in character than the lipoma, and lack any aggregation of uni-vacuolated fat cells.

Treatment and Prognosis

Treatment of laryngeal lipomas involves complete surgical removal of the lesion to a margin of normal tissue. Most pediatric associated lipomas are removed via an external surgical approach. Recurrence is rare.

Neural Tumors

Granular Cell Tumor

First described in 1926, the granular cell tumor was originally classified as a myoblastoma and thought to be a tumor of muscle origin.[122] Subsequent investigations have shown that the tumor is of neural derivation and most likely of Schwann cell origin.[123] Laryngeal granular cell tumors are rare in the pediatric population[124,125,126,127,128] and most head and neck lesions will in fact involve the tongue. When the larynx is involved, the true vocal cord, posterior third, is the most commonly affected site.[124]

The granular cell tumor is slow growing, and the most common presenting symptom for laryngeal tumors is hoarseness. However, other symptoms including cough, dyspnea, dysphagia, hemoptysis and stridor have also been reported in pediatric age patients.[122,123,124,125,126,127,128]

Pathologic Features

Grossly, granular cell tumors tend to be rubbery to firm, often yellowish appearing growths. Most tumors will be less than 2 cm in greatest dimension. Histologically, tumors will be encapsulated and composed of large round to polygonal cells with an oval hyperchromatic central nucleus and small nucleolus. Pseudoepitheliomatous hyperplasia of the overlying laryngeal epithelium is frequently present. (Figure 15.26) The cytoplasm of the tumor cells is typically granular and

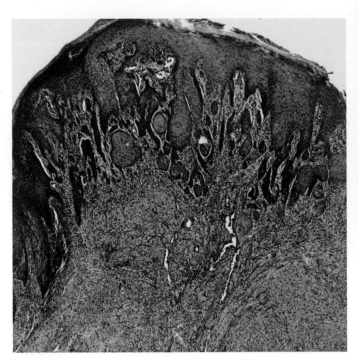

Figure 15.26 Granular cell tumor. Note the characteristic pseudoepitheliomatous hyperplasia of overlying squamous epithelium.

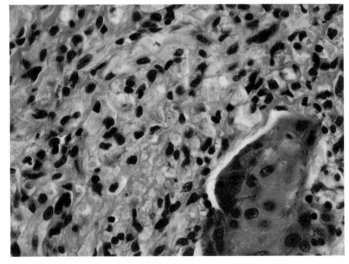

Figure 15.27 Large round to polygonal tumor cells with an oval hyperchromatic central nucleus and small nucleolus characterize this granular cell tumor. The cytoplasm of the tumor cells is typically granular and eosinophilic and cell borders are ill-defined.

eosinophilic and cell borders tend to be ill-defined (Figure 15.27). Electron microscopic examination of tumor cells will demonstrate granular cells with lysosomal membrane bound autophagic vacuoles containing mitochondria, myelin figures, rough endoplasmic reticulum and myelinated and non-myelinated axon like structures.[129] Tumor cells usually grow in a trabecular, syncytial or nested pattern.

Tumor cells stain positively for S100 protein, neuron specific enolase and vimentin, and negatively for cytokeratin, muscle markers, glial fibrillary acidic protein or neurofilament protein. Molecular analysis has shown that some tumors contain osteoponin (OPN) mRNA. Malignant granular cell tumors have been documented but no malignant tumors have been reported in the pediatric age group in a laryngeal location.

Treatment and Prognosis

Complete surgical excision of the tumor can be accomplished endoscopically when small tumors are encountered. An external surgical approach may be required for large tumors. Patient prognosis is excellent although recurrence can range as high as 10 percent.

Nerve Sheath Tumors

Laryngeal Schwannoma and *neurofibroma*, the two most commonly occurring benign nerve sheath neoplasms are quite rare in pediatric age patients.[130] Most nerve sheath tumors in this location, when seen in children, will be associated with neurofibromatosis type 1 and 2.[133] Chinn et al. in a 2014 review of the world literature, documented only 62 pediatric neurofibromas ever reported in this location.[134] The vast majority of either Schwannomas or neurofibromas originate as supraglottic tumors that arise from the medial ramifications of the internal branch of the superior laryngeal nerve. Favored supraglottic sites include the aryepiglottic fold, and the false vocal folds. The subglottic region is uncommonly involved. True vocal cord involvement is also quite rare.[135,136]

Symptomatology can include dysphonia and progressive dyspnea. Rare asphyxiation has been reported.[134] The histopathology of neurofibroma and Schwannoma are discussed in detail in Chapter 2 of this text.

Treatment and Prognosis

Depending on their size and location, Schwannoma and neurofibroma can be treated using either minimally invasive endoscopic resection or open surgical extirpation with tracheotomy.[137] Recurrence, although uncommon, can be a complicating factor.

Laryngeal Paraganglioma

Laryngeal paragangliomas are benign neuroendocrine tumors that originate from extra-adrenal, neural crest-derived superior or inferior paraganglia in the larynx.[138] Very few reported cases of pediatric age head and neck paragangliomas exist in the literature, and the mean age of occurrence for all tumors is just under 50.[139,140,141,142] Most laryngeal paragangliomas, whether in adults or children, occur in the supraglottic larynx, and females are most often affected. Rarely, tumors can be multicentric.

Hoarseness and respiratory obstruction, including stridor can be encountered in children with a laryngeal paraganglioma but such symptomatology is rare. MRI is typically used to define the anatomic limits of the tumor, while CT of the neck will commonly show an enhanced lobulated mass.

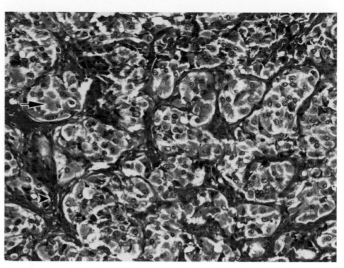

Figure 15.28 Laryngeal paraganglioma. The tumor is composed of an alveolar cluster of chief cells (arrow) that are surrounded by spindle shaped sustentacular cells (arrowhead).

Pathologic Features

The histologic features of laryngeal paragangliomas are identical to those seen in other anatomic sites. Tumors will display a hallmark "zellballen" pattern of growth. Round or oval chief cells with abundant eosinophilic, granular or clear cytoplasm and round or oval nuclei with a dispersed chromatin pattern are characteristically identified (Figure 15.28). Chief cells will be marginated by *sustentacular cells* spindle shaped modified Schwann cells that will be strongly S100 protein reactive. The collagenous interstitium of the tumor is generally richly vascular. Chief cells will stain positively for neuroendocrine markers including synaptophysin and chromogranin. Both tumor cell types will stain negatively for epithelial and mesenchymal markers. Principal microscopic differential diagnoses include carcinoid or atypical carcinoid.[138,139,140,141,142]

Treatment and Prognosis

Laryngeal paragangliomas are treated by surgical resection using an external approach rather than an endoscopic one. Patient prognosis is excellent, however, local recurrence anywhere from 1 to 15 years after initial surgery, will occur in 15 to 20 percent of patients.

Benign Muscle Tumors

Rhabdomyoma

Benign tumors of skeletal muscle origin can be divided into cardiac and extracardiac subtypes. Extracardiac tumors can further be classified as adult, fetal and genital.[144,145] Most rhabdomyomas in children are cardiac associated and occur as a component of tuberous sclerosis.[145] Only recently has a rare case of a pediatric patient with tuberous sclerosis and a laryngeal fetal cellular rhabdomyoma been reported.[144] Individuals with laryngeal rhabdomyomas most often present with

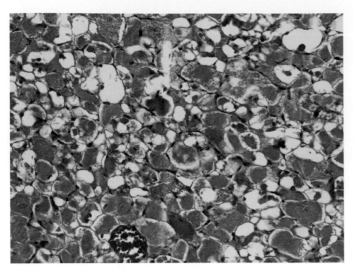

Figure 15.29 Adult rhabdomyoma. Note the closely packed polygonal eosinophilic cells with one or more round to oval nuclei, and prominent nucleoli and the abundant eosinophilic vacuolated cytoplasm that is glycogen rich.

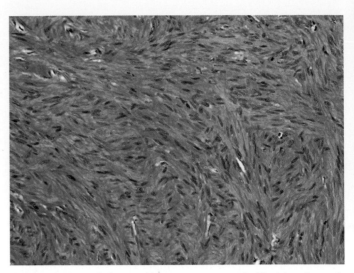

Figure 15.30 Simple laryngeal leiomyoma composed of fascicles of smooth muscle fibers with no evidence of necrosis or mitoses. Tumor cells have blunt ended nuclei and richly eosinophilic cytoplasm.

symptoms of stridor, although dyspnea, dysphasia and hoarseness can also be encountered.

Pathologic Findings

Grossly, tumors tend to be lobulated and well circumscribed. On microscopic examination, fetal rhabdomyomas will be composed of small immature muscle cells, with round to spindle shaped nuclei and minimal cytoplasm. Eosinophilic strap cells with striations will be few in number, and necrosis, mitosis and pleomorphism will not be seen. Adult rhabdomyomas in contrast, will be composed of closely packed polygonal eosinophilic cells that contain one or more round to oval nuclei and prominent nucleoli (Figure 15.29). The cytoplasm will be glycogen rich and tumor cells can appear vacuolated after formalin fixation, giving cells a spider web like appearance. Rod shaped crystals may also be present within the cytoplasm of tumor cells.

Fetal rhabdomyomas will stain diffusely positive for desmin, myoglobin, smooth muscle actin calponin and muscle specific actin. Focal positivity for MYF-4, S100 protein and vimentin may also be seen. Tumor cells will stain negatively for pancytokeratin, CD1a, GFAP, chromogranin and synaptophysin.

Treatment and Prognosis

Rhabdomyomas are benign tumors with no malignant potential. Laryngeal tumors in pediatric age patients are generally treated by endoscopic resection. Recurrence is rare.

Leiomyoma

Laryngeal leiomyomas occur very rarely. Just over 40 cases have been reported in the literature since 1966.[147,148] Most cases reported in the pediatric age group have been in adolescents.[147,148,149] Tumors in this location are theorized to arise from the smooth muscle within the walls of blood vessels, or from aberrant undifferentiated mesenchyme.[150]

Laryngeal leiomyomas can be supraglottic, glottic or subglottic. Most reported cases have been in a supraglottic location,[151,152] and patient symptoms can range from dyspnea to extreme tenderness and pain, to stridor.

Pathologic Features

Three histologic subtypes of leiomyoma occur in the larynx: simple, vascular (angioleiomyomatous) and epithelioid. Simple leiomyomas will be composed of fascicles of smooth muscle fibers with no necrosis or mitoses, while vascular leiomyomas will have a rich capillary or cavernous vascular supply integrated within the tumor's concentric layers of smooth muscle fibers (Figure 15.30).[147,148,149,152] Simple tumors will be composed of cells that have blunt ended nuclei, and tumor cells will be rich in eosinophilic cytoplasm. Epithelioid tumors will be made up of nests and cords of cells with round to oval nuclei, and epithelioid cells will be admixed with spindle cells. Tumor cells in all subtypes will stain positively for the muscle markers SMA, MSA, calponin and desmin.

Treatment and Prognosis

Conservative surgical removal, employing either endoscopic excision or with an external approach is the modality of choice for treating leiomyomas in children. Recurrence and persistence have been reported.

Inflammatory Myofibroblastic Tumor (IMT, Inflammatory Pseudotumor)

IMT, first described by Keen et al.[153] and further defined by Wenig et al.[154] is an inflammatory pseudotumor composed of myofibroblastic cells with an associated admix of collagen and chronic inflammatory cells. The etiology of the tumor is

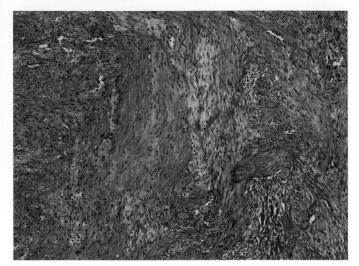

Figure 15.31 IMT composed of loosely arranged spindle to ovoid or epithelioid appearing myofibroblasts arranged in a storiform or fascicular pattern.

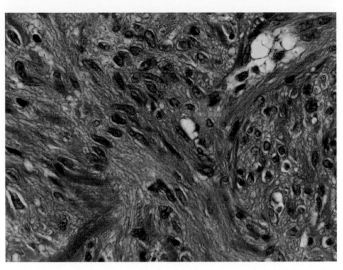

Figure 15.32 High power photomicrograph of tumor cells highlighting the mature collagenous stroma and the eosinophilic cytoplasm of tumor cells in an IMT.

unclear; although the tumor is considered by most investigators to be a reactive process, initiated by immunologic events, trauma or infection.[156]

Less than 50 cases have been reported in the literature since 1995,[156] with eight of those cases occurring in pediatric age group patients. Laryngeal tumors have been identified in the supraglottic, glottic and subglottic areas with the glottis representing the most common laryngeal site. Patient symptoms can range from hoarseness to stridor. In addition to laryngeal sites, tumors have also been documented in the oral cavity, the maxillary sinus and the parapharyngeal space. Males are more often affected than females.

Pathologic Features

On gross inspection, the IMT will have a polypoid, multi-nodular or nodular appearance, be fleshy in consistency and range from 1 to 4 cm in greatest dimension. Microscopically, tumors will be subepithelial in their presentation and be composed of loose spindle to stellate cells, and sometimes slender axonal or epithelioid appearing myofibroblasts arranged in a storiform or fascicular pattern. Tumor cells will have ovoid to oblong nuclei with prominent nucleoli and basophilic fibrillar cytoplasm (Figure 15.31). Intranuclear inclusions may also be seen. The tumor stroma varies from myxoid to collagenous (Figure 15.32) and the tumor's vascular component can be quite variable. Admixed within the tumor there will be prominent collections of mature lymphocytes, plasma cells, eosinophils, histiocytes and fibroblasts. Tumor cell nuclear pleomorphism is not seen and mitosis is rare, although reactive cellular atypia may be seen.

Tumor cell myofibroblasts are immunoreactive (cytoplasmically) to vimentin. Smooth muscle actin, muscle specific actin and calponin show variable reactivity. Occasional desmin positivity may be seen. Tumor cells will stain negatively for S100 protein, myoglobin, myogenin, CD117, HMB-45, MyoD1 and CD34.

ALK gene rearrangement and expression has been reported in IMT tumor cells themselves, but not in the inflammatory component, particularly in children and young adults.[158] The chromosomal rearrangement occurs cytogenetically at chromosome 2p23.

Histologic differential diagnoses can include contact ulcers of the larynx, pyogenic granuloma, nodular fasciitis, fibrosarcoma and spindle cell SCC. Laryngeal spindle cell carcinoma is exceedingly rare in children. It will lack the myxoid pattern of IMT, and demonstrate no cytologic atypia. Cytokeratin immunoreactivity will be seen 75 percent of cases. The marked inflammatory component of IMT often mandates excluding infectious diseases such as atypical mycobacterium, by special stains. The cytologic atypia characteristic of fibrosarcoma will be absent in IMT.

Treatment and Prognosis

The most common treatment modality for the IMT is conservative surgical excision using laser or microlaryngoscopic techniques. The use of steroids and non-steroidal anti-inflammatory drugs as a treatment modality has been associated with regression in some, but not all patients. IMT can be recurrent in as great as 20 percent of patients. Tumors rich in an inflammatory component may have a better prognosis than those that are purely spindle cell in their character. Tumors that are p53 expressive with DNA aneuploidy are thought to be more biologically aggressive.

Benign Salivary Gland Tumors

Benign salivary gland tumors of the larynx are rare in all age groups. The most common benign salivary gland tumor encountered in pediatric age group patients is the pleomorphic adenoma. A complete discussion of the pathobiology of pleomorphic adenoma can be found in Chapter 10 of this text.

Malignant Laryngeal Neoplasms

Pediatric Laryngeal Squamous Cell Carcinoma (Laryngeal SCC)

Laryngeal SCCs occur infrequently in pediatric age group patients, representing less than 1 percent of all pediatric tumors.[160] Fewer than 100 cases have been reported in the world's literature, and most head and neck SCCs in pediatric age patients occur in the oral cavity and oropharynx. Nearly a third of the 100 reported cases have occurred as a result of malignant transformation of JORRP.[161,162,163] Irradiation of RRP, HPV infection, passive or active smoking and asbestos exposure have all been implicated in the etiology of pediatric laryngeal SCC.[164]

Most children and adolescents with laryngeal SCC will present with non-specific symptoms that can also be encountered in benign conditions, including hoarseness, cough, respiratory infections and voice changes. While laryngeal SCC in adults is essentially a life-style related disease, most often resulting from long term tobacco use, pediatric age group SCC is more often HPV associated, or associated with prior radiation therapy for RRP.

The vocal folds are the most common site for tumors to arise, followed by supraglottic and subglottic tissues.[165,166] Laryngeal examination will generally show a polypoid lesion or a mass that in many instances may be thought to represent benign papillomatosis.

The biological behavior of Laryngeal SCC in the pediatric population is, on the whole, a more aggressive one than that seen in SCC in the adult population.[167] The most common HPV types that are associated with SCC transformed juvenile papillomatosis are the 6 and 11 genotypes, particularly HPV 11, although HPV 13, 16, 18, 31 and 33 have also been found to be associated with disease transition.

The histopathology of laryngeal SCC is similar to that encountered in adults, and most pediatric age group patients will present with conventional well differentiated SCCs, in which sheets, nests and cords of neoplastic squamous cells ramify throughout a chronically inflamed connective tissue stroma (Figure 15.33). Tumors will generally show a pattern of local spread that is similar to that seen in adult SCCs.[166]

Apart from the conventional SCC, other subtypes of SCC, including verrucous carcinoma, spindle cell carcinoma and basaloid, acantholytic and clear cell carcinomas, are not well documented in the pediatric literature.

Treatment and Prognosis

The management of laryngeal squamous cell cancer in children is challenging and can prove to be more difficult than in adults. In addition to being more biologically aggressive, SCC in pediatric age patients tends to present at a more advanced stage. Long term complications, including recurrence and psychological sequelae are common to the disease process.[161]

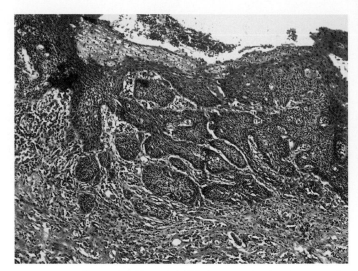

Figure 15.33 Conventional laryngeal SCC demonstrating invasive nests of malignant squamous cells into a chronically inflamed connective tissue stroma.

Management usually consists of total laryngectomy with or without postoperative radiation and or chemotherapy. HPV testing is mandatory for the proper early recognition and treatment of laryngeal SCC in pediatric age patients.

Pediatric Laryngeal Sarcomas

Approximately 40 percent of rhabdomyosarcomas (RMS) are localized to the cervico-cephalic region. Among the importantly occurring sarcomas of childhood and adolescence, RMS is by far the most common malignancy to arise in the larynx. Nonetheless, Ferlito et al. in an extensive review of the literature, found only 47 documented malignant laryngeal neoplasms in children and adolescents. Embryonal RMS accounted for 20 cases in that study, followed by three cases of synovial sarcoma, two cases of malignant fibrous histiocytoma (anaplastic pleomorphic sarcoma) and single cases of chondrosarcoma, Ewing sarcoma/PNET, Fibrosarcoma, malignant Schwannoma and "mixed" sarcoma.

The ensuing discussion will center on the two most common sarcomas of the larynx to be found in pediatric age patients: RMS and synovial sarcoma. The histopathologic features of additional significant sarcomas common to the head and neck region of children and adolescents are discussed elsewhere in this textbook in association with their presentation in specific anatomic locations, however, in this chapter we discuss Rhabdomyosarcoma and Synovial sarcoma.

Rhabdomyosarcoma (RMS)
Clinical Features

RMS of the larynx accounts for less than 3 percent of all RMSs that occur in the cervico-cephalic region.[170,171] The first case of laryngeal RMS in a child was described in 1944 by Glick.[172] Since that original description, no more than two dozen laryngeal RMSs have been reported in pediatric age group patients.

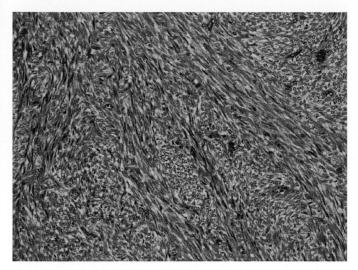

Figure 15.34 Synovial sarcoma. Monophasic synovial sarcoma showing spindle cells arranged in a fascicular fashion.

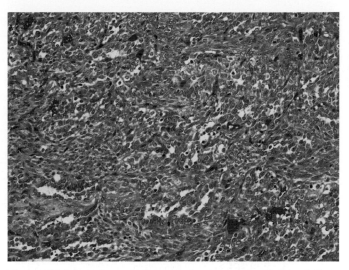

Figure 15.35 Biphasic synovial sarcoma showing ovoid epithelial cells that form glandular spaces associated with spindle cells arranged in fascicles.

Affected individuals have ranged in age from 1 to 18, and all laryngeal locations (supraglottic, glottic and subglottic) have been documented as anatomic sites of origin for the tumor. Symptoms can range from hoarseness to stridor in patients laryngeal RMS.[172,173,174]

Pathologic Features

Histologically, most laryngeal RMSs are *embryonal* (ERMS), and will be composed of malignant round to oval cells with scant cytoplasm and hyperchromatic nuclei or truncated spindle cells with an elongated nucleus. Mitoses will be common and the tumor stroma will range from fibrous to myxoid. A loss of heterozygosity of the short arm of chromosome 11 (11p15.5) characterizes ERMS cytogenetically.[174] Alveolar RMS of the larynx in pediatric age patients accounts for 15 percent of tumors while the *pleomorphic* form of the disease is rarely, if ever, encountered in the pediatric age group. A complete discussion of pathobiology and the special stains required to the diagnosis of ERMA along with a discussion of the cytogenetics of the disease can be found in Chapter 2 of this text.

Treatment and Prognosis

The principal mode of treatment for laryngeal RMS is surgery (partial to total laryngectomy) although combined chemotherapy and radiation therapy have been employed in both a primary and adjuvant role. Vincristine, actinomycin and cyclophosphamide are the most commonly employed chemotherapeutic agents used in the treatment of RMS. The overall five-year survival rate for children with tumors in this site is about 60 percent.[171]

Synovial Sarcoma

Synovial sarcoma is an aggressive malignant soft tissue neoplasm that is genetically characterized by a t(X: 18) (p11.2;q 11.2) balanced translocation. Synovial sarcoma most commonly affects the extremities. The head and neck region is an uncommon site with less than 4 percent of cases presenting in this anatomic region. Less than a dozen cases have been documented in the pediatric population.[175,176,177,178,179] Tumors are most often exophytic or pedunculated masses that involve the endolarynx or hypopharynx. The most common presenting symptomatology is dyspnea or hoarseness.

Pathologic Features

Histologically, laryngeal synovial sarcoma, as in all other anatomic sites, can present as a monophasic or biphasic tumor. Monophasic tumors will be largely composed of malignant appearing spindle cells; whereas biphasic synovial sarcoma will be composed of spindle cells admixed with a glandular epithelial cell component in variable proportions.

The spindle cell component of the tumor will typically be composed of uniform spindle to ovoid cells with pale staining nuclei and ill-defined cell borders (Figure 15.34). Nucleoli will be inconspicuous. Mitoses are usually scant except in poorly differentiated tumors, where they can increase significantly. An epithelial component will be lacking. The tumor stroma can range from fibrotic to myxoid to microcystic.

Biphasic tumors will contain both a spindle cell (synoviocytic) and epithelial (glandular) component. The epithelial component will consist of glands with lumina that may contain mucin. (Figure 15.35) The glandular epithelial lining is often papillary. Glandular lining cells can appear cytologically atypical or quite bland.

Squamous metaplasia and keratinization may occur within the tumor and large areas of calcification can also be present. Most synovial sarcomas will exhibit cytokeratin, CK7 and CK19 positivity in the epithelial component of the tumor, with rare positive foci staining in the spindle cell component. The epithelial component of the tumor can also be EMA reactive.

BCL2 is diffusely expressed in all synovial sarcomas particularly in the spindle component. Focal positive staining for S100 protein, CD99 and desmin may be present. Vimentin staining will be absent in the spindle cell component of the tumor.

Treatment and Prognosis

Treatment experience related to laryngeal synovial sarcoma is limited in the pediatric population, but typically includes total laryngectomy and adjuvant chemotherapy and radiation therapy. Local regional recurrence is common and is usually seen early (within two years of treatment), in the follow-up period.

Malignant Salivary Gland Tumors

Rare malignant salivary gland tumors involving the larynx have been reported in the pediatric population including mucoepidermoid carcinoma, malignant mixed tumor and adenocarcinoma NOS. The characteristic histopathology of these tumors is discussed in detail in Chapter 11.

References

Introduction

1. Hartnick CJ, Cotton RT. Syndromic and other congenital anomalies of the head and neck. *Otolaryngol Clin North Am* 2003; 33:1293–1308.

2. Wyatt ME, Hartley BEJ. Laryngotracheal reconstruction in congenital laryngeal webs and atresia. *Otolaryngol Head Neck Surg* 2005; 132:232–238.

3. Tucker GF, Tucker JA, Vidic B. Anatomy and development of the cricoid: serial section whole organ study of perinatal larynges. *Ann Otol Rhinol Laryngol* 1977; 86:766–769.

4. Zaw-Tun HI. Development and congenital laryngeal atresia and clefts. *Ann Otol Rhinol Laryngol* 1988; 97:353–358.

5. Holinger LD, Lusk RP, Green CG. *Pediatric Laryngology and Bronchoesophagology*. Philadelphia: Lippencott-Raven 1997.

Laryngomalacia

6. Jackson C, Jackson CL. Laryngomalacia. In: *Diseases and Injuries of the Larynx*. New York: Macmillan 1942: 63–69.

7. Wiatrak BJ. Congenital anomalies of the larynx and trachea. *Otolaryngol Clin North Am* 2000; 33:91–110.

8. Daniel SJ. The upper airway: congenital malformations. *Pediatr Respir Rev* 2006; 7:S260–263.

Vocal Cord Paralysis

9. Daya H, Hosni A, Bejar-Solar I, et al. Pediatric vocal cord paralysis: a long term retrospective study. *Arch Otolaryngol Head Neck Surg* 2000; 126:21–25.

10. Parikh S. Pediatric vocal fold immobility. *Otolaryngol Clin N Am* 2004; 37:203–215.

11. Holinger LD, Holinger PC, Holinger PH. Etiology of bilateral abductor vocal cord paralysis. *Ann Otol Rhinol Laryngol* 1976; 85:428–436.

12. Mace M, Williamson E, Worgan D. Autosomal dominantly inherited adductor laryngeal paralysis – a new syndrome with suggestion of linkage to HLA. *Clin Genet* 1978; 14:265–270.

13. Manaligod JM, Skaggs J, Smith RJ. Localization of gene for familial laryngeal abductor paralysis to chromosome 6Q16. *Arch Otolaryngol Head Neck Surg* 2001; 127:913–917.

14. King E, Blumin J. Vocal cord paralysis in children. *Curr Opin Otolaryngol Head Neck Surg* 2009; 17:483–487.

15. Sipp A, Keschner J, Braune N, Hartnick C. Vocal cord medialization in children. Injection laryngoplasty, thyroplasty, or nerve innervation. *Arch Otolaryngol Head Neck Surg* 2007; 133:767–771.

16. Cohen M, Mehta D, Maguire R, Simons J. Injection medialization laryngoplasty in children. *Arch Otolaryngol Head Neck Surg* 2011; 137:264–268.

17. Lewy RB. Response of laryngeal tissue to granular Teflon in situ. *Arch Otolaryngol* 1966; 83:355–359.

18. Laccourreye O, Papon JF, Kania R, et al. Intracordal injection of autologous fat in patients with unilateral laryngeal nerve paralysis: long term results from the patient perspective. *Laryngoscope* 2003; 113:541–545.

19. Milstein CF, Akst LM, Hicks D, et al. Long term effect of micronized AlloDerm injection for unilateral vocal cord paralysis. *Laryngoscope* 2005; 115:1691–1696.

20. Hughes RG, Morrison M. Vocal cord medialization by transcutaneous injection of calcium hydroxyapatite. *J Voice* 2005; 19:674–678.

21. Schramm VL, May M, Lavarato AS. Gelfoam paste injection for vocal cord paralysis: temporary rehabilitation of glottic incompetence. *Laryngoscope* 1978; 88:1268–1273.

22. Tanna N, Zalkind D, Glade RS, Bielamowicz SA. Foreign body reaction to calcium hydroxyapatite vocal fold augmentation. *Arch Otolaryngol Head Neck Surg* 2006; 132:1379–1382.

Laryngeal Cysts

23. Ramesar K, Albizzati C. Laryngeal cysts: clinical relevance of modified working classification. *J Laryngol Otol* 1988; 102:923–925.

24. Abercrombie J. Congenital cyst in the larynx. *Trans Pathol Soc London* 1881; 32:33–34.

25. DeSanto LW, Devine KD, Weiland LH. Cysts of the larynx – classification. *Laryngoscope* 1970; 80:145–176.

26. Prowse S, Knight L. Congenital cyst of the infant larynx. *Int J Pediatr Otorhinolaryngol* 2012; 76:708–711.

27. Ku ASW. Vallecular cyst: report of four cases-one with coexisting laryngomalacia. *J Larngol Otol* 2000; 114:224–226.

28. Sands NB, Anand SM, Manoukian JJ. Series of congenital vallecular cysts: a rare yet potentially fatal cause of upper airway obstruction and failure to thrive in the newborn. *J Laryngol Head Neck Surg* 2009; 38:6–10.

29. Wenig B. *Atlas of Head and Neck Pathology. Non Neoplastic Lesions of the Larynx.* ed 2, Ed. Wenig B. Philadelphia: Saunders / Elsevier Inc. 2008: 417–418.

30. Ward RF, Jones J, Arnold JA. Management of congenital saccular cysts of the larynx. *Ann Otol Rhinol Laryngol* 1995; 104:707–710.

Laryngocele

31. Ruthka J. Laryngocele: a case report and review. *J Otolaryngol* 1983; 12:389–392.

32. Tawalbeh M, Nawasreh O, Husban A, Momani O. Laryngocele: a case report. *JRMS* 2003; 10:54–57.

33. Civantos FJ, Holinger LD. Laryngoceles and saccular cysts in infants and children. *Arch Otolarngol Head Neck Surg* 1992; 118:296–300

34. Donegan JO, Strife JL, Seid AB, et al. Internal laryngocele and saccular cyst in children. *Ann Otol Rhinol Laryngol* 1980; 89:409–413.

Subglottic Stenosis

35. Choo K, Balakrishnan A. Subglottic stenosis in infants and children. *Singapore Med J* 2010; 51:848–852.

36. Fearon B, Crysdale WS, Bird R. Subglottic stenosis of the larynx in the infant and child. Methods of management. *Ann Otol Rhinol Laryngol* 1978; 87:645–648.

37. Mcdonald IH, Stocks JG. Prolonged nasotracheal intubation. A review of its development in a pediatric hospital. *Br J Anaesthes* 1965; 37:161–173.

38. Choi SS, Zalzal GH. Changing trends in neonatal subglottic stenosis. *Otolaryngol Head Neck Surg* 2000; 122:61–63.

39. Walner DL, Loewen MS, Kimura RE. Neonatal subglottic stenosis-incidence and trends. *Laryngoscope* 2001; 111: 48–51.

40. Holinger PH, Johnson KC, Schiller F. Congenital anomalies of the larynx. *Ann Otol Rhinol Laryngol* 1954; 63: 581–606.

41. Hartnick CJ, Cotton RT. Syndromic and other congenital anomalies of the head and neck. *Otolaryngol Clin North Am* 2003; 33:1293–1308.

42. Wiatrak BJ. Congenital anomalies of the larynx and trachea. *Otolaryngol Clin North Am* 2000; 33:91–110.

43. Myer CM III, O'Conner DM, Cotton RT. Proposed grading system for subglottic stenosis based on endotracheal tube sizes. *Ann Otol Rhinol Laryngol* 1994; 108:319–323.

Laryngeal Web

44. Benmansour N, Remacle M, Matar N, et al. Endoscopic treatment of anterior glottis webs according to Lichtenberger technique, and results in 18 patients. *Eur Arch Otorhino Laryngol*, 2012; 269:2075–2080.

45. Chong ZK, Jawan B, Poon Y, Lee JH. Unsuspected difficult intubation caused by laryngeal web. *Br J Anaesth* 1997; 79:396–397.

46. Tewfik TL, Sobol SE. Congenital anomalies of the larynx. In: *Diagnosis and Treatment of Voice Disorders*. Eds. Sataloff RT, Korovin GS. Thompson JS, Rubin D. NY: Plural Publishing inc. 2003.

47. Nabi N, Chaudhary S, Ahuia S, Geol A. A rare case of laryngeal webexcision by CO2 laser in a child: an anaeasthetic challenge. *J Anaesthesiol Clin Pharmacol* 2011; 27:119–120.

48. Liu DB, Zhong JW, Huang ZY, et al. Diagnosis and treatment of laryngeal web in infants. *ZhinghuaEr Bi Yan HouTou Jing WaiKeZaZhi* 2006; 41:120–122.

Laryngeal Atresia

49. Hartnick CJ, Cotton RT. Syndromic and other congenital anomalies of the head and neck. *Otolaryngol Clin North Am* 2003; 33:1293–1308.

50. Decou JM, Jones DC, Jacobs HD, et al. Successful ex utero intrapartum treatment (EXIT) procedure for congenital high airway obstruction syndrome (CHAOS) owing to laryngeal atresia. *J Pediatr Surg* 1998; 33: 1563–1565.

51. Onderoglu L, Karamursel BS, Bulun A, et al. Prenatal diagnosis of laryngeal atresia. *Prenat Diagn* 2003; 23: 277–280.

52. Wyatt ME, Hartley BEJ. Laryngotracheal reconstruction in congenital laryngeal web and atresia. *Otolaryngol Head Neck Surg* 2005; 132:232–238.

Vocal Cord Nodules

53. Senturia BH, Wilson FB. Otorhinolaryngologic findings in children with voice deviation. *Ann Otol Rhino Laryngol* 1968; 77:1027–1041.

54. Gray DS, Smith ME, Schneider H. Voice disorders in children. *Pediatr Clin North Am* 1996; 43:1357–1384.

55. Maddern BR, Campbell TF, Stool S. Pediatric voices disorders. *Otolaryngol Clin North Am* 1991; 24:1125–1140.

56. Dobres R, Lee L, Stemple J, et al. Description of laryngeal pathologies in children evaluated by otolaryngologists. *Journal of speech and hearing disorders* 1990; 55:526–532

57. Pannbecker M. Treatment of voice nodules: options and outcomes. *Am J Speech-Language Pathol* 1999; 8: 209–217.

58. Shah R, Woodnorth GH, Glynn A, Nuss R. Pediatric vocal cord nodules: correlation with perceptual voice analysis. *Int J Pediatr Otorhinolaryngol* 2005; 69:903–909.

59. Roy N, Kellianne I, Redmond S, Muntz H. Behavioral characteristics of children with vocal fold nodule. *J Voice* 2007; 21:157–168.

60. Wohl D. Non surgical management of pediatric vocal fold nodules. *Arch Otolaryngol Head Neck Surg* 2005; 131:68–70.

61. Hartnick CJ. Validation of pediatric voice quality-of-life instrument: the pediatric voice outcome survey. *Arch Otolaryngol Head Neck Surg* 2002; 128:919–922.

62. Handler SD. Direct laryngoscopy in children: rigid and flexible fiberoptic. *Laryngoscope* 2002; 112:559–564.

63. Hirschberg J, Dejonckere PH, Hirano M, et al. Voice disorders in children. *Int J Pediatr Otorhinolaryngol* 1995; 32: S109–S125.

64. Tillman B, Rudert H, Schunke M, et al. Morphological studies on the pathogenesis of Rcineke's edema. *Eur Arch Otorhinolaryngol* 1995; 252:469–474

65. Barnes LF. *Diseases of the Larynx, Hypopharynx and Trachea in Surgical Pathology of the Head and Neck*, ed 3, New York, NY: CRC Press 2008.

Contact Ulcers

66. Jackson C. Contact ulcers of the larynx. *Ann Otol Rhinol Laryngol* 1928; 37: 227–230.

67. Jackson C, Jackson CL. Contact ulcers of the larynx. *Arch Otolaryngol*, 1935; 22:1–15.

68. Beham AW, Pucllman K, Laird R, et al. A TNF-regulated recombinatorial macrophage immune receptor implicated in granuloma formation in tuberculosis. *PLOS Patho* 2011; Nov 7(11):e 1002375.

69. Delima Pontes PA, DeBiase NG, Gadelha EC, et al. Clinical evolution of contact granuloma: treatment and prognosis. *Laryngoscope*, 1999; 109:289–294.

70. Havas TE, Priestly J, Lowinger DS. A management strategy for vocal process

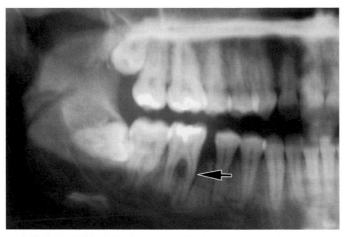

Figure 16.9 Widening of the periodontal ligament space in osteosarcoma of the posterior mandible (arrow).

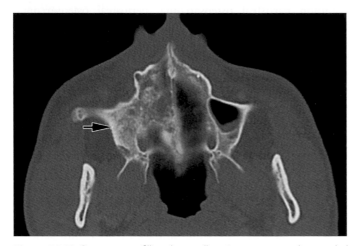

Figure 16.10 Osteosarcoma filling the maxillary sinus as a somewhat mottled mixed radiolucent and radiopaque mass.

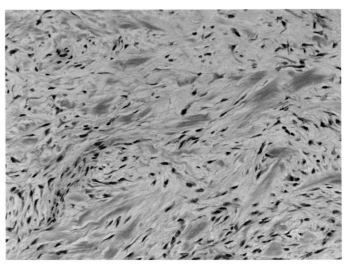

Figure 16.11 Fibroblastic osteosarcoma composed of fibroblastic appearing spindle cells and malignant osteoid product. Spindle cells that are cytologically atypical can be seen.

osteosarcoma. Osteosarcoma can prove to be quite radiodense when it arises in a sinus cavity (Figure 16.10).

Vertebral Osteosarcomas

Vertebral osteosarcomas in children are quite rare. The vast majority of such lesions will arise in adults following radiation therapy for Paget's disease. However, vertebral osteosarcomas have been reported in patients ranging in age from 3 to 70.[50,51] The classic presenting symptom associated with cervical vertebral osteosarcoma is pain. Patients may also present with sensory or motor deficits, or with the presence of a rare palpable mass. Most osteosarcomas involving the cervical vertebral result in radiolucent destruction of the vertebrae, and in most instances, tumor will ultimately extend beyond the bony vertebral margins and into soft tissue.[45,52]

Pathologic Features

Grossly, osteosarcomas in pediatric age group patients will tend to be firm, gritty, tan or somewhat myxoid in their appearance. Tumors generally range in size from 2 to 10 mm. Extra osseous lesions will typically show soft tissue extension of the neoplasm beyond its bony compartment. Osteosarcomas that affect the craniofacial complex of children, as with adults, are typically classified as: 1) osteoblastic, 2) chondroblastic, 3) fibroblastic and 4) telangiectatic. The small cell osteosarcomas, low grade central osseous osteosarcomas and high grade cortical surface osteosarcomas that are seen in adults rarely occur in children.[53,54,55] Two special forms of osteosarcoma, parosteal and periosteal osteosarcoma, which both occur as cortical bone surface-based neoplasms rather than lesions of the medullary compartment do occur with some frequency in children and will be discussed under a separate heading.

Osteosarcoma, Histologic Subtypes

Most osteosarcomas, when all age groups are considered, will be *osteoblastic*, and represent neoplasms that will be made up largely of malignant tumor osteoid and reactive, necrotic or sclerotic bone. Chondroblastic osteosarcoma, in which the tumor is made up largely of malignant cartilage is the second most frequent histological subtype identified. *Fibroblastic* or *fibrohistiocytic* osteosarcoma is typically made up of fibroblastic appearing spindle cells that will be interlacing and cytologically atypical (Figures 16.11, 16.12, 16.13). Fibroblastic osteosarcomas will typically show a classic interlacing herring bone pattern within the tumor. A pattern that may be difficult to distinguish from pleomorphic undifferentiated sarcoma (malignant fibrous histocytoma). *Telangiectatic* osteosarcoma will be histologically composed of cystic blood filled spaces that are intersected by bony septa cytologically atypical spindle cells (Figures 16.14 & 16.15) and malignant tumor osteoid.

Osteoblastic osteosarcoma will be composed of such significant amounts of malignant tumor osteoid that normal bone

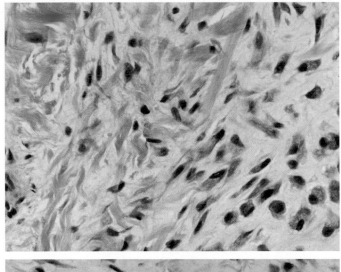

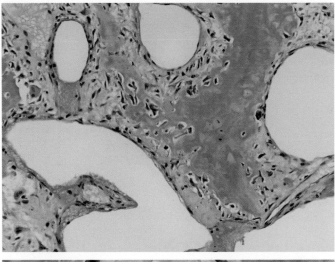

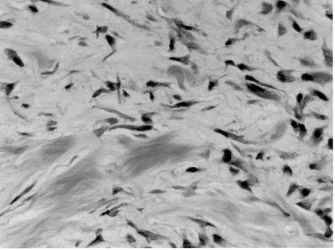

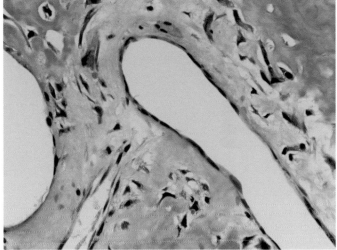

Figures 16.12 (top) & 16.13 (bottom) Two photomicrographs, in which wispy malignant osteoid is also evident.

Figures 16.14 (top) & 16.15 (bottom) Telangiectatic osteosarcoma rich in vascular spaces that are intersected by malignant bony septa and atypical spindle cells.

may not be identified (Figure 16.16). *Chondroblastic osteosarcoma* will display chondroid material or a cartilaginous matrix that may be arranged in nodular patterns throughout the tumor mass (Figures 16.17 & 16.18). Enchondral ossification may occur as well. Multinucleated giant cells may also be prominent throughout the tumor matrix regardless of the tumor's histologic subtype. None of the histologic patterns seen in osteosarcoma will be pure and when one reviews multiple sections of osteosarcoma, a wide variation in histologic patterns will typically be seen such that an admixture of osteoblastic, chondroblastic, telangiectatic and fibroblastic components may be identified. The variable histologic pattern of osteosarcoma of the craniofacial complex in children, however, may not allow for standard histologic grading of that tumor, except for those instances in which well differential low grade central osseous osteosarcoma is recognized.

Since multinucleated giant cells are common to osteosarcomas in children, osteosarcomas in pediatric age group

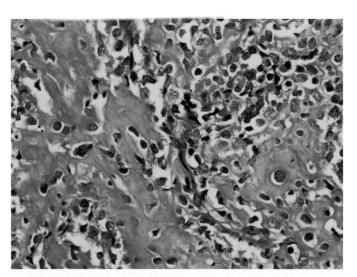

Figure 16.16 Osteoblastic osteosarcoma composed of malignant tumor osteoid. The osteoid product surrounds hyperchromatic cytologically atypical nuclei.

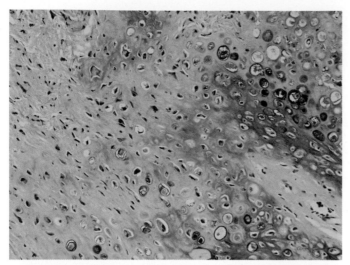

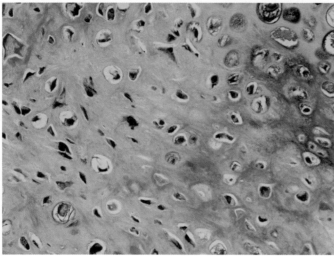

Figures 16.17 (top) & 16.18 (bottom) Chondroblastic osteosarcoma displaying a cartilaginous matrix that is marginated by a malignant osteoid product at intermediate and high power.

patients must be distinguished from central giant cell granuloma (tumor) (CGCG), which can also be rich in multinucleated giant cells. Those osteosarcomas whose histology is dominated by osteoclasts will always demonstrate, in some component of the tumor, malignant cartilage or malignant osteoid. In order to accurately determine that such an osteoclastic or giant cell tumor is indeed an osteosarcoma, all tissue samples that are reviewed must be representative samples. Small biopsies may in fact lead to misinterpretation. Osteosarcomas can also be histologically separated from CGCG because of the abundance of atypical mitotic activity and necrosis that will generally be present in osteosarcoma.

Data comparing the histologic, molecular and immunohistochemical characteristics of pediatric osteosarcoma of the jaws to either extremity osteosarcoma or adult jaw osteosarcoma is limited.[43] Jasnau et al. examined 25 head and neck osteosarcoma cases for p53, MDM2, CDK4, PCNA and Ki67 expression. Among those cases, four tumors were in pediatric

age patients. No definitive immunohistochemical features were identified that could help distinguish pediatric tumors from those in adults.

Electron microscopic evaluation of osteosarcomas has demonstrated that most tumor cells, regardless of the tumor's sub classification, will demonstrate interlacing and anastamosing rough endoplasmic reticulum in association with hydroxyapatite crystals set within an intracellular matrix of collagen.[56] Cox-2 has been used as a valuable marker in distinguishing between osteosarcoma and osteoblastoma. Osteosarcomas tend to be Cox-2 negative, whereas osteoblastomas tend to be Cox-2 reactive or positive. Osteocalcin also tends to be significantly higher in osteoblastomas than in osteosarcomas, and osteosarcoma will tend to be CD99 reactive unlike osteoblastoma. One important key to rendering a proper diagnosis of osteosarcoma of the craniofacial region is to refrain from attempting to render a diagnosis based upon small biopsies. Interpretation of tumor histology must be made in conjunction with clinical and radiographic findings. If all of these factors are not taken into consideration, osteosarcoma may easily be confused with osteoid osteoma, osteoblastoma or even cementoblastoma of odontogenic origin.

Osteosarcomas in pediatric age group patients are usually classified as either low, intermediate or high grade tumors. Regardless of the histological subtype of the tumor, most tumors that affect the jaw bones of children will be high grade. High grade tumors tend to be richly cellular with a large number of spindle or polygonal cells and minimal bone formation, while low grade tumors tend to be less atypical in appearance cytologically and display more bone formation.

While all of the common histologic subtypes of osteosarcoma (*osteoblastic, chondroblastic, fibroblastic and telangiectatic*) can be seen in the head and neck region in children, chondroblastic osteosarcomas are the most common, followed by osteoblastic and rare fibroblastic tumors. Telangiectatic osteosarcomas are exceedingly uncommon in the head and neck region of children and adolescents.

Cytogenetically, osteosarcoma will demonstrate a high incidence of mutations in the oncogenes P53, Rb and MDM-2. Rb1 mutation has been reported in as high as 40 percent of osteosarcomas.[58,59,60,61] Biegel et al.[62] have reported finding a series of complex karyotypes in pediatric osteosarcomas, reporting modal numbers in the hypodiploid, triploid and hypertetraploid ranges. Reportedly, 17p11.2-p12 is the most common region of chromosomal aberrancy in osteosarcoma, showing up typically as an amplification.[63]

Differential Diagnosis

From a differential diagnostic standpoint, osteoblastoma, chrondrosarcoma, FD and even an immature fracture callus can resemble osteosarcoma. An adequate tissue sample that is representative of the tumor is therefore mandatory in order to differentiate osteosarcoma from the aforementioned lesions. Osteoblastoma can be distinguished from osteosarcoma because in most instances that tumor will present as a well circumscribed mass with a sclerotic border, whereas osteosarcoma will grow as an infiltrative lesion without margination by bone. Histologically, osteoblastoma will also feature bony trabeculas that are thicker or broader than those seen in the osteosarcoma. Finally, osteoblastoma will also tend to show significant bone remodeling without evidence of the tumor cell pleomorphism or atypical mitoses that are common to osteosarcoma.

Osteoid osteoma tends to generally be a very small lesion, rarely attaining a diameter size of more than 1.5 cm, rarely showing lesional progression, and unlike osteosarcoma, osteoid osteoma will not demonstrate an infiltrative pattern.

FD will lack the malignant tumor osteoid that characterizes osteosarcoma histologically, and radiographically FD will present more often than not as a lesion that has a ground glass or orange peel appearance. Additionally, FD will tend to resorb or uniformly melt away the bony cortex of the bone involved. This radiographic feature can be quite helpful in separating FD from osteosarcoma.

Unlike osteosarcoma, a fracture callus will usually demonstrate endochondral ossification with a proliferation of some cartilaginous elements. A thorough clinical patient history, should typically lead one toward a diagnosis of a fracture rather than osteosarcoma.

Osteosarcoma Variants

Periosteal Osteosarcoma

Periosteal osteosarcoma is a rare form of osteosarcoma that is most often identified in the second decade of life. In the head and neck region, periosteal osteosarcoma is more common in the mandible than the maxilla, and the vast majority of such tumors in the craniofacial complex never attain a size greater than 3.5 cm in greatest dimention.[63,64] Unlike periosteal osteosarcoma of long bones, where a radiating radiographic pattern of osseous spicules along the bony cortex is common, tumors affecting the craniofacial complex will show no specific radiographic pattern.

Pathologic Features

Grossly, periosteal osteosarcoma will display no specific or characteristic appearance other than that of a well circumscribed lobular mass. Tumors tend to be gray, with a glistening somewhat chondroid cut surface. Histologically, the tumor will consist of spindle shaped malignant, mesenchymal cells resembling fibroblasts admixed with malignant cartilaginous tissue that is most often high grade. Aggregates of malignant osteoblastic and fibroblastic cells can be identified within the tumor, but they will be encountered much less frequently than the far more common malignant cartilaginous matrix. The tumor may show normal ossification near the cortical bone that it abuts, or in the region where it intersects with or invades soft tissue. In order to render a diagnosis of periosteal osteosarcoma, the tumor being assessed must directly abut a thickened

cortex and at the same time show limited bony invasion. Periosteal osteosarcoma will lack the cytologically atypical fibroblastic stroma of parosteal osteosarcoma and the tumor will also fail to demonstrate the interlacing seams of malignant tumor osteoid that are typical of parosteal osteosarcoma.

Bridge et al. in a review of 73 osteosarcomas, found that periosteal osteosarcomas showed a consistent trisomy 17 karyotypic structural change.[65]

Parosteal Osteosarcoma

Parosteal osteosarcoma is a tumor that is most commonly identified in adults. The majority of patients with parosteal osteosarcoma will develop their tumor well beyond the second and third decades of life. That demographic alone serves to separate parosteal osteosarcoma from periosteal osteosarcoma, the latter being a neoplasm that is far more common in children. When the rare parosteal osteosarcoma does occur in the head and neck region of a child or adolescent, the most common sites of presentation will be the mandible, the maxilla and the bones of the cranium.[66-69]

Parosteal osteosarcoma will usually present as a painless, slow growing mass that develops along the surface of bones (most often the femur), as either a broad-based mass or a lobular excrescence. Tumors, because of their rapid proliferation will cause thickening of the underlying bony cortex. Radiographically, a zone of cleavage or separation may be identified between the tumor mass and the underlying cortical bone, resulting in a "juxtacortical" appearance. The tumor may resemble an osteoid osteoma radiographically, such that the central portion of the tumor will be radiolucent and the peripheral margins of the tumor quite ossified and radiopaque. Invasion of the underlying bone is rare but will sometimes be identified.

Parosteal osteosarcoma will not demonstrate any direct histologic communication between the neoplasm and the underlying medullary bone. Kumar et al. have reported that the vast majority of parosteal osteosarcomas will range in size from 2 to 5 cm in greatest dimention.[67]

Grossly, parosteal osteosarcoma will consist of a nodular tumor mass which may have a marginating fibrous capsule. On cut section the tumor can have a gelatinous, fibrous or gritty to granular appearance. The peripheral margins of the tumor may in fact be rubbery or fleshy, and depending on the length of time the tumor has been developing, the tumor mass may be as dense and as hard as cortical bone.

Microscopically, most parosteal osteosarcomas will be composed of well formed osseous trabecula set in a hypercellular collagenous stroma. Tumors display only minimal cellular atypia. The stroma of the tumor can resemble that of a fibrosarcoma, or it may appear cytologically as bland as the stroma seen in a benign fibroma or even a mature FD. The bone that is found within the tumor will tend to be composed of interlacing aggregates of neoplastic trabecular bone arranged in parallel, lattice-like aggregates. The tumor will lack the cytologically atypical fibroblastic stromal elements of a conventional osteosarcoma and the spaces or zones between malignant osseous trabeculae will generally be filled with normal fibrous connective tissue.

Parosteal osteosarcomas contain cartilaginous aggregates in well over 50 percent of cases, and although parosteal osteosarcomas have been histologically graded by some investigators in a manner similar to that of conventional osteosarcoma (grades I, II and III), the vast majority of parosteal osteosarcomas are low-grade, with no more than 15 percent of tumors in any age group, showing high grade differentiation.

Differential Diagnosis

Several lesions can resemble parosteal osteosarcoma histologically, including periosteal osteosarcoma, actively growing FD, myositis ossificans and Ewing sarcoma (ES) or Primitive Neuroectodermal Tumor (PNET). Histologically, myositis ossificans will be composed of woven bone elements or it will be a totally ossified process composed of normal appearing lamellar bone, while parosteal osteosarcoma will be composed of spindle cells and an osteoid product set in a fibro-osseous stroma that shows cytologic atypia. On occasion, osteochondroma may be interpreted to represent a parosteal osteosarcoma, however, osteochondroma will have a cartilaginous cap of benign cartilage, while parosteal osteosarcoma, although it may show histologic remnants of a cartilaginous cap, will always be characterized by the cytologic hallmarks of malignancy. In addition, the fibrous stroma of a parosteal osteosarcoma will be quite proliferative, whereas the stroma of osteochondroma will consist of normocellular marrow. On a molecular level, parosteal osteosarcoma can be distinguished from the more common central osseous osteosarcoma largely based upon the fact that *RB1 mutations* will be absent in parosteal osteosarcoma.[70] PNET will generally lack the large pleomorphic tumor cells of an osteosarcoma even when smaller malignant appearing round cells are present.

Extraskeletal Osteosarcoma

Extra skeletal osteosarcomas are rare in pediatric age patients and most tumors will occur in patients in the fifth and sixth decades of life. Less than 5 percent of all extra skeletal osteosarcomas occur in patients younger than 30 years of age.[43, 71] Tumors can arise as a result of prior radiation therapy or de novo, and fewer than 5 percent of all tumors will arise in the head and neck region. Extra skeletal osteosarcoma, which must be differentiated microscopically from myositis ossificans and peripheral fibroma with ossification, will show significant anaplasia and cytologic atypia, features that are not generally encountered in myositis ossificans or the peripheral fibroma with ossification. Osteosarcoma will show a high incidence of Rb, p53 and MDM2 oncogenic mutations as will pleomorphic undifferentiated sarcoma.[43]

Treatment and Prognosis for Osteosarcoma

Osteosarcomas in the head and neck region are treated by marginal resection of the tumor, most often in concert with multidisciplinary treatment that includes combined pre-surgical adjuvant chemotherapy and more rarely 3D conformed radiotherapy. Maxillary and extragnathic tumors are inherently difficult to resect due to their close proximity to the orbit and intercranial nerves. Mandibular tumors are somewhat more amenable to wide resection.[43, 73] Complete surgical resection will produce the most predictive outcome for osteosarcoma.

Overall survival for patients with osteosarcoma in the craniofacial region is much worse for those patients with extragnatic tumors. Jasnau et al.[43] report that while chemotherapy improves the prognosis for individuals with extremity osteosarcomas dramatically, its impact on craniofacial osteosarcomas remains controversial. However, the use of chemotherapy as part of multimodality therapy for craniofacial osteosarcoma in a multi-institutional setting appears to be more effective for craniofacial osteosarcomas than any single therapeutic modality alone.[43]

The five year survival rates for osteosarcoma of the craniofacial region in children and adolescents ranges from 25 to 50 percent with mandibular lesions having a somewhat better prognosis than maxillary lesions.[48,49] The prognosis for vertebral osteosarcomas in children is poor, with most patients dying within one year of their diagnosis.[52] Parosteal osteosarcoma has a much better prognosis than conventional central medullary osteosarcoma and five year survival rates for parosteal osteosarcoma can range as high as 80 percent. Ten year survival rates will be somewhat less. Wide surgical excision is the treatment of choice for parosteal osteosarcoma. Periosteal osteosarcoma in the craniofacial region in both children and adults is reported to have a prognosis that is better than conventional central osseous osteosarcoma, but somewhat worse than parosteal osteosarcoma.[63,64,72] Extra skeletal osteosarcomas, which tend to be high grade tumors, occur primarily in the cervical spine region. If head and neck tissues are involved, the majority of patients will survive less than three years following diagnosis.[47]

Benign Neoplasms of Cartilage

Chondroma

Chondroma (enchondroma) involving the craniofacial skeleton, and bones of the head and neck region are rare. Matsuzaka et al. in a review of 32,625 cases seen by the Departments of Clinical Patholophysiology and Pathology at the Tokyo Dental College between the years of 1966 and 2001 identified 569 lesions that involved the formation of bone, cartilage or cementum.[74] Only one chondroma, which arose in the premolar region in a male in the third decade of life, was accessioned in that study. The aggregated studies of Huvos et al.[75] Unni et al.[76] Schajowicz,[77] Mirra[78] and Inwards[79] documented only four chondromas in the head and neck region in a compilation of nearly 1,250 chondromas that were evaluated by these investigators.

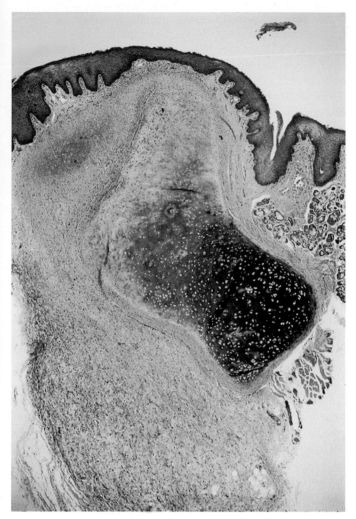

Figure 16.19 Chondroid choristoma of the tongue demonstrating chondroid metaplasia within the deep connective tissue of the tongue. (Reprinted from Marx R, Stern D. *Oral and Maxillofacial Pathology: A Rationale for Diagnosis and Treatment* with permission from Quintessence Publishing Company).

Chondromas can present as central osseous lesions of bone or as lesions that involve the soft tissues of the head and neck region. Chondromas have been reported in almost all bones of the head and neck, including the mandible, maxilla, the nasal cartilages, the paranasal sinuses, the ear, the larynx and in cervical vertebrae. Those chondromas that have been reported in soft tissue are thought by some investigators to represent choristomas rather than true neoplasms (Figure 16.19).

In children, chondromas have been documented in patients as young as eight.[80] Tumors are most commonly encountered between the second and fourth decades of life when they are present in the head and neck region.[76,77,78] Fu and Perzin and Kirby and Aubegaokar, in their investigations of chondromas in the nasal, paranasal sinuses and nasopharynx reported finding only seven chondromas in patients ranging from 10 to 46 years of age. Craniofacial chondromas have also been reported in children and adolescents in association with Mafucci's syndrome and Ollier's disease.[82,83]

Pediatric aged patients generally do not complain of significant clinical symptoms early on in the development of a chondroma. However, as lesions grow, neurologic symptoms tend to predominant, which, depending on the location of the lesion can include paresthesia, nerve palsy, loss of vision, tinnitus, facial numbness or hoarseness. Radiographically, most chondromas will present as unilocular or multilocular growths that may display focal radiopacities within them.

Pathologic Features

Grossly, chondromas will present as either single or multiple yellow, white or opalescent appearing nodular growths. Chondromas tend to grow in a lobulated pattern such that tumor masses are sometimes pseudopod-like.

Histologically, chondromas will be composed of uniform and often lobular aggregations of hyaline cartilage, that will be made up of chondrocytes with nuclei that will tend to be quite hyperchromatic. Rare multinucleate chondrocytes may be seen within lacunar spaces. Chondromas can sometimes contain bone or an osteoid product. Lesions that are histologically suggestive of a chondroma, and which contain bone should be sectioned extensively since such an admixture of bone and cartilage can be sometimes actually be representative of a low grade osteosarcoma.

Chondromas in pediatric age group patients tend to be more cellular than similar lesions in adults. Thus isolated binucleate features seen in a chondroma in a child or adolescent are not necessarily worrisome. Nonetheless, any accumulation of binucleate and open-face nuclei with associated mitoses should cause one to consider the possibility of a low-grade chrondrosarcoma.

The most significant biologic risk for any individual in the pediatric age group with a chondroma of the head and neck region, or with multiple enchondromas of long bones will be in those patients who have either Ollier's disease or Maffucci's syndrome.[84,85] Both disorders carry with them an increased risk for malignant change in their disease associate chondromas. Malignant transformation has been reported to occur in between 15 percent and 50 percent of chondromas in individuals in a setting of either Maffucci's syndrome or Ollier's disease. Mutations in PTH/PTHrP type I receptor are thought to be important in contributing to Ollier's disease in some patients.[86]

One of the significant problematic issues related to the diagnosis of cartilaginous tumors in the head and neck region remains the difficulty that is associated with separating benign cartilaginous neoplasms from those that are malignant. Most authorities, including the authors of this text, are in agreement with the diagnostic concepts espoused by Gnepp,[87] who takes the position that all symptomatic cartilaginous lesions in the craniofacial region should be managed as if they were a chondrosarcoma and considered to be malignant until proven otherwise.

The histologic presence of atypical mitoses, enlarged or binucleate chondrocytes and proof of radiographic extension of a cartilaginous neoplasm into bony medullary or trabecular spaces, even in a pediatric age patient favor a diagnosis of chondrosarcoma.

Treatment and Prognosis

Chondromas are managed in nearly all instances as if they were low-grade chondrosarcoma. The treatment therefore involves marginal tumor resection with a 1 cm peripheral margin of normal tissue. In instances of multiple chondromatosis, or Ollier's disease, chondromas are managed most appropriately by long-term radiographic and clinical evaluation. Multiple enchondromas in children are generally considered to be benign unless they show rapid growth or expansion. Enchondromas are usually treated surgically if the patient's chief complaints increase or if there is a cosmetic deformity. Defects can be treated by grafting bone, however, since patients who develop Ollier's disease will have multiple lesions throughout the body, surgery and grafting must, of necessity, be selective. In those instances in which patients have multiple pathologic fractures related to their Ollier's disease, or in those cases in which malignant transformation is suspected, surgery can be employed. Patients with Ollier's disease are managed by life-long monitoring of their disease, because of the risk of malignant transformation of their disease associated enchondromas.

Osteochondroma

Although osteochondromas are most often classified as benign tumors that are derivatives of both bone and cartilage, they are in fact more than likely hamartomatous growths rather than true neoplasms.[88] Most tumors will arise from endochondral bones and therefore most osteochondromas occur in long bones. Less than 1 percent of all osteochondromas occur in the head and neck region. Those lesions that occur in the head and neck region tend to present at least a decade later than osteochondromas in long bones. Despite its rarity, the solitary osteochondroma is the most common benign cartilaginous tumor of pediatric age group patients, accounting for nearly one half of all benign cartilaginous tumors of childhood.

Multiple hereditary exostosis (MHE) will account for 15 percent of all osteochondromas in children,[89,90] although MHE is rare in the head and neck region of children. Osteochondromas that do occur in the head and neck region typically involve the cervical spine, with more than half of all reported cases occurring in that location. Other common head and neck sites include the mandibular condyle and the coronoid process.[89,90] Osteochondromas that arise in the spine will most often involve the posterior portions of spinous processes, however, osteochondromas can involve the vertebral bodies, or the anterior portions of the spinous processes.

Most solitary osteochondromas in the head and neck region occur in patients in the second decade of life, and males are affected twice as often as females. Although osteochondromas are considered by most investigators to represent hamartomatous growths, recent genetic studies have demonstrated chromosomal and genetic mutations involving the EXT1 gene in osteochondromas. Thus there remains support for the premise that osteochondromas may represent true neoplasms.[90]

In children, osteochondromas have been reported to develop after radiation therapy, and a small percentage of osteochondromas do undergo malignant transformation. Three to five percent of osteochondromas that occur as part of MHE syndrome are subject to malignant transformation.[91,92]

Most osteochondromas that occur in the head and neck region of children and adolescents represent asymptomatic lesions that are identified incidentally. However, lesions involving the coronoid process of condyle may be associated with a dull ache or pain. The bony expansion resulting from an osteochondroma, depending on the tumor's location, can cause neurologic symptoms, including dysphasia, facial asymmetry, malocclusion and even trismas, especially if the mandibular condyle is involved. Osteochondromas may or may not be palpable clinically and it is possible that lesions may not be readily observed on routine radiographs because of the length of time that is required for an osteochondroma to impinge on what is most often an otherwise radiolucent space.

Lesions that involve the coronoid process and condyle will show a remarkably reproducible radiographic appearance. Condylar lesions when viewed on CT will most often appear radiopaque and tapered with an anteriomedial extension into the lateral pterygoid tendon.[93] (See Figure 16.20.) Two additional imaging presentations are common to CT scans, either of a radiopaque mass arising from the medial pole of the condyle with extension along the lateral pterygoid tendon, or of a radiopaque mass arising solely from the lateral pole of a condyle.[93]

Marx has reported that most osteochondromas that involve the coronoid process will be located on the medial edge of that process where the temporalis tendon attaches.[93] Joint spaces may demonstrate tumor associated satellite radiopacities in this site. Tumors that display enlargement and irregular peripheral margins, or display multiple ossifications within the tumor mass or pain, may be undergoing possible sarcomatous transformation.[92] Thus, one of the clinicoradiographic criteria that has been used to separate osteochondroma from a possible osteosarcoma, from a differential diagnostic standpoint, is the fact that osteosarcoma will generally demonstrate a thickened cartilaginous cap while osteochondromal will not. This finding, while demonstrable on CT imaging, is not pathognomonic of either a benign or malignant process, especially in a child where the cap may show little wear, and generally remains quite thick. Scintigraphic studies and MRI imaging have been used to attempt to identify tumor associated metabolic activity as well as arterial and venous compromise that may be associated an osteochondroma.[94,95] However, these investigative methods are not definitively diagnostic of the process.

Most osteochondromas in the head and neck region will be 1 to 3 cm in diameter and rarely will tumors attain a size greater than 7 cm.[90] While synovial chondromatosis can

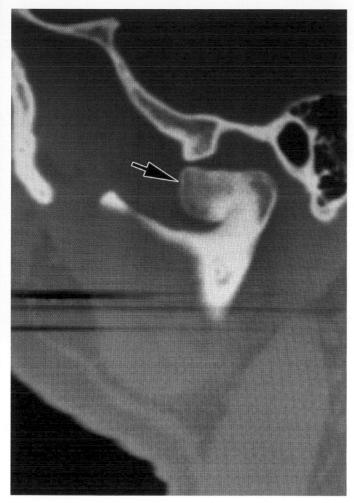

Figure 16.20 Osteochondroma of the condyle demonstrating a tapered radiodense lesion.

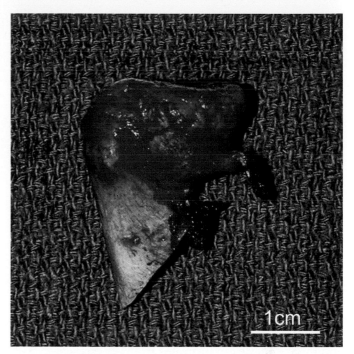

Figure 16.21 Osteochondroma, gross specimen. A nodular mass is evident just above the condylar neck resection margin. The tumor mass encompasses the lateral pterygoid tendon. (Reprinted from Marx R, Stern D. *Oral and Maxillofacial Pathology: A Rationale for Diagnosis and Treatment* with permission from Quintessence Publishing Company).

resemble osteochondroma clinically, the diffuse, painful multiple radiopacities and condylar enlargements that are typically seen in the temporomandibular joint (TMJ) space in synovial chondromatosis will tend to separate that disorder from osteochondroma. Finally, the tendon extension that is generally identified in an osteochondroma will be absent in synovial chondromatosis.[93]

Pathology

On gross inspection, osteochondromas tend to be either pedunculated or sessile masses that extend from their bony origin to a point where they are marginated by a thin glistening (cartilaginous) cap (Figure 16.21). That overlying cartilaginous cap may appear undulating, papillary or smooth. The cartilaginous cap of an osteochondroma in a child will tend to be much thicker than the cartilaginous cap in an adult, and in a child, thickened zones of apparent cartilage, when identified grossly will tend to be highly suggestive of osteochondroma. In those cases where the condylar cap thickness is greater than 2 cm on gross inspection, the possibility of osteosarcoma should be entertained.[96]

Histologically, the peripheral, outer margin or head of an osteochondroma will be made up of benign hyaline cartilage, delineated at its periphery by perichondrium that is continuous with the periosteum of the underlying bone. The tumor's cartilaginous cap will consist of normal appearing chondrocytes that will display a solitary dark blue staining nucleus within their lacunae. While binucleotide chondrocytes may be observed in pediatric age patients, these nuclei tend to be of less concerning in terms of an atypical cytopathology, than in an adult, where chondrosarcoma would be a more likely consideration in the differential microscopic diagnosis.

Chondrocytes in an osteochondroma tend to be laid down in linear parallel strands, columns or cords. In a child where the bone is typically still growing, the chondrocyte lacunar spaces will tend to be quite large where they interface with bone. The underlying bone will be richly vascularized especially where the bone marginates cartilage. Deeper bone will tend to be more mature, partially ossified or rich in marrow. From a differential diagnostic standpoint, the presence of bone marrow in a specimen will tend to favor a diagnosis of osteochondroma, whereas the absence of marrow elements tends to be more consistent with what can be seen histologically in osteosarcoma or chondrosarcoma. Since 1 to 2 percent of all osteochondromas will give rise to chondrosarcoma, recognition of such a telling histologic feature is important. Observation of these classic histologic features in concert with a genetic aberrancy, demonstrating a loss of heterozygosity at the EXT1 locus in certain lesions, may also prove to

405

be helpful in separating osteochondroma from osteosarcoma and chondrosarcoma.[97,98,99]

Treatment

The treatment of choice for osteochondroma is local surgical excision for those lesions occurring in the head and neck region. Osteochondromas in other sites, depending on their associated symptomatology and the surgical risk involved in their management, may not immediately be managed surgically. Spinal cord compression is reported to occur in as high as 4 percent of osteochondromas of the cervical spine.[100] Alterations in the thickness of the cartilaginous cap surrounding a suspected osteochondroma may mandate obligatory surgical excision regardless of the site of the tumor, even in a child. When the mandibular condyle is involved, condylectomy at the neck is most appropriate. The resulting surgical defect can be treated by a costochondral graft or reconstruction with alloplastic replacement. In cases when an alloplastic reconstruction procedure is entertained, a titanium plate with condylar replacement is recommended.[93]

Those osteochondromas that arise solely from the lateral pole of the condyle can be treated by direct excision. In such instances a large portion of the condyle is retained and lateral pterygoid function is maintained.[93] In those instances where the coronoid process is involved, coronoidectomy is the treatment of choice. This procedure will result in surgical extension into the temporalis tendon, but no reconstruction of the coronoid process is required.[93]

Recurrence of an osteochondroma in the pediatric age patient is rare and in those instances when a recurrence is reported, it is likely that the recurrence represents transformation of the osteochondroma to either an osteosarcoma or chondrosarcoma. Malignant transformation of osteochondromas in MHE tends to be higher than with solitary osteochondromas and such recurrences have been reported to be as high as 25 percent.[93] The risk of an osteochondroma in a child progressing to chondrosarcoma or osteosarcoma is real but uncommon.[101,102]

Chondromyxoid Fibroma

Chondromyxoid fibroma is an uncommon benign tumor, first characterized by Jaffe and Lichenstein in 1948.[103] The tumor, which accounts for less than 1 percent of all bone tumors, has an overall slight male predominance. Chondromyxoid fibromas typically involve lower extremity bones with the metaphysis of the tibia being involved in over one third of all reported cases.[104] Approximately 2 percent of chondromyxoid fibromas will involve the bones of the skull and jaws.[105] A gender predilection has not been documented for those lesions that involve craniofacial region.[106]

Chondromyxoid fibromas that involve the craniofacial region of children and adolescents are exceedingly rare, accounting for less than 1 percent of all bone tumors in children.[107] Hammad et al. in a review of 20 gnathic chondromyxoid fibromas, found that seven occurred in children and adolescents, with the youngest patient being ten and the oldest sixteen. Five patients in the Hammad et al. study were male and two were female. The most commonly affected craniofacial sites for chondromyxoid fibroma in children are the mandible, maxilla and temporal bone.[104,105,106,107,108,109,110]

Chondromyxoid fibromas will most commonly develop at or near active or mature secondary centers of ossification in most of the skeleton. However, lesions that occur in the mandible and maxilla must of necessity develop in a different fashion, since those two bones ossify in fibro-membranous tissue that does not have a cartilaginous association. Therefore some investigators have suggested that chondromyxoid fibromas of the maxilla and mandible might be more appropriately classified as simply a variant of a chondroma.[112]

The vast majority of chondromyxoid fibromas that occur in the bones of the head and neck region will present as slowly enlarging swellings. Lesions tend to be lobular, often somewhat eccentrically placed, solitary lytic lesions of bone. Less commonly, the chondromyxoid fibroma can appear as multilocular or polycystic radiolucent lesion with peripheral bony margins that can range from poorly defined, to well defined, to scalloped. The chondromyxoid fibroma can be a destructive enough lesion to erode its marginating bony cortex, and pain may therefore become a prominent symptom.[113] Differential radiographic diagnoses may include chondroblastoma, central giant cell tumor (granuloma) chondrosarcoma or a benign odontogenic neoplasm. Intra lesional calcified matrix is a rare radiographic finding in chondromyxoid fibroma.

Pathologic Features

Most chondromyxoid fibromas will be submitted as gritty, granular somewhat myxoid tumor currettments. The tumor will be composed histologically of a lobular admixture of fibrocartilage set in a fibromyxoid stroma. Tumors will tend to display a variable degree of cellularity and most tumors are richly vascular. Individual tumor cells will consist of pleomorphic, angular and stellate appearing fibroblastic cells. (Figure 16.22) The nuclei of the tumor cells are often stippled and mitotic figures may be identified. Those areas of the tumor that are highly myxoid, or chondromyxoid will often show a retraction of the stroma from associated chondroid cells, giving the tumor a pseudoglandular appearance (Figure 16.23). The chondromyxoid fibroma will lack any evidence of true hyaline cartilage matrix of the type seen in enchondromas or chondrosarcoma. Mitotic activity is quite rare in chondromyxoid fibroma, and much more common to chondrosarcoma.

Differential Diagnosis

Differential microscopic diagnoses for chondromyxoid fibroma can include chondrosarcoma and chondroblastoma. Chondroblastoma will typically be characterized histologically by so-called chicken-wire calcifications, a feature that will be absent in chondromyxoid fibroma. Chondromyxoid fibroma will also lack a hyaline cartilage matrix and the tumor will fail

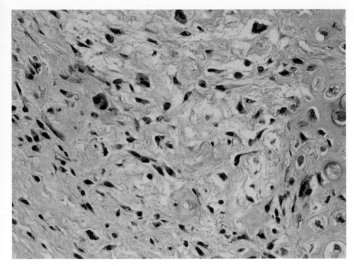

Figure 16.22 Chondromyxoid fibroma composed of fibrocartilage set in a fibromyxoid stroma.

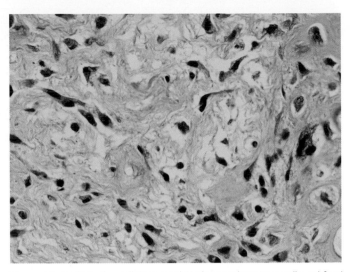

Figure 16.23 Note the stellate somewhat pleomorphic tumor cells and focal retraction of the stroma from chondroid cells at the tumor's periphery.

to demonstrate significant extension into surrounding bone. In long bones, chondromyxoid fibroma has been reported to occur in association with the ABC, especially in children, but no such association has been documented with tumors involving the craniofacial region.

Chondromyxoid fibroma is one of only two neoplasms that arise from incompletely differentiated cartilage. The only other tumor to do so is chondroblastoma. Safar et al.[114] have proposed a specific genetic indicator or linkage for chondromyxoid fibroma, the pericentric inversion of the 6[inv(6)(p25q13)] chromosome and Justin et al.[115] have shown phenotypic pattern of diversity in chondromyxoid which mimics fetal cartilage canal development.

Treatment and Prognosis

The suggested therapeutic approach to managing a chondromyxoid fibroma in the craniofacial region of a child is total excision of the lesion to healthy tumor free margins.[113] Curettage has been employed in the management of these tumors, however, such treatment results in tumor being left behind in a high percentage of cases, prompting recurrence.[116] Among the seven chondromyxoid fibromas involving the jawbones reported by Hammed,[107] either enucleation of the tumor or resection was employed. Three of the seven tumors treated by enucleation recurred within a period of two years. No instances of recurrences, where resection was employed, were reported after a similar two-year follow-up. Radiotherapy is contraindicated in the management of this tumor and reports of malignant transformation of chondromyxoid fibroma in the absence of radiotherapy remains largely unconvincing.

Chondroblastoma

Chondroblastoma is a rare benign tumor of immature chondroblasts. The tumor, first described by Jaffe and Lichenstein in 1942,[117] accounts for no more than 1 percent of all primary bone tumors. Chondroblastoma is thought by most investigators to be a tumor that arises from secondary centers of ossification.[118] Most osteoblastomas originate from the epiphyses of long bones, predominantly the proximal and distal portions of the femur and the proximal humerus and tibia, and most tumors will affect individuals in the second decade of life, most often individuals in the 15 to 25 year age group. In an evaluation of 87 chondroblastomas that were studied in a pediatric population, Sailhan[119] found no tumors in the head and neck region.[119]

Chondroblastomas that involve the skull and facial bones tend to arise in patients who are a decade older than those patients with chondroblastomas of the axial skeleton. In a Mayo Clinic study that included 495 cases of chondroblastoma, 6.9 percent of the tumors evaluated were located in the skull or facial bones.[120] Eighty-three percent of tumors occurred in patients 30 years of age or older.[120] Bertoni et al.[121] in a review of chondroblastomas of skull and facial bones, found that 21 of the 30 tumors that were studied involved the temporal bone, and that the next most common site of presentation was the mandible.[121]

Chondroblastomas of the TMJ are exceedingly rare. Nwoku et al.[122] reported only seven chondroblastomas of the TMJ in a review of 32,000 patients with head and neck tumors who were treated at their institution.

Most pediatric age patients with a chondroblastoma that involves a craniofacial bone will present with a chief complaint of pain. Pain may be present in concert with a localized swelling, or if the tumor involves the TMJ, a restricted oral opening or malocclusion.[123]

Chondroblastomas affecting bones of the head and neck region of children will generally range up to 4 cm in maximum size. Radiographically, tumors tend to present as round radiolucent lesions that are marginated by sclerotic bone. Tumors involving the bones of the craniofacial complex will often cause erosion or destruction of peripheral marginating bone, and as many as one half of all cases of chondroblastoma that present in the head and neck region will manifest radiographically as multiple aggregates of calcification within a central radiolucent zone.[124,125]

Pathologic Features

On gross inspection, chondroblastomas will be made up of aggregates of granular, gritty and sometimes friable or hemorrhagic accumulations of red, tan or brown tissue. Tumors will be composed histologically of an accumulation of chondroblasts that are cytologically uniform. Tumor cells will display definitive cytoplasmic borders and clear to eosinophilic cytoplasm, and tumor cells will be cytologically bland with one to two nuclei. In contradistinction to chondroblastomas that involve the axial skeleton, chondroblastomas in the head and neck region may show slightly more mitotic activity.[124] The nuclei of tumor cells in a chondroblastoma are often clefted or grooved and tumors may show a characteristic lattice-like or "chicken wire" pattern with central zonal necrosis, dystrophic calcifications and giant cells.[121,125] Craniofacial tumors will typically show histologic evidence of a chondroid matrix and a transition from cellular areas within the tumor to areas that are more cartilaginous.

The predominance of true chondroid matrix, which is quite typical of chondroblastoma of axial bones in pediatric patients tends to be lacking in chondroblastomas of the head and neck region.[125] Accumulations of pigmented macrophages, central zones of pseudocyst formation and prominent hyaline cartilage formation are more frequent in craniofacial chondroblastoma than in axial lesions.

Stefansson et al.[126] and Nakamura, et al.[127] have demonstrated that S-100 protein can be used as a useful diagnostic marker for chondroblastoma, especially in those instances in which the tumor contains numerous multinucleated giant cells and a diagnosis of CGCG is being entertained.

Differential Diagnosis

While chondroblastoma can resemble osteoblastoma histologically, osteoblastoma tends to be a much more richly vascular neoplasm than chondroblastoma, and cartilage production will typically be absent in osteoblastoma. In those instances in which a chondroblastoma shows significant multinucleated giant cell reactivity and in those tumors in which chondroblastic tumor cells appear histiocytic, a differential diagnosis of Langerhans cell histiocytosis may be considered. CD1a immunohistochemical staining can prove quite helpful in separating the two entities. In rare instances, chondroblastoma can demonstrate a distinctly clear cell pattern, in which case the tumor may need to be differentiated from metastatic disease. Areas of ossification within clear cell zones will tend to favor metastatic disease, as most chondroblastomas will not display significant ossification within the central body of the tumor. On occasion, odontogenic myxoid can resemble a chondroblastoma. However, the myxoid tumor matrix of an odontogenic myxoma

will dominate the tumor histology, and odontogenic epithelium may also be identified within the tumor.

Treatment and Prognosis

Chondroblastomas of the craniofacial skeleton are usually treated by aggressive surgical curettage, or if they involve the mandibular condyle, either condylectomy or en bloc resection. Recurrences following therapy are reported to be in the 10 to 15 percent range.[120,121] Malignant change in chondroblastomas has been reported, either as a result of prior radiation therapy or as a spontaneously developing neoplasm.[128]

Synovial Chondromatosis

Synovial chondromatosis is a metaplastic condition in which hamartomatous nodular and progressive benign cartilaginous lesions occur in synovial membranes and tendon sheaths. Most cases of synovial chondromatosis will affect the knee joint, with the elbow, hip and shoulder joints representing the next most commonly involved sites. Lesions occur most commonly in teenagers and young adults, with approximately 3 percent of cases occurring in the craniofacial region. The most frequent site for synovial chondromatosis to occur in the craniofacial region is the TMJ. The disorder has a slight male predilection, when it involves the TMJ, and the right TMJ is more often affected than the left. Lesions of the TMJ can progress beyond the glenoid fossa to extend into and destroy the middle cranial fossa, ear canal and mandibular condyle. The most common presenting clinical signs of synovial chondromatosis are pain and swelling in the TMJ area. When there is significant TMJ destruction, crepitus is common. Facial pain, swelling and a limited mouth opening are frequent symptoms as well. Patients may also complain of occlusal changes involving the teeth and it is not uncommon for various disorder associated symptoms to last anywhere from two to five years before there is intervention.[129,130,131]

When synovial chondromatosis affects the TMJ, the synovium will become hyperplastic, proliferate and ultimately undulate into a series of villous folds. Subsynovial surface cells will then typically undergo a form of nodular cartilaginous metaplasia. It is these nodules that eventually work their way through the synovial surface to become free-floating joint mites. In cases of long standing disease, the process may result in complete ossification of the nodules within the joint or bone, and rarely to joint ankylosis.

MRI imaging is the most effective method of visualizing the loose calcified material or so-called rice bodies that occur within the TMJ. However, both MRI and CT imaging are recommended in order to establish a reliable diagnosis of synovial chondromatosis.[132,133,134,135] CT findings can define the size, shape and location of loose bodies within the joint, but the bodies must be calcified if they are to be detected. Synovial chondromatosis has been subclassfied into three stages on the basis of MRI and CT imaging.[135] Stage one lesions show metaplastic synovium without loose bodies. Stage two lesions will show metaplastic synovium with loose "rice" bodies, and stage three lesions will show only loose "rice" bodies within the joint.[136]

From a clinical differential diagnostic standpoint, degenerative joint disease, rheumatoid arthritis, chondroblastoma and chondrosarcoma should be considered when entertaining a diagnosis of synovial chondromatosis. Patients with degenerative joint disease will typically have radiographic studies that show osteophyte formation, significant narrowing of the joint space and even subchondral sclerosis. Since juvenile rheumatoid arthritis can demonstrate the type of hyperplasic synovial proliferation that is seen in association with the lengthy, acute and chronic inflammation, typical of synovial chondromatosis, laboratory studies, including a rheumatoid factor are mandatory in order to separate juvenile rheumatoid arthritis from synovial chondromatosis. Chondrosarcoma, unlike synoial chondromaotisis will typically invade and destroy the surrounding bone.[136]

Pathology

Grossly, tissue samples will consist of cartilaginous nodules that are either embedded within connective tissue of subsynovial origin, or individual or loosely aggregated calcified bodies. Histologically the calcified bodies (joint mites) will be composed of multiple aggregates of metaplastic degenerative chondroid tissue with an associated dystrophic calcification of the synovial membrane.

Differential Diagnosis

In children, the one disease that must be differentiated from synovial chondromatosis is osteochondrosis dissecans, a disorder that can also result in loose calcified bodies in the TMJ. Osteochondrosis dissecans, however, is traumatic in origin, and a history of trauma to the TMJ will always be a component of the disease process.

Pigmented villonodular synovitis (PVS), most often diagnosed in the knee, can also occur in the TMJ, and it must be differentiated from synovial chondromatosis histologically. PVS is a slowly progressive fibrohistiocytic proliferation in which multinucleated giant cells, lymphocytes and lipid-laden macrophages will be identified within the joint space. This microscopic pattern of giant cell aggregation, chronic inflammation, histocytic proliferation and lipid-laden macrophages is not a histologic pattern that is typical of synovial chondromatosis.

Treatment and Prognosis

The treatment of choice for synovial chondromatosis is navigational TMJ surgery, employing arthroscopy synovectomy to remove disease associated loose bodies and involved synovial membrane during the diagnostic exploratory biopsy.[137] Postoperative physical therapy and anti-inflammatory drug management will be required in most patients.

In some instances synovial chondromatosis is a self-limiting disease, and management with non-invasive procedures using non-steroidal anti-inflammatory drugs can prove as affective as surgical intervention in such cases.

Malignant Neoplasms of Cartilage

Chondrosarcoma

Chondrosarcoma is an uncommon malignant neoplasm of bone that most often occurs in adults. Most tumors arise in long bones of the extremities and the osseous pelvis. Chondrosarcoma accounts for less than 5 percent of all primary malignant skeletal tumors that present in the first two decades of life.[138] Chondrosarcomas in children and adolescents, regardless of their site of origin, generally arise as solitary neoplasms. However, childhood chondrosarcomas can arise in a setting of syndromic multiple hereditary chondromas.[138] Twenty to thirty percent of individuals who have Maffucci's syndrome and Ollier's disease will have their chondromas transition to chondrosarcoma. Such malignant transition is much more common in children and adolescents than adults.[139,140,141,142]

Chondrosarcoma of the jaws and craniofacial skeleton accounts for slightly less than 12 percent of all cases of chondrosarcoma; the most common site being the maxilla.[139] The mandible and sinonasal region are the next most frequent sites for chondrosarcoma to arise in children. Pontes et al.[139] in a retrospective clinicopathologic analysis of head and neck chondrosarcomas that included 680 patients world-wide, were able to identified only 11 chondrosarcomas in individuals in the pediatric age group. Rare head and neck sites for chondrosarcoma include the cervical vertebra, orbit and nasopharynx.[141]

Most chondrosarcomas in children and adolescents will present as a painless swelling, although loosening of teeth, nasal obstruction, pain and diplopia have been reported.[140]

The radiographic appearance of chondrosarcomas that involve the head and neck region of children and adolescents will generally be that of an aggressively erosive lesion of bone. (Figure 16.24) Lesions involving the jawbones may display a widening of the periodontal ligament space radiographically, a feature that has also been well described in cases of osteosarcoma.[143] Diagnostic studies, including CT and MRI are usually employed to delineate the extent of the tumor and determine if there is soft tissue expansion. While rings and crescents of calcified product tend to be a common and somewhat characteristic radiographic feature of the neoplasm, the degree of calcification in any one chondrosarcoma will vary.

Among standard forms of chondrosarcoma of the head and neck region in pediatric age patients, three basic histopathologic patterns: 1) mesenchymal, 2) myxoid and 3) clear cell, can be identified. *Mesenchymal chondrosarcoma* is the most common tumor subtype to be identified in children, and accounts for between 20 and 30 percent of all chondrosarcomas in the head and neck region of pediatric age patients. Approximately one third of all mesenchymal chondrosarcomas that occur in the head and neck region will arise as extra osseous lesions.[144] Mesenchymal chondrosarcoma occurs most

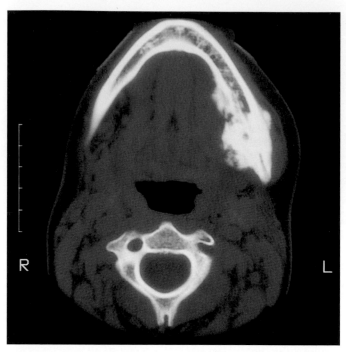

Figure 16.24 The extracortical sunburst pattern of bone formation is not specific for chondrosarcoma and can be seen in a host of rapidly growing malignancies of children, including osteosarcoma and ES. (Reprinted from Marx R, Stern D. *Oral and Maxillofacial Pathology: A Rationale for Diagnosis and Treatment* with permission from Quintessence Publishing Company).

frequently in the second decade of life, although rare congenital examples of this form of chondrosarcoma have been reported.[145]

The maxilla and mandible are the most common sites for mesenchymal chondrosarcoma, although the bones of the skull, cervical vertebra, ethmoid sinuses and nasal pharynx can be affected. The most common presenting symptom associated with mesenchymal chondrosarcoma as well as clear cell chondrosarcoma in a child or adolescent will be pain, swelling or the presence of a bone eroding mass. *Myxoid chondrosarcoma* is a tumor that most often affects extra skeletal sites. This form of chondrosarcoma is exceedingly rare in the head and neck region, and in a review of 14 myxoid chondrosarcomas in the intracranial region, Gonzales-Lois et al.[146] identified only three cases in children or adolescents. Myxoid chondrosarcomas will generally present initially as a painless swelling. Radiographically, tumors may or may not have central calcifications within them.

Laryngeal chondrosarcoma represents the most infrequently identified subtype of head and neck chondrosarcoma to be seen all age groups. Rarely do laryngeal tumors occur in patients less than 30 years of age.[147] When childhood tumors do occur, they tend to be less than 2 cm in maximum dimension, and a palpable mass may or may not be evident upon clinical examination of the patient.[147] CT scans may demonstrate calcifications within a larger radiolucent tumor mass. Most laryngeal chondrosarcomas tend to be low grade neoplasms histologically, with little cytologic atypia, and thus they

may be difficult to distinguish from a benign chondroma. Therefore the surgical pathologist must evaluate the process, especially in instances of an incisional biopsy, judiciously, and render a definitive diagnosis only when the entire lesion can be examined.

Pathologic Features

Most chondrosarcomas of the conventional variety will be submitted to the laboratory as lobular, gray, glistening pieces of tissue which may contain a granular, gritty calcified product or show areas of myxoid, mucoid or cystic degeneration. *Extra skeletal (myxoid) chondrosarcomas* will tend to be grossly gelatinous or mucoid lesions. Mesenchymal chondrosarcomas will be gray tan on gross inspection and somewhat firmer than extra skeletal (myxoid) chondrosarcomas. They will tend to therefore more closely resemble conventional chondrosarcomas grossly. Clear cell chondrosarcomas have no distinctive gross appearance that would enable one to distinguish them from a conventional chondrosarcoma.

Conventional chondrosarcoma in children and adolescents can be histologically graded as: either low grade (grade 1), intermediate grade (grade 2) or high grade (grade 3). Grade 1 lesions typically resemble normal benign cartilage, and they will display a somewhat lobular histologic appearance in which cartilaginous cells are quite uniform. There may be a minimal amount of increased cellularity in grade 1 tumors however, atypical mitoses are rare. Grade 2 tumors will frequently demonstrate areas that are myxoid, with a prominent myxoid stroma and a matrix of hyaline cartilage. Grade 2 tumors tend to show an increased cellularity when compared with grade 1 tumors, and tumor cell nuclei that are binucleate and multinucleate can be identified within the lacuni of cartilaginous cells (Figures 16.25, 16.26 & 16.27). Atypical mitoses will be more common in grade 2 tumors than grade 1 tumors. Grade 3, or high grade tumors show significant pleomorphism of tumor cells and the tumor stroma will display a high degree of cellularity. Grade 3 lesions as a whole tend to be poorly differentiated, and frequently do not contain normal appearing cartilage. Grade 3 tumors will display an exceedingly high mitotic index and the tumor may display focal areas of necrosis. High grade tumors are exceedingly rare in children and as a whole chondrosarcomas in children tend to be low grade neoplasms.

Chondrosarcoma, regardless of histologic grade will contain intermittent areas of bony calcification, and typically the neoplasm will infiltrate osseous trabecula in a manner that shows normal bone interfacing with the malignancy. This pattern is quite different from what is typically seen in benign chondromatosis where individual enchondromas remain separated from surrounding bone. Solitary enchondromatosis is exceedingly rare in the jawbones, and solitary lesions that are cartilaginous in nature and which display any cellular atypia should be examined microscopically with the knowledge that such lesions are frequently malignant. The cartilage that is seen in the chondromas associated with Ollier's disease and

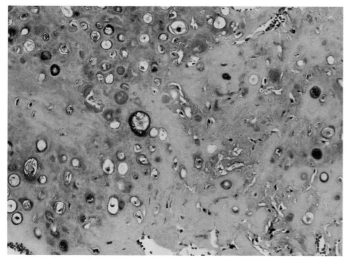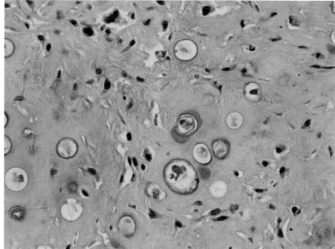

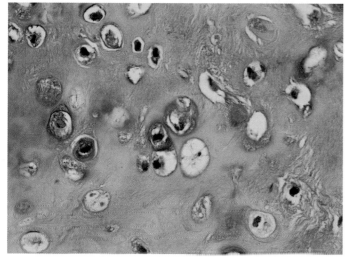

Figures 16.25 (top left), 16.26 (top right) & 16.27 (bottom)
Chondrosarcoma. This chondroid malignancy features increased cellularity, with associated nuclear pleomorphism and hyperchromasia. Note the binucleate cells in all three photomicrographs.

Maffucci's syndrome tends to be hypercellular and mitotically active, however, such a cytologic finding may not be representative of malignant neoplasia and clinicopathologic correlation is mandatory when examining all such lesions histologically.

Differential Diagnosis

Chondrosarcoma can be difficult to distinguish from chondroblastic osteosarcoma histologically. Osteosarcoma must of necessity show a clear origin of the neoplastic process from primitive malignant osteoid, while chondrosarcoma will arise from a cartilaginous matrix that will lack a malignant osteoid component. *Clear cell chondrosarcoma* can occasionally be seen in children and it may be difficult to distinguish from osteosarcoma.[148] This histologic variant of chondrosarcoma will be characterized by an accumulation of granular/or clear cells set in a primitive chondroid matrix. Multinucleated giant cells are common to this form of chondrosarcoma, as are aggregates of reactive bone. The bone seen in the tumor will however represent a lesional background component and the tumor is not one that arises from malignant osteoid.

Mesenchymal chondrosarcoma generally shows a biphasic histologic pattern in which undifferentiated round or spindle shaped primitive mesenchymal cells that have a sarcomatous appearance will be admixed with aggregates of well differentiated cartilaginous tumor cells or a recognizable chondroid product. The tumor stroma will generally contain an abundant vascular component that may in some instances mimic the staghorn shaped spaces typical of a hemangiopericytoma (Figure 16.27.1). The cartilaginous component of the tumor will be composed of hyaline cartilage-like zones that may show cytologic atypia (Figure 16.27.2). Small round cells that are strongly Sox 9 and vimentin reactive, but typically CD56, CD57 and neuron enolase negative can be identified within the hyaline cartilage component of the tumor. Mesenchymal chondrosarcoma will tend to stain negatively for type 2 collagen, S-100 protein, epithelial membrane antigen, cytokeratins and CD34, but will be CD99 reactive.[149]

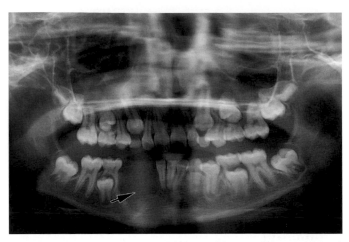

Figure 16.28 Large, destructive radiolucency of the mandible in a child with fibrosarcoma (arrow). (Reprinted from Marx R, Stern D. *Oral and Maxillofacial Pathology: A Rationale for Diagnosis and Treatment* with permission from Quintessence Publishing Company).

Most fibrosarcomas will arise in soft tissue, and the head and neck region is the most common soft tissue site. When tumors arise in association with bone, periosteal tumors are much more common than central osseous forms of the disease. Most bone associated tumors will involve the mandible, with the posterior mandible being more often affected than the anterior mandible. Tumors can also arise within the bones of the skull, the nasal bones and bones of the cervical spine.[167]

The most common presenting symptom for the child or adolescent with fibrosarcoma of bone will be a swelling which may be associated with pain or paresthesia. Loose teeth, ulceration of the mucosa, bony erosion (Figure 16.28) and abscess formation may also be present at the time of diagnosis. Central osseous fibrosarcoma will tend to present as an expansile moth eaten radiolucency often without a limiting bony margin.[167,168,169] Radiographically fibrosarcomas are generally evaluated using CT scans, plain film radiology and MRI scanning. Positive electron transmission scanning (PET scans) can prove valuable in ruling out metastatic disease.

Fibrosarcomas of bone were at one time thought to be relatively common. However, the subclassification of biologically aggressive fibrous tumors into 1) pleomorphic undifferentiated sarcoma, 2) fibromatosis, 3) fibroblastic osteosarcoma, 4) nodular fasciitis and 5) infantile fibrosarcoma has greatly reduced the number of true bony fibrosarcomas that are diagnosed. The etiology of fibrosarcoma has not been identified and although trauma has been implicated as a possible causal factor in some cases, there is no indication that trauma plays an etiologic role in development of fibrosarcoma in infants or children. Etiologically, a characteristic translocation, t(12;15)(p13;q25) with an ETV6-NTRK3 gene fusion is a specific finding in the tumor, as are gains in chromosomes 8, 11, 17 and 20.[170]

Pathologic Features

Fibrosarcoma will grossly consist of gray, tan, rubbery aggregates of tumor tissue or present as an intact rubbery gray tan tumor mass. Histologically tumors are classified as low, intermediate or high grade.[169] There is no difference in histologic appearance between those tumors that are classified as infantile fibrosarcoma and those tumors that occur as adolescent or adult neoplasms. Most infantile forms of fibrosarcoma, whether they arise in soft tissue or bone, will be low grade tumors.

Low grade (grade 1) fibrosarcoma will typically show a classic herringbone pattern of spindle cells arranged in fascicles. Grade 1 tumors will tend to have only minimal cellular pleomorphism, little cellular atypia, a low mitotic rate and little or no evidence of necrosis. The tumor matrix will be composed predominantly of mature collagen or streaming fibroblasts. High grade (grade 3) tumors tend to show marked cellularity, an increased rate of atypical mitoses, cellular necrosis and significant cellular pleomorphism. A stromal collagen matrix will be minimal or absent in grade 3 tumors, and a herringbone pattern will be lacking. Intermediate (grade 2) tumors will tend to demonstrate a histologic pattern that is intermediate between that of grade 1 and grade 3 tumors, with evidence of cytologically atypical fibroblasts, spindle cells and some degree of a herringbone pattern. (Figures 16.29 & 16.30).

From a differential diagnostic standpoint, infantile fibrosarcoma of bone should be differentiated from pleomorphic undifferentiated sarcoma, juvenile fibromatosis, leiomyosarcoma, spindle cell squamous cell carcinoma and mucosal melanoma. While monophasic synovial sarcoma can also resemble infantile fibrosarcoma histologically, that tumor will typically show a t(X;18) translocation, which will be absent in fibrosarcoma.

Fibromatosis (desmoid-type fibromatosis, aggressive fibromatosis) can resemble fibrosarcoma of bone histologically, especially if the fibrosarcoma is low grade. However, fibromatosis will generally lack a herringbone histologic pattern, the tumor will show almost no mitoses, and the tumor will be histologically composed of mature collagen to a far greater extent than that seen in infantile fibrosarcoma.

Leiomyosarcoma, like fibrosarcoma will be composed of interlacing fascicles of cells, but tumor cell nuclei, unlike those of fibrosarcoma, will tend to be blunt ended rather than sharp ended and there will typically be perinuclear clearing around the nuclei of leiomyosarcoma tumor cells.

Fibrosarcoma will consistently stain negatively for actin, desmin, S-100 protein, Bcl2 and cytokeratins 7 and 19, and the tumor will be vimentin reactive. These immunohistochemical findings should help to exclude a more immunohistochemically reactive spindle cell carcinoma of epithelial origin and leiomyosarcoma from fibrosarcoma. On rare occasions melanoma arising from the oral mucosa can resemble fibrosarcoma, especially if there is no tumor pigment present, or if the tumor takes on a spindle type pattern. However, melanoma markers, including C-KIT will be positive in mucosal melanoma, unlike fibrosarcoma.

Pleomorphic undifferentiated sarcoma can resemble fibrosarcoma histologically.[171] However, the tumor can be

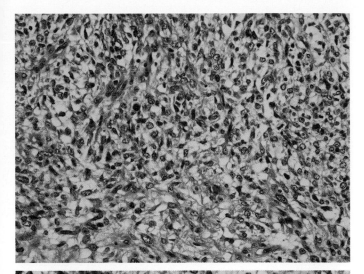

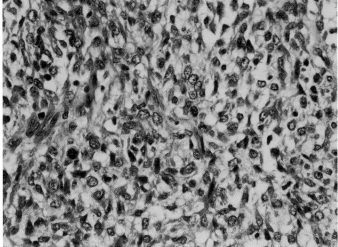

Figures 16.29 (top) & 16.30 (bottom) Highly cellular fibrosarcoma with a minimal fascicular growth pattern are seen in these low and intermediate power photomicrographs. Individual tumor cells are pleomorphic with only small amounts of streaming eosinophilic cytoplasm.

distinguished from fibrosarcoma because of its storiform proliferation of fibroblasts, its admix of pleomorphic mononuclear cells resembling histocytes, the tumors significant mitotic rate and the presence of multinucleated giant cells.

Treatment and Prognosis

Fibrosarcoma of bone in the pediatric population rarely metastasizes and the tumor generally has a natural history that is similar to juvenile fibromatosis.[172,173] The prognosis for pediatric age patients with fibrosarcoma will largely be related to the histologic grade of the neoplasm and the success of surgical resection.[167,168,169] When metastases occur, they occur via a vascular route and most often any distant tumor spread that occurs will be to the lungs. Neoadjuvant chemotherapy has been used in the treatment of some cases of fibrosarcoma but surgical resection with a wide margin of

uninvolved tissue is the most often employed treatment for fibrosarcoma in children.[174]

Benign Fibro-Osseous Diseases of Bone

Fibrous-Osseous Lesions of the Jaws and Craniofacial Skeleton

Fibro-osseous lesions of the jaws and craniofacial skeleton, which occur quite commonly in childhood and adolescence, represent a varied group of bone and connective tissue proliferative processes that result in an aberrant proliferation of a mineralized product and collagen. These lesions, whether they are developmental, true neoplasms or dysmorphic and dysplastic lesions of bone can produce a myriad of clinical and radiographic findings. Fibro-osseous lesions of the craniofacial skeleton tend not to have a single or specific histopathology. Rather, the lesions that occur in this site represent a group of pathologic processes that require significant clinicopathologic correlation on the part of the clinician and pathologist if an appropriate diagnosis is to be arrived at. Perhaps nowhere in pathology is it more important to integrate clinical, radiographic and pathologic findings, in order to establish a diagnosis.

Fibrous Dysplasia

FD is a non-inherited fibro-osseous disorder that affects both medullary and cortical bone, and a disease that is characterized by abnormal bone maturation and remodeling. On a genetic level, FD is a non-malignant condition that is caused by activating mutations in the *GNAS* gene. Mutations in that gene do not allow for either the differentiation of, or proliferation of bone forming stromal cells. In patients with FD, normal bone and bone marrow are replaced by a disorganized or otherwise poorly organized matrix of immature woven bone and fibrous connective tissue. The FD phenotype is variable and may be isolated to a single skeletal site or multiple sites.[1] Extra skeletal manifestations of FD are common, predominantly characterized by skin and/or endocrine organ abnormalities.[175]

FD has classically been separated into four distinct clinical subtypes: 1) monostotic FD, 2) craniofacial FD, 3) polyostotic FD of the Jaffe–Lichtenstein type and 4) polyostotic FD of the McCune–Albright type.[175,176,177,178,179,180,181,182,183,184]

Monostotic FD, in which a single bone is involved, accounts for 75 percent of FD cases, regardless of site. When the monostotic form of the disease occurs in the jaws, the mandibular body and the premolar/molar region of the maxilla are the most frequently involved sites.

Polyostotic forms of FD are a less common, accounting for between 25 and 30 percent of all FD cases. Most cases of polyostotic FD present before the age of ten.[175] When polyostotic FD affects endocrine organs, resulting in endocrine abnormalities and skin pigmentation, most often unilateral café-au-lait macules, the disease is classified as McCune–Albright syndrome.

Individuals affected by the Jaffe–Lichenstein form of FD will characteristically have the polyostotic form of the disease

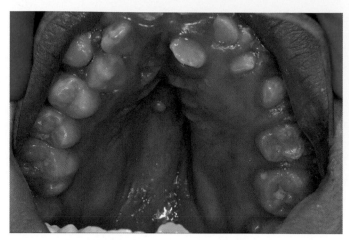

Figure 16.31 FD of the maxilla in a child. Note the bilateral elliptical expansion of the maxillary alveolus. (Reprinted from Marx R, Stern D. *Oral and Maxillofacial Pathology: A Rationale for Diagnosis and Treatment* with permission from Quintessence Publishing Company).

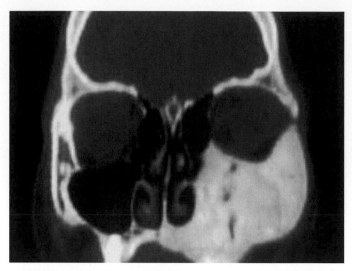

Figure 16.32 Craniofacial FD characteristically involves the maxilla zygoma, vomer and frontal bones. (Reprinted from Marx R, Stern D. *Oral and Maxillofacial Pathology: A Rationale for Diagnosis and Treatment* with permission from Quintessence Publishing Company).

without skin pigmentation or endocrine abnormalities.[175] The most common endocrinopathies that are associated with the McCune–Albright form of FD include precocious puberty in female patients and more rarely hyperthyroidism. Other endocrine abnormalities include hyperparathyroidism, Cushing's syndrome, hyperprolactinemia and gynecomastia.[185,186]

McCune–Albright syndrome is much more common in females than males and the syndrome is thought to account for approximately 5 percent of all bone lesions seen in children. However, the true incidence of this form of FD is not readily available, since a host of patients are asymptomatic and do not present from evaluation or management.

FD of the craniofacial region, which can be either polyostotic or monostotic, is characterized by the involvement of two or more bones of the jaw, mid-face, skull complex in continuity. Nearly 50 percent of individuals with polyostotic FD will present with involvement of the craniofacial skeleton,[178] whereas only 25 percent of individuals with monostotic FD will have the bones of the their face, jaws, and skull affected.[178]

FD is a disorder of growing bones and a developmental disorder that generally becomes apparent between the ages of 5 and 15. The disorder initiates in the embryonic stage at which point either a GNSA mutation, or a deletion occurs. This gene, which encodes for intercytoplasmic transducer protein, also has a general overall responsibility for bone maturation. Once intercytoplasmic transducer protein is lost, subsequent daughter cells will produce an immature bone matrix made up of benign dysplastic bone, the hallmark of FD.

Aberrant or abnormal daughter cells that lack signal transducer protein do not always migrate to bone. Occasionally these cells will migrate to primordia of both skin and endocrine glands. As a result of this migration, McCune–Albright syndrome or the Jaffe–Lichtenstein form of FD, with their unique polyostotic manifestations of the disease may eventuate.

Clinical Features

The location and type of FD that is identified in the pediatric age patient will dictate the patient's signs and symptoms. The signs and symptoms of the disease as it presents in the craniofacial region can vary from facial deformity and asymmetry to visual changes, hearing impairment, nasal congestion and/or obstruction, pain, paresthesia and malocclusion.[175] The vast majority of all patients with craniofacial FD will be diagnosed during the first two decades of life.[179,180,181,182]

Asymmetry and swelling are the most frequent complaints associated with FD when it is identified in the maxilla, mandible and facial skeleton. (Figure 16.31) When FD involves the sinuses, the most commonly involved site will be the sphenoid sinus, followed by the ethmoid and maxillary sinuses.[175] Sinus infection in FD is not uncommon and the source of such infections is often related to obliteration of the sinus and destruction or elimination of the sinus lining Schneiderian membrane. There is no indication however, that a history of sinusitis and facial pain or headaches will correlate with the amount of the craniofacial disease that is discovered in a patient. It has been suggested that an excess production of growth hormone can be associated with significant FD involvement of the sinonasal region, but such a correlative occurrence is quite rare.[183]

Café-au-lait macules and precocious puberty will be absent in the pure form of *craniofacial FD*. This form of FD will most often involve the maxillofacial apparatus. (Figure 16.32) The sphenoid bone, temporal bone, nasal concha and clivus can be affected singularly in craniofacial FD but far less commonly. FD involving the skull base may result in compression of cranial nerves, and a resultant visual impairment or hearing loss, while FD involvement of the temporal bones can result in occlusion of the bony ear canals and the formation of cholesteatomas.

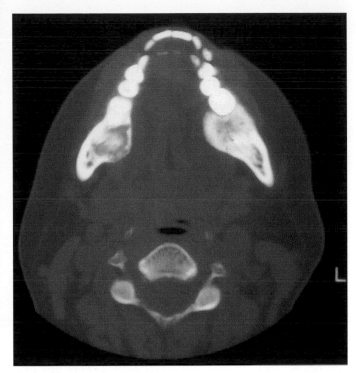

Figure 16.33 FD. CT scan demonstrating bilateral elliptical mottled and largely radiodense lesions of the mandible.

The radiographic findings that are seen in FD are variable and will to some extent be based on the patient's age. The radiographic appearance of FD on plain films was at one time categorized as either 1) *ground glass-like*, 2) *sclerotic* or 3) *cystic*. The availability of CT scanning has demonstrated, however, that the vast majority of FD cases in children are quite homogeneous lesions that tend to show a finely trabecular pattern of bone filling in the normal medullary compartment. Thus, lesions that would otherwise be classified as either cystic or sclerotic lesions on plane film evaluation are in fact quite rare. Nonetheless, in the absence of CT, the most common presentation of FD will be that of a relatively fusiform, ground glass appearing growth (Figure 16.33) that is poorly demarcated from the surrounding uninvolved bone. FD will tend to blend into normal bone, often replacing the cortices so that lesions, especially those involving the maxilla and mandible, will demonstrate the complete absence of a bony cortex. Soft tissue growths, most commonly intramuscular myxomas, have been reported in association with FD, (Mazabraund syndrome); however, such growths are rare in children.[187]

Clinical Differential Diagnoses

It is often difficult to distinguish FD from ossifying fibroma, the lesion with which FD is most frequently confused clinically. Ossifying fibromas tend to be well delineated or well demarcated, typically spherical lesions, rather than fusiform shaped lesions radiographically. However, both processes can cause cortical expansion of the bone and both can demonstrate a medullary replacement pattern that can be quite

heterogeneous. Radiographically, ossifying fibromas will tend to appear totally radiolucent, entirely radiopaque or radiographically mixed in their appearance, while FD will appear poorly demarcated, ground glass-like, or radiodense and fusiform rather than spherical. FD will replace the bony cortices or resorb them rather than expand them as ossifying fibroma does. Eighty percent of all craniofacial dysplasia cases are diagnosed within the first two decades of life, whereas ossifying fibroma, except for the "juvenile active" form of the disease will occur in patients beyond the second decade of life. Finally, as high as 70 percent of patients with polyostotic FD will present with an elevation of alkaline phosphatase. Patients with ossifying fibroma will not demonstrate this abnormality in their bone chemistry.

Although the single most important disorder that FD must be distinguished from is ossifying fibroma, a host of other disorders can simulate FD, including chronic sclerosing osteomyelitis and osteosarcoma. Osteosarcoma is typically a biologically aggressive lesion that will invade and erode cortical bone to extend into the soft tissue in a rapidly progressive fashion. Such a clinically aggressive growth pattern is not part of the pathology of FD.

Chronic sclerosing osteomyelitis is a painful infective process that is most often associated with a prior endodontic therapy, and an associated long-term local infection or periapical abscess. In most instances, *actinomyces species* and *eikenella corrodens* can be isolated from chronic sclerosing osteomyelitis. Chronic sclerosing osteomyelitis will also, unlike FD, demonstrate areas of intact normal cortical bone without generalized cortical resorption, and bony expansion will tend to be minimal.

Garré osteomyelitis may be confused with FD; however, this disorder will cause bone to proliferate in an extracortical periosteal fashion radiographically and histologically (Figures 16.34, 16.35, 16.36 & 16.37). Garré osteomyelitis is also nearly always associated causally with a non-vital cariously involved tooth, most often the first molar tooth, a feature that is uncommon in FD.

Pathologic Features

Biopsied tissue from FD will tend to be gritty, granular or rubbery in texture. Histologically FD will be composed of a haphazard arrangement of both trabecular and/or woven bone that is set in a matrix of collagen which ranges from immature to mature (Figures 16.38 & 16.39). The histologic appearance of FD will vary, largely based on the length of time that FD has been present. In long standing lesions, the supporting fibrous stroma may be quite mature and significant amounts of lamellar bone and bony trabecula may be arranged in a typical parallel fashion. In more immature lesions, bony trabeculae will tend to be thin, haphazard and script or puzzle-like in their arrangement as they attempt to blend into a collagenous stroma (Figures 16.40 & 16.41). Although the bony trabeculae that are seen in FD are often described as lacking osteoblastic rimming, such a finding is not always present and in many FD

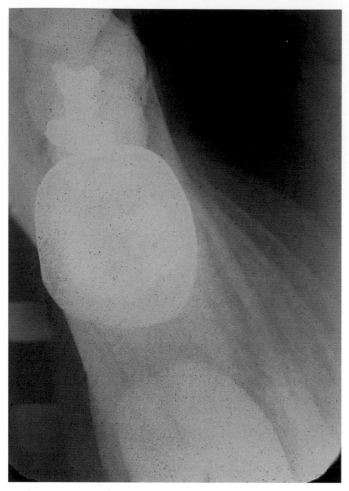

Figure 16.34 Onion skin layering of periosteum in Garres osteomyelitis.

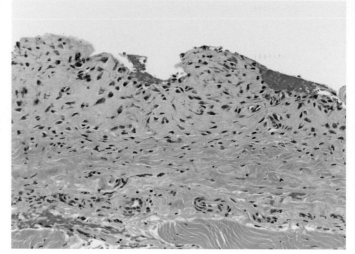

Figure 16.35 Garres osteomyelitis demonstrating proliferative periostitis.

lesions, osteoblastic rimming of trabeculae will be quite prominent. One key histologic feature that is common to FD is the so-called feather-like appearance of the bone that can be seen in the disease, and the tendency of such bone to blend directly into a primitive collagenous stroma. Multinucleated giant cell forms can commonly be seen within the stromal elements of FD, and osteoclasts can be variably present, depending on the stage at which FD is biopsied. A host of ancillary tests can be performed to complete the diagnosis of FD including molecular studies that will show missense mutations in the *GNAS-1* gene. These ancillary tests, although often quiet valuable in terms of management of a specific FD patient are not necessary in order to render a diagnosis of FD.

Differentiating FD from ossifying fibroma can sometimes prove to be a difficult diagnostic challenge. GNAS mutations in FD can be identified in all cases, whereas no GNAS mutations will be identified in ossifying fibroma cases. GNAS mutations at the Arg codon can thus prove to be helpful in the differential diagnosis of the two lesions.[188]

Treatment and Prognosis

The treatment of FD involves close and judicious follow-up of the patient. In most instances surgical intervention is not required. Lesions that are small and asymptomatic at the time of diagnosis will tend to remain as such. Marx et al.[188] have suggested that the preferred approach to the treatment of both maxillofacial monostotic FD and craniofacial FD is most often no treatment. Some children however, do not adapt well psychologically to any degree of facial expansion and deformity and those patients may therefore require treatment. The most effective management modality for craniofacial FD is osseous recontouring of the bone. Such recontouring is most effective as patients approach adulthood, a period during which the disease tends to show some modification in, and slowing of its growth pattern.

FD can be a persistent disease and in those instances of craniofacial FD in which growth is dramatic and/or functionally compromising, surgery can be employed as soon as possible following the diagnosis. Approximately 25 percent of patients who are initially treated surgically in any juvenile FD age group will show a recurrence.[188] Regrowth of craniofacial FD following biopsy tends to occur most commonly in patients who have had a biopsy or a surgical recontouring procedure done prior to 21 years of age. FD is episodic in its growth pattern and although episodic, that growth tends to be relatively steady.

Some reports in the literature suggest that surgical intervention will stimulate the growth of FD, however, it is more likely that such episodic post-surgical growth occurs as part of the natural history of the disease rather than because of some external form of stimulation such as surgery.[188] When FD is in the process of undergoing an episodic expansion, surgery is contraindicated until a time when such expansion stops. That timeframe is generally considered to be a period of three months after the active FD growth phase becomes quiescent.[188] Resection is rarely, if ever, indicated for craniofacial FD, except in those instances where extreme expansion results in airway obstruction, vision impairment or a hearing deficit.

Malignant degeneration of FD is rare. Most instances in which such a transition has been reported have occurred in

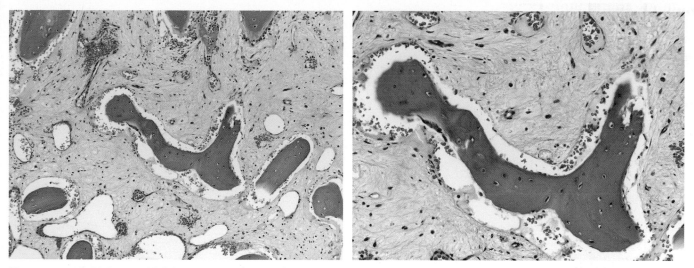

Figures 16.36 (left) & 16.37 (right) Aggregates of reactive bone are evident in these intermediate and high power photomicrographs.

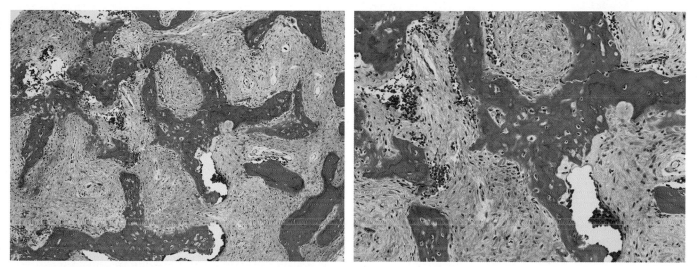

Figures 16.38 (left) & 16.39 (right) FD characterized by woven bone set in a collagen matrix. Associated osseous trabeculae resemble Chinese script.

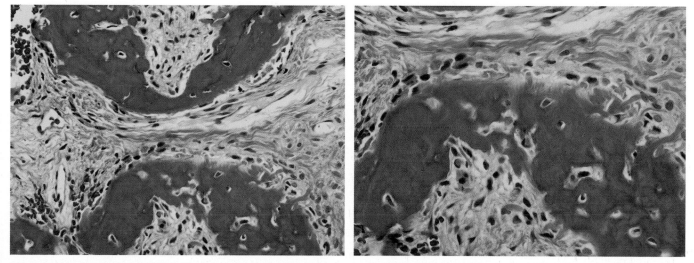

Figures 16.40 (left) & 16.41 (right) FD. High power photomicrographs showing U-shaped woven bone that attempts to blend into a collagenous stroma at the margins are seen in these intermediate and high power photomicrographs.

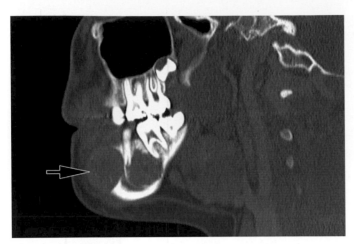

Figure 16.42 CT scan showing a well circumscribed largely radiolucent conventional ossifying fibroma of odontogenic origin. (Reprinted from Marx R, Stern D. *Oral and Maxillofacial Pathology: A Rationale for Diagnosis and Treatment* with permission from Quintessence Publishing Company).

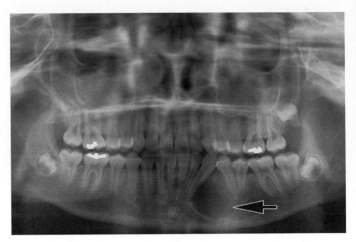

Figure 16.43 Conventional ossifying fibroma presenting as a well demarcated radiolucency of the mandible on a panoramic radiograph.

patients who have been treated with radiation therapy for their FD.[188,189] The most common malignancies that have been reported in association with FD, (fibrosarcoma, chondrosarcoma and pleomorphic undifferentiated sarcoma) can take up to 35 years to develop. FD has also been reported to occur less frequently in association with ABCs, mucoceles and osteomyelitis.[175] Since sarcomatous transformations of FD can indeed occur, long term follow-up of all FD patients is mandatory and biopsy of any lesion displaying an atypical clinical or radiographic change is warranted.

Segmental odontomaxillary dysplasia (SOD) is a disorder that can simulate FD. SOD is typically seen in patients between the ages of 5 and 19. The etiology of the disorder is not known. SOD characteristically affects the maxilla and will result in a markedly thickened gingiva which will overlie the underlying bony disease process and the expansion of the maxilla. This clinical finding will be in contrast to FD in which the gingiva and overlying oral tissues appear normal. SOD patients have also been reported to show external root resorption and enlarged pulp chambers, features that are not typically seen in FD.[188] Distinction of SOD from FD must be made on the basis of clinicopathologic evaluation, since biopsies are not pathognomonic.

Ossifying Fibroma and its Variants

Ossifying fibroma is a benign, generally slow growing, fibro-osseous lesion that can affect any of the bones of the craniofacial skeleton. The mandible is that most common site for ossifying fibroma, with the posterior molar region of the mandible most often affected.[191,192,193,194] Ossifying fibromas are far more common in the jaws than long bones, largely due to the large amount of mesenchymal induction that takes place in the jaw bones. This inductive effect results in the formation of not only bone but also cementum and periodontal ligament, providing a rich mileau for genetic errors and tumor development that is not present in long bones. Ossifying fibroma can

be divided into three distinct subtypes: *conventional ossifying fibroma of odontogenic origin, juvenile ossifying fibroma* and finally, *extra gnathic ossifying fibroma* of the skull, a disorder that affects only adults.

Ossifying Fibroma of Odontogenic Origin (Conventional Ossifying Fibroma)

Ossifying fibromas of odontogenic origin arise as benign neoplasms that involve the jawbones only. The World Health Organization (WHO)[195] suggests that since these lesions can only be found in the tooth-bearing areas of the mandible and maxilla, ossifying fibromas of odontogenic origin are most likely a derivative of cells that reside within the periodontal ligament.[195]

Clinical Findings

Ossifying fibroma of odontogenic origin, occasionally referred to as cemento-ossifying fibroma, will most often present as a painless spherical or ovoid expansion of the jaw. This tumor is much more common in the mandible than the maxilla, and the lesion has a peak incidence in second, third and fourth decades of life. There is a distinct female predilection for the tumor, reported to be as great as 5:1.[195]

Radiographically, lesions that involve the mandible will typically cause a characteristic thinning of the anterior border of the mandible on radiographs or CT scans.[193,194] (Figure 16.42) Lesions can present radiographically as either radiolucent, radiopaque or mixed radiographic growths. (Figure 16.43) Since ossifying fibromas are of periodontal ligament origin, they can have extensive mesenchymal cellular induction of bone, cementum and fibrous connective tissue, which can result in the tumor often demonstrating a transitional opaque/lucent radiographic appearance.

Traiantafillidou et al.[194] in a review of 14 cases of ossifying fibroma of the jaws in which patients ranged in age from 7 to 55 years, found that bone swelling or expansion was the most common presenting symptom regardless of age. Displacement of teeth adjacent to the tumor is also common and on surgical

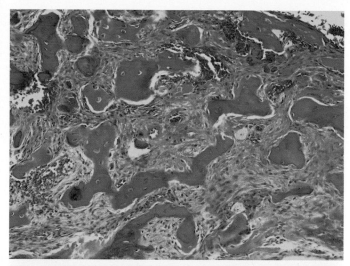

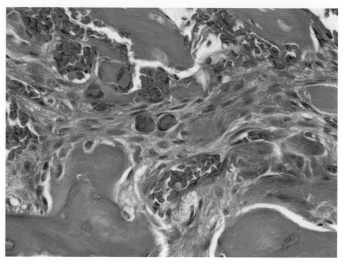

Figure 16.46 High power photomicrograph of bony trabeculae in a conventional ossifying fibroma. Osteoblastic and osteoclastic activity can be seen marginating the bone.

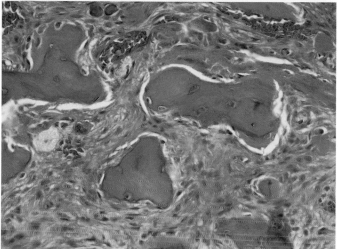

Figures 16.44 (top) & 16.45 (bottom) Conventional ossifying fibroma showing osseous trabeculae set in a well vascularized collagenous matrix at low and medium powers.

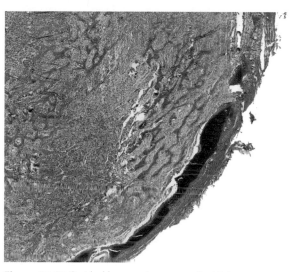

Figure 16.47 Residual bony cortex, as seen in this low power photomicrograph of an ossifying fibroma, tends to favor that diagnosis over FD.

exploration of the tumor mass, the tumor will often show either a separation or a distinct demarcation from the surrounding bone. A connective tissue tumor capsule is however, not always readily identified radiographically or clinically.

Pathologic Features

Grossly, ossifying fibroma of the conventional variety will be a dense spherical mass that is composed of fibrous tissue and bone. Histologically, ossifying fibromas of odontogenic origin will be composed of two readily identifiable components: 1) a fibrous stroma and 2) bone that demonstrates varying degrees of maturation. The tumor stroma can range from loosely aggregated primitive fibrous connective tissue that is rich in fibroblasts, to mature dense collagen. Within this collagenous matrix, bony ossicles, bone trabecula, and immature osteoid or mature bone can be identified (Figures 16.44 & 16.45). These calcified aggregates will often coalesce or anastomose and frequently they will take on a cementicle-like appearance similar to the type of cementicles that can routinely be observed in the periodontal ligament. Woven and lamellar bone aggregates will be quite common throughout the tumor stroma. These bony aggregates can be marginated by either osteoblasts or osteoclasts. (Figure 16.46)

From a differential diagnostic standpoint, ossifying fibroma of odontogenic origin can be difficult to separate from FD. Although such separation can be problematic histologically, the presence of a normal bony cortex or remnants thereof, (Figure 16.47) and the presence of rounded calcified ossicles within the tumor stroma, tends to favor a diagnosis of ossifying fibroma.

Differential Diagnosis

Ossifying fibroma of odontogenic origin is generally a lesion that can be shelled out or easily enucleated or curetted. Unlike

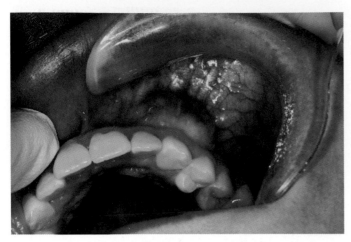

Figure 16.48 Juvenile ossifying fibroma presenting as a nodular maxillary expression. (courtesy of Dr. John Hildebrant).

FD, ossifying fibroma of odontogenic origin will typically have a nodular rather than an elliptical growth pattern. The ossifying fibroma of odontogenic origin also is a tumor that predominantly affects adults rather than children, whereas FD is largely a lesion of childhood. Conventional ossifying fibroma should be distinguished from focal cemento-osseous dysplasia (condensing osteitis) of the jaws with which it can be confused clinically and histologically. While conventional ossifying fibroma will typically show no attachment relationship to, or directly abut the apex of any involved teeth, focal cemento-osseous dysplasia will show such a relationship, with the root or roots of teeth involved of teeth in 85 percent of cases. In addition, nearly all patients with focal cemento-osseous dysplasia will be asymptomatic. Finally, focal cemento-osseous dysplasia shows a peak incidence in the fourth or fifth decades of life, presenting a decade later than most patients who have conventional ossifying fibroma.[196]

Treatment and Prognosis

The vast majority of conventional ossifying fibromas are treated by surgical excision that is conservative in nature. Typically such surgery will involve curettage and eburnation of the surrounding bone. In the studies of Traiantafillidou et al.[194] in which 14 conventional ossifying fibromas in pediatric age group patients were managed, curettage was the initial treatment of choice. Only one patient in that study required subsequent partial maxillectomy, and all patients were free of disease as long as 17 years after their initial surgery.

Juvenile Ossifying Fibroma

Juvenile ossifying fibroma is a unique type of ossifying fibroma that can be separated into two distinct clinicopathologic subtypes, *trabecular* and *psammomatoid*. The trabecular juvenile ossifying fibromas will present as nodular expansile lesion that will predominantly affect the jaws (Figure 16.48), whereas psammomatoid juvenile ossifying fibromas are largely expansile lesions that affect the frontal, ethmoid and periorbital bones.[197,198,199]

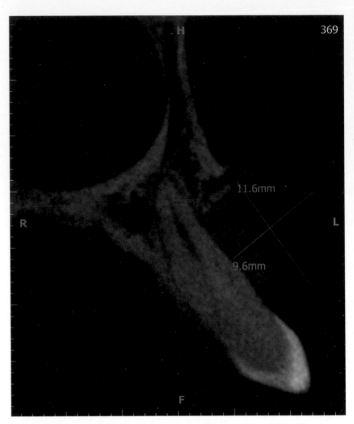

Figure 16.49 CT scan showing encapsulated trabecular ossifying fibroma.

Trabecular Juvenile Ossifying Fibroma

Most patients with juvenile ossifying fibroma of the trabecular variety are under the age of 15 years when diagnosed, however patients can range in age from 3 months to 72 years.[197,198,199,200,201] Males outnumber females with the trabecular form of the disorder and trabecular lesions tend to occur in the maxilla somewhat more frequently than the mandible. Trabecular ossifying fibromas can occur in extragnathic sites, however occurrence in those sites is quite rare.[199,200,201,202]

On radiographic examination trabecular juvenile ossifying fibromas tend to be expansile lesions that can have either a radiolucent, (Figure 16.49) ground-glass or totally radiopaque appearance. The rapidity of the tumor's growth will often result in perforation of the cortex or at least thinning of the surrounding cortical bone. The tumor can also more rarely have a honeycombed or multilocular radiographic appearance.

Pathologic Features

The trabecular juvenile ossifying fibroma will consist grossly of a spherical bony mass that is marginated by a connective tissue capsule (Figure 16.50). Histologically, the tumor will be composed of a stroma composed of loosely arranged immature collagen that will show a significant proliferation of spindle cell fibroblast or polyhedral cells. Ramifying throughout this collagen matrix, there will be aggregates of poorly mineralized bone, cellular osteoid, osteoid strands and occasionally cementicle particles (Figure 16.51). Aggregates of osteoclast-like giant

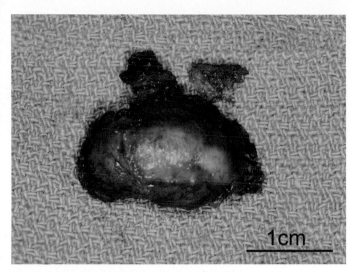

Figure 16.50 Gross specimen. Juvenile ossifying fibroma, trabecular variant. The tumor is marginated by a collagenous capsule.

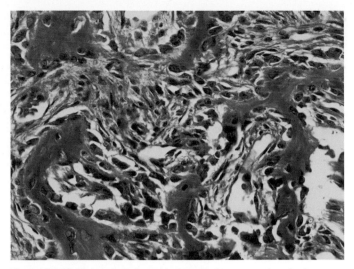

Figure 16.52 High power photomicrograph of osseous trabeculae in a trabecular ossifying fibroma. Note the cell rich stroma and occasional osteoclasts.

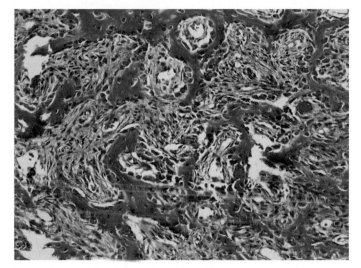

Figure 16.51 Trabecular juvenile ossifying fibroma composed of osseous trabeculae that are immature, and set in a spindle cell proliferation of fibroblasts.

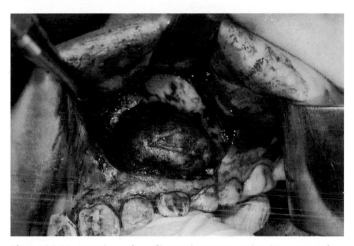

Figure 16.53 Juvenile ossifying fibroma being resected with a margin of normal bone.

cells will be common to the tumor as well (Figure 16.52). Mitotic activity is typically minimal, but may indeed be present. The coexistence of ABCs or CGCGs with trabecular juvenile ossifying fibromas has been reported.[202]

Treatment and Prognosis

The initial treatment of choice for trabecular juvenile ossifying fibroma, a lesion that is often a recurrent one, is complete surgical excision (Figure 16.53). Slootweg et al.[9] reported a recurrence rate of 30 percent in 33 patients they studied. All of the recurrent cases that were then followed up by that investigative team, were cured by means other than radical surgical excision. However, Chang et al.[203] as well as Guriel et al.[204] report that that more than 30 trabecular juvenile ossifying fibromas they encountered, showed an aggressive biologic behavior that required radical surgical excision.

Psammomatoid Juvenile Ossifying Fibroma

Psammomatoid juvenile ossifying fibroma is a rare entity that most often affects extragnathic bones of the craniofacial skeleton. The maxilla and mandible are thus rarely affected. The bones that are most often involved include the frontal ethmoid, and periorbital bones. First described by Gogl et al.[205] the psammomatoid variant of ossifying fibroma was initially identified in the nose and the paranasal sinuses. The tumor has often been confused with the far more common central osseous ossifying fibromas of the gnathic region, and it has therefore been difficult for some authorities to accept that the lesion represents a true and separate entity. Johnson et al.[200] originally reported the lesion as "juvenile active ossifying fibroma," in light of its biological aggressiveness and unique histopathology.

Psammomatoid juvenile ossifying fibromas are tumors that most often affect children and adolescents; however, affected

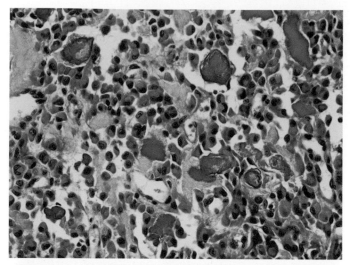

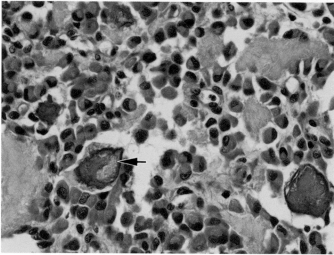

Figures 16.54 (top) & 16.55 (bottom) Medium and high power photomicrographs of a psammomatoid juvenile ossifying fibroma composed of relatively uniform small ossicle-like (psammomatoid bodies) (arrow) and an immature bone matrix.

individuals tend to be somewhat older than those with the trabecular form of the tumor. Psammomatoid lesions tend to have an aggressive biologic behavior and a high recurrent rate.

Radiographically psammatoid lesions are characterized by bony expansion that may cause nasal obstruction, tosis and even blindness. The vast majority of tumors will present as well defined and well demarcated round lesion that may show a central area of osseous sclerosis or a central ground glass appearance. As with the trabecular form of the tumor, psammomatoid juvenile ossifying fibromas can be multilocular.[200] Lesions tend to be well circumscribed masses when they present on CT scans and they will typically show an area of radiodensity that is marginated by a thick capsule of bone.

Pathologic Features

The psammomatoid juvenile ossifying fibroma will be characterized histopathologically by a proliferation of ossicles or psammomatoid bodies that are set in a richly vascularized, highly proliferative fibroblastic stroma. Psammomatoid bodies within the tumor tend to be round to sometimes trabecular and they are most often basophilic (Figures 16.54 & 16.55). The psammomatoid bodies will often take on a so-called cementicle-like pattern, however the lesions arise in sites where teeth do not develop and therefore these psammomatoid aggregates are clearly not of odontogenic origin. The tumors are often marginated by a peripheral capsule of bone that shows significant osteoblastic and osteoclastic activity. Psammomatoid juvenile ossifying fibromas, like the trabecular form of the tumor, have been reported to occur in association with ABCs and giant cell granulomas.

From a differential diagnostic standpoint, the psammomatoid and trabecular ossifying fibroma can be separated from one another on the basis of their site of anatomic presentation. Genetic assessments of trabecular and psammomatoid juvenile ossifying fibromas have shown that the psammomatoid tumor variant will demonstrate chromosomal void points that are non-random at the Xq26 and 2q33 chromosomal break points.[206] Dal Cin et al. have reported 2q31-32, q35-36 deletions in the conventional form ossifying fibroma of odontogenic origin.[207] These genetic findings can prove helpful in separating the three common forms of ossifying fibroma from one another.

Treatment and Prognosis

Psammomatoid juvenile ossifying fibromas are treated by complete surgical excision. Recurrence rates for the tumor are reported to be in the 30 to 58 percent range.[194] Although multiple recurrences are common for both the trabecular and psammomatoid types of juvenile ossifying fibroma, neither tumor type has shown a tendency to undergo malignant transformation.

Central Giant Cell Granuloma (Central Giant Cell Tumor)

Since its initial identification, CGCG has been known by a host of names including giant cell reparative granuloma, giant cell lesion of bone and giant cell tumor of bone. WHO prefers the term CGCG to describe this benign rarely aggressive idiopathic central osseous lesion of bone that occurs almost exclusively in the jaws.[208] We will use the term CGCG throughout this discussion with the caveat that the term granuloma is not used in its strictest sense, and with the knowledge that the term "central giant cell granuloma" is so engrained in the world's literature that continued usage is appropriate.

The CGCG accounts for approximately 7 percent of all benign tumors of the jaws.[209] Tumors occur predominantly in the first three decades of life, although Kruse-Losler et al.[210] report that nearly 77 percent of the lesions they identified in a series of 26 cases, occurred in patients younger than 30 years of age, and 50 percent occurred in patients between the ages of 1 and 11. This finding is consistent with most reports in the

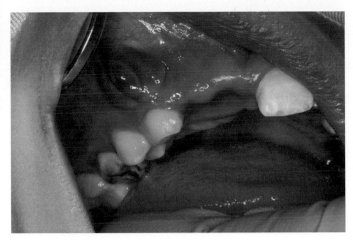

Figure 16.56 Localized soft tissue and bony expansion of the anterior maxilla in a child with a CGCG. (Courtesy of Dr. Thomas Borris).

literature which indicate that approximately one-half of all CGCGs that are identified are seen in patients less than 19 years of age.

CGCG shows a significant female preponderance, with approximately two thirds of all cases affecting females. Lesions occur more frequently in the mandible than the maxilla and CGCGs tend to be unifocal as opposed to multifocal. Tumors are generally confined to the tooth bearing areas of the jaws and can present as expansile, cortex thinning unilocular or multilocular lesions. Tumors will often appear to have a blue hue clinically due to their rich vascularity (Figure 16.56). The anterior mandible is the favorite site of presentation.

CGCGs are tumors that are characterized by cells that have an osteoclastic phenotype,[211] and although the jawbones are most frequently affected, tumors are not exclusive to the jaws and may involve the sphenoid and temporal bones with some frequency. Although most tumors are typically well defined and generally do not show invasion through the bony cortex, rapidly growing biologically aggressive tumors have been reported.

MRI imaging of a giant cell granuloma will generally show a lesion that is hypointense on both T1 and T2 weighted images. Plain film radiographs will demonstrate a well marginated unilocular or multilocular radiolucent lesion (Figure 16.57), while CT scans will typically show bony expansion with remodeling of adjacent bone and associated lytic bone destruction.

Pathologic Features

Giant cell granulomas tend to have a relatively characteristic and clastic gross and microscopic histopathology. Grossly, the tumors are typically composed of aggregates of granular, gritty highly hemorrhagic soft tissue (Figure 16.58).

Histologically, tumors tend to be unencapsulated masses that will be composed of aggregates of multinucleated osteoclast like giant cells that are set in a stroma that is well vascularized. Stromal cells generally consist of: 1) osteoclast-

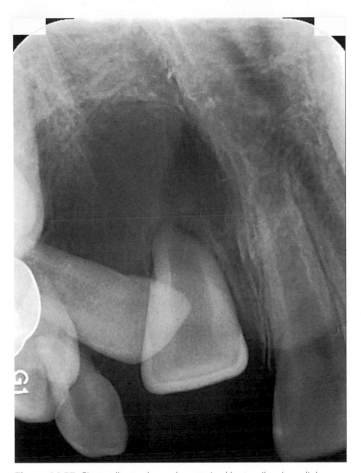

Figure 16.57 Giant cell granuloma characterized by a unilocular radiolucency of the anterior maxilla. (Courtesy of Dr. Thomas Borris).

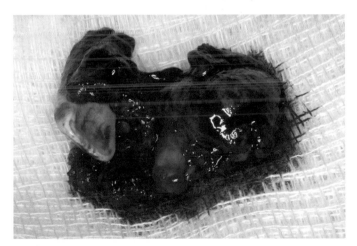

Figure 16.58 Gross surgical specimen of CGCG. Note the bulbous hemorrhagic nature of the tumor as it surrounds maxillary anterior teeth. (Courtesy of Dr. Thomas Borris).

like giant cells that are of macrophage origin, which may present as individual cells or be arranged in clusters around small capillaries; and 2) fibroblast-like cells that tend to be elongated and spindle shaped (Figures 16.59 & 16.60). The giant cells that are identified in the CGCG are identical to

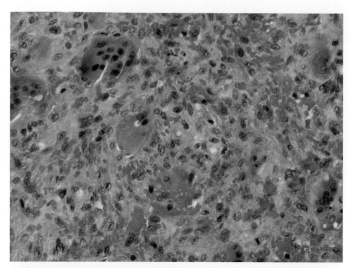

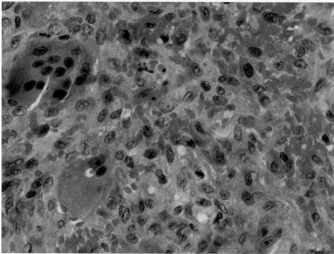

Figures 16.59 (top) & 16.60 (bottom) Characteristic histopathology of a CGCG, showing hemorrhagic stromal elements and multinucleated giant cells, in these intermediate and high power photomicrographs.

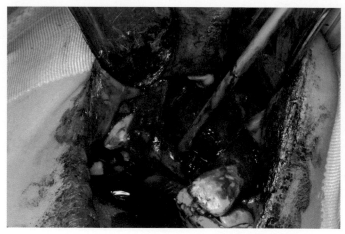

Figure 16.61 Remaining bony defect after enucleation of a giant cell granuloma in a child. (Courtesy of Dr. Thomas Borris).

those seen in Cherubism, foreign body giant cell reactions, the brown tumor of hyperparathyroidism and ABCs.[212]

Giant cell granulomas, will frequently demonstrate areas of hemorrhage, hemosideron pigment and fibrosis. Multinucleated giant cells will typically be strongly immunoreactive for CD68, which suggests a histiocytic or macrophage origin for the tumor. No specific molecular pathogenesis for the CGCG has been identified; however, Ardekian et al. have demonstrated a novel *NFI* splice mutation that results in deletion of the GTPase-activating domain of neurofibromin in CGCG. This finding however, has only been found in patients with CGCG and neurofibromatosis.[213] Heterozygous and homozygous mutations in the calcium sensing receptor (CARS) gene have also been identified in giant cell granulomas as well as in primary hyperparathyroidism.[214]

Attempts have been made to distinguish between histologically aggressive and non-aggressive forms of CGCG using Ki67 stains. It appears that Ki67 expression is similar in both

biologic variants of the disease and its expression does not lead to any meaningful distinction between aggressive and non-aggressive tumors.

Assessment of p53 protein reactivity also does not allow one to discriminate between those tumors that may be aggressive and those that will not. Finally, some investigators have suggested that the over secretion of RANKL, a receptor activator of nuclear factor B ligand, may be responsible for channeling the aggressiveness of CGCGs.[215]

Increased expression of *WWOX* messenger RNA transcriptional levels in giant cell lesions of the jaws has been reported in non-aggressive giant cell granulomas of the jaws using both quantitative reverse transcription PCR and immunohistochemical analysis.[216] Similar findings have been observed in peripheral giant cell granulomas and in Cherubism. Interestingly, WWOX protein has been detected exclusively in the cytoplasm of the multinucleated giant cells of giant cell lesions of the jaws.[216]

Treatment and Prognosis

CGCGs of the jaw are most often treated by curettage with aggressive eburnation of the surrounding bone. (Figure 16.61) Recurrence rates range from 10 to 33 percent and secondary curettage, after the initial therapy, is often required to fully eradicate a lesion. En-bloc resection is sometimes necessary to eradicate CGCGs. When employed, the bony tumor margin should be 1 cm from the margins of the central bony lesional defect. Non-surgical alternatives to therapy include the use of intra lesional cortical steroid injection, treatment with antiangiogenic interferon alpha and subcutaneous calcitonin injection.[217,218,219]

"True" Giant Cell Tumor of Bone

True giant cell tumors of bone are as a distinct rarity in children as well as in adults. When the jaws are involved, the majority of true giant cell tumors are associated with Paget's disease. Most individuals with true giant cell tumors of the jaws and skeletal bones will be older than 50 years of age and there is a slight female predilection for the tumor. In contra distinction to the far more common CGCG, the jawbones are rarely involved by true giant cell tumors, and most true giant cell tumors of bone affect the frontal, temporal and occipital bones when they occur in the head and neck region. Rarely, tumors can also involve the thyroid cartilage.[220] Most tumors, regardless of site, will present as poorly delineated radiolucencies, or on occasion as a soft tissue mass.

Histopathologically, the true giant cell tumor of bone will be composed of multinucleated giant cells set in a spindle cell stroma similar to that seen in a CGCG. Tumors may have a prominent fibroblastic stroma, a feature that can occasionally help to distinguish the true giant cell tumor of bone from CGCG. Mitotic figures are more common in true giant cell tumors of bone than in CGCGs. Large vascular spaces that are sinusoidal in nature are also a more common component of true giant cell tumors of bone than CGCGs of bone. Necrosis tends to be a feature of true central giant cell tumors of bone more often than with CGCGs.[221]

However, the aforementioned histologic features are not absolutes, and in many instances true giant cell tumors will show no distinctive histology that is in anyway different from that of a CGCG. True giant cell tumors of bone must in the end be distinguished on a clinicopathologic basis from CGCG, brown tumor of hyperparathyroidism, Cherubism and foreign body giant cell granulomas.

Treatment and Prognosis

Most true central giant cell tumors of bone will affect the bones of the skull and most tumors will tend to behave as aggressive lesions biologically. Tumors are most often treated by surgical excision with post-operative radiation therapy. Malignant transformation has been reported but is quite rare.

Aneurysmal Bone Cyst

The ABC is a lesion that typically involves the long bones or vertebra. The ABC tends to occur in individuals who are younger than 20 years of age and an approximately 2 percent of all ABCs will present in the head and neck region, with the mandible being the most commonly affected site.[222] The temporal bone, the occipital bones, the frontal bone and the orbital bones represent the most common extragnathic sites. Craniofacial ABCs will typically have two clinicopathologic presentations. They will present as a primary, solitary and distinctive pathologic process; or occur in association with other benign and malignant conditions including, CGCGs, ossifying fibroma, chondroblastoma, osteoblastoma and osteosarcoma.[223,224] Many investigators consider the ABC to be simply a CGCG with large blood filled vascular spaces.

Most ABCs will present radiographically as slowly growing, unilocular or multilocular cystic appearing lesions. In contrast to CGCG, a large number of ABCs will be associated with pain or swelling. Biologically aggressive lesions in the head and neck region often occur as cortex rupturing or

blow-out lesions. Depending on the site of occurrence, such lesions can cause blurred vision, blindness, paresthesia or numbness.

Pathologic Features

Most ABCs will present grossly as granular, gritty or hemorrhagic lesions that frequently have a sac-like honeycomb appearance. ABCs can range from spongy to quite firm.

Microscopically, ABCs are typically composed of aggregates of spindle cells, multinucleated giant cells, hemorrhage and numerous large sinusoidal spaces (Figures 16.61.1, 16.61.2 & 16.61.3). The cystic spaces are often separated by bony or collagenous septae. Tumors will frequently contain an abundance of reactive or woven bone, along with areas of calcification and occasionally zones of chondroid metaplasia. The most significant microscopic features of the ABC that allow its separation for CGCG will be the presence of large sinusoidal spaces filled with red cells, and the septal-like histopathology of the ABC. Although giant cell granulomas can on occasion display the same histopathologic features, the large sinusoidal spaces that are seen in ABCs tend to lack smooth muscle or elastic fibers, which will be common to the blood vessels of the CGCG.

ABCs have a somewhat more destructive biologic behavior than CGCGs and the genetics of the ABC have been linked to a t(16;17)(q22;p13) chromosomal tranlocation in tumors.[225] Yet Pringle et al.[226] have demonstrated that ABCs have an oncogene translocation of TRE17/USP6, which regulates TRE17 and which is necessary for GTPase binding.[226] This oncogenic alteration may also be responsible for the biologic aggressiveness of these lesions.

Treatment and Prognosis

Most ABCs are treated by aggressive curettage regardless of their site of origin. ABCs of the jaws have a recurrence rate of approximately 19 percent.[227] One of the factors that lead to their recurrence is incomplete removal of the lesion initially. Some investigators[228] have suggested that increased numbers of mitoses in an ABC can be a predictor of that tumors recurrence probability. Malignant transformation of ABCs has been reported, but such transformation is rare.[229,230]

Hyperparathyroidism

Primary hyperparathyroidism is a common endocrinopathy that is most often associated with a parathyroid adenoma. Characterized by multinucleated giant cell aggregates histologically, and caused by oversecretion of parathyroid hormone, the disorder can result in a hypercalcemia that causes radiolucent osteolytic defects of bone known as "brown tumors."[231,232,233,234,235,236] Brown tumors of hyperparathyroidism are exceedingly rare in children. When tumors involve the craniofacial skeleton the most common sites are the temporal bone, the nasal cavity and the paranasal sinuses. Radiographically lesions will present as multilocular radiolucencies

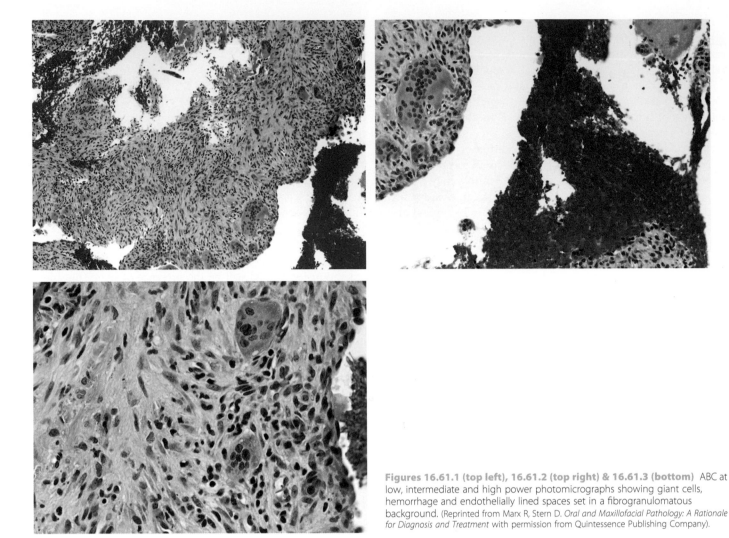

Figures 16.61.1 (top left), 16.61.2 (top right) & 16.61.3 (bottom) ABC at low, intermediate and high power photomicrographs showing giant cells, hemorrhage and endothelially lined spaces set in a fibrogranulomatous background. (Reprinted from Marx R, Stern D. *Oral and Maxillofacial Pathology: A Rationale for Diagnosis and Treatment* with permission from Quintessence Publishing Company).

of the jaw and can thus mimic an ABC, CGCG or Cherubism. Treatment for a brown tumor of hyperparathyroidism usually involves removal of the causative parathyroid adenoma or parathyroid carcinoma and appropriate therapy for the metabolic bone disease.

Cherubism

Clinical Features

Cherubism is an autosomal dominant genetic disease with a variable phenotypic expression.[237] The disorder occurs as a result of normal mandibular and maxillary bone being replaced by a fibrovascular stroma containing giant cells. Cherubism will involve only the embryologic maxilla and mandible. The condyle is always spared, as the condyle develops from a separate primordial focus, independent from Meckle's cartilage. The orbital floor and middle turbinate are involved in severe cases of Cherubism since they represent portions of the maxilla. Forty percent of Cherubism cases are sporadic, and the parents of affected individuals may not

necessarily have a history of the disease. The disorder is caused by presumed gain of function mutations in the SH3BP2 gene transcript.[238]

Children first develop signs of Cherubism between 2.5 and 5 years of age and thereafter more rapidly develop the full genetic expression of the disease, a painless expansion of the mandible and sometimes the maxilla with associated multilocular radiolucencies. In severe cases, mouth breathing occurs which can lead to an open bite.

After complete development of the disorder, clinicians may recognize three levels of disease expression,[239] typically classified as types I, II or III Cherubism. Type I Cherubism, which will involve only the rami of the mandible bilaterally, may go unnoticed. In fact, individuals with type I disease are often described as simply having chubby cheeks, until a panoramic or cone beam CT scan is taken that demonstrates radiolucencies in each ramus.

Type II Cherubism is well recognized clinically because of its greater expansion of, and extension within, the mandible as far anteriorly as the mental foramen. The maxilla will also be

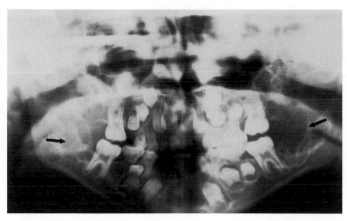

Figure 16.62 Type III Cherubism demonstrating multilocular symmetric expansion of the mandible, and all components of the maxilla with sparring of the condyles. (Reprinted from Marx R, Stern D. *Oral and Maxillofacial Pathology: A Rationale for Diagnosis and Treatment* with permission from Quintessence Publishing Company).

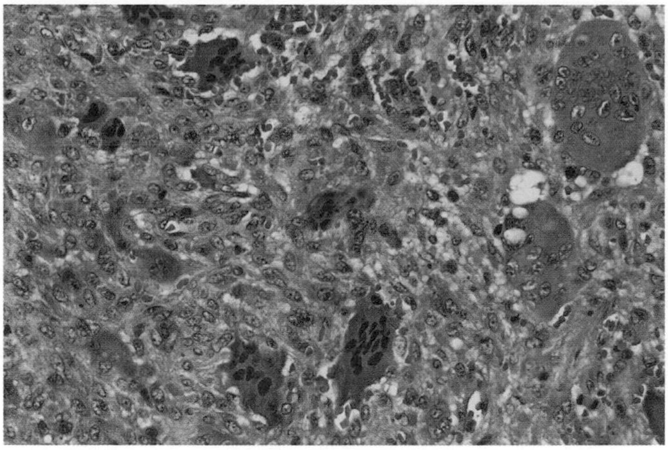

Figure 16.63 Cherubism characterized by foreign body type giant cell aggregates set in a richly vascularized fibrous stroma.

involved in type II disease, but only in the molar areas. This maxillary and mandibular involvement adds to a more noticeable clinical expansion.

Type III Cherubism will involve the entire mandible, crossing the midline and sparing each condyle. The entire maxilla will be involved as well in type III disease, including the orbital floor and middle turbinate, and the bony expansion will be greater than that seen in Type II Cherubism. Involvement of the orbital floors will cause the globes to turn upward, resulting in an excessive scleral show that gives the eyes the appearance of looking toward the heavens. Hence the name Cherubism, which was originally applied to the disease process as a comparative reference to the paintings of renaissance art in which Cherubs consistently "looked toward the heavens."

Radiographs of a child with Cherubism will show a symmetrical expansile multilocular involvement of the mandible and/or maxilla depending on the type of Cherubism (I, II or III) (Figure 16.62). In all individuals with the disorder, the condyle and upper condylar neck will appear normal. Multiple unerupted teeth and agenesis of teeth are frequently noted radiographically.

Expansile multilocular radiolucent lesions of the mandible and maxilla may be seen in several syndromes that can mimic Cherubism, including Noonan's syndrome, Jaffe–Campanacci syndrome, and Ramon syndrome. Additionally, Langerhan cell histiocytosis, rare primary hyperparathyroidism in a child, and the multiple odontogenic keratocysts than can be part of the basal cell nevus syndrome can all resemble Cherubism radiographically.

A family history and a thorough clinical examination, coupled with detailed radiographic assessment or CT scans are all that is usually necessary to diagnose Cherubism. No laboratory test is diagnostic of the disorder, except for expert genetic testing which is usually unnecessary to confirm the disorder.

Pathologic Features

Typically, the surgical specimen from an individual with Cherubism will consist of friable mottled red-brown, sometimes gritty tissue that on cut section may show a whorled or lobulated pattern. Microscopically, the appearance will be that of an admixture of loosely arranged fibrous connective tissue, multinucleate giant cells and occasional fragments of poorly mineralized bone. Giant cells of the type seen in giant cell granulomas are a predominant feature of the process (Figure 16.63). Thin-walled vessels are often prominent throughout the supporting lesional stroma, and in many cases, giant cells tend to aggregate around small vascular spaces. Hemosiderin may also be prominent within the tumor. When the lesions are mature, the histologic features are often those of mature interlacing collagen fascicles, with only scant giant cells.

Several lesions can appear histologically identical to Cherubism, including CGCG, the giant cell lesions seen in Noonan's syndrome which is sometimes linked to Cherubism and the brown tumor of hyperparathyroidism. Thorough patient histories and adequate clinical work-up are absolutely mandatory if one is to distinguish these lesions from the other. When an appropriate familial history is demonstrable, in concert with the classic disease histopathology, a diagnosis of Cherubism can usually be established.

Treatment and Prognosis

Cherubism is not a curable disease. The natural course of the disease is one of gradual enlargement of the jaws that continues to puberty and then subsides. The clinician should therefore resist the urge to resect bone. Osseous contouring, if necessary, is best accomplished after there is evidence of growth cessation or in the later teenage years. Osseous contouring accomplished at this age can be expected to retain the bony reduction obtained.[240] If accomplished earlier, however, while the Cherubism is still active, the expansion will redevelop within 12 to 18 months. When employed, any osseous contour procedure may result in significant blood loss. Although the vasculature in cherubic bone is not under arterial pressure, an oozing type of blood loss over a large surface area will occur at

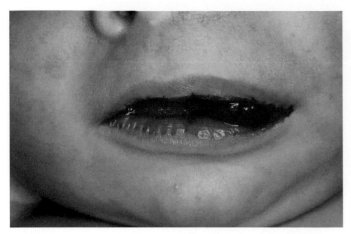

Figure 16.64 MNTI presenting as a hemorrhagic anterior maxillary mass. (Reproduced with permission from Cambridge University Press).

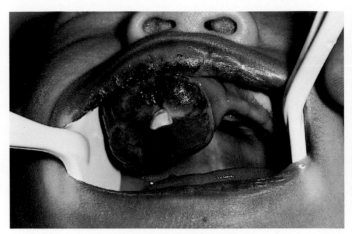

Figure 16.65 A second nodular hemorrhagic MNTI with a central incisor tooth erupting from the tumor mass. (Reprinted from Marx R, Stern D. *Oral and Maxillofacial Pathology: A Rationale for Diagnosis and Treatment* with permission from Quintessence Publishing Company).

surgery. Therefore, the surgeon must prepare for possible transfusions and have local hemostatic measures such as Surgicel®, Gelfoam® or Avitene® available and prepared.

Most individuals with Cherubism will have their Cherubism cease to grow at approximately 15 years of age and from there on undergo a gradual involution of the expansion, leaving unerupted teeth and radiolucencies as an aftermath.[241]

The prognosis for an individual with Cherubism is good, but will often necessitate prosthodontic replacement of teeth subsequent to disease resolution. Dental implants remain a treatment option, but residual pockets of Cherubic bone often mandate their removal and local grafting to prepare the involved site to receive an implant.

Genetic counseling is recommended for teenage patients, who must realize that even if they have a sporadic form of the disease, they now will pass on the Cherubic inheritance to 75 percent of their own offspring.

Rare Childhood Tumors of Bone

Melanotic Neuroectodermal Tumor of Infancy (MNTI)

MNTI is a rare pigmented osteolytic neoplasm that will most often involve the jaws of newborn infants. Although 90 percent of all lesions occur in the head and neck region, other rare sites including the epididymis, femur, skin, mediastinum and brain can be affected. First described in 1918 by Krompecher,[241] the tumor is thought to be of neural crest origin. Most tumors will present clinically as an anterior maxillary or premaxillary mass (Figure 16.64 & 16.65) with a subjacent radiolucency in infants younger than one year of age. Tumors occur in males and females in a ratio that is nearly equal.[242]

Occasionally teeth will be entrapped within the tumor (Figure 16.66) and they will float freely in space in a radiographic matter similar to that seen in Langerhan's cell histiocytosis. Tumors can also resemble neuroblastoma and retinoblastoma radiographically.[242,243,244] Most tumors will range in size from 2 to 4 cm in diameter and they may contain

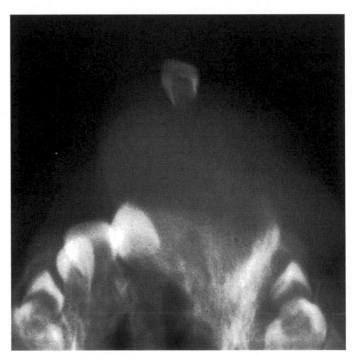

Figure 16.66 MNTI with irregular bony margins. The tumor has displaced adjacent teeth laterally and a central incisor inferiorly. (Reprinted from Marx R, Stern D. *Oral and Maxillofacial Pathology: A Rationale for Diagnosis and Treatment* with permission from Quintessence Publishing Company).

calcifications, although tumors can appear totally radiolucent without any associated calcifications or tooth entrapment. Occlusal radiographic films can be quite helpful in demonstrating calcifications within the tumor. Patients with a MNTI will frequently show elevated urinary vanilmandelic acid levels as well as serum alpha fetoprotein elevation.[245]

Pathologic Features

The melanotic neuroectodermal tumor will separate quite readily from surrounding bone, but is typically however, only partially encapsulated. On cut section, the tumor will usually

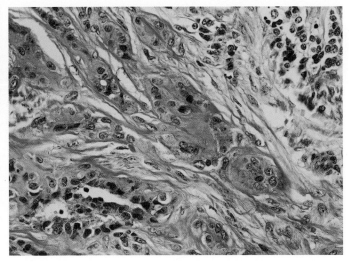

Figure 16.67 Biphasic melanotic neuroectodermal tumor composed of large polygonal pigmented cells and small non-pigmented cells that resemble lymphocytes.

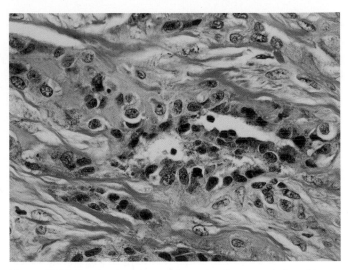

Figure 16.68 The alveolar pattern of the melanotic neuroectodermal tumor cells can be seen prominently in this high power photomicrograph.

present as a firm, lobular or multilobular, glistening, gray to white mass that may have speckles or streaks of black pigmented material distributed throughout it. Entrapped tooth buds may also be seen within the tumor mass. The lesion can also present as a multilobular or nodular mass and not as a single tumor mass.

Histologic examination of the tumor will reveal a biphasic neoplasm that is composed of large polygonal pigmented cells and smaller non-pigmented cells (Figure 16.67). The larger cells will tend to be arranged in sheets, or appear at the margins of smaller cells that are lymphocytic or neuroblastic in appearance. The tumor's smaller cells will tend to fill alveolar spaces, and the smaller cells will have dark staining nuclei and minimal cytoplasm. The tumor's larger cuboidal pigmented cells will contain pigmented or melanotic granules whereas smaller non-pigmented cells will not (Figure 16.68). Occasional spindle-shaped pigmented cells can be seen within the tumor as well.

Target polygonal tumor cells will generally stain positively for HMB-45, keratin and neuron specific enolase. Tumors will also be S-100 protein negative, CD99, and desmin positive. Differential diagnoses should include other small round blue cell tumors including rhabdomyosarcoma, neuroblastoma, and lymphoma. Cytogenetic studies of the melanotic neuroectodermal tumor have demonstrated an amplification of the MYCN gene and a 1p deletion along with t(11;22) (q24;q12) and t(11;22) (13p;q12) translocations.[246]

Treatment and Prognosis

Conservative surgical excision with a 0.5 mm margin of normal bone is generally curative for the MNTI. Recurrences do occur however, and are reported to be in the 15 percent range.[247] Rare malignant variants have been documented;[248] however, some reported cases were likely neuroblastomas.

Neoplasms of Uncertain Histogenesis

Ewing Sarcoma/Peripheral Primitive Neuroectodermal Tumor

ES represents a component of a primitive neuroectodermal spectrum of exceedingly rare sarcomas (ES, atypical ES, peripheral primitive neuroectodermal tumor [pPNET]) that affect both bone and soft tissue. Although generally classified as a bone tumor, ES/PNET can occur in soft tissue alone. Ewing's sarcoma represents one end of a histopathologic continuum of disease in which a malignant neoplasm results from chromosomal translocation at chromosomes 11 and 22, at their respective q24 and q12 loci, resulting in a t(11;22) (q24:q12) translocation which fuses the ESs gene of chromosome 22 to the FLI1 gene of chromosome 11.[249]

This family of tumors accounts for approximately 8 percent of all pediatric cancers that are broadly in pediatric patients classified as non-rhabdomyosarcomatous soft tissue sarcomas (NRSTS).[250] Among this primitive neuroectodermal class of tumors, neuroblastoma and central nervous system small round cell tumors that include meduloblastoma are also commonly included. pPNET is often used to describe the entire class of small round, blue cell head and neck tumors.

It is often difficult to distinguish ES from members of the larger family of peripheral primitive neuroectodermal tumors, based purely on the histomorphology of a particular tumor. However, tumors can be generally distinguished individually based upon electron microscopic findings and immunohistochemical analysis. In a general sense, ES tends to demonstrate less neural phenotypic differentiation and will typically lack the neurotubules, neurofilaments and neurosecretory granules that are seen in PNET.[249,251,252,253]

ES/PNET will typically present in patients who are younger than 20 years of age. Eighty-five percent of tumors arise in bone, while 15 percent arise in deep soft tissues as extra skeletal

431

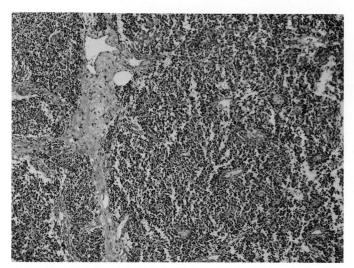

Figure 16.69 ES composed of sheets of small round blue cells.

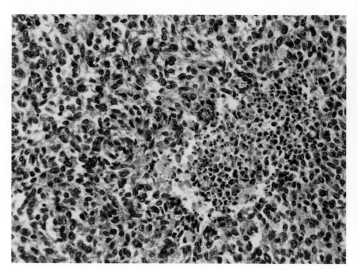

Figure 16.70 ES. Tumor cells display course chromatin, hyperchromatic nuclei and atypical mitoses. Note the central area of tumor cell necrosis.

lesions. As a rule, tumors that are composed of larger cells with prominent nucleoli are generally considered to be part of the Ewing spectrum of the disease, whereas tumors that are composed of smaller cells are considered to be within the pPNET spectrum of disease. While pPNETs seldom occur in the head and neck region and rarely involve bone, ES will more commonly affect the head and neck region, presenting as a tumor of bone that expands into soft tissue.[254] Substantively ES and pPNET differ only in their degree of morphological differentiation and the extent of their neuroectodermal phenotype.

ES/PNET is exceedingly rare in blacks, and males are more often affected than females. Patients with ES/PNET will often present with pain, fever and occasionally leukocytosis. Thus, when bone is primarily involved, patients are often initially thought to have an osteomyelitis that is suppurative in nature. As lesions grow and become more destructive of either soft tissue or bone they can resemble fibrosarcoma, neuroblastoma, Hodgkin lymphoma or metastatic carcinoma.

CT scans and radiographs of classic ES will most frequently show an ill-defined irregular destructive lesion involving bone, and in so-called classic cases of Ewing's sarcoma there will often be a periosteal deposition of bone that is in fact a proliferative periostitis. This periostitis which is often described radiographically as "onion skinning," generally involves the jaws, most often the mandible, but the pattern can also be seen in other craniofacial bones. The tumor can be destructive radiographically or produce the type of sunray radiologic pattern that is commonly identified in osteosarcoma of bone or chondrosarcoma of bone. On MRI imaging the tumor is often of low to intermediate signal intensity on T1 weighted images and high signal intensity on T2 weighted images. All-in-all, markedly diverse CT and MRI findings can be seen in patients with ES/PNET.

When tumors originate in soft tissue they often demonstrate an ill-defined soft tissue mass or lobular masses that spread aggressively into adjacent anatomic sites. Calcifications are rare findings in ES/PNETs and almost never reported in head and neck tumors. ES/PNETs will often show necrosis and therefore it can be difficult to obtain a representative biopsy specimen. ES/PNET is a tumor that foremost lends itself to cytogenetic testing, in order to be properly classified and diagnosed.

Pathologic Features

James Ewing first identified the tumor that is named after him, classifying it as an "endothelioma of bone." Microscopically he described the tumor as a small round cell neoplasm that even today favorably meets that histologic criterion.[255] Histopathologically, classic ES will tend to develop in bone and present as an undifferentiated tumor, whereas PNET tends to more frequently involve soft tissue and present histopathologically as a tumor with more phenotypically neuroendocrine features than ES. Seven various PNET (pPNET) histologic subtypes are recognized: 1) classic ES, 2) large cell ES, 3) PNET, 4) Adamanthonoma fibroma-like ES, 5) spindle cell sarcoma-like ES, 6) sclerosing and 7) vascular forms of ES.

Grossly ES/PNETs are polypoid lobular lesions that may appear ulcerative or hemorrhagic, especially those of soft tissue in origin. Lesions that arise primarily within bone will often have a gritty, granular consistently. Regardless of which end of the Ewing family of tumor's continuum the neoplasm develops along, all lesions will appear histologically to be small round blue cell neoplasms that will be made up of a lobular arrangement of uniform sheets of small to medium size round cells with sparse vacuolated cytoplasm (Figure16.69). Tumor cells are typically 2 to 3 times the size of lymphocytes. The chromatin of tumor cells will be coarse, the nucleoli quite small and necrosis common (Figure 16.70). Mitotic figures will be seen but tend not to be prominent, and a filigree pattern may be observed as tumor cells infiltrate through a supporting thin fibrous connective tissue stroma. Occasionally, so-called Homer-Wright or perivascular pseudo rosettes can be appreciated. Tumor cells can show a significant degree of pleomorphism and pleomorphic giant cells may be seen. Rich in glycogen, tumor cells will stain PAS positively. Most tumor cells will also express CD99 and vimentin. Neuron-specific enolace and synaptophysin will be expressed in a high percentage of tumors but not all tumors. FLI1 will be positive as well as caveolin1.

The gene fusion product EWS/FLI-1 can be identified using immunohistochemical methods, which is supportive of a human marrow mesenchymal stem cell as the tumor's cell of origin. The chromosomal translocations common to ES/pPNET, t(11;22) (q24;q12) or t(21;22) (q22;q12) can be readily identified using PCR or FISH in 85 percent of cases. Rare histologic variants of the ES/PNET in which the tumor cells can appear spindle-like, quite large and adenomatous, or sclerosing will all show similar cytogenetic findings. Therefore genetic assessment of any tumor suspected of being an ES/pPNET requires cytogenetic assessment in order to distinguish it from other rare malignant neoplasms.[256]

Differential microscopic diagnoses can include most of the small round cell neoplasms that can occur in the head and neck region of children including lymphoma, melanoma, olfactory neuroblastoma, rhabdomyosarcoma, pituitary adenoma and undifferentiated carcinoma. Since many of these lesions can also arise in both bone and soft tissue, accurate microscopic assessment can prove quite difficult. Lymphomas can be separated from the Ewing's family of tumors based upon a lymphoma panel of immunohistochemical stains. Olfactory neuroblastomas will tend to have a stromal background that is neurofibrillary. In addition, the olfactory neuroblastoma will be CD56 positive and typically CD99 negative. Melanoma will mark positively with S-100 protein and will

also be HMB-45 positive and melan-A positive. On occasion, mesenchymal chondrosarcomas can resemble the ES/PNET; however, that tumor will tend to show a proliferation of either S-100 protein positive chondroid or a malignant osteoid matrix.

Treatment and Prognosis

ES/PNET is treated with radiation therapy and combined chemotherapy. In those instances in which the tumor arises within bone, most commonly the jaw, tumors are initially treated by surgery that most often creates a continuity defect that will require subsequent reconstructive management. Tumor stage is one of the most important considerations for patients when dealing with an ES/PNET. Those patients who have disseminated disease at the time of presentation typically have a 30 percent survival rate, whereas patients who have no disseminated disease have a 65 percent survival rate after five years.[257] The single modality of treatment that has vastly improved disease free survival rate for ES/PNET has been the use of chemotherapy. High dose chemotherapy, including vincristine, adramycin, ifosfamide, cyclophosphamide and doxorubicin have enhanced survival significantly, pushing five-year survival rates to as high as 68 percent in patients undergoing such treatment regimens.[258,259] Lesions that are initially unresectable and lesions that show a poor response to chemotherapy will most often undergo a radiotherapy regimen.

Overall the Ewing's family of tumors have a relatively good prognosis if the disease has not metastasized at the time of initial diagnosis. Tumors with the least favorable prognosis include those in which there is a direct extension of the tumor mass into soft tissue, tumors that demonstrate aneuploidy and tumors that are multi focal.

References

Osteoma

1. Matsuzaka K, Shimono M, Uchiyama HN, et al. Lesions related to the formation of bone, cartilage, or cementum arising in the oral area: a statistical study and review of the literature. *Bull Tokyo Dent Coll*, 2002, 43: 173–180.

2. Larrea-Oyarbide N, Valmaseda-Castellon, Berini-Ayte's L. Osteomas of the craniofacial region: review of 106 cases. *J Oral Pathol Med*, 2008, 37: 38–42.

3. Samy LL, Mostafa H. Osteomata of the nose and paranasal sinuses with a report of 21 cases. *J Laryngol Otol*, 1971, 85: 449–469.

4. Smith ME, Calcaterra TC. Frontal sinus osteoma. *Ann Otol Rhinal laryngeal*, 1989, 98: 896–900.

5. Nielson GP, Rosenberg E. Update on bone forming tumors of the head and neck. *Head Neck Pathol*, 2007, 1: 87–93.

6. Halawi AM, Maley JE, Robinson RA, et al. Craniofacial osteoma: clinical presentation and patterns of growth. *Am J Rhinol Allergy*, 2013, 27: 120–133.

7. Earwaker J. Paranasal sinus osteomas. A review of 46 cases. *Skeletal Radiol*, 1993, 22: 417–423.

8. Kaplan I, Nicolaou Z, Hateul D, et al. Solitary central osteoma of the jaws. A diagnostic dilemma. *Oral Surg Oral Med Oral Pathol Oral Radiol Endodo*, 2008, 106: e22–e29.

9. Derniciaro E. Gardner's syndrome. *Dermatol Clin*, 1995, 13: 51–56.

10. McHugh JB, Mukherji SK, Lucas DR. Sino-orbital osteoma: a clinicopathological study of 45 surgically treated cases with emphasis on tumors with osteoblastic-like features. *Arch Pathol Lab Med*, 2009, 133: 1587–1593.

Osteoblastoma

11. BoKhari K, Hameed My, Ajmal M, et al. Benign osteoblastoma involving maxilla: a case report and review of the literature. *Case Reports in Dentistry*, 2012, doi 10.1155/2012/351241.

12. Alvares Capelozza AL, Giao Dezottl MS, Casati Alvares L, et al. Osteoblastoma of the mandible: systemic review of the literature and report of a case. *Dentomaxillofac Radiol*, 2005, 34: 1–8.

13. Loizaga JM, Calvo M, Lopez Barea F, et al. Osteoblastoma and osteoid osteoma. Clinical and morphological features of 162 cases. Pathol Red. *Pract*, 1993, 189: 33–41.

14. Jones AC, Prihoda TJ, Kacher JE, et al. Osteoblastoma of the maxilla and mandible: report of 24 cases, review of the literature and discussion of its relationship to osteoid osteoma of the

jaws. *Oral Surg, Oral Med, Oral Pathol, Oral Radiol Endod*, 2006, 102: 639–650.

15. Lucas DR, Unni KK, McLeod RA, et al. Osteoblastoma: Clinicopathologic study of 306 cases. *Human Pathol*, 1994, 25: 117–134.

16. Berry M, Mankin H, Gebhardt M, et al. Osteoblastoma: a 30 year study of 99 cases. *J Surg Oncology*, 2008, 98: 179–183.

17. Nielsen GP, Rosenberg AE. Update on bone forming tumors of the head and neck. *Head and Neck Pathology*, 2007, 1: 87–93.

18. Della Rocca C, Huvos AG. Osteoblasoma. Varied histological presentations with a benign clinical course. An analysis of 55 cases. *Am J Surg Pathol*, 1996, 20: 841–850.

19. Kiyohara H, Sawatsubashi M, Matsumoto N., et al. Benign Osteoblastoma of the ethmoid sinus. *Auris Nasus Larynx*, 2013, 40: 338–341.

20. Ahmed MS, Nwoky AL. Benign Osteoblastoma of the mandibular ramus. Review of the literature and report of a case. *J Oral Maxillofac Surg*, 2000, 58: 1310–1317.

21. Kulkarni MM, Shah AK, Ahire S. Aggressive Osteoblastoma of the mandible: a case report. *Int J Contemp Dent*, 2011, 2: 135–138.

22. Manjunatha BS, Sunit P, Amit, M, et al. Osteoblastoma of the jaws: a report of a case and review of the literature. *Clinics and Practice*, 2011, 118: 256–258.

23. Unni KK. *Dahlin's Bone Tumors: General Aspects and Data on 11,087 Cases*, Ed 5, Philadelphia, Lippincott-Raven, 1996.

24. Ohkubo T, Hernandez JC, Goya K, et al. "Aggressive" osteoblastoma of the maxilla. *Oral Surg, Oral Med, Oral Pathol, Oral Radiol, Endodo*, 1989, 68: 69–73.

25. Dal Cin P, Sciot R, Samson J, et al. Osteoid osteoma and osteoblastoma with clonal chromosome changes. *Br J Cancer*, 1994, 78: 344–348.

26. Mascarello JT, Krous HF, Carpenter DM. Unbalanced translocation resecting in the loss of the chromosome 17 short arm in osteoblastoma. *Cancer Genet Cytogenet*, 1993, 69: 65–67.

27. Bertoni F, Unni KK, Lucas DR, et al. Osteoblasoma with cartilagninous matrix an unusual morphologic

presentation in 18 cases. *Am J Surg Pathol*, 1993, 17: 69–74.

28. Ahmed MS, Nwoky AL. Benign osteoblastoma of the mandibular ramus. Review of the literature and report of a case. *J Oral Maxillofac Surg*, 2000, 58: 1310–1317.

Osteoid Osteoma

29. Nielsen GP, Rosenberg AE. Update on bone forming tumors of the head and neck. *Head and Neck Pathol*, 2007, 1: 87–93.

30. Zwimpfer JJ, Tucker WS, Faulkner JF. Osteoid osteoma of the cervical spine. Case reports and review of the literature. *Can J Surg*, 1982, 25: 637–641.

31. Pettine KA, Klassen RA. Osteoid-osteoma and osteoblastoma of the spine. *J Bone Joint Surg Am*, 1986, 68A: 354–361.

32. Frassica FJ, Waltarip RL, Sponseller PD, et al. Clinicopathologic features and treatment of osteoid osteoma and osteoblastoma in children and adolescents. *Orthop Clin North A*, 1996, 27: 559–574.

33. Gitelis S, Schajowiet F. Osteoid osteoma and osteoblastoma. *Orthop Clin North Am*, 1989, 20: 313–325.

34. Greenspan A. Benign bone-forming lesions: osteoma, osteoid osteoma, and osteoblastoma. Clinical imaging, pathologic and differential considerations. *Skeletal Radiol*, 1993, 22: 485–500.

35. Raskas DS, Graziano GP, Herzenberg FJ, et al. Osteoid osteoma and osteoblastoma of the spine. *J Spinal Disor*, 1992, 5: 204–211.

36. Scheine NJ, Malone M, Ashworth MA, Jacques TS. *Diagnostic Pediatric Surgical Pathology*. Churchill Livingstone, Elsevier, 2000, p. 231.

37. Gamba JL, Martinez S, Apple J, et al. Computed tomography of axial skeletal osteoid osteomas. *AJR Am Roent Genol*, 1984, 142: 769–772.

38. O'Connell JS, Nanthakumar SS, Nielsen GP, et al. Osteoid ostoma: the uniquely innervated bone tumor. *Mod Pathol*, 1998, 11: 175–180.

39. Rosenthal DI, Hornicek FJ, Wolfe MW, et al. Percutaneous radiofrequency coagulation of osteoid osteoma compared with operative treatment. *J Bone Joint Surg Am*, 1998, 80: 815–821.

Osteosarcoma

40. Nielsen GP, Rosenberg AE. Update on bone forming tumors of the head and neck. *Head and Neck Pathol*, 2007, 1: 87–93.

41. Garrington GE, Scofield HJ, Cornyn J, et al. Osteosarcoma of the jaws. Analysis of 56 cases. *Cancer*, 1967, 20: 377–391.

42. Saito Y, Miyajima C, Nakao K, et al. Highly malignant submandibular extra skeletal osteosarcoma in a young patient. *Auris Nasus Larynx*, 2008, 35: 576–578.

43. Jasnau S, Meyer U, Potratz J, et al. Craniofacial osteosarcoma: experience of the cooperative German-Austrain-Swiss osteosarcoma study group. *Oral Oncology*, 2008, 44: 286–294.

44. Huh WW, Holsinger FC, Levy A, et al. Osteosarcoma of the jaw in children and young adults. *Head and Neck*, 2012, 34: 981–984.

45. Kim HJ, McLawhorn AS, Boland PJ. Malignant osseous tumors of the pediatric spine. *J Am Acad Orthopedic Sufg*, 2012, 20: 646–656.

46. Salvati M, Ciappeta P, Raco A. Osteosarcoma of the skull. Clinical remarks on 19 cases. *Cancer*, 1993, 71: 2210–2216.

47. Lei YY, Vantassel P, Nauert C, et al. Craniofacial osteosarcomas plain film, CT and MRI findings in 46 cases. *AJR Am J Roentgerol*, 1988, 150: 1397–1402.

48. Bertoni F, Dallera P, Bacchini P, et al. The insituto Rizzoli-Beretta experience with osteosarcoma of the jaws. *Cancer*, 1991, 68: 1555–1563.

49. Clark JL, Unni KK, Dahlin DC, et al. Osteosarcoma of the jaw. *Cancer*, 1983, 51: 2311–2316.

50. Shives TC, Dahlin DC, Sim FH, et al. Osteosarcoma of the spine. *J Bone Joint Surg Am*, 1986, 86A: 660–668.

51. Barwick KW, Huvos AG, Smith J. Primary osteogenic sarcoma of the vertebral column: a clinicopathologic correlation of ten patients. *Cancer*, 1980, 46: 595–604.

52. Kebudi R, Ayan I, Darendelier F, et al. Primary osteosarcoma of the cervical spine. A pediatric case report and review of the literature. *Med Pediatr Oncol*, 1994, 23: 162–165.

Chondroma

53. Chan CW, Kung TM, Ma L. Telangietic osteosarcoma of the mandible. *Cancer*, 1986, 58: 2110–2115.

54. Giangaspero F, Stracca V, Visona A, et al. Small cell-osteosarcoma of the mandible. *Case report. Appl Pathol*, 1984, 2: 28–31.

55. Kurt AM, Unni K, McLeod RA, et al. Low grade intraosseous osteosarcoma. *Cancer*, 1990, 65: 1418–1438.

56. Garbe LR, Monges GM, Pellegrin FM, et al. Ultrastructural study of osteosarcomas. *Hum Pathol*, 1981, 12: 891–896.

57. Badawi-EL ZH, Muhammad EM, Noaman HH. Role of immunohistochemical cyclo-oxygenase-2 (COX-2) and osteocalcin in differentiating between osteoblastomas and osteosarcomas. *Mallays J Pathol*, 2012, 34: 15–23.

58. Araki N, Uchida A, Kimura T, et al. Involvement of the retroblastoma gene in primary osteosarcomas and other bone and soft tissue tumors. *Clin Orthop Relat Res*, 1991, 271–277.

59. Reissman PT, Simon MA, Lee WH, et al. Studies of the retinoblastoma gene in human sarcomas. *Oncogene*, 1989, 4: 839–843.

60. Wadayama B, Toguchida J, Shimizy T, et al. Mutation spectrum of the retroblastoma gene in osteosarcomas. *Cancer Res*, 1994, 54: 3042–3048.

61. Biegel JA, Womer BA, Emanuel BS. Complex karyotypes in a series of pediatric osteosarcomas. *Cancer Genet Cytogenet*, 1989, 38: 89–100.

62. vanDaniel M, Hulsebos TJ. Amplification and over expression of genes 17p 11.2-p1c in osteosarcoma. *Cancer Genet Cytogenet*, 2004, 153: 77–80.

63. Minio AJ. Periosteal osteosarcoma of the mandible. *Int J Oral Maxillofac Surg*, 1995, 24: 226–228.

64. Patterson A, Greer RO, Howard D. Periosteal osteosarcoma of the maxilla. A case report and review of literature. *J Oral Maxillofac Surg*, 1990, 48: 522–526.

65. Bridge JA, Nelson M, McComb F, et al. Cytogenetic findings in 73 osteosarcoma specimens and review of the literature. *Cancer Genet Cytogenet*, 1997, 95: 74–87.

66. Millar BG, Browne RM, Flood TR. Juxtacortical osteosarcomas of the jaws. *Br J Oral Maxillofac Surg*, 1990, 28: 73–79.

67. Kumar R, Moser P, Madewelll JF, et al. Parosteal osteosarcoma arising in cranial bones. Clinical and radiologic features in eight patients. *AJR Am J Roentgerol*, 1990, 155: 113–117.

68. Longhi A, Errani C, Pepaolis M, et al. Primary bone osteosarcoma in the pediatric age. State of the art. *Cancer Treat Rev*, 2006, 32: 423–436.

69. Daw, NC, Mahmoud HH, Meyer WH, et al. Bone sarcomas of the head and neck in children. The St. Jude Children's Research hospital Experience. *Cancer*, 2000, 88: 2172–2180.

70. Unni KK. Parosteal osteosarcoma. In Fletcher CDM, Unni KK, Mertens F (eds) *Pathology and Genetics of Tumours of Soft Tissue*. France, IARC Press, 2002, pp. 279–281.

71. Lee JS, Fetsch JF, Wasdhal DA, et al. A review of 40 patients with extra skeletal osteosarcoma. *Cancer*, 1995, 76: 2253–2259.

72. Rieske P, Bartkowiak JK, Szadowska AM, et al. A comparative study of p53/MDM2 genes alterations and p53/MDM2 proteins immunoreactivity in soft tissue sarcomas. *J Exp Clin Cancer Res*, 1999, 18: 403–416.

73. Kebudi R, Ayan I, Darendeliler E, et al. Primary osteosarcoma of the cervical spine. A pediatric case report and review of the literature. *Med Pediatr Oncol*, 1994, 23: 162–165.

74. Matsuzaka K, Shimono M, Uchiyama et al. Lesions related to the formation of bone, cartilage or cementum arising in the oral area: a statistical study and review of the literature. *Bull Tokyo Dent Coll*, 2002, 43: 173–180.

75. Huvos AG. *Bone Tumors. Diagnosis, Treatment and Prognosis*, Ed 1, Phildelphia, WB Saunders, 1991.

76. Dahlin DC, Unni KK. *Bone Tumors: General Aspects and Data on 8,542*, Charles C Thomas Publishers, Springfield, Ed 4, 1986.

77. Schajowicz F. *Tumors and Tumor-Like Lesions of Bone. Pathology, Radiology and Treatment*, Ed 2, New York, Springer-Verlag, 1994.

78. Mira JM. *Bone Tumors. Clinical Radiologic and Pathologic Correlations*. Philadelphia Lea & Febiger, 1989.

79. Inwards CY. Update on cartilage forming tumors of the head and neck. *Head and Neck Pathol*, 2007, 1: 67–74.

80. Fu Y-S, Perzin KH. Non-epithelial tumors of the nasal cavity, paranasal sinuses and nasopharynx: a clinicopathologic study. III. Cartilaginous tumors (chondromas, chondrosarcomas) *Cancer*, 1974, 34: 453–463.

81. Kilby D, Ambegaokar A. The nasal chondroma: 2 case reports and a survey of the literature. *J Laryngol Otolgy*, 1977, 91: 415–426.

82. Ghogawala Z, Moore M, Strand R, et al. Clival Chondroma in a child with Ollier's disease. Case report. *Pediat Neuro Surg*, 1991, 17: 53–56.

83. Rathore PK, Mandal S, Meher R, et al. Giant ossifying chondroma of the skull. *Int J Pediatr Otorhinolaryngol*, 2005, 69: 1709–1711.

84. Kosaki N, Yabe H, Anazawa U, et al. Bilateral multiple malignant transformation of Ollier's disease. *Skeletal Radiol*, 2005, 34: 477–484.

85. Cook PL, Evans PG. Chondrosarcoma of the skull in Maffucci's syndrome. *Br J Radiol*, 1977, 50: 833–836.

86. Hopyan S, Gokgoz N, Poon R, et al. A mutant PTH/PTHrP type I receptor in enchondromatosis. *Nat Genet*, 2002, 30: 306–210.

87. Gnepp DR. *Diagnostic Surgical Pathology of the Head and Neck*, Ed 2, Philadelphia, Saunders Elsevier, 2009, p. 743.

Osteochondroma

88. Saglik Y, Altay M, Unai VS, et al. Manifestations and management of osteochondromas: a retrospective analysis of 382 patients. *Acta Orthop*, 2006, 72: 748–755.

89. Dahlin DC. *Bone Tumors: General Aspects and Data on 6,221 Cases*, Ed 3, Charles C Thomas, Springfield, IL, 1978.

90. Khurana J, Abdul-Karim F, Boree JVMG. Osteochondroma. In Fletcher CDM, Unni KK, Metens F. (eds) *World Health Organization Classification of Tumors. Pathology and Genetics of Tumors of Soft Tissue and Bone*. Lyon, France, IRAC, 2002, pp. 234–236.

91. Canella P, Gardin F, Borriani S. Exostosis: development, evolution and relationships to malignant

degeneration. *Ital J Orthop Traumatol*, 1981, 7: 293–298.

92. Niedzwiecka M, Kaczmarek P, Krawczy, T. Benign but fatal. A case of a newborn with congenital osteochondroma. *Bone*, 2013, 54: 169–171.

93. Marx RE, Stern D. *Oral and Maxillofacial Pathology. A Rationale for Diagnosis and Treatment*, Ed 1, Chicago. Hanover Park, IL, Quintessence Publishing Company, 2012.

94. Shore RM, Pozanski AK, Anandappa EC, et al. Arterial and venous compromise by osteochondroma. *Pediatr Kadiol*, 1994, 24: 39–40.

95. Mehta M, White LM, Knapp T, et al. MR imaging of symptomatic osteochondromas with pathologic correlations. *Skeletal Radio*, 1998, 27: 427–436.

96. Garrison RG, Uni KK, McLeod RA. Chondrosarcoma arising in osteochondroma. *Cancer*, 1982, 49: 1890–1897.

97. Ahn J, Ludecke H-J, Lidow S, et al. Cloning of the putative suppressor gene for hereditary multiple exostoses (EXT1) *Nat Genet*, 1995, 11: 137–143.

98. Zak BM, Crawford BE, Esko JD. Hereditary multiple exostoses and heparin sulfate polymerization. *Biochim Biophys Acta*, 2002, 1573: 346–355.

99. Feeley MG, Boehm AK, Bridge RS, et al. Cytogenetic and molecular cytogenetic evidence of recurrent 8q 24.1 loss in osteochondroma. *Cancer Genet Cytogenet*, 2002, 137: 102–107.

100. Ostuk C, Tezer M, Hamzaoglu A. Solitary osteochondroma of the cervical spine causing spinal cord compression. *Acta Orthop Belg*, 2007, 73: 133–136.

101. Chiurco AA. Multiple exostoses of bone with fatal spinal cord compression, report of a case and brief review of the literature. *Neurology*, 1970, 20: 275–278.

102. Kitsoulis P, Vassiliki G, Kallopi S, et al. Osteochondromas: review of the clinical radiological and pathological features. *In Vivo*, 2008, 22: 633–646.

Chondromyxoid Fibroma

103. Jaffe HL, Lichtensteen L. Chondromyxoid fibroma of bone: a distinctive benign tumor likely mistaken for chondrosarcoma. *Arch Pathol*, 1948, 45: 541–551.

104. Rahimi A, Beabout JW, Ivins JC, et al. Chondromyxoid fibroma: a clinicopathologic study of 76 cases. *Cancer*, 1972, 30: 726–736.

105. Huvos AG. *Bone Tumors: Diagnosis Treatment and Prognosis*. Philadelphia, W.B. Saunders, 1991, pp. 319–330.

106. Batsakis JG, Raymond AK. Pathology consultation: chondromyxoid fibroma. *Ann Otol Rhinol Laryngol*, 1989, 98: 571–572.

107. Hammad H, Hammond HL, Kurago ZB. Chondromyxoid fibroma of the jaws: case report and review of the literature. *Oral Surg Oral Med Oral Radiol Oral Pathol and Endod*, 1998, 85: 293–300.

108. Khatana S, Singh V, Gupta A. Unilocular anterior mandibular swelling. *Int J Pediatr Otolargol*, 2013, 77: 964–971.

109. Oh N, Korsandi AS, Scheri S, et al. Chondromyxoid fibroma of the mastoid portion of the temporal bone. MRI and PET/CT findings and their correlation with histology. *Ear Nose Throat J*, 2013, 92: 201–203.

110. Gupta S, Heman-Ackah SE, Harris JA, et al. Chondromyxoid fibroma of the temporal bone. *Oto Neuro Fol*, 2012, 33: e71–e72.

111. Sharma M, Velho V, Ginayake R, et al. Chondromyxoid fibroma of the temporal bone: a rare entity. *Neurosci*, 2012, 7: 211–214.

112. Aegerter E, Kirkpatrick JA. *Orthopedic Diseases. Physiology Radiology*. Phildaelphia, W.B. Saunders, 1963, pp. 580–587.

113. Fotiadis E, Akritopoulos P, Samoladas E. Chondromyxoid fibroma. A rare tumor with an unusual location. *Arch Orthop Trauma Surg*, 2008, 128: 371–375.

114. Safar A, Nelson M, Neff JR, et al. Recurrent anomalies of 6[inv(6) (p25q13] in chondromyxoid fibroma. *Human Pathol*, 2000, 31: 306–311.

115. Justin J, Akpalo H, Gambarotti M, et al. Phenotypic diversity in chondromyxoid fibroma reveals differentiation pattern of tumor mimicking fetal cartilage canals development. *Am J Pathol*, 2010, 177: 1072–1078.

116. Durr HR, Liehemann, Nerlich A, et al. Chondromyxoid fibroma of bone. *Arch Orthop Trauma Surg*, 2000, 120: 42–47.

Chondroblastoma

117. Jaffe H, Lichtenstein L. Benign chondroblastoma of bone. A reinterpretation of the so called calcifying or chondromatous giant cell tumor. *Am J Pathol*, 1942, 18: 969–991.

118. Springfield DS, Capanna R, Gherlinzoni F, et al. Chondroblastoma. A review of seventy cases. *J Bone Joint Surg Am*, 1985, 67: 748–755.

119. Sailhan F, Chotel F, Parot R. Chondroblastoma of bone in a pediatric population. *J Bone Joint Surg Am*, 2009, 91: 2159–2168.

120. Kurt AM, Unni KK, Sim FH, et al. Chondroblastoma of bone. *Hum Pathol*, 1989, 20: 965–976.

121. Bertoni F, Unni KK, Beabout W, et al. Chondroblastoma of the skull and facial bones. *Am J Clin Pathol*, 1987, 88: 1–9.

122. Nwoku AL, Koch H. Temporomandibular joint. A rare localization for bone tumors. *J Maxillofac Surg*, 1974, 2: 113.

123. Kondoh T, Hamada Y, Kamei K, et al. Chondroblastoma of the mandibular condyle. Report of a case. *J Oral Maxillofac Surg*, 2002, 60: 198–203.

124. Turwtto, RE, Kurt AM, Sim FH, et al. Chondroblastoma. *Hum Pathol*, 1993, 24: 944–949.

125. Edel G, Ueda Y, Nakanishi J, et al. Chondroblastoma of bone. A clinical, radiological, light and immunohistochemical study. *Virhows Arch*, 1992, 421: 355–366.

126. Wolff DA, Stevenson S, Goldberg VM. S-100 protein immunostaining identifies cells expressing a chondrocytic phenotype during articular cartilage repair. *J Orthop Res*, 1992, 10: 49–57.

127. Nakamura Y, Becker LE, Marks, A. S-100 protein in tumors of cartilage and bone. *Cancer*, 1983, 52: 1820–1825.

128. Kyriakos M, Land VJ, Penning HL, et al. Metastatic chondroblastoma. Report of a fatal case with a review of the literature on atypical, aggressive, and malignant chondroblastoma. *Cancer*, 1985, 55: 1770–1789.

Synovial Chondromatosis

129. Hohlweg B, Metzger MC, Bohin J, et al. Advanced image findings and complete-assisted surgery of suspected synovial chondromatosis in the temporomandibular joint. *J Magnetu*

Resonance Imaging, 2008, 28(5): 1251–1257.

130. Van Arx DP, Simpson MJ, Batman P. Synovial chondromatosis of the temporomandibular joint. *Br. J Oral Maxillofac Surg*, 1988, 26: 297–305.

131. Koyama J, Ito J, Hayashi T, et al. Synovial chondromatosis in the temporomandibular joint complicated by displacement and calcification of the articular disk: report of two cases. *AJNR Am J Neuroradiol*, 2001, 22: 1203–1206.

132. Chen A, Wong LY, Sheu CY. Distinguishing multiple rice body formation in chronic subacromial-subdeltoid bursitis from synovial chondromatosis. *Skeletal Radiol*, 2002, 31: 119–121.

133. Kim HG, Park KH, Huh JK. Magnetic resonance imaging characteristics of synovial chondromatosis of the temporomandibular joint. *J Orofac Pain*, 2002, 16: 148–153.

134. Voge TJ, Abolmaalin N, Maurer J. Neoplasms of the temporomandibular joint (TMJ). Diagnosis, differential diagnosis and intervention. *Radiology*, 2001, 41: 760–771.

135. Guarda-Nardini L, et al. Synovial chondromatosis of the temporomandibular joint: a case description with systemic review of the literature. *Int J Oral Maxillofac Surg*, 2010, 39: 745–755

136. Fujita S, Yoshida H, Tojyo I, et al. Synovial chondromatosis of the temporomandibular joint. Clinical and immunohistopathological considerations. *Br J Oral Maxillofac Surg*, 2004, 42: 259–260.

137. Hohlweg Majert B, Schon R, Schmelzeisen R, et al. A navigational maxillofacial surgery using virtual models. *World J Surg*, 2005, 29: 1530–1538.

Chondrosarcoma

138. Chou P, Mehta S, Gonzalez-Crussi F. Chondrosarcoma of the head in children. *Pediatr Pathol*, 1990, 10: 945–958.

139. Pones HAR, Pontes FSC, deAbreu MC, et al. Clinicopathological analysis of head and neck chondrosarcoma: three case reports and literature review. *Int J Oral Maxillofac Surg*, 2012, 41: 203–210.

140. Prado Ornellas F, Nishimoto IN, deCruz Perez, DE. Head and neck chondrosarcoma: analysis of 16 cases. *Br J Oral Maxillofac Surg*, 2009, 47: 555–557.

141. Huvos AG, Marcove RC. Chondrosarcoma in the young. A clinicopathologic analysis of patients younger than 25 years of age. *Am J Surg Pathol*, 1987, 11: 930–942.

142. Liu J, Hudkins PG, Swee RG et al. Bone sarcomas associated with Ollier's disease. *Cancer*, 1987, 59: 1376–1385.

143. Garrington GE, Scofield HJ, Cornyn J, et al. Osteosarcoma of the jaws: analysis of 56 cases. *Cancer*, 1967, 20: 377–391.

144. Gupta S. Mesenchymal chondrosarcoma of maxilla: a rare case report. *Med Oral Pathol Oral Cir Bucal*, 2011, 16: e493–e496.

145. Turner S, Kebudi R, Peksayor G, et al. Congenital mesenchymal chondrosarcoma of the orbit. Case report and review of the literature. *Ophthalmology*, 2004, 111: 1016–1022.

146. Gonzales-Lois C, Cuevas C, Abdullah O, et al. Intracranial extra skeletal myxoid chondrosarcoma: case report and review of the literature. *Acta Neurochir*, 2002, 144: 735–740.

147. Devaney KS, Ferlito A, Silver CL. Cartilaginous tumors of the larynx. *Otol Phinol Laryngol*, 1995, 104: 251–255.

148. Slootweg PJ, Clear-cell chondrosarcoma of the maxilla. Report of a case. *Oral Surg, Oral Med, Oral Pathol*, 1980, 50: 233–237.

149. Pang ZG, He XZ, Wu, LY, et al. Clinicopathologic and immunohistochemical study of 23 cases of mesenchymal chondrosarcoma. *Zhonghu Bing Xue Za Zhi*, 2011, 40: 368–372.

150. Meis-Kundblom JM, Bergh P, Gunterberg B, et al. Extra skeletal myxoid chondrosarcoma. A reappraisal of its morphologic spectrum and prognostic factors based on 17 cases. *Am J Surg Pathol*, 1999, 23: 636–650.

151. Antonseon CR, Argani P, Erlandson RA, et al. Skeletal and extra skeletal myxoid chondrosarcoma: a comparative clinicopathologic ultra structural and molecular study. *Cancer*, 1998, 83: 1504–1521.

152. Tarkkauren M, Wiklend T, Virolainen M, et al. Differentiated chondrosarcoma with t(9;22) (q34; q11-12). *Genes Chromosomes. Cancer*, 1994, 9: 136–140.

153. Stehman G, Anderson H, Mandahl N, et al. Translocation of t(9;22) (q22;q12) is a primary cytogenetic abnormality in extraskeletal myxoid chondrosarcoma. *Int. J. Cancer*, 1995, 62: 398–402.

154. Szuhai K, Cleton-Hansen A-M, Pancras GW, et al. Molecular pathology and its diagnostic use in bone tumors. *Cancer Genetics*, 2012, 205: 193–204.

155. Gadwal SR, Fanburg-Smith, JC, Gannon FH, et al. Primary chondrosarcoma of the head and neck in pediatric patients. A clinicopathologic study of 14 cases with review of the literature. *Cancer*, 2000, 88: 2181–2188.

156. Angiero F, Vinci R, Sidoni A, et al. Mesenchymal chondrosarcoma of the left coronoid process. Report of a unique case with clinical histopathologic and immunohistochemical findings, and a review of the literature. *Quintessence Int*, 2007, 38: 349–355.

Chordoma

157. Dahlin DC, MacCarty CS. Chordoma: a study of 59 cases. *Cancer*, 1952, 5: 1170–1178.

158. Raffel C, Wright DC, Gutin PH, Wilson CB. Cranial chordomas: clinical presentation and results of operative and radiation therapy in twenty-six patients. *Neurosurgery*, 1985, 17: 703–710.

159. Borba LA, Al-Mefty O, Mrak RE, Suen J. Cranial chordoma in children and adolescents. *J Neurosurg*, 1996, 84: 584 591.

160. Omerod R. A case of chordoma presenting in the nasopharynx. *J Laryngol Otol*, 1960, 74: 245–254.

161. Whelan MA, Reede DL, Meisler W, Bergeron RT. CT of the base of the skull. *Radiol Clin North Am*, 1984, 22: 177–217.

162. Erdem E, Engardo C, Antuaco MD. Comprehensive review of intracranial chordoma. *Radiographics*, 2003, 23: 995–1009.

163. Suba Z, Hauser P, Garami M, Martonffy K, et al. Skull base chordoma mimicking a preauricular neoplasm in a child: clinicopathological features and biological behaviour. *J Craniomaxillofac Surg*, 2007, 35: 35–38.

164. Pamir MN, Ozduman K. Analysis of radiological features relative to histopathology in 42 skull-base

chordomas and chondrosarcomas. *Eru J Radiol*, 2006, 58(3): 461–470.

165. Chugh R. Chordoma. The non-sarcoma primary bone tumor. *Oncologist*, 2007, 12: 1344–1350.

166. Oakley GJ. Brachyury, Sox-9 and podoplanin, new markers in skull base chordomas vs chondrosarcoma differential. A tissue array-based comparative analysis. *Mod Path*, 2008, 21: 1461–1469.

Fibrosarcoma

167. Gosau M, Draenert FG, Winter WA. Fibrosarcoma of the childhood mandible. *Head and Face Medicine*, 2008, 4: 21–23.

168. Pereira CM, Jorge J, Hipolito LP, et al. Primary intraosseous fibrosarcoma of the jaw. *Int J Oral Maxillofac Surg*, 2005, 34: 579–581.

169. Kahn LP, Vigorita V. Fibrosarcoma of bone. In Fletcher CDM, Unni KK, Mertens F, (eds) *World Health Organization Classification of Tumours. Pathology and Genetics of Tumors of Soft Tissue and Bone.* Lyon France, IARC Press, 2002, pp. 289–290.

170. Knezevich SR, McFadden DE, Tao W., et al. A novel ETV-6-NTRK3 gene fusion differentiates congenital fibrosarcoma from other childhood spindle tumors. *Am J Surg Pathol*, 2000, 24:937–946.

171. Fletcher CDM, Unni KK, Mertens I. *World Health Organization Classification of Tumors, Pathology and Genetics of Soft Tissue and Bone: So-called Fibrohistocytic Tumors.* Lyon, IARC Press, 2002, 120–125.

172. Wanebo HJ, Koness RJ, MacFarlane JK. Head and neck sarcoma: report of the head and neck sarcoma registry. Society of head & Neck Surgeons Committee on Research. *Head and Neck*, 1992, 14: 1–7.

173. Gorsky M, Epstein JB. Head and neck and inter-oral soft tissue sarcomas. *Oral Oncol*, 1998, 34: 292–296.

174. Nagler RM, Malkin L, Ben-Arieh Y, et al. Sarcoma of the maxillofacial region, follow-up of 25 cases. *Anticancer Res*, 2000, 20: 3735–3742.

Fibrous Dysplasia

175. Lee JS, Fitz Gibbon EJ, Chen YR. Clinical guidelines for management of craniofacial fibrous dysplasia. *Orphanet J Rare Dis*, 2012, doi: 10.1186/1750-1172-7-51-52.

176. Tsai EC, Santorreneos S, Rutka JT. Tumors of the skull bone in children: review of tumor types and management strategies. *Neuro Surg Focus*, 2002, 12: e1.

177. Riminucci M, Liu B, Corsi A., et al. The histopathology of fibrous dysplasia of bone in patients with activating mutations of the Gsa gene: site-specific patterns and current histological hallmarks. *J Pathol*, 1999, 187: 249–258.

178. Parekh SG, Donthineni-Rao R, Ricchetti E., et al. Fibrous dysplasia. *J Am Acad Orthop Surg*, 2004, 12: 305–313.

179. Valentini V, Cassoni A, Marianetti TM, et al. Craniomaxillofacial fibrous dysplasia: conservative treatment or radical surgery? A retrospective study of 68 patients. *Plastic and Reconstructive Surg*, 2009, 123: 653–660.

180. Michael CB, Lee AG, Patrinely JR. Visual loss associated with fibrous dysplasia of the anterior skull base. Case report and review of the literature. *J Neurosurg*, 2000, 92: 350–354.

181. Dian E, Morris DE, Lo LJ, et al. Cyst degeneration in craniofacial fibrous dysplasia. Clinical presentation and management. *J Neurosurg*, 2007, 107: 504–508.

182. Kelly MH, Brillante B, Collins MT. Pain in fibrous dysplasia of bone: age-related changes and anatomical distribution of skeletal lesions. *Osteoporos Int*, 2008, 19: 57–63.

183. Sciarretta V, Pasquini E, Frank G., et al. Endoscopic treatment of benign tumors of the nose and paranasal sinuses. Report of 33 cases. *Am J Rhinol*, 2006, 20: 64–71.

184. Long JJ, Jung HH, Lee HM, et al. Monostatic fibrous dysplasia of temporal bone. Report of two cases and review of its characteristics. *Acta Otolaryngol*, 2005, 125: 1126–1129.

185. Chung KF, Alaghband-Zadeh J, Guz A. Acromegaly and hyperprolactinemia in McCune-Albright syndrome. Evidence of hypothalamic dysfunction. *Am J Dis Chil*, 1983, 137: 134–136.

186. Aarkkog D, Tveteraas E. McCune-Albright's syndrome following adrenalectomy for Cushing's syndrome in infancy. *J Pediatr*, 1968, 73: 89–96.

187. Aoki T, Kouho H, Hisaoka M., et al. Intramuscular myxoma with fibrous dysplasia: a report of two cases with a

review of the literature. *Path Int*, 1995, 45: 65–171.

188. Shi RR, Zue-Fen L, Zang R, et al. GNAS mutational analysis in differentiating fibrous dysplasia and ossifying fibroma of the jaw. *Modern Pathology*, 2013, 26: 1023–1031.

189. Marx KE, Stern D. *Oral and Maxillofacial Pathology: A Rational for Diagnosis and Treatment*, Ed 2, Chicago, Quintessence Publishing Company, 2010, p. 791.

190. Ruggieri P, Sim, FH, Band JR, et al. Malignancies in fibrous dysplasia. *Cancer*, 1994, 73: 1411–1424.

Ossifying Fibroma

191. Eversole LR, Leider AS, Nelson K. Ossifying fibroma: a clinicopathologic study of sixty-four cases. *Oral Surg, Oral Med, Oral Pathol, Oral Radio, Endod*, 1985, 60: 505–511.

192. Mintz S, Velez I. Central ossifying fibroma: an analysis of 20 cases and review of the literature. *Quintessence Int*, 2007, 38: 222–227.

193. Waldron CA. Fibro-osseous lesions of the jaws. *J Oral Maxillofac Surg*, 1993, 51: 828–835.

194. Traiantafillidou K, Venetis G, Karakinaris G., et al. Ossifying fibroma of the jaws: a clinical study of 14 cases and review of the literature. *Oral Surg Oral Med Oral Pathol Oral Radiology Endod*, 2012, 114: 193–199.

195. Slootweg PJ, El-Mofty SK. Ossifying fibroma. In Barnes, L Everson JW, Reichart P, Sidransky D (eds) *Pathology and Genetics Head and Neck Tumors.* Lyon, France, IARC Press, 2005, pp. 319–320.

196. Su L, Weathers DR, Waldron CA. Distinguishing features of focal cemento-osseous dysplasia and cemento-ossifying fibromas. II A clinical and radiographic spectrum of 316 cases. *Oral Surg Oral Med Oral Pathol Oral Radiol Endod*, 1997, 84: 540–549.

197. El-Mofty S. Psammomatoid and trabecular juvenile ossifying fibroma of the craniofacial skeleton. Two distinct clinicopathologic entities. *Oral Surg Oral Med Oral Pathol Oral Radiol Endod*, 2002, 93: 296–304.

198. Slootweg PJ, Muller H. Juvenile ossifying fibroma. Report of four cases. *J Craniomaxillofac Surg*, 1990, 18: 125–129.

199. Slootweb PJ, Panders AK, Loopmans R., et al. Juvenile ossifying fibroma. An analysis of 33 cases with emphasis on histopathological aspects. *J Oral Pathol Med*, 1994, 23: 385–388.

200. Johnson LC, Youseti TN, Heffiner DK et al. Juvenile active ossifying fibroma; its nature dynamics and origin. *Acta Otolaryngol Sluppl* 1991, 448: 1–40.

201. Thankappan S, Nair S, Thomas KP et al. Psammomatoid and trabecular varients of juvenile ossifying fibroma-two case reports. *Indian J Radiol Imaging*, 2009, 19: 116–119.

202. Kaplan I, Manor R, Yahalom R, et al. Giant cell granuloma associated with central ossifying fibromas of the jaws: a clinicopathologic study. *Oral Surg Oral Med Oral Pathol Oral Radiol Endod*, 2007, 103: e35–e41.

203. Chang CC, Hung HY, Chang JX. Central ossifying fibroma: a clinicopathologic study of 28 caes. *J Formos Med Assoc*, 2008, 107: 288–294.

204. Guriel M, Uckan N, Guler N, et al. Surgical and reconstructive treatment of a large ossifying fibromas of the mandible. A retrognathic patient. *J Oral Maxillofac Surg*, 2001, 59: 1097–1100.

205. Gogl H. Das Psammo-osteoid-fibroma der nas und ihreso neben humohlen. *Monatsschr Ohrenheilk Lar Rhin*, 1949, 83: 1–10.

206. Sawyer JR, Tryka AF, Bell JM, et al. Non random chromosome break-points at Xq26 and 2q33 characteristic cemento ossifying fibromas of the orbit. *Cancer*, 1995, 76: 1853–1859.

207. Dal Cin P, Sciot R, Fossion E, et al. Chromosomal abnormalities in cemento ossifying fibroma. *Cancer Genet Cytogenet*, 1993, 71: 170–172.

Central Giant Cell Granuloma

208. Barnes L, Everson JW, Reichart et al. *Pathology and Genetics. Head and Neck Tumors. WHO Classification of Tumors.* Lyon, IARC Press, 2005.

209. Stauropoulos J, Katz J. Central giant cell granuloma; a systematic review of the radiographic characteristics with addition of 20 new cases. *Dentomaxillofac Radiol*, 2002, 31: 213–217.

210. Kruse-Losler B, Raihanatou D, Gaetner C, et al. Central giant cell granuloma of the jaws: a clinical, radiologic and histopathologic study of 26 cases. *Oral Surg Oral Med Oral Pathol Oral Radiol Endod*, 2006, 101: 346–354.

211. Liu B, Yu SF, Li TJ. Multinucleated giant cells in various forms of giant cell containing lesions of the jaws express features of osteoclasts. *J Oral Pathol Med*, 2003, 32: 367–375.

212. Huvos AG. *Bone Tumors. Diagnosis, Treatment and Prognosis*, Ed 2, Philadelphia, WB Saunders 1991.

213. Ardekian L, Manor R, Peled M, et al. Bilateral central giant cell granulomas in a patient with neurofibromatosis. Report of a case and review of the literature. *J Oral Maxillofac Surg*, 1999, 57: 869–872.

214. Catani F, Pardi E, Borsari S., et al. Molecular pathogenesis of primary hyperthyroidism. *J Endocraniol Invest*, 2011, 34: 35–39.

215. Itonaga I, Hussein I, Kudo O, et al. Cellular mechanisms of osteoclast formation and lacunar resorption in giant cell granuloma of the jaw. *J Oral Pathol Med*, 2003, 32: 224–231.

216. Amaral FR, Diniz GM, Bernardes VF. WWOX expression in giant cell lesions of the jaws. *Oral Surg, Oral Med, Oral Pathol, Oral Radio*, 2013, 116: 210–213.

217. Sezer B, Koyuneu B, Gomel M, et al. Interlesional corticosteroid inject for central giant cell granuloma. A case report and review of the literature. *Turk J Pediat*, 2005, 47: 75–81.

218. O'Regan M, Gibb DH, Odell, W. Rapid growth of giant ell granuloma in pregnancy treated with calcitonin. *Oral Surg Oral Med Oral Pathol Oral Radiol Endod*, 2001, 92: 532–538.

219. Kaban LB, Troulis MJ, Ebb D, et al. Antiangiogenic therapy with interferon alpha for giant cell lesions of the jaws. *J Oral Maxillofac Surg*, 2002, 60: 1103–1113.

220. Wieneke JA, Gannon KH, Heffner DK, et al. Giant cell tumor of the larynx. A clinicopathologic study of eight cases and a review of the literature. *Neurosurgery*, 2001, 48: 424–429.

221. Ayclair PL, Cucnin P, Kratochuil FJ, et al. A clinical and histomorphologic comparison of the central giant cell granuloma and the giant cell tumor. *Oral Surg Oral Med Oral Pathol*, 1988, 66: 197–208.

Aneurysmal Bone Cyst

222. Gingell JC, Levy BA, Beckerman T, et al. Aneurysmal bone cyst. *J Oral Maxillofac Surg*, 1984, 42: 527–534.

223. Martinez V, Sissions HA. Aneurysmal bone cyst. A review of 123 cases including primary lesions and those secondary to other bone pathology. *Cancer*, 1988, 61: 2291–2304.

224. Lee HL, Cho KS, Choi KU. Aggressive aneurysmal bone cyst of the maxilla confused with telangiectic osteosarcoma. *Auris Nasus Larynx*, 2012, 39: 337–340.

225. Panoutakopoulous G, Pandis N, Kyrlazoglou I, et al. Recurrent t(16;17) (q22; p13) in aneurysmal bone cysts. *Genes Chromosomes. Cancer*, 1999, 26: 265–266.

226. Ye Pringle, LM, Lau AW, et al. TRE 17/USP6 oncogene translocation in aneurysmal bone cyst indices matrix metalloproteinase production via actiuation of N7-Kappa B. *Oncogene*, 2010, 29: 3619–3629.

227. Vergel DeDios AM, Bond JR, Shives TC, et al. Aneurysmal bone cyst. A clinicopathologic study of 238 cases. *Cancer*, 1992, 69: 2921–2931.

228. Ruiter DJ, van Rijssel JG, van der Velde EA. Aneurysmal bone cysts. A clinicopathological study of 105 cases. *Cancer*, 1977, 39: 2231–2235.

229. Briadley GW, Greene JF, Jr, Frankel LJ. Case reports: malignant transformation of aneurysmal bone cysts. *Clin Orthop Relat Res*, 2005, 438: 282–287.

230. Kryiakos M, Hardy D. Malignant transformation of aneurysmal bone cyst with analysis of the literature. *Cancer*, 1991, 68: 1770–1780.

Hyperparathyroidism

231. Goshen O, Aviel-Ronen S, Dori S, Talmi YP. Brown tumour of hyperparathyroidism in the mandible associated with atypical parathyroid adenoma. *J Laryngol Otol*, 2000, 114: 302–304.

232. Guney E, Yigibasi OG, Bayram F, et al. Brown tumor of the maxilla associated with primary hyperparathyroidism. *Auris Nasus Larynx*, 2001, 28: 369–372.

233. Watanabe T, Tsukamoto F, Shimizu T, et al. Familial isolated hyperparathyroidism caused by single adenoma: a distinct entity different from multiple endocrine neoplasia. *Endocr J*, 1998, 45: 637–646.

234. Yamazaki H, Ota Y, Aoki T, et al. Brown tumor of the maxilla and mandible: progressive mandibular brown tumor after removal of

parathyroid adenoma. *J Oral Maxillofac Surg*, 2003, 61: 719–722.

235. Scott SN, Graham SM, Sato Y, Robinson RA. Brown tumour of the palate in a patient with primary hyperparathyroidism. *Ann Otol Rhinol Laryngol*, 1999, 108: 91–94.

236. Jebasingh F, Jubbin J, Shah A, et al. Bilateral maxillary brown tumours as a first presentation of primary hyperparathyroidism. *Oral Maxillofac Surg*, 2008, 12: 97–100.

Cherubism

237. Jones WA. Familial multilocular cystic disease of the jaws. *Am J Cancer*, 1933, 17: 946.

238. Ueki Y, Tiziani V, Santanna C, Fukai N, et al. Mutations in the gene encoding c-Ab1-binding protein SH3BP2 cause Cherubism. *Nat Genet*, 2001, 28: 125–126.

239. De Lange J, Van den Akker HP. Clinical and radiological features of central giant-cell lesions of the jaw. *Oral Surg Oral Med Oral Pathol Oral Radiol Endod*, 2005, 99: 464–470.

240. Kozakiewicz M, Percynska-Partyka W, Kobos J. Cherubism – clinical picture and treatment. *Oral Dis*, 2001, 7: 123–130.

Rare Childhood Tumors of Bone

241. Krompecher Z. Zur histogenese and morpjologic den adamantinome and sonstiger kiefergeschwulste. *Beitr Pathol Anat*, 1918, 64: 165–197.

242. Barrett AW, Morgan M, Ramsay AD, Farthing PM, Newman L, Speight PM. A clinicopathological and immunohistochemical analysis of melanotic neuroectodermal tumor of infancy. *Oral Surg Oral Med Oral Pathol Oral Radiol Endod*, 2002, 93: 688–698.

243. Siddiqui TH, Amin MR, Bashar MA, Ahmed Z, et al. Melanotic neuroectodermal tumour of infancy. *Mymensingh Med J*, 2011, 20: 312–315.

244. Agarwal P, Saxena S, Kumar, GLupta R. Melanotic neuroectodermal tumor of infancy: Presentation of a case affecting the maxilla. *J Oral Maxillofac Pathol*, 2010, 14: 29–32.

245. Borello ED, Gorlin RJ. Melanotic neuroectodermal tumor of infancy – a neoplasm of neural crese origin. Report of a case associated with high urinary excretion of vanilmandelic acid. *Cancer*, 1966, 12: 196–206.

246. Khoddami M, Squire J, Zielenska M, Thorner P. Melanotic neuroectodermal tumor of infancy: a molecular genetic study. *Pediatr Dev Pathol*, 1998, 1: 295–299.

247. Kaya S, Unal OF, Sarac S, Gedikoglu G. Melanotic neuroectodermal tumor of infancy: report of two cases and review of literature. *Int J Pediatr Otorhinolaryngol*, 2000, 52: 169–72.

248. Dehner LP, Sibley RK, Sauk JJ. Malignant neuroectodermal tumor of infancy. A clinical, pathologic, ultrastructural and tissue culture study. *Cancer*, 1979, 43: 389–410.

Neoplasms of Uncertain Histogenesis

Ewing Sarcoma/PNET

249. deAlva E, Pardo J. Ewing's tumor. Tumor biology and clinical application. *Int J Surg Pathol*, 2001, 9: 7–17.

250. Ries, LAG, Smith MA, Garney JG, et al. *Cancer Incidence and Survival among Children and Adolescents. United States SEER Program. 1975–1995, NIH Pub.*
No 99-4649. Bethesda, National Cancer Institute SEER Program, 1999.

251. Linnoila RI, Trokos M, Triche TJ, et al. Evidence for neural origin and PAS positive variants of the malignant small cell tumor of thoraco-pulmonary region. (Askin tumor). *Am J Surg Pathol*, 1985, 10: 124–133.

252. Carvajal R, Meyers P. Ewing's sarcoma and primitive neuroectodermal family of tumors. *Hematol Oncol Clin North Am*, 2005, 19: 501–525.

253. Windfuhr JP. Primitive neuroectodermal tumor of the head and neck: incidence, diagnosis and management. *Ann Otol Rhinol Laryngol*, 2004, 113: 533–543.

254. Dick EA, McHugh K, Kimber C, et al. Imaging of non-central nervous system primitive neuroectodermal tumors. Diagnostic features and correlation with outcome. *Clin Radiol*, 2001, 56: 205–215.

255. Ewing J. Diffuse endothelioma of bone. *Proc NY Pathol Soc*, 1921, 21: 17–24.

256. Folpe AL, Goldblum JR, Rubin BP, et al. Morphologic and immunophenotype diversity in Ewing family tumors. A study of 66 genetically confirmed cases. *Am J Surg Pathol*, 2005, 29: 1025–1033.

257. Cangir TJ, Vietti EA, Gehan G, et al. Ewing's sarcoma metastatic at diagnosis. *Cancer*, 1990, 55: 887–893.

258. Vaccani JP, Forte V, deJong AL, et al. Ewing's sarcoma of the head and neck in children. *Int J Pediatric Otorhinolaryngol*, 1999, 48: 209–216.

259. Van Doominck JA, Schaub B, et al. Current treatment protocols have eliminated the prognostic advantage of type 1 fusions in Ewing sarcoma. A report from Children's Oncology Group. *J Clin Oncol*, 2010, 28: 1989–1994.

Disorders of the Ear

Sherif Said

Developmental Anomalies of the Ear

Introduction

The ear is the site of many congenital malformations which can be encountered either in isolation or present in association with other anomalies, syndromes and malformations, and all of which can impact the well being of infants and children through adolescence and into adult life. Developmental conditions that are encountered by the pathologist in a surgical setting either in the form of a biopsy, or as a resected specimen are the principal focus of this discussion.

Accessory Tragus (Supernumerary Tragi/Heterotrophic Tragi)

At the end of the fifth week of embryonic life, the auricle forms from tissue derived from the first and second branchial arches.[1] Three surface irregularities initially appear on each arch. The arches then move dorsally and develop further to ultimately fuse and form the auricle.[1,2] It is along this line of fusion that the accessory tragus can occur.

This anomaly may occur as an isolated condition or in association with other congenital malformations including cleft lip or palate, mandibular hypoplasia or in concert with a host of syndromes including Goldenhar syndrome, Townes–Brocks syndrome, Treacher–Collins syndrome, VACTRAL syndrome and Wolf–Hirschhorn syndrome.[2]

The prevalence of the solitary accessory tragus is estimated at 1 to 10 occurrences per 1000 live births.[3] Bilateral lesions have a prevalence of approximately 9 to 10 occurrences per 100,000.[2,3,4,5]

Clinical Features

The accessory tragus will present as a sessile or pedunculated nodule arising on or near the tragus along a line extending between the tragus and angle of mouth, or along the anterior border of the sternomastoid mucocele. (Figure 17.1) Accessory tragus tissue has also been reported in a middle ear location.[6] Clinical differential diagnoses include skin tag, epidermoid cyst, lipoma, adnexal skin tumors and branchial cysts.

Pathologic Findings

Microscopic Features

On microscopic examination, the accessory tragus will be covered by cutaneous epithelium that overlies subjacent dermal tissue with adnexal structures. A central core of mature cartilage and fibroadipose tissue characterize the histopathology of the lesion in most cases, although cartilage is not seen in all variants (Figure 17.2).

Treatment and Prognosis

Simple excision is the definitive treatment. Audiometry is recommended for children with an accessory tragus, as decreased hearing in affected patients has been reported.[2]

Choristoma (Heterotopia) of the Middle Ear and Mastoid

Choristomas represent the presence of histologically normal tissue in an ectopic anatomic site. The middle ear is one of the locations where both salivary gland and neuroglial heterotopias can be encountered in pediatric patients.

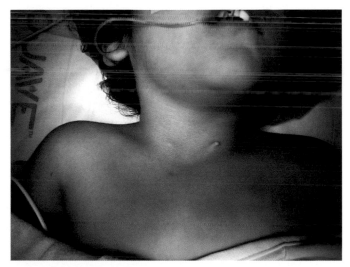

Figure 17.1 Accessory tragus seen low in the neck at the inferior and anterior border of the sternomastoid muscle rather than in the more common preauricular location. (photo courtesy of Dr. Vincent Eusterman).

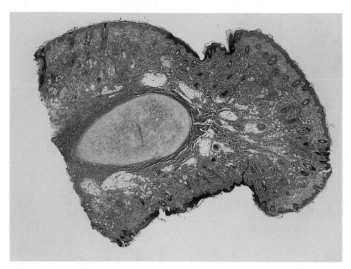

Figure 17.2 Accessory tragus with a central core of benign cartilage that is surrounded by skin adnexal structures and fibroadipose tissue and covered superiorly by cutaneous epithelium.

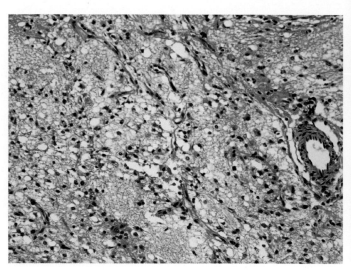

Figure 17.3 Neuroglial choristoma of the middle ear, isolated within the middle ear of a child with conductive deafness. The tissue was not contiguous with the brain tissue, ruling out the possibility of an encephalocele.

The *salivary gland choristoma* was initially described by Taylor and Martin in 1961.[7] Since that original description salivary gland choristomas have been further described and well documented in the literature.[8] *Neuroglial middle ear choristomas*, are less frequently encountered.[9]

Salivary gland choristomas in children and adolescents are usually associated with abnormalities in the ossicular chain and/or the facial nerve.[10,11] Most such choristomas of the middle ear develop just prior to, or during the fourth month of gestation. Although the exact mechanism of their formation is not known, the associated abnormalities in the ossicles and facial nerve are thought by some investigators to be related to concomitant embryologic failure of the second branchial arch to properly develop.[10,12] Most lesions will involve the patient's left side.[13]

Neurological choristomas in children are considered to develop as a result of a congenital defect in the overlying temporal bone tegmen tympani, allowing herniation of brain tissue into the subsequent defect.[14] The defect may heal or further develop as a neural crest remnant.[15]

Sebaceous choristomas of the middle ear have been reported in pediatric age group patients, however, they are quite rare.[16]

Clinical Features

Affected pediatric aged patients may be asymptomatic or demonstrate evidence of conductive deafness, otitis media (OM) or earache. On otoscopic examination, a mass may be seen behind the tympanic membrane with or without middle ear inflammatory changes and tympanic membrane retraction. A CT or MRI scan will generally confirm the presence of a middle ear mass.

Pathologic Findings

Histologic examination of *salivary gland choristomas* will reveal an admixture of mucoserous glands and adipose tissue,

while the *neuroglial choristoma* will demonstrate glial cells, histiocytes and reactive inflammatory changes (Figure 17.3). Microscopic differential diagnoses include inflammatory space occupying lesions of the middle ear including encephalocele, teratomas, ganglioma, meningioma, neuroma, adenocarcinoma and hamartoma.

Treatment and Prognosis

Conservative surgical removal is the treatment of choice.[17] Incomplete removal of the choristomas tends however, to not accompanied by recurrence.[18] In rare instances salivary gland tumors have been reported to arise within middle ear choristomas.[18,19]

First Branchial Cleft Anomalies

First branchial cleft anomalies involving the ear constitute less than 10 percent of all branchial clefts defects.[20,21] Most such anomalies will present clinically with an associated concurrent infection.

First branchial cleft anomalies are caused by incomplete closure of the ectodermal portion of the first branchial cleft, resulting in fistulas, sinuses or cysts, depending on the degree of tissue closure.[20,21]

These anomalies can be divided into two groups:[22,23,24] 1) anomalies that are located medial, inferior or posterior to the concha and pinna, and which form sinuses at the level of the mesotympanum, and 2) anomalous lesions that present at a point just below the angle of the mandible in association with a fistula or sinus tract. These fistulae or tracts may extend over the angle of the mandible and through the parotid gland parenchyma toward the external auditory canal (EAC). Mixed anomalous lesions demonstrating a combination of these anatomic locations and clinical findings have also been reported.[25] The majority of such anomalies, (68 percent), occur as cysts.

Sinuses or sinus tracts, also referred to as "periauricular pits," and fistulas account for the remainder of cases.[21,26]

Pathologic Findings

Histologically, first branchial cleft Type I anomalies will be lined by keratinizing squamous epithelium that will be supported by a collagenous base that lacks adnexal structures (Figure 17.4). Type II anomalies will consist of both ectodermal and mesodermal components. Ectodermally derived keratinized squamous epithelium will line a potential space or sinus tract that will be marginated by connective tissue that contains adnexal structures, and occasionally cartilage (Figure 17.5).

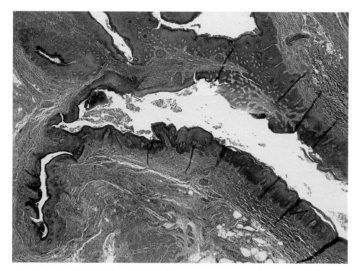

Figure 17.4 This first branchial cleft Type I anomaly presented medial to the pinna as a sinus tract. Note the keratinized squamous epithelial lining and the lack of adnexal structures in the marginating connective tissue.

Treatment and Prognosis

Treatment involves complete surgical excision. Type II anomalies can sometimes be surgically challenging due to their passage through the parotid parenchyma and their close approximation to facial nerve branches.

Acquired Diseases and Lesions of the Ear
External Ear
Exostosis of the External Ear Canal

Exostoses involving the external ear canal of the pediatric patient typically present as nodular, pedunculated, mound like or flat topped elevations.

These lesions, which are usually multiple and bilateral, occur primarily in children and adolescents who engage in aquatic activity.[27,28,29,30,31] Affected individuals will usually remain asymptomatic until approximately 80 percent of the meatus is obstructed by the exostosis and there is resultant wax retention. Conductive hearing loss, tinnitus and chronic inflammation are common to the condition.[32]

Pathologic Findings

Exostoses are usually covered by epithelium and a periosteal layer, unless they become denuded during surgical canaloplasty. Lesions will be composed of laminated compact bone that will sometimes display a prominent "onion skin" appearance on cross section (Figure 17.6).

The most common differential microscopic diagnosis will normally include osteoma, a lesion with a similar histologic appearance, but a lesion that is typically unilateral, nearly always pedunculated and one that tends to occur predominantly along suture lines (Figure 17.7).[33]

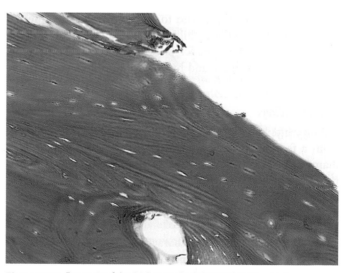

Figure 17.6 Exostosis of the EAC. Note the laminated "onion skin" appearance of the bone and a single focus of fibrovascular tissue.

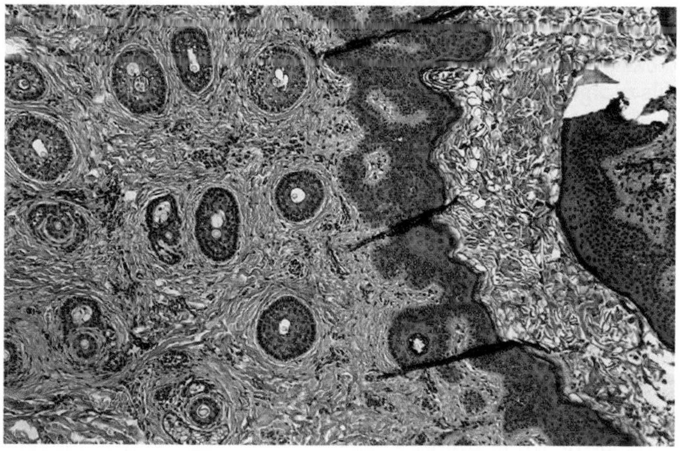

Figure 17.5 This first branchial cleft Type II anomaly presented inferior to the pinna as a sinus tract. Note the tract's keratinized squamous epithelial lining and surrounding adnexal structures (hair follicles and sebaceous glands) which are present within the marginating connective tissue.

Clinical Features

Pediatric patients usually present with a spontaneously occurring intensely painful papule with central ulceration, which will involve the helix or antihelix of the ear.[58,59] Most lesions will be less than 1 cm in size. The surface epithelium, in addition to frequently being ulcerated, will also often be crusted over.

Pathologic Findings

On microscopic examination, juvenile CNHC will demonstrate ulceration that extends to include the underlying elastic cartilage. The ulcer base will be filled with granulation tissue, and areas of fibrinoid necrosis that will be infiltrated by neutrophils and chronic inflammation cells. The process will typically involve the underlying perichondrium and auricular cartilage, and stromal fibrosis is common. The epithelium adjacent to the ulcer will typically show pseudoepitheliomatous hyperplasia.

Treatment and Prognosis

Surgical excision is the treatment of choice for juvenile CNHC, including soft tissue wedge resection and cartilage removal alone. Less commonly, conservative non-surgical approaches have been employed successfully,[60] including the use of a doughnut shaped pillow[61] and carbon dioxide laser therapy.[62]

Keratosis Obturans (KO)

KO generally results from abnormal self-cleansing of the ear and lateral extrusion of keratin into the EAC with a resultant accumulation of keratin debris within the canal and subsequent canal obstruction by either keratin or a resultant inflammatory response. The etiology of KO remains undetermined. The disorder, common in children and adolescents, can cause conductive hearing loss, pressure ulceration and occasionally pain. Secondary infection is common. Histologically the process will consist of an accumulation of keratin debris, cholesterol clefts, chronic inflammation and occasional epithelial ulceration. Treatment consists of debridement of the affected area.

Angiolymphoid Hyperplasia with Eosinophilia (ALHE, Epitheloid Hemangioma)

First described by Wells and Whimster in 1969,[63] ALHE is a benign idiopathic condition that presents either as a single nodule, plaque, papule, or as an aggregation of multiple nodules or plaques in variable anatomic sites throughout the body. The disease which occurs equally in all races, tends to be more common in females, and is not associated with peripheral eosinophilia, increased IgE levels or lymphadenopathy. ALHE has a predilection for the head and neck region, including the external ear (auricle/preauricular area and EAC).[63,64]

Clinical Features

The disorder is most prevalent in the young to middle aged adults but can be seen as well in the pediatric age group.[64]

Trauma, infection and reactive or reparative processes have all been suggested as possible causes. Vaccination has also been proposed as a possible etiologic factor in childhood cases.[65,66,67] It has been suggested that ALHE may represent a low grade T-cell lymphoproliferative disorder;[68] however, there is no definite proof that it is, and the process often regresses spontaneously.[69,70]

Pathologic Findings

On microscopic examination, ALHE will present as a well circumscribed nodular non-encapsulated vascular proliferation with a surrounding dense lymphohistiocytic infiltrate that is rich in eosinophils. The process will involve the dermis and subcutaneous tissues, such that a prominent infiltrative appearing vascular proliferation rich in endothelial cells that appear "epitheloid" predominates. The capillaries to medium sized arteries and veins that are lined by the plump epithelioid or histocytic appearing endothelial cells with eosinophilic cytoplasm and pleomorphic hyperchromatic nuclei which are seen in ALHE can on occasion appear malignant (Figures 17.11 & 17.12). Endothelial cell nuclei may protrude in to the lumen of vascular spaces in hobnail fashion in ALHE, therefore important differential diagnoses to be considered include hemangioma, angiosarcoma, papillary endothelial hyperplasia and Kimura disease.

Kimura disease can resemble ALHE, in that clinically and microscopically both diseases can result in a disease associated similar nodularity, lymphadenopathy and eosinophilia. However, the lesions of Kimura disease present with deeper involvement of the connective tissue than those of ALHE. The disorder is also associated with peripheral eosinophilia, increased IgE levels and typically, significantly greater lymphadenopathy than ALHE. In Kimura disease a lymphocytic infiltrate will dominate lesional histopathology, and unlike ALHE, the process will always show a prominent population of eosinophils and minimal epithelioid changes in vascular lining endothelial cells. [69,70] (See Figures 17.13 & 17.14.)

Treatment and Prognosis

Local excision of ALHE is most often curative; however, recurrences do occur. Laser therapy has also been employed to treat both ALHE and Kimura disease. Corticosteroid therapy has also been used to treat both disorders, and although not curative, steroid treatment can help to alleviate symptoms.

Idiopathic Cystic Chondromalacia of the Auricular Cartilage

Clinical Features

Idiopathic cystic chondromalacia, when seen in pediatric age group patients is also known as "pseudocyst of the auricle," The disorder is encountered most often in adolescents and individuals in their late teens.[71,72,73] Males are more often affected than females. The etiology of this benign cystic degenerative disease process is unknown; although trauma has been

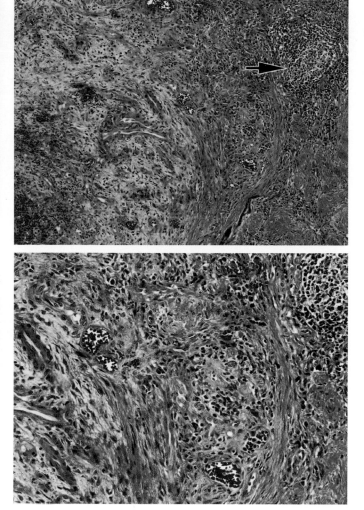

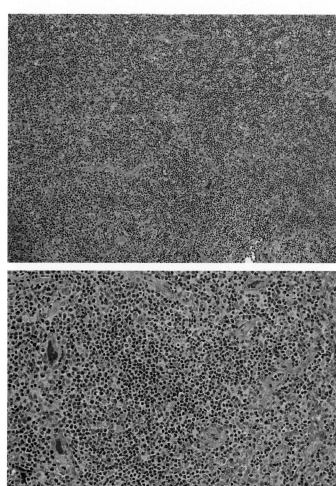

Figures 17.11 (top) & 17.12 (bottom) ALHE demonstrating a lymphocytic infiltrate forming a germinal center (arrow) an eosinophilic infiltrate, and prominent blood vessels (Figure 17.12). Higher power photomicrograph showing the histologic components of ALHE, including blood vessel formations with plump endothelial cells, eosinophils, lymphoid tissue and streaming fibroblasts in the background.

Figures 17.13 (top) & 17.14 (bottom) Low power photomicrograph showing a dense inflammatory cellular infiltrate consisting of small lymphocytes, plasma cells and numerous eosinophils. Thin-walled blood vessels lined by flattened endothelial cells are prominent (Figure 17.14). Higher power photomicrograph showing flattened endothelial cells and lymphocytes.

suggested as a possible initiating factor.[74] Ischemic necrosis of the cartilage or abnormal lysosomal enzymatic release by chondrocytes has also been proposed as a causal factor. The scaphoid fossa of the auricle is the most common site of occurrence, the process can be unilateral or bilateral and lesions can range up to 3 cm in diameter. Symptoms most often include unilateral focal asymptomatic swelling of the auricular cartilage.

Pathologic Findings

On gross inspection, the process will present as a glistening generally intact intracartilaginous cyst that contains clear or olive-oil like fluid. Histologically, the pseudocystic lumen will be marginated by irregular intracartilaginous fibrous tissue, degenerated cartilage, and occasionally granulation tissue. A true epithelial lining will not be present. The histologic

findings can be similar to those seen in CNCH, which, however, is not pseudocystic, and in relapsing polychondritis (RP), which results in cartilage necrosis.

Treatment and Prognosis

Complete surgical excision is curative. Other treatment modalities, including needle aspiration and incision and drainage have shown varying degrees of success. Steroid injection has proven to be unsuccessful as a management modality.

Pediatric Onset Perichondritis, (Relapsing Polychondritis)

Clinical Features

RP is a rare multi-body system disease that is characterized by widespread, destructive and inflammatory cartilaginous lesions,[75,76,77] including most often bilateral chondritis of the ears. The nose, larynx, eye joints and respiratory tract can also be involved. The disorder usually presents in episodic painful flares. The process, when it is chronic and involves the ears, can lead to cauliflower/floppy ears. Saddle nose, and laryngotracheal stenosis are common in other head and neck sites that are affected.

RP occurs primarily in the fourth to fifth decades of life and is seldom encountered in the pediatric age group.[75, 78,79,80] Unlike adults however, children with RP will have a family history of autoimmune disorders including, Sjögren's syndrome, SLE, inflammatory bowel disease, Hashimoto thyroiditis, rheumatoid arthritis and myelodysplasia. A genetic predisposition for RP has been proposed,[75,81] but no definitive evidence to support such an origin for the disorder has been proven. The disease is clearly known however, to be an inflammatory autoimmune disorder against type II collagen.

The episodic nature of RP, coupled with the rarity of the condition and the fact that the condition is a systemic one that can involve multiple sites, sometimes results in a delayed diagnosis. Initial symptoms can include chondritis of the ears, nose and larynx, as well as inflammatory arthritis, aphthosis, erythema nodosum, a maculopapular rash and purpura.[75] MAGIC syndrome, Goodpasture syndrome, Henoch Schönlein purpura and juvenile monomyelocytic leukemia can occur in children with RP, as can type I dermatomyositis, and inflammatory arthritis.

Differential diagnoses include otitis externa, acute infectious polychondritis and systemic vasculitides, including Wegner's Granulomatosis.

Pathologic Findings

A biopsy of ear cartilage will demonstrate only non-specific perichondrial inflammation and erosion of cartilage,[75] thus diagnosis of the disorder is generally based on clinical criteria being met, in concert with lesional histopathology. Granular deposits of immunoglobulins and the C3 component of complement can be found within perichondral blood vessels, and at the chondrofibrous junction and may prove helpful in establishing a diagnosis.[82] Patients may also demonstrate anti-type II collagen antibodies, and mild anemia.

Treatment and Prognosis

The primary treatment for RP involving the ear includes the use of non-steroidal anti-inflammatory drugs, corticosteroid therapy and immunosuppression, depending on the severity of the condition. The prognosis in children is variable and episodic relapses can occur.

The Middle Ear
Otitis Media (OM)

Acute and chronic inflammation of the middle ear, or OM, is one of the most common global causes of health care visits for children. One hundred million cases a year are reported, with 22.6 percent of such cases occurring in children under five years of age.[83] Fifty thousand OM associated deaths per year are documented worldwide in children less than five years of age.[83,84] OM tends to peak during the winter months with the onset of increased respiratory tract infections in children.

Acute OM can be clinically classified as either: 1) acute otitis (AOM) or 2) Otitis media with effusion (OME).[85] Chronic otitis media (COM) is defined as OM that persists beyond three months, and chronic suppurative otitis media (CSOM) represents a form of OM that is characterized by the presence of purulent otorrhea with chronic tympanic membrane perforation that persists for more than six weeks despite appropriate treatment for an initial AOM.[83]

Risk factors associated with the development of OM include atopy, chronic sinusitis, ciliary dysfunction, craniofacial abnormalities such as cleft palate, genetic conditions including Down's syndrome, immune incompetence and a patient age of less than two years.

Dysfunction or blockage of the eustachian tube is recognized as the primary mechanism initiating OM.[86] This dysfunction or blockage leads to negative middle ear cavity pressure with resultant aspiration of nasopharyngeal contents into the middle ear. Inflammation of the middle ear lining with effusion will typically ensue. OM associated eustachian tube dysfunction or blockage occurs in children as a result of viral infection in 75 percent of cases.[83] Viruses that are commonly encountered include *respiratory syncytial virus, parainfluenza (types 1, 2, 3) and influenza (A and B) adenovirus, and coronavirus*.[83,87] *Parechovirus and Human Metapneumonia virus (hMPV)* have also been identified in OM.[83]

Although viral infections are most often causal, bacterial infections enhance the risk of bacterial coinfection in OM. *Streptococcus pneumoniae, Haemophilus influenzae, Moraxella catarrhalis* and less commonly *Staphylococcus aureus* are frequently identified in OM.[88] In a case of CSOM, the most common bacterial pathogens are *P. aeruginosa, other enteric gram negative bacilli, and S. aureus* including *MRSA*.[83]

Clinical Features

Initial clinical symptoms in AOM include fever, otalgia, conductive hearing loss, usually accompanied by or preceded by an upper respiratory tract infection and allergic rhinitis. Otoscopic examination will reveal a hyperemic, opaque, bulging tympanic membrane with impaired motility, possible perforation and purulent otorrhea.

OME will generally cause few symptoms apart from hearing loss, while CSOM will tend to be characterized clinically by a perforated tympanic membrane with an associated chronic purulent discharge.

Pathologic Findings

Acute OM is usually treated by conservative non-invasive management; thus microscopic examination of tissue is uncommon. However, when tissue is obtained and examined, a mixed inflammatory infiltrate, congestion and edema with

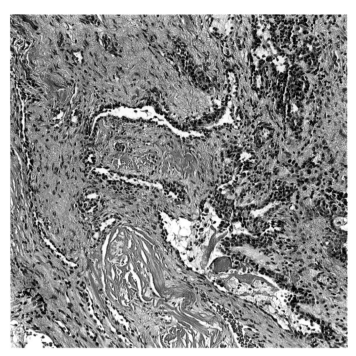

Figure 17.15 Thickened, fibrotic and folded middle ear lining mucosa with a mixed inflammatory cellular infiltrate can be seen in OM.

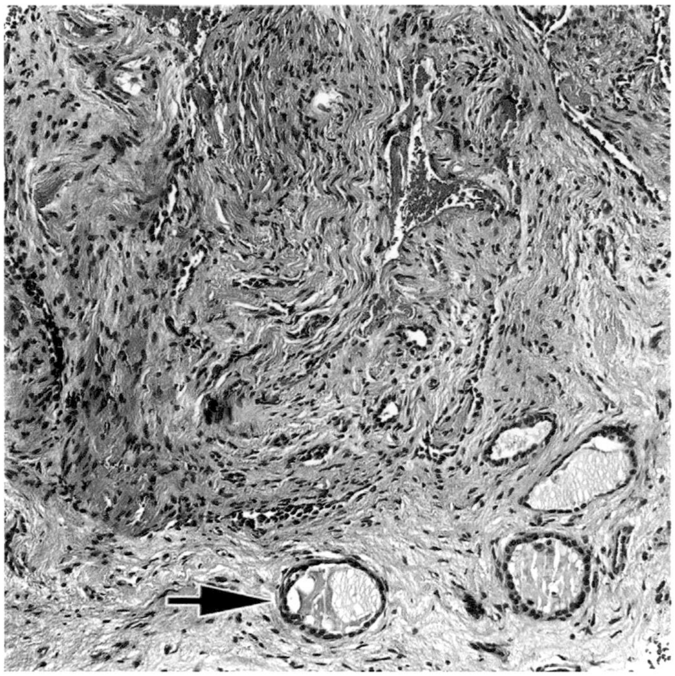

Figure 17.16 "Adenomatoid metaplasia" of the chronically inflamed middle ear epithelium in OM. Notice the pseudoglandular formations caused by invagination of the surface epithelium into the edematous underlying stroma (arrow).

polypoid mucosal thickening will be seen (Figure 17.15). Associated destruction of middle ear ossicles with scarring, fibrosing osteitis and sclerotic bone formation, are less common.

Chronic OM tends to demonstrate a more chronic inflammatory infiltrate histologically, including the accumulation of foreign body type giant cells. Glandular metaplasia (adenomatoid metaplasia) of the middle ear lining epithelium may also be seen (Figure 17.16) and can be a cause for concern as this transition may be confused with a glandular neoplasm. Fibrosis, granulation tissue accumulation, cholesterol granuloma formation, sclerosis of bone and tympanosclerosis may also be seen (Figure 17.17).

Treatment and Prognosis

The use of high dose Amoxicillin to treat initial episodes of non-severe OM is recommended.[85] Amoxicillin-Clavulanate can be used for patients with severe disease. Children with persistent OME as well as those patients who are at risk for developmental delay, or middle ear damage typically require insertion of a tympanostomy tube.[89]

Otic Polyp (Aural Polyp)
Clinical Findings

The otic polyp is a benign polypoid proliferation of chronically inflamed granulation tissue that arises from middle ear mucosa secondary to a long-standing middle ear infection, most often in children with chronic OM. Otic polyps can extend as a mass into the EAC in cases where there is tympanic membrane perforation.[90,91] Symptomatology can include

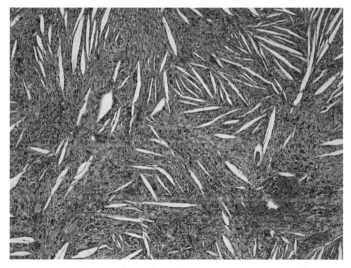

Figure 17.17 Cholesterol granuloma formation in COM. Note the fibrotic stroma with hemosiderin deposition and a background of chronic inflammation and numerous cholesterol clefts with surrounding giant cells and histiocytes.

otalgia, bleeding, conductive hearing loss or a sense on the part of the patient that an ear mass is present. CT scans can be employed to exclude neoplasia.

Pathologic Findings

On gross inspection aural polyps tend to be soft, nodular and rubbery in consistency. Microscopically, lesions are generally composed of edematous granulation tissue that is rich in

Benign Middle Ear Tumors

Middle Ear Adenoma (MEA)

MEA is an uncommon benign glandular neoplasm that will show variable morphologic, cytologic and IHC differentiation along neuroendocrine and mucin secreting pathways.[210,211,212,213] MEAs occur in all age groups, including the pediatric age group, where adolescents between 13 and 18 are favored.[214,215,216] The tumor accounts for less than 2 percent of ear tumors. No known tumor associated etiologic factor has been identified, and while some investigators theorized that the tumor is derived from enterochromaffin cells of the foregut,[217] others have suggested that these tumors are derived from epithelial stem cells that are capable of differentiating into both endocrine and non-endocrine cells.[218]

Clinical Features

The most common presenting symptom seen in patients with a MEA is unilateral conductive hearing loss and a reported feeling of fullness in the ear. Tinnitus and dizziness and bleeding may also be encountered. On otoscopic examination, the tympanic membrane is usually intact. Computerized CT scans will typically demonstrate opacification of the middle ear, and depending on the extent of the tumor, opacification of the mastoid. MRI will demonstrate and enhance middle ear mass.[219] Occasionally OM or a cholesteatoma may accompany the tumor. The tumor can be locally aggressive and may invade adjacent vital structures.

Pathologic Findings

On gross inspection, the MEA will most often to be a grey to red-brown, rubbery nodule or mass that will separate easily from associated bony structures. On microscopic examination, the tumor will be encapsulated, and composed of tumor aggregates that have an architecture that can be solid, cystic, trabecular or papillary in its presentation (Figure 17.32).

Ductal appearing spaces will be lined by eosinophilic cytoplasm, or by basaloid cuboidal or columnar cells. No myoepithelial layer will be identified surrounding glandular spaces. Tumor cells may appear plasmacytoid on occasion.[220] No significant mitotic activity will be seen in tumor cells and glandular lumena usually contain periodic acid Schiff and Alcian blue positive mucinous material.

Cytokeratin stains, including AE1/AE3, epithelial membrane antigen (EMA) and CK7 are usually reactive, while CK20 may be focally weak staining or negative. Depending on the degree of neuroendocrine expression; chromogranin, synaptophysin (Figure 17.33), neuron specific enolase (NSE), serotonin and human pancreatic polypeptide stains may be reactive in varying degrees. Desmin and Actin stains will be negative, however, S100 protein stains may be focally positive.[213,215] Electron microscopic analysis will[211] show basally situated cells containing neuroendocrine granules and apically situated dark cells containing mucous granules.

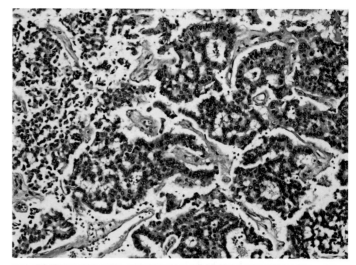

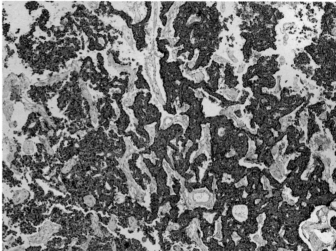

Figures 17.32 (top) & 17.33 (bottom) MEA. Cuboidal tumor cells line glandular spaces in this MEA (17.33). Strong synaptophysin expression, indicating neuroendocrine differentiation is demonstrated in a MEA.

Differential diagnoses include COM associated glandular metaplasia of the middle ear lining, ceruminal gland adenoma, paraganglioma, acoustic neuroma (AN), meningioma, endolymphatic sac papillary tumor (ESPT) and RMS.

Treatment and Prognosis

Surgical excision that includes the ossicular chain is the treatment of choice for the MEA, with simple excision being employed if the tumor is small and confined to the middle ear. More radical mastoidectomy has been employed for larger, more expansive tumors. Recurrence may occur due to incomplete tumor resection, and can be seen in 15 percent of patients.[213]

Paraganglioma (Glomus Jugulare/Tympanicum)

Naturally occurring glomus bodies can be found along the course of the tympanic branch of the glossopharyngeal nerve as it progresses from the jugular fossa to the promontory of the middle ear and Jacobson nerve.[221] From a radiographic standpoint the glomus jugulotympanium and the glomus tympanicum are distinctive lesions; however, they are histologically identical.

Paragangliomas arising along this nerve were first described in 1945 by Rosenwasser.[222] These tumors are exceedingly rare in pediatric age group patients,[223,224,225,226,227,228,229,230] but have been reported in children as young as six months of age.[223,224,225,226,227,228]

Glomus tympanicum can also present as a familial tumor with an autosomal dominant pattern of inheritance. Two affected genetic loci have been identified (11q13.1 and 11q22.3-q23).[231] Tumors in the pediatric age group can be associated with multiple endocrine neoplasia syndrome II or with von Hippel–Lindau disease.

Tumors arise from chemoreceptor paraganglial cells. In addition to being familial in origin, tumors can also be multicentric and bilateral. Only 10 percent of tumors occur in children.

A variable range of symptoms has been repeated in pediatric age group patients, ranging from OM with ear discharge, to pulsating tinnitus, to pain and conductive deafness. Twenty five percent of pediatric cases have been shown to secrete vasoactive endocrine substances in comparison to only 3 percent of adult cases. Thus, routine analysis of urine for catecholamines, and VMA levels in children with suggestive symptoms is warranted.[224,226] The tumor can be multifocal in 25 percent of cases,[224,227,228] resulting in multi-site glomus jugulare and glomus tympanicum tumors. Pediatric glomus tympanicum can be a biologically aggressive tumor.

Otoscopic examination in uncomplicated cases will show a red pulsatile mass behind an intact tympanic membrane. In complicated cases OM will generally also be seen with associated erosion of the mastoid, and rarely conductive deafness. CT with contrast or MRI will demonstrate the presence of a vascular mass in nearly all cases.

Tumors can be classified and staged according to size[232] as type I to IV tumors. Type I tumors tend to be small and involve the jugular bulb and middle ear, whereas Type IV tumors may well demonstrate mastoid involvement and intracranial extension.

Mutations at the germline level have been identified and include mutations in subunits of the juccinate-ubiquinone oxidoreductase gene.

Pathologic Findings

On gross inspection, the glomus tumor will be a red friable mass. On microscopic examination, the tumor will be composed of Zellballen nests of "chief cells" with round to oval or spindle shaped nuclei. Chromatin will be coarse and dispersed and tumor cells will have abundant eosinophilic granular cytoplasm. Chief cell nests will be surrounded by spindle-shaped sustentacular cells which represent modified Schwann cells (Figure 17.34). FNA will show three cell types: small polyglonal cells, spindle cells and large strap cells.

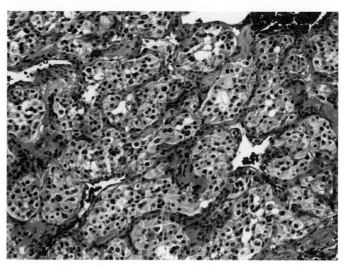

Figure 17.34 Glomus tympanicum tumor. Cell nests composed of chief cells showing neuroendocrine features are evident. Cells have abundant eosinophilic cytoplasm and nuclei with "salt and pepper" appearing chromatin. Tumor cell nests are surrounded by spindle shaped sustentacular cells.

Sustentacular cells will be S100 protein positive, while chief cells will be positive for neuroendocrine markers including chromogranin and synaptophysin, and negative for pancytokeratin.

Differential diagnoses include MEA, AN and meningioma. S100 protein stains will verify a diagnosis of AN whereas meningioma will demonstrate psammoma bodies and EMA reactivity. The MEA will be unique among the three lesions in that it will display a glandular appearance.

Treatment and Prognosis

Complete surgical excision is the treatment of choice for paragangliomas. Tympanotomy can be employed as can mastoidectomy. Preoperative embolization has been advocated as a method of decreasing the vascularity during the operative procedure. The invasiveness of these tumors may preclude complete tumor excision and radiotherapy has been used as an adjuvant form of therapy. Tumors in the pediatric age group can be biologically aggressive and even fatal due to the proximity of the tumor to anatomic structures that are vital.[224,225,226,227,228]

Mucosal Papillomas of the Middle Ear

Mucosal papillomas that involve the middle ear of children and adolescents are rare.[233] Etiologically these lesions are related to embryological migration of schneiderian mucosa into the middle ear, followed by chronic mucosal irritation and ultimate tumor production.[234,235]

Symptoms vary, and range from COM preceding the onset of a middle ear papilloma to conductive hearing loss, and otorrhea.[233,234,235,236] The tympanic membrane may be either intact or perforated in instances of middle ear papillomas or papillomatosis. *Microscopically*, lesions in this site are similar to sinonasal schneiderian papillomas of the inverted and cylindrical type

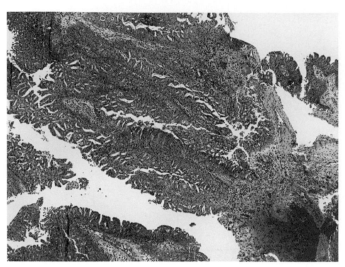

Figure 17.35 Schneiderian oncocytic type papilloma of middle ear showing both inverted and exophytic growth patterns.

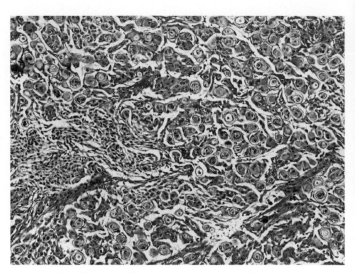

Figure 17.36 Meningothelial meningioma of the middle ear. Note the absence of psammoma body formation in the tumor. Syncytial cells with round to oval nuclei are arranged in cellular whorls.

(Figure 17.35). Microscopic *differential diagnoses* include MEA, glomus tympanicum and endolymphatic sac adenocarcinoma. The treatment of choice for a middle ear papilloma is surgical excision of the lesion. Recurrence is uncommon.

Other Benign Tumors of the Temporal Bone

Extracranial Meningiomas

Meningiomas represent benign neoplasms that arise from the arachnoid cells that form the arachnoid villi, and although they are a common intracranial tumor, pediatric cases are rare and account for no more than 1.5 percent of all intracranial meningiomas. Primary extracranial meningiomas, including those of the ear and temporal bone of pediatric age individuals have been cited even more sporadically in the literature.[237,238,239,240,241,242]

Extracranial meningiomas can affect the external ear, the middle ear and other temporal bone sites including the internal auditory canal, jugular foramen, geniculate ganglion, roof of eustachian tube or sulcus of the greater petrosal nerve.[237,238,239,240,241,242] Cerebellopontine angle meningiomas can also extend into the internal ear canal.[243]

The association of neurofibromatosis type II (NF-2) with meningiomas, is well documented in the adult population, but that association has not been reported in the pediatric population where the ear is involved.[244]

Clinical Features

Symptoms will vary according to the site of the tumor, to include conductive or sensorineural hearing loss, headaches, vertigo, and dizziness, loss of balance, cranial nerve abnormalities and OM as the most common symptoms in children.

CT and MRI will reveal a soft tissue density with variable vascularity, and associated temporal air space cell opacification, bone erosion, sclerosis or hyperostosis.

Pathologic Findings

On gross examination, the tumor is typically a lobular, rubbery to firm or occasionally gritty mass.

Microscopically the extracranial meningioma will be composed of nests of epithelioid appearing tumor cells. Tumor cells will typically have a syncytial pattern of arrangement. Four histologic variants may be identified, with the meningothelial or syncytial variant being most common variant seen in pediatric age patients. (Figure 17.36) Fibroblastic, transitional and angioblastic variants have of the tumor are rare in children. No relationship has been observed that links histologic subtype to tumor behavior.

Tumor cells will generally be arranged in lobules and tumor cell nuclei will tend to have a delicate chromatin pattern. Intranuclear inclusions and calcifications in the form of psammoma bodies, typically less common than they are in extracranial meningiomas may be seen. Synchronous meningomas and cholesteatomas have been observed but they are extremely rare in children.[238] Tumors will be EMA, keratin and CAM5.2 positive and only weakly positive for S100 protein. Chromogranin and synaptophysin will be non-reactive.

Differential diagnoses include MEA, jugulotympanic paraganglioma and AN.

Treatment and Prognosis

Complete surgical excision is the treatment of choice for the extracranial meningioma.[238] Malignant change can occur and has been reported in children in a cerebellopontine angle location.[243] Tumors recur approximately 20 percent of the time and the five-year survival rate is in the 75 to 80 percent range.

Acoustic Neuroma (Schwannoma)

AN is a benign nerve sheath neoplasm that is in fact a schwannoma that most often arises from the vestibulocochlear nerve within the internal auditory canal. The majority of such tumors involve the vestibular division of the eighth nerve rather than its cochlear division. The tumor is extremely rare in children,[245,246,247,248,249] and arises most often along the so-called Rednik–Obersteiner line or the neuroglial/neurolemmal junction, which is usually located immediately inside the internal auditory meatus. Arising from schwann cell origin, the tumor has no definitive causation, although loud noise and trauma have been suggested as possible etiologies.

Clinical Features

ANs account for 6 to 10 percent of all intracranial tumors and they can occur as sporadic tumors and arise as unilateral lesions,[245] or they can be found in pediatric age patients in association with neurofibromatosis-II in which bilateral ANs represent a hallmark of the syndrome.[246]

Most neurofibromatosis-II patients with AN tend to be in their teens and most will present with sensorineural hearing loss, tinnitus and disequilibrium with gait instability. If the tumor enlarges it can affect adjacent cranial nerves (V, VII, IX, X, XI) leading to facial paresis and other cranial nerve deficits. Increased intracranial pressure symptomotology and signs, including headache, vomiting, papilledema and even death can occur when there is secondary tumor extension associated herniation of the brain stem. The duration of symptoms can be variable, ranging from a few weeks to five years in some cases.[245]

MRI is considered to be a sensitive tool in the radiological identification of AN and will usually show widening or erosion of the internal auditory canal with intense enhancement in the porus acustius region. CT scans will often show internal auditory canal widening.[250]

Pathologic Findings

On gross examination, ANs are usually firm, white to grey or yellow tan in color and they are often cystic. Tumors generally range in size from 10 to 60 mm in diameter.[245]

Microscopic inspection of the tumor will show the characteristic appearance of a schwannoma with alternating Antoni-A spindle cells, and Antoni-B eosinophilic hypocellular zones (Figure 17.37). Characteristic Verocay bodies may also be seen. Tumor cell nuclei tend to be elongated and twisted or wavy. Degenerative changes are common, including cystic changes, hyalinization, hemorrhage, dystrophic calcifications and necrosis. Rare mitotic activity may be seen, but does not confer a diagnosis of malignancy.

Schwannomas typically stain positively for S100 protein and negatively for keratins and neuroendocrine markers.

Differential diagnoses include MEA, Jugulotympanic paraganglioma and meningioma, and solitary fibrous tumor. Meningiomas will have a whorled appearance and will often contain psammoma bodies whereas AN will not. The solitary fibrous tumor will be CD34 and BCL–2 immunoreactive.

Treatment and Prognosis

Complete surgical excision with functional preservation of the facial nerve and cochlear function using a translabyrinthine or

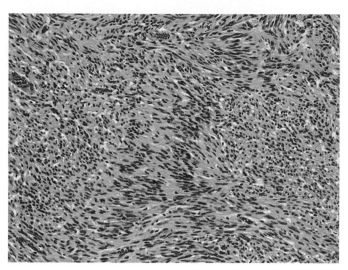

Figure 17.37 Schwannoma of the internal acoustic meatus. Notice the highly cellular (Antoni A) spindle cell component, and the acellular eosinophilic (Antoni B) zones.

retrosigmoid approach[251,252] represent the treatments of choice for AN in pediatric age patients, most of whom will be NF-2 patients. Embolization of the tumor has been employed in children in an attempt to reduce tumor vascularity and the associated risk.[247] New neurosurgical techniques with improved imaging, cranial nerve monitoring and neuroanesthesia have reduced the need for embolization.[251] Malignant change in AN is exceedingly rare. Patients will have a very good prognosis and the tumor is rarely recurrent.

Mesenchymal Tumors

Mesenchymal tumors of the middle ear include hemangioma, lipoma, osteoblastoma, chondroblastoma, teratoma and osteoma. The histopathology and pathobiology of these tumors are discussed elsewhere in this text.

Tumors of Indeterminate Biologic Behavior and Malignant Tumors of the Ear

Tumors of indeterminate biologic behavior and malignant ear tumors are extremely rare entities that are seldom encountered in pediatric patients. RMS, a neoplasm that can be encountered in all areas of the head and neck, is the most common offender.

Tumors of Indeterminent Biologic Behavior

ESPT, first described by Heffner in 1988[253] is a rare low grade locally aggressive papillary neoplasm that causes extensive bony destruction and invasion. The tumor arises from the pars rugosa of the endolymphatic sac[254] and has been reported in pediatric age group in patients as young as four years.[253,254,256] Many cases have been identified in association with von Hippel–Lindau disease (VHL) [255,257]

Clinical Findings

Symptoms will most often include unilateral sensorineural hearing loss together with tinnitus, vertigo, ataxia and cranial nerve paresis or paralysis, particularly of the facial nerve. Serous OM or an epitympanic mass may be seen.

CT scan and MRI will show a lytic bone lesion and the tumor will tend to invade posteriorly toward the cerebellopontine angle or anterolaterally to the temporal bone.[254]

The diagnosis of ESPT should prompt evaluation of the patient for VHL, an autosomal dominant disorder with variable expression caused by mutations of the von Hippel–Lindau tumor suppressor gene.[255,256]

Pathologic Findings

On microscopic examination, the tumor will show complex papillary structures and cystic areas that will be lined by a single layer of uniform flat or cuboidal to columnar epithelial cells. These lining cells will have eosinophilic to clear cytoplasm and generally indistinct cell borders (Figure 17.38). Nuclear pleomorphism, if present, will be minimal and in some instances crowded cystic or glandular appearing areas will contain eosinophilic colloid-like material. An intervening hypervascular stroma in which degenerative changes, are common, including dystrophic calcifications, psammoma bodies and cholesterol granulomas will be seen.

Periodic acid Schiff stains with and without diastase will positively stain intracytoplasmic and the colloid like secretions. On rare occasion, mucicarmine stains may be focally positive for mucin. Tumor cells will be strongly positive for cytokeratins and variably positive for EMA, S100 protein, NSE, Synaptophysin, Ber-EP4 and GFAP. Thyroglobulin and TTF-1 stains will be non-reactive.

Differential diagnoses include, MEA, choroid plexus papilloma, ceruminal gland adenocarcinoma and metastatic adenocarcinoma.

Treatment and Prognosis

The management of ESPT is primarily surgical through a transtemporal approach or by the use of suboccipital craniotomy

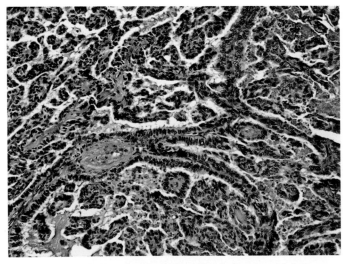

Figure 17.38 ESPT. Note the arborized papillary formations with lining cuboidal cells.

to gain exposure. Complete removal is essential, as recurrence will almost certainly occur if the tumor is incompletely removed. Postoperative radiation may be used in cases where complete resection is not possible. The ESPT which is quite aggressive, biologically, can show widespread infiltration and destructive, and can eventually result in death if left untreated.

Malignant Tumors

Malignant epithelial tumors of the ear that are commonly seen in adults including squamous cell carcinoma and ceruminal gland adenocarcinoma are exceedingly rare in children. RMS, however, represents a commonly encountered malignancy in this site in children. Chondrosarcoma and osteosarcoma can also be encountered in the ear. Cutaneous malignancies, including basal cell carcinoma melanoma, dermatofibrosarcoma protuberans, merkel cell carcinoma and pleomorphic undifferentiated sarcoma which can involve the ear are described in Chapters 2 and 4 of this textbook.

Rhabdomyosarcoma

RMS is the third most common sarcoma of childhood[258] with 35 percent of cases occurring in the head and neck region.[259,260] Ear involvement by RMS is uncommon,[261,262,263] but well documented. Most affected individuals will be under the age of 20, and the embryonal histologic subtype of the tumor is most common. Males are more often affected than females and the auditory canal and middle ear are the most common site of origin.

Clinical Findings

Most pediatric age patients with RMS will present with nonspecific aural symptoms that include chronic aural discharge, unresponsiveness to repeated OM antibiotic therapy, otalgia, aural polyposis, and facial nerve paresis or paralysis. Paralysis of other cranial nerves including II, V, VI and XII and unilateral dearness can also occur. Larger neglected tumors may sometimes present as an aural fungating mass with associated regional deformity. Growth disturbance has been encountered in some children affected by the tumor.[263] CT scans will show a mass consistent with an expansile growth.

Pathologic Findings

Details concerning the microscopic diagnosis and histologic features of RMS are discussed in Chapter 2 of this textbook. Among the four histologic types of tumors (embryonal, alveolar, pleomorphic and botryoid), embryonal RMS is the most common type to be encountered in the ear in pediatric age group patients. Embryonal RMS is characterized by the proliferation of rhabdomyoblasts that display eosinophilic cytoplasm with cellular elongation toward a so-called tadpole pattern (Figure 17.39). The stroma of the tumor will generally be myxomatous in appearance and markedly edematous. Differential diagnoses include aural polyp, lymphoma and fetal rhabdomyoma.

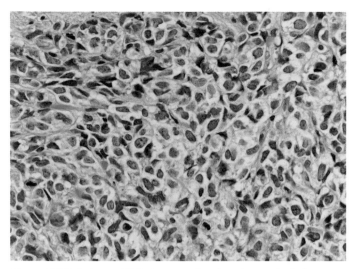

Figure 17.39 Embryonal RMS demonstrating abundant cytologically malignant rhabdomyoblasts.

Treatment and Prognosis

Although RMS has historically carried a poor prognosis, the advent of multimodal treatment by a multidisciplinary team has greatly improved the outcome for many pediatric age patients.[263,264,265] Davidson, in 1966, reported a mean survival rate of 11 months for ear tumors.[266] The international society of pediatric oncology[264] now reports complete remission with modern chemotherapeutic and radiation therapy treatment modalities in 91 percent of patients diagnosed initially with non-metastatic disease.

Younger patients with PAX7-FKHR gene mutation tumors which are less locally aggressive fair better, as do patients with smaller tumors.

Metastasis occurs in 20 percent of cases to regional lymph nodes, or distant hematogenous metastasis will occur to the lungs, bone marrow, brain, liver, pancreas and heart.[263]

Basal Cell Carcinoma

Basal cell carcinomas in children are extremely rare entities and are usually seen in association with basal cell nevus syndrome,[267] xeroderma pigmentosum,[268] nevus sebaceus[269] or following high dose radiotherapy. Sporadic de novo, idiopathic cases involving the ear have been reported.[270,271,272]

Due to the low index of suspicion on the part of practitioners, and the rarity of these lesions in children, delayed diagnosis can be quite problematic. The histopathology of basal cell carcinoma is discussed in more detail in Chapter 4 of this textbook.

Other Tumors

Malignant salivary gland tumors of the parotid gland can occasionally involve the ear due to the glands' proximity to the ear. Ceruminal gland malignancies including adenoid cystic carcinoma, mucoepidermoid carcinoma, adenocarcinoma and squamous cell carcinoma are rarely seen in pediatric age patients.

References

Accessory Tragus

1. Wood-Jones F, Chuan IW. The development of the external ear. *J Anat* 1933–1934; 68:525–533.

2. Jansen T, Romiti R, Altmeyer P. Accessory Tragus: report of two cases and review of the literature. *Pediatr Dermatol* 2000; 17:391–394.

3. Melnick M, Myrianthopolos NC. External ear malformations: epidemiology, genetics, and natural history. *Birth defects* 1979; 15:1–138.

4. Weichmann A. Briecht uber die in den jahren bis 1893 bis juli 1912 in der koniglichen universitats-Poliklinik ohern-, nasen- und halskrankheiten in Gottingen beobachtenen angeborenen missidungen des ohers (dissertation). *Gottengen* 1912.

5. Guszman J. Beitrage Zur Lehre der branchiogenen ohr-und halsanhange. *Z Ges Anat* 1926; 81: 554–562.

6. Chintalapati K, Gunasekaran S, Frewer J. Accessory tragus in the middle ear: A rare congenital anomaly. *Int. J Pediatr Otorhinolaryngol* 2010; 74:1338–1339.

Middle Ear Choristoma

7. Taylor GD, Martin HF. Salivary gland tissue in the middle ear. A rare Tumor. *Arch Otolaryngol.* 1961; 73:651–657.

8. Ha SL, Shin JE, Yoon TH. Salivary gland choristoma of the middle ear: a case report and review of the literature. *Laryngoscope* 1984; 94: 228–230.

9. Farneti P, Balbi M, Foschini MP. Neuroglial choristoma of the middle ear. *Acta Otorhinolaryngologica Italica* 2007; 27:94–97.

10. Kartush JM, Graham MD, Arbor A. Salivary gland choristoma of the middle ear: A case report and review of the literature. *Laryngoscope* 1984; 94:228–230.

11. Morimotot N, Ogawa K, Kanzaki. Salivary gland choristoma in the middle ear. A case report. *Am J Otolaryngol* 1999; 20: 232–235.

12. Patten BM. *Human Embryology.* 3rd Ed. New York NY: McGraw-Hill 1986.

13. Enoz M, Suoglu Y. Salivary gland choristoma of the middle ear. *Laryngoscope* 2006; 116:1033–1034.

14. Gyure AJ, Glasscock ME, Pensak ML. A clinicopathologic study of 15 patients with neuroglial heterotopias and encephaloceles of the middle ear and mastoid region. *Laryngsocope* 2000; 110:1731–1735.

15. Plontke SK, Preyer S, Pressler H, Mundiger PM, Plinkert PK. Glial lesion of the infratemporal fossa presenting as a soft tissue middle ear mass – rudimentary encephalocele or neural crest remnant? *Int. J Pediatr Otorhinolaryngol* 2000; 56:141–147.

16. Nelson EG, Kratz RC. Sebaceous choristoma of the middle ear. *Otolaryngol Head Neck Surg* 1993; 108:372–373.

17. Lee DK, Kim JH, Cho YS, et al. Salivary gland choristoma of the middle ear in an infant: a case report. *Int J Pediatr Otorhinolaryngol* 2006; 70:167–170.

18. Saeed YM, Bassis ML. Mixed tumor of the middle ear. A case report. *Arch Otolaryngol* 1971; 93:433–434.

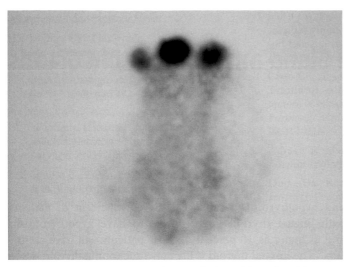

Figure 18.2 A (131I) radionucleotide scan of a lingual thyroid nodule. Note the intake. The patient had no thyroid gland in the neck. (Reprinted from Marx R, Stern D. *Oral and Maxillofacial Pathology: A Rationale for Diagnosis and Treatment* with permission from Quintessence Publishing Company).

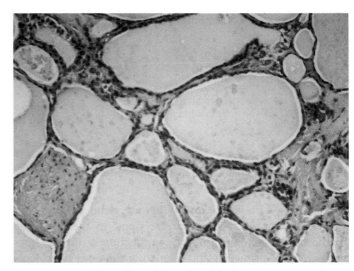

Figure 18.3 Histology of lingual thyroid nodule demonstrating normal thyroid glandular tissue. (Reprinted from Marx R, Stern D. *Oral and Maxillofacial Pathology: A Rationale for Diagnosis and Treatment* with permission from Quintessence Publishing Company).

bundles and can appear infiltrative, although the process is benign. Thyroid follicular cells will generally appear histologically normal or occasionally atrophic. Parathyroid tissue may also be identified incorporated within the nodular architecture of the persistent lingual thyroid. Mutations in transcription fermination factor-2 (TTF2) and PAX8 as well as mutations in thyrotropin (TSH) receptor genes have been reported in a small percentage of children with dysgenesis of the thyroid.[8] However, these findings have not been reported in instances of ectopic thyroid tissue.

Treatment and Prognosis

Since the majority of patients with persistent lingual thyroid tissue are asymptomatic, biopsy of a suspected lingual thyroid nodule is typically not undertaken until a diagnosis of persistent lingual thyroid gland is ruled out, and no treatment should be undertaken in patients with suspected lingual thyroid nodules until an 131I radioisotope scan has been done in order to determine whether or not the patient has adequate normal thyroid tissue in the neck. In those children who are symptomatic and who have appropriate thyroid tissue in the neck, surgical excision of the lingual thyroid can be contemplated. In most cases however, the lingual thyroid nodule should not be surgically removed, given the surgical risk of hemorrhage or infection. In addition, it is possible to induce a thyroid storm, resulting in the release of copious amounts of thyroid hormone into the vascular system when a surgical procedure is undertaken. Thyroid ablation with radioactive iodine can be used to eradicate functioning ectopic thyroid tissue if necessary. On rare occasions, children with lingual thyroid nodules, who also have entrapped parathyroid tissue within the nodule, may develop tetany if the thyroid tissue is removed.

Lingual thyroid tissue has the same inherent potential to develop pathologies as normal thyroid tissue does, including carcinoma, adenomas and goiter.[9,10,11,12,13] The vast majority of reports in the literature where such transitions have occurred in children have occurred in males.[14,15,16,17,18,19] Thyroid carcinoma of any type arising from a lingual thyroid is rare. It is important to recognize that 75 percent of patients with infantile hypothyroidism who present with thyroid tissue as a mass in the tongue will indeed not have thyroid carcinoma.[6]

Ectopic/Heterotopic Thyroid Tissue and Parasitic Thyroid Nodules

Heterotopia, the presence of normal thyroid tissue in an abnormal location is uncommon.[1,2,3] The most common sites of occurrence aside from lingual thyroid tissue are the sella turcica, submandibular region, larynx and trachea, esophagus, liver, gall bladder and common bile duct, mediastinum, pancreas, adrenal gland and retroperitoneum and ovarian tissue (struma ovarii) (Figure 18.4). Histologically, the ectopic tissue will consist of normal thyroid tissue.

A "parasitic thyroid nodule" is a thyroid nodule that is anatomically separated from the main thyroid gland. These nodules usually result from the formation of colloid or hyperplastic thyroid tissue that grows and gradually shifts its position to a site that is rather than midline, more lateral in the neck. The nodule can either lose its connection with the thyroid gland or maintain a tenuous attachment to the main thyroid gland. Malignant change in heterotopic thyroid tissue can occur, but occurs primarily in adults, and only rarely in pediatric age group patients.

Thyroglossal Tract Cyst (Thyroglossal Duct Cyst)

The thyroglossal tract cyst represents a cystic dilatation of the thyroglossal duct in the midline of the neck. The cyst occurs most often above the level of the thyroid isthmus and below the level of the hyoid bone. Although most cysts occur in the

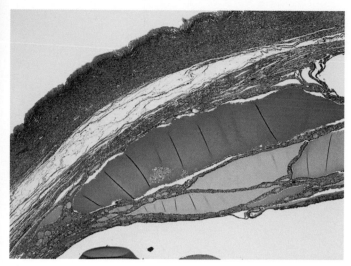

Figure 18.4 Struma ovarii. This photomicrograph demonstrates benign thyroid tissue partially surrounded by ovarian tissue.

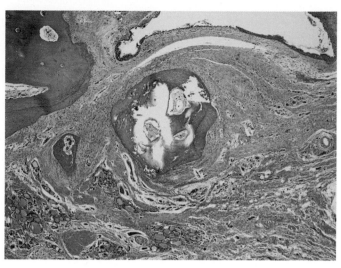

Figure 18.6 Thyroglossal tract cyst. Hyoid bone segments are seen with an intervening thyroglossal duct cyst that is lined by respiratory type epithelium. Benign thyroid follicles can be seen where the thyroglossal tract cyst perforates the hyoid bone.

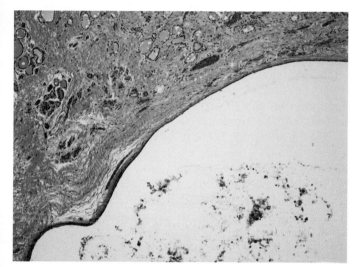

Figure 18.5 Thyroglossal tract cyst. A large cystic space lined by thin squamous epithelium and marginated by benign thyroid follicles set in fibrous tissue characterize this thyroglossal tract cyst.

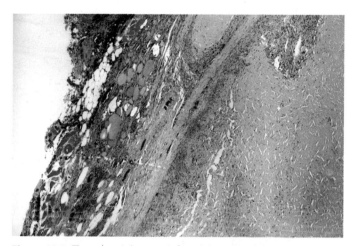

Figure 18.7 Thyroglossal duct cyst. Infected thyroglossal duct cyst containing central basophilic debris and marginated by histiocytes and chronic inflammatory cells.

midline, rare instances of lateral thyroglossal duct cysts can also occur.[20,21,22,23,24,25]

The thyroglossal cyst is usually connected to the hyoid bone and rarely the cyst may perforate that bone. Most lesions will present as an asymptomatic neck mass unless infected, when they often will present as tender midline swelling. The cyst will move up and down with deglutition and moves upwards when the tongue is protruded.

In children, lesions of significant size can cause respiratory compromise or even obstruction with cyanosis.[23]

Pathologic Features

Histologically, the thyroglossal duct cyst will be lined by respiratory or squamous epithelium (Figure 18.5). The wall of the cyst will generally contain benign thyroid tissue in the

majority of cases, although the thyroid tissue can appear hyperplastic or even neoplastic. Cysts can penetrate the hyoid bone (Figure 18.6) or become infected (Figure 18.7). Malignant change can occur in thyroglossal duct cysts in children[25] (Figure 18.8); however, such changes are rare.

Differential diagnoses include thymic cyst, dermoid cyst, laryngocele, branchial cleft cyst and metastatic thyroid carcinoma.

Treatment and Prognosis

The treatment of choice for the thyroglossal tract cyst is en bloc resection of the cyst with the central portion of the hyoid bone.[26] A further discussion of thyroglossal tract cyst can be found in Chapter 7, odontogenic and non-odontogenic cysts.

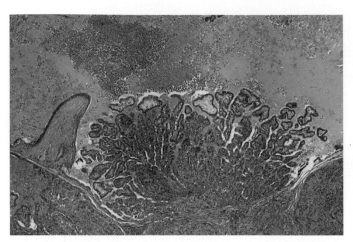

Figure 18.8 Thyroglossal duct cyst demonstrating a papillary thyroid carcinoma (PTC) developing within the epithelial lining.

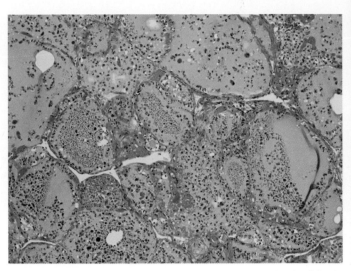

Figure 18.9 Black thyroid. Note the black pigment entrapped within follicular cells and also the colloidal component of the associated glandular tissue.

Thyroid Inclusions in Lymph Nodes

Thyroid inclusions in lymph nodes can represent a controversial finding, largely because the presence of such a finding triggers the question of whether or not a true malignancy might not exist. Investigators who accept thyroid inclusions in lymph nodes as a true pathologic entity report strict criteria for its diagnosis:[27,28,29] (1) The lymph node should be located in midline or medial to the jugular vein; (2) The identified thyroid tissue must be located in the nodal capsule and cannot otherwise replace lymphoid parenchyma; (3) The thyroid inclusions must be cytologically bland with evidence of atypia and (4) There must be absence of a primary thyroid cancer.

The diagnosis of benign thyroid inclusion should be made with extreme care even if the above criteria are met. Principal differential diagnoses most often include metastatic tumor, and Hashimoto's thyroiditis, in which thyroid nodularity may appear in concert with lymphoid tissue containing germinal centers. Studies of BRAF mutations in thyroid inclusion nodules have shown an absence of mutations in up to 69 percent of Hashimoto's thyroiditis cases. This finding is in contrast to those seen in papillary thyroid carcinoma (PTC), where BRAF mutations are far more common.[4] Thus, this molecular assessment can prove valuable in distinguishing a thyroid inclusion from cancer.

Thyroid Pigment and Crystal Deposition

The term "black thyroid" has been used to describe a condition in children and adults who have taken minocycline, with the resultant deposition of a dark brown to black pigment in the apex of the follicular cells and in the colloid of the thyroid gland.[30,31] (See Figure 18.9.) Black thyroids show no functional abnormalities. Crystals can also appear in the thyroid gland during childhood. Chief among these is calcium oxalate crystal deposition.[32]

Autoimmune Thyroid Disease

Chronic Lymphocytic Thyroiditis (Hashimoto's Thyroiditis)

Hashimoto's thyroiditis is an autoimmune disorder characterized most commonly by hypoparathyroidism, due to cell and antibody mediated immune mechanisms.

The disease, which is five to seven times more common in women than men, typically affects individuals in the 30 to 45 year age group. However, Hashimoto's thyroiditis does affect pediatric age individuals, primarily female teenagers as the most common cause of thyroid disease in children and adolescents. Individuals otherwise at risk include patients with a family history of disorders of the thyroid. Aberrancy in the HLA-DR5 gene and the cytotoxic T-lymphocyte antigen 4 gene puts individuals further at risk.

Chronic lymphocytic thyroiditis (CLT) accounts for approximately 40 percent of goiters in adolescents. Most patients with CLT are diagnosed between the ages of 10 and 12. Lesions typically present as smooth, nodular enlargements. The vast majority of patients will be euthyroid or asymptomatic at the time of diagnosis. Less than 5 percent of patients will have thyrotoxicosis. The etiology of the disorder has not been fully delineated but it is suspected that t-cell mediated cytotoxicity in which there is cytokine immune surveillance loss in a toxicity that is directed again follicular epithelial cells. CLT in children tends to sporadic. The disorder can be associated with chronic juvenile arthritis, lupus erythematosus, Sjogrens syndrome and mixed connective tissue disease. Most tumors are diagnosed on the basis of a final needle aspiration biopsy.

Clinical Findings

Pediatric age group patients can present with an enlarged, firm, lobulated thyroid gland, or they may present with minimal changes in the thyroid, such that no lesion is palpable.[41] The

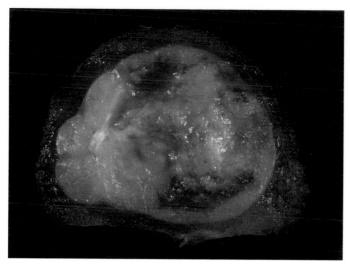

Figure 18.10 Hashimoto's thyroiditis. Gross photograph.

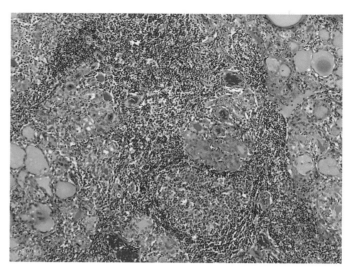

Figure 18.11 Hashimoto's thyroiditis. Classic features of Hashimoto's thyroiditis showing a dense lymphoplasmacytic infiltrate with the formation of germinal centers, glandular atrophy and Hürthle cell metaplasia are seen in this photomicrograph.

disease can be further classified as either *classic* or *fibrous* although four histologic variants of the disease are common. The classic form of the disease, and the most common, occurs in children most often due to a goiter or due to iodine deficiency in iodine replete areas of the globe.[37,38,39,40] Females are more often affected than males (10:1). The fibrous end stage variant occurs in only 10 percent of cases. Children can present with no signs or symptoms or with a goiter in which bilateral diffuse enlargement of the thyroid may be seen. Decreased thyroxine (T4) levels and rarely decreased thyroid stimulating hormone (T3) levels will be seen, but most patients are euthyroid.

Hashimoto's thyroiditis and atrophic thyroiditis are the most common subtypes of chronic lymphocytic thyroiditis to cause juvenile hypothyroidism.[33] The disease shows a female predilection and occurs most frequently in patients with a family history of autoimmune thyroid disease. Patients with insulin dependent diabetes and autoimmune polyglandular syndrome, Down's syndrome, Turner syndrome and Klinefelter syndrome are most commonly affected.[34,35,36] At the onset of disease, patients may be euthyroid or hyperthyroid before reverting to a hypothyroid state.

The disease can be further confirmed clinically by detecting antibodies to TG and particularly TPO which are detectable in most patients with chronic lymphocytic thyroiditis and are used as markers for the disease.

Pathologic Features

Grossly, the gland will appear firm, enlarged with nodular mass or masses (Figure 18.10) or in late stages a more atrophic mass. The thyroid capsule will generally be intact. Hashimoto's thyroiditis is characterized histologically by the presence of a dense lymphocytic glandular infiltrate that can form lymphoid follicles (Figure 18.11). The infiltrate will be rich in lymphocytes and overly rich in plasma cells. Most lymphoid follicles had a well defined germinal center and mantle zone with an absent marginal zone. Focal to complete effacement of the

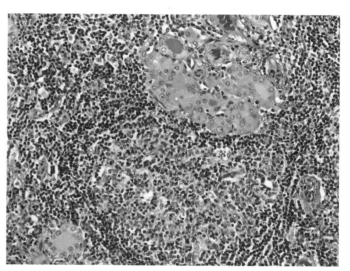

Figure 18.12 High power photomicrograph demonstrating Hürthle cell metaplasia and a lymphocytic infiltrate forming germinal centers.

architecture of the gland with localized fibrosis and nodule formation or atrophy of thyroid follicles will be seen. Focal to extensive Hürthle cell metaplasia (Figure 18.12) will be seen. These eosinophilic cells with granular cytoplasm will marginate atrophic colloid zones. Atypical nuclear features can be seen in follicular lymphocytic cells. Squamous metaplasia can also be seen (Figure 18.13).

Histologic variants of Hashimoto's thyroiditis include: a fibrous variant, a fibrous atrophy variant, a juvenile variant and a cystic variant. Most patients with Hashimoto's associated thyroiditis will remain hypothyroid.

Treatment and Prognosis

Levothyroxine treatment is the most common management modality for Hashimoto's thyroiditis. This drug has been

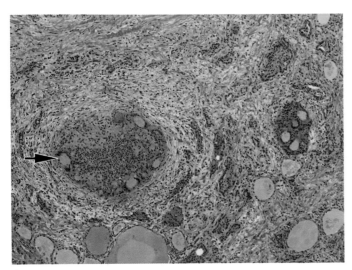

Figure 18.17 Granulomatous thyroiditis (De Quervain's thyroiditis) demonstrating granuloma formation with residual acute and chronic inflammation and giant cell formation (arrow).

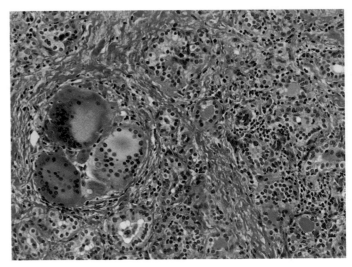

Figure 18.18 Small granulomas with giant cells and mild chronic inflammation can be seen in this example of palpation thyroiditis.

and supportive, while prednisone is generally employed in severe cases.

Other less common causes of granulomatous forms of thyroiditis include fungal, mycobacterial infections, sarcoidosis and syphilis.

Palpation thyroiditis occurs due to thyroid trauma or significant palpation of the gland. Histologically a follicle or a small group of follicles will be affected in association with follicular epithelial loss. Colloid will spill into the parenchyma of the gland and granuloma formation and foreign body giant cell aggregation will ensure. (Figure 18.18)

Neonal hypothyroidism

Neonatal Hypothyroidism

The worldwide incidence of *congenital hypothyroidism* is not definitively known but is thought to be more than 1 in 2500 infants.[54,55,56,57] The diagnosis of hypothyroidism must be made early within the first few days of life in order to prevent the development of many of the disorder's harmful effects, chief among them, mental retardation. Measurement of T4 and/or serum TSH concentrations represents the most important of screening strategies.[54,55,58,59] TSH levels will be elevated in primary hypothyroidism or compensated hypothyroidism.

Hypothyroidism in neonates can be permanent or transient. The causes of permanent neonatal hypothyroidism include 1) thyroid dysgenesis,[60,61] 2) Inborn errors of thyroid hormone production including, low TSH responsiveness, low or absent iodide concentration, defective organification of iodide, defective thyroglobulin synthesis and transport, and abnormal iodotyrosine deiodinase activity.[62] Additional causes include central TSH deficiency, or decreased T4 action, primarily due to thyroid hormone receptor beta molecular defect, and inadequate transport of or a defect in T4 to T3 conversion.

The causes of primary transient neonatal hypothyroidism include iodine deficiency or excess, maternal use of antithyroid medications, maternal TSH blocking antibodies or monoallelic mutations in DUOX2.

Central transient hypothyroidism can be caused by prenatal exposure to maternal hypothyroidism, prematurity and drugs.

The common features of hypothyroidism (lethargy, hypotonia, large tongue, facial puffiness, cold hands and feet) are usually subtle in the neonatal period and difficult to detect. The patient may represent with non-specific findings including feeding difficulties, hypothermia, unconjugated hyperbilirubinemia and large fontanelles.

Detection of the disorder can be based on clinical signs and symptoms alone, including elevated birth weight, constipation, jaundice, noisy respirations and a horse cry. However, less than 10 percent of infants with hypothyroidism are diagnosed based on clinical signs and symptoms. *Acquired hypothyroidism* in pediatric patients, which typically has an insidious onset, is generally due to an asymptomatic goiter.

Treatment and Prognosis

Thyroid hormone replacement therapy should be started as soon as possible following confirmatory laboratory test. Although mental retardation associated with this condition has been eradicated in parts of the world that employ newborn screening, subtle cognitive behavioral deficits have been reported in some affected children.[55,63,64]

Therapeutic goals include thyroid function normalization and elimination of any signs and symptoms of the disease. Levothyroxine is the most commonly employed drug used to treat hypothyroidism. Twenty percent of children will recover to a euthyroid state and will not require long term thyroid replacement therapy.

Neonatal Hyperthyroidism

Neonatal hyperthyroidism, which is most often transient, occurs due to the passage of maternal stimulating TSH receptor antibodies transplacentally to the unborn child before birth. This occurs primarily from mothers with Graves's disease.[65] Neonatal hyperthyroidism may also rarely occur as a consequence of a child being born to hypothyroid mother with no thyroid function. This occurs due to prior thyroid surgery or radiation, or an autoimmune destructive process in the mother.[66,67]

Although the onset of neonatal hyperthyroidism may be delayed until the TSH blocking antibodies are removed from the circulation; more commonly the disorder is present early, in the first week of life. The newborn will usually exhibit tachycardia, poor weight gain, eye prominence and nervousness, hyperactivity or goiter. Other findings can include hepatosplenomegaly or jaundice. More serious consequences include arrhythmia and cardiac failure, which may arise if there is a delay in diagnosis. Long term problems including developmental delays and cranial stenosis may occur. Neonatal hyperthyroidism last on average for two to three months. Hyperthyroidism can appear later in children and adolescents and will most often be a result of Graves' disease. Thyrotoxicosis and opthalmopathology are the most common clinical findings in this group of patients. Identification of elevated T4 and TSH levels in a child with or without a goiter is generally confirmatory of the disease.

Treatment and Prognosis

The treatment for neonatal hyperthyroidism includes antithyroid drug therapy using propylthiouracil, methimazole or carbimazole to the mother and to the new born infant after birth. Iodine can be used to block thyroid hormone release as well. In children and adolescents who have Graves' disease, surgery following the employment of antithyroid medications is the treatment of choice.

Benign and Malignant Tumors of the Thyroid Gland

Follicular Adenoma

Follicular adenomas represent encapsulated thyroid tumors of follicular cell differentiation. Etiologically, follicular adenomas have been linked largely to prior irradiation and an iodine deficient diet.[68]

Tumors can be associated with inherited syndromes including Carney complex and multiple hamartoma syndrome (Cowden disease). Tumors most often affect adults and are rare in pediatric age group patients. Any portion of the thyroid gland can be involved. Females are most often affected and most lesions will present as a painless asymptomatic thyroid mass or nodule, although large tumors may cause difficulty in swallowing.

Radiographic and CT findings can be non-specific and ultrasound tends to be a much more definitive and diagnostic

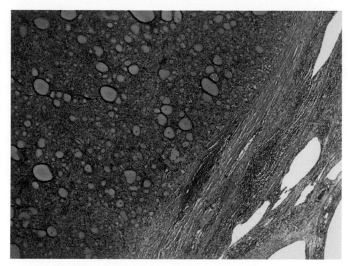

Figure 18.19 Follicular adenoma displaying a well defined capsule.

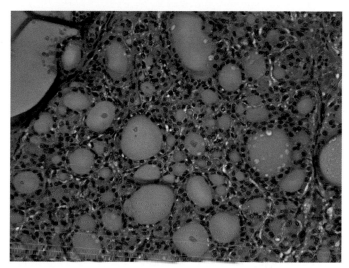

Figure 18.20 This high power photomicrograph shows a mixture of microfollicles and normal size follicles together with a macrofollicle in the upper left hand corner. This mixed follicular pattern is typical of the follicular adenoma.

imaging study. Ultrasound can identify and separate true tumor from a thyroid nodule by demonstrating a homogenous mass in the case of tumor – a mass that will generally demonstrate an isolated echo. Most pediatric patients will be euthyroid and only rarely are follicular adenomas functional.

Pathologic Findings

The follicular adenoma will typically present as a well circumscribed tumor mass that will be surrounded by a well defined capsule. Occasionally tumors arise in the background of nodular hyperplasia. Tumors are most often 1 to 3 cm in diameter and grossly, the cut surface will appear hemorrhagic or cystic.

Follicular adenomas can be histologically classified as *embryonal* or *solid*, *micro-follicular* or *fetal* and *simple*.[68,69,70,71,72,73,74,75] (See Figures 18.19 & 18.20.) Occasionally tumors will demonstrate a trabecular pattern

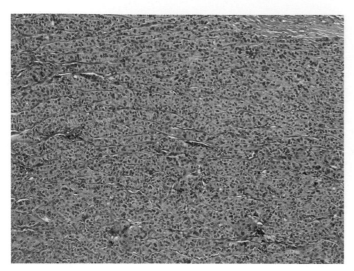

Figure 18.21 Follicular adenoma. This adenoma exhibits a trabecular pattern. Notice the parallel rows of cells with an intervening thin supporting parenchyma that is rich in blood vessels.

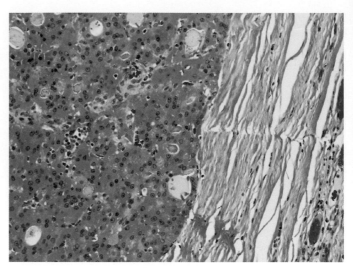

Figure 18.22 Follicular adenoma (oncocytic adenoma) composed of Hürthle cells. The tumor has a thick capsule and a microfollicular pattern.

(Figure 18.21). The encapsulated tumor will be composed of tumor cells that are cuboidal, columnar or polygonal. Nuclei will be round and dark or hyperchromatic. Mitoses are extremely rare. Degenerative changes may occur within the tumor including myxoid change, stromal edema, cystic change, fibrosis, hyalinization, hemorrhage, calcification or infarction. The tumor stroma will consist of well vascularized but thin collagen. Rare oncocytic adenomas (Hürthle cell tumors)[69] have been reported in children (Figure 18.22). Follicular adenomas that display papillary hyperplasia featuring cystic areas in association with papillary formations are particularly common in children and adolescents.[70]

Cytologic Findings

Fluorescence in situ hybridization (FNA) is commonly employed to help assess and diagnose follicular thyroid adenomas and the solitary thyroid nodule. Although FNA cannot be used to separate carcinoma from a nodule or an adenoma, in the case of follicular adenoma, epithelial cells will tend to show microfollicular structures which favor a diagnosis of a *follicular adenomatous lesion*.

Immunohistochemically, follicular adenomas will stain positively for keratins, TTF-1 and thyroglobulin. CK19, neuroendocrine markers and calcitonin will be negative. Differential diagnoses include adenomatoid nodules, which will be composed of morphologically similar follicular aggregates to those of a follicular thyroid adenoma but will lack a capsule. Minimally invasive follicular carcinoma can be differentiated from follicular adenomas based on follicular carcinoma's ability to demonstrate invasion.

RAS gene mutations have been detected in some follicular adenomas, but not in the toxic form of the disease.[76] Mutations in the TSH receptor gene and genes encoding GTP-binding protein have been described in hyperfunctioning adenomas.[77] Clonal aberrations have been detected in

45 percent of thyroid adenomas, and Trisomy 7 is a frequent aberration in these tumors. Translocations involving 19 (19q13) and the short arm of chromosome 2 (2p21) are commonly identified in the tumor,[78] as well as deletions of chromosome 13.

Treatment and Prognosis

The management of follicular adenomas involves lobectomy of the affected thyroid lobe. Levothyroxine has been employed to suppress TSH, a management modality that may decrease nodule size, but which is not curative. Patients have an excellent prognosis following surgery, although standardized assessments of thyroid nodules in children have confirmed a higher cancer prevalence than in adults.[79]

Hyalinizing Trabecular Tumor

The hyalinizing trabecular tumor (HTA) is a neoplasm of follicular origin that exhibits a trabecular growth pattern with intratrabecular hyalinization. Classically defined as an adenoma, the tumor may in fact represent a variant of papillary carcinoma. Investigators have recently shown that the tumor exhibits RET/PTC rearrangements and a nuclear morphology similar to that of PTC.[80,81] Rare lymph node metastasis have also been reported.[82,83,84,85] The etiology is unknown; however, a history of prior radiation exposure has been suggested as an etiologic source.

The HTA accounts for less than 1 percent of primary thyroid gland neoplasms. It is rarely seen in individuals younger than 30, but has been reported in children. Females are most often affected and the tumor will usually present as an asymptomatic non-palatal lesion.

Imaging studies employed as diagnostic aids usually include scintigraphy which will commonly show a *cold* nodule, and ultrasound which will demonstrate a solid nodule that is hyperechoic or heterogeneous in its echo pattern.

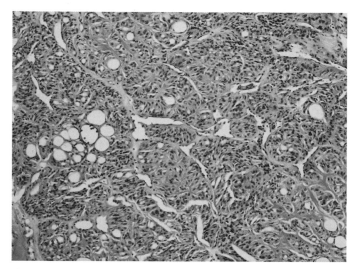

Figure 18.23 Hyalinizing trabecular tumor. Note the trabecular growth pattern with intervening hyalinized basement membrane.

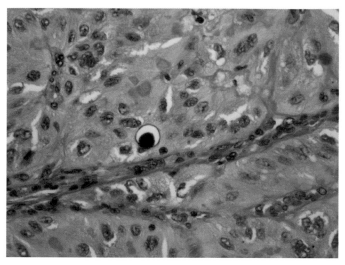

Figure 18.25 Photomicrograph showing psammoma body formation in an HTA.

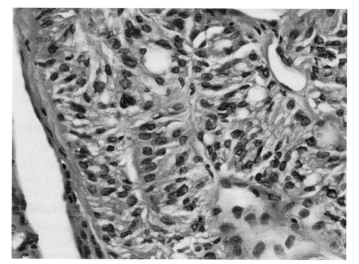

Figure 18.24 High power view showing tumor cells that appear fusiform, ovoid, polygonal and spindle, and show grooves, an irregular nuclear membrane, fine chromatin and occasional pseudoinclusions similar to those seen in papillary carcinoma.

Pathologic Findings

HTA will be identified on gross inspection as a well circumscribed or thinly encapsulated nodule that on cut section is solid and most often yellow tan. Tumors rarely attain a size of greater than 2 cm. Histologically, the tumor will be encapsulated and show a trabecular or nested growth pattern in which tumor cells have an alveolar arrangement. PAS positive hyalinized basement membrane material will present throughout a dense tumor stroma and colloid will rarely be seen. Tumor cells tend to be fusiform or polygonal with amphophilic, eosinophilic or clear cytoplasm (Figures 18.23 & 18.24).

Tumor cell nuclei will be oval or elongated, and may demonstrate prominent grooves and occasional pseudoinclusions. Round yellow appearing paranuclear cytoplasmic

bodies and psammoma bodies can also frequently be seen (Figure 18.25).

Immunohistochemically, tumor cells will be TTF-1 and thyroglobulin reactive. Tumors will be non-reactive for calcitonin, NSE, chromogranin A or synaptophysin and S100 protein.

Follicular thyroid carcinoma (FTC), and medullary thyroid carcinoma (MTC), which will show cytologic atypia in tumors cells, must be excluded from a differential diagnostic standpoint.

Treatment and Prognosis

Most hyalinizing trabecular adenomas will behave in a non-consequential fashion and patient prognosis is excellent. However, rare tumors have been reported to metastasize. Thus the HTA is regarded by some investigators to be a tumor that has rare, but real malignant potential. The standard treatment for the tumor is thyroid lobectomy.

Thyroid Hyperplasia

Hyperplasia of the thyroid in children is rare. When there is evidence of significant hyperplasia of the thyroid, the disorder can be associated with thyrotoxicosis or hyperthyroidism.[86] Children can develop simple goiters of the thyroid gland, a disorder that is most common in adolescence and is much more frequently seen in females than males.[87,88] Colloid goiters, which are a form of thyroid hyperplasia, tend to be multinodular in their presentation or sometimes diffuse (Figure 18.26). Histologically, the follicles that are seen in colloid goiters will vary in size and will frequently show the formation of colloid cysts. The cysts will be flanked by follicular nodules that are rimmed by aggregates of connective tissue. Hemorrhage will often be common throughout the tissue sample. From a differential diagnostic standpoint, the lesion must be distinguished clinically and microscopically from

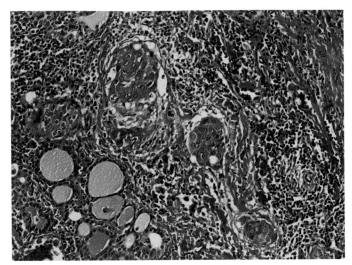

Figure 18.34 Squamous metaplasia is prominent in this sclerosing FTC variant.

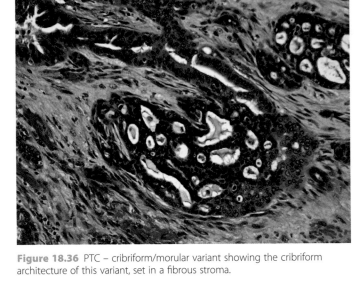

Figure 18.36 PTC – cribriform/morular variant showing the cribriform architecture of this variant, set in a fibrous stroma.

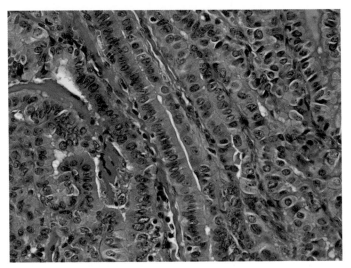

Figure 18.35 PTC – tall cell variant. In the tall cell variant, the cell length is about three to four times its width, and the cytoplasm is usually quite eosinophilic, however, the nuclei show characteristic papillary carcinoma features. Another feature of the tall cell variant is the tendency to form long follicles that collapses to ultimately have the appearance of railroad tracks.

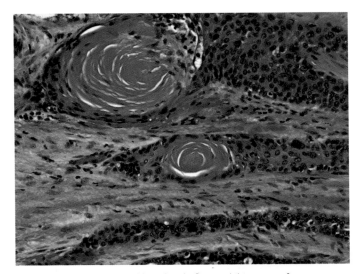

Figure 18.37 The tumor, although cribriform, exhibits areas of squamous differentiation.

will show large cells with enlarged nuclei that will demonstrate nuclear folds or grooves. There will be a high nuclear cytoplasmic ratio to tumor cells with nuclear crowding and overlapping nuclear chromatin that will generally be clear. Thickened colloid aggregates with rare psammoma bodies may be seen.

Immunohistochemical examination of PTC will usually show strong TTF-1, CK19, HBME-1, gelectin-3, CK7 and thyroglobulin positivity. Cytogenetically, tumors will show RET/PTC1 rearrangements which are due to a (10) (q11.2: q21) inversion. Point mutations in the BRAF and RAS genes can also be identified cytogenetically.

Differential Diagnoses

From a differential diagnostic standpoint, MTC, follicular carcinoma and diffuse hyperplasia of the thyroid must be considered when a diagnosis of PTC is entertained. Diffuse thyroid hyperplasia will not show the atypical cytologic nuclear features of PTC and, in addition, in cases of hyperplasia, the entire thyroid gland will be involved. MTC will lack colloid, a distinguishing diagnostic feature of MTC, while follicular carcinoma will demonstrate a classic follicular thyroid architecture pattern without evidence of papillary structures. Rarely, adenomatoid nodules can resemble PTC. Such nodules will lack the atypical nuclear features of PTC, they will be multifocal within the gland and the process will tend not to be encapsulated.

Treatment and Prognosis

PTC is treated by either surgery or radiation therapy. Surgery is by far the most common management modality and will typically include some form of thyroid lobectomy. When

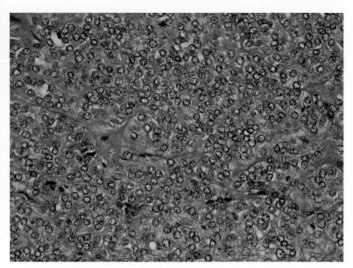

Figure 18.38 PTC – solid variant. Solid sheets and aggregates of tumor cells are seen in this variant.

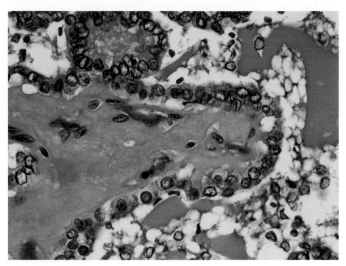

Figure 18.40 High power view of the tumor seen in Figure 18.39, showing the features of PTC.

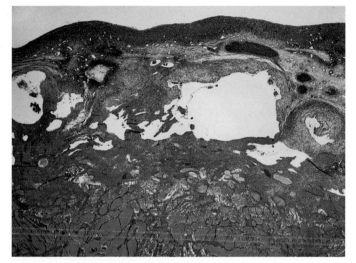

Figure 18.39 PTC in struma ovarii. Low power view showing papillary carcinoma arising in struma ovarii. The upper pole of the photomicrograph shows ovarian tissue, while the lower pole shows the tumor.

radiation therapy is employed, radio ablative iodine therapy, 131I, is used. This form of treatment is usually reserved for pediatric age group patients with extensive cervical node involvement, distant metastasis or when vital organs are at risk. PTC in children has an excellent prognosis with 95 to 98 percent survival rate after 20 years. Tumors that are problematic typically spread by lymphoid channels and will metastasize to regional lymph nodes. Tumors that are RET/PTC3 positive tend to show a worse prognosis than those which are negative.[116]

Follicular Thyroid Carcinoma

FTC represents the second most common form of malignancy of the thyroid, accounting for 10 to 12 percent of all primary thyroid malignancies.[117,118,119] FTC is an exceedingly rare tumor in pediatric age group patients. Classically characterized by a proliferation of thyroid epithelial follicular cells that will not demonstrate the nuclear atypical or papillary features of papillary carcinoma, FTC have often been associated with certain familial syndromes in close to 5 percent of cases. Those syndromes include Werner syndrome, Cowden disease and Carney syndrome or complex. Most tumors are thought to be related to iodine deficiency or radiation exposure, and FTC shows a very specific developmental pattern in which 15 to 20 percent of all patients who develop the neoplasm will have pre-existing thyroid disease including, adenomatoid nodules, or a thyroid adenoma.

The vast majority of affected patients are in the fifth or sixth decades of life when they develop FTC; however, lesions in all age groups typically appear as a nodule within the thyroid.[120] Most pediatric age group patients will be girls who may present with hoarseness, dysphasia or dyspnea. Strider can occur but is rare and a palpable thyroid mass may or may not be evident. As a whole, FTCs in children tend to be larger than PTCs.

In individuals with FTC, thyroid function tests are usually normal. Ultrasound will most often demonstrate a mass that is solid and hypo echoic, and scintigraphy will highlight a nodule that will be "cold."

Pathologic Features

When examined grossly, FTC will be an irregularly but thickly encapsulated nodular growth. Histologically, tumors are characterized by the formation of colloid filled follicles that are rimmed by cells that will demonstrate a greater cellularity than a typical thyroid follicle. Tumor cell nuclei are usually irregularly shaped, with coarse chromatin. Nuclei can be hyperchromatic and tumor cells will have a variable degree of eosinophilic or amphophilic cytoplasm. The connective tissue stromal component of the tumor will tend to be relatively thick and composed of well formed collagen.

487

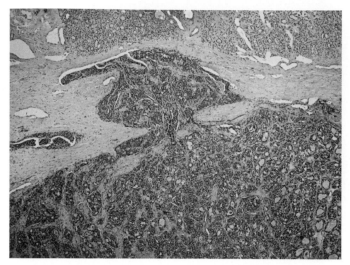

Figure 18.41 Minimally invasive FTC demonstrating capsular invasion.

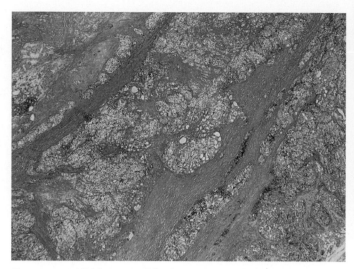

Figure 18.43 Widely invasive follicular carcinoma. Low power view of widely invasive infiltrating FTC.

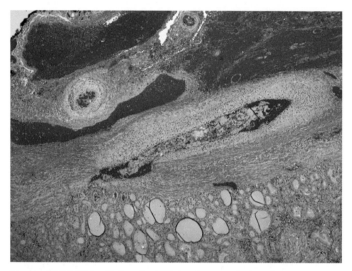

Figure 18.42 Minimally invasive FTC showing vascular invasion.

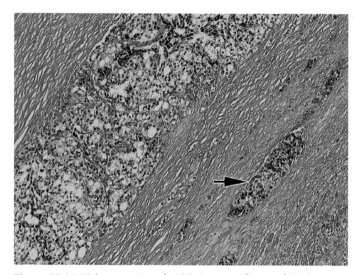

Figure 18.44 High power view of widely invasive infiltrating follicular carcinoma with a focus of vascular invasion (arrow).

Tumors can be histologically classified as 1) minimally invasive or low grade carcinomas (Figures 18.41 & 18.42), 2) widely invasive carcinomas, 3) oncocytic carcinomas, 4) clear cell carcinomas and 5) signet ring carcinomas.

Widely invasive tumors will display significant capsular and vascular invasion (Figures 18.43 & 18.44), while oncocytic tumors will feature large polygonal cells with granular cytoplasm. Clear cell tumors will be made up of 70 to 80 percent glycogen rich clear cells, and signet ring tumors will be composed of cells with large vacuoles in the cytoplasm. Capsular invasion is defined as penetration of the tumor into one-half the thickness of the marginating capsule. When vascular invasion is identified, vessels that are within the marginating capsule will show invasion. Invasion cannot be identified within the tumor cell nests themselves. Tumors that are widely invasive will typically show a so-called mushroom pattern of invasion in which the capsule may be totally lost or impossible to identify.

FNA cytology will show groups of follicular cells that form structures that have a ring-like or circular quality. Colloid will be sparse and enlarged cuboidal cells can be seen. Oncocytic tumors will demonstrate large round cells with granular cytoplasm.

Immunohistochemically, FTCs will be TTF-1, CK7 and thyroglobulin positive. HBME-1, CITED-1 and galectin-3 will be also positive. Molecular cytogenetic findings will show a rearrangement of the peroxisome proliferator activated receptor gamma gene (PPAR).

From a differential diagnostic standpoint, follicular adenoma, adenomatoid nodules and PTC should to be considered. FTC will not show the atypical nuclear features that are classic for PTC, and FTC will generally not show the multinodularity of an adenomatoid nodule. FTC will lack the colloid that is classically identified in MTC.

Treatment and Prognosis

FTCs are treated by surgery and radiation, using radio ablative iodine therapy.[121] Surgery usually includes lobectomy or thyroidectomy. When radio ablative iodine therapy is used, it is employed only in those cases in which there is not a total thyroidectomy. Patients have an excellent prognosis with 95 percent of patients with minimally invasive disease having a 20-year survival. Widely invasive tumors however, are much more aggressive biologically and only 50 percent of the patients will have a 20-year survival.

Medullary Thyroid Carcinoma (MTC)

MTC is a rare form of thyroid cancer that originates from the parafollicular C cells. MTCs account for 5 to 10 percent of all thyroid cancers in the pediatric age group. Two types of MTC exist; those that are sporadic and those that are familial or inherited.[122,123,124,125] Sporadic cases are usually seen in adults, while pediatric MTC tends to be associated with familial forms of the disease that are due to point mutations in the RET proto-oncogene.[125,126,127,128] MTC occurs in pediatric age group patients as a part of multiple endocrine neoplasia syndrome, type 2A (Sipple syndrome)[128] in which patients have hyperparathyroidism, medullary carcinoma of the thyroid, adrenal pheochromocytoma and endocrine tumors of the pancreas; or as MEN2B (Wegenmann–Froboese syndrome) that will include in addition to the aforementioned tumors, mucosal and soft tissue neoplasms.[127]

MEN type 2A tends to occur late in adolescence to early adult life, whereas MEN type 2B is most often a disorder of infancy and childhood. Females are slightly more often affected than males in either of the syndrome types, and tumors will usually present as soft tissue nodules involving the upper lobe or middle lobes of the thyroid gland.[8] Tumors can range up to 2 cm in diameter.[130]

Patients with sporadic disease may present with symptoms of pain, hoarseness or simple cervical lymph node swellings. In those instances in which patients have a familial or inherited disease association, constitutional symptoms often develop that include sweating, headache, diarrhea, multiple oral mucosal neuromas and Cushing symptoms. Imaging analysis will generally show a "cold" mass on scintigraphy and a definable mass on ultrasound assessment. CT scans can be employed to demonstrate the degree of lymph node disease. Tumors in children can sometimes be large enough to replace an entire lobe of the thyroid.

Pathologic Features

On gross examination, the tumor will tend to appear yellow/tan on cut section and the surface will be rubbery and firm. Calcifications can sometimes be seen within the tumor mass and tumors may be gritty or granular as well. Hemorrhage and necrosis are rare within cut sections.

Histologically, the tumor will consist of nests or lobules of tumor cells that often show a trabecular or organoid pattern.

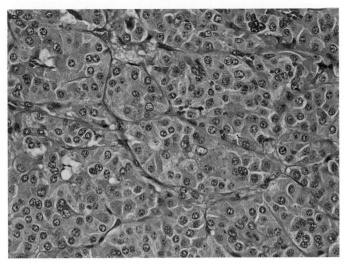

Figure 18.45 MTC demonstrating a solid nesting pattern with epithelioid nuclei that exhibit a neuroendocrine pattern (salt and pepper appearance).

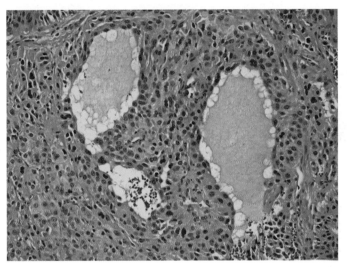

Figure 18.46 Photomicrograph showing a solid and follicular pattern.

Tumor cells will tend to be oval, spindle or plasmacytoid in their appearance and the cytoplasm of tumor cells is typically eosinophilic, granular or clear and oncocytic. Tumor cell nuclei will frequently have a neuroendocrine appearance with a stippled chromatin pattern (Figure 18.45). Intranuclear inclusions may be seen. Tumor cell nests can display a solid, follicular or spindle cell pattern (Figures 18.46 & 18.47).

Tumor cells may show a moderate degree of pleomorphism and multinucleated giant cells can also be identified. The stromal component of the tumor will typically be composed of collagen that is thick and hyalinized, and an amyloid product can be seen in two-thirds of cases. Histologic variants of the tumor also include oncocytic forms of the disease, papillary and pseudo papillary forms, and glandular giant cell. These rare histologic variants, which required immunohistochemical (IHC) confirmation, can be separated from other primary

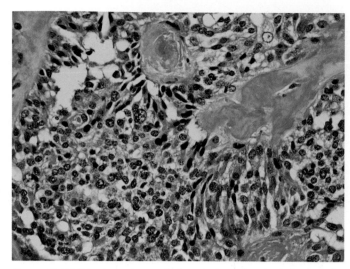

Figure 18.47 This photomicrograph shows polygonal and spindle shaped cells together with amyloid in the background stroma.

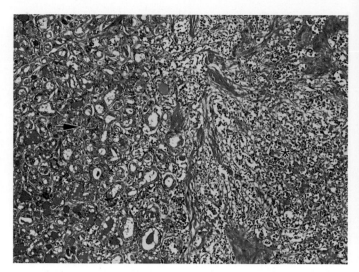

Figure 18.49 A mixed tumor showing medullary carcinoma on the right hand side of the photomicrograph (arrow) and the follicular variant of papillary carcinoma on the left (asterisk).

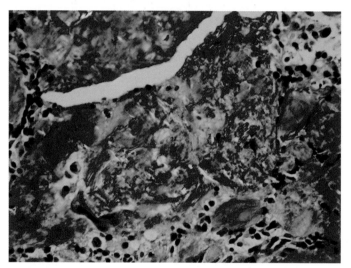

Figure 18.48 Congo-red stain showing apple green birefringence of MTC tissue.

tumors or secondary tumors that closely resemble them, on the basis of IHC staining patterns and reactivity.

MTC tissue, when stained appropriately, will usually show strong Congo-red positivity for amyloid with light green birefringence by polarization (Figure 18.48). From a differential diagnostic standpoint, FTC, papillary carcinoma, paraganglioma and metastatic carcinoma all need to be entertained in the differential diagnosis of MTC. Mixed medullary and papillary thyroid carcinomas have been reported but are rare in children (Figure 18.49).

While IHC will generally show calcitonin reactivity, chromogranin CEA-P cytologic examination of tissue can be difficult to evaluate, but will typically show oval to polygonal tumor cells with a plasmacytoid appearance and associated aggregates of amyloid. Tumor cell nuclei will be hyperchromatic with intranuclear inclusions.

Treatment and Prognosis

MTC is usually treated by a thyroidectomy before twelve months of age in patients with germ line RET mutations.[131,132,133] Partial thyroidectomy is usually employed if the carcinoma is part of a heritable disease. Adjuvant therapies include radiation therapy, chemotherapy and targeted molecular therapy using tyrosine kinase inhibitors.[134] The prognosis for the MTC patient is quite good with a survival rate over a ten-year period of 75 percent.[130,134] The most predictive measurement of outcome is the stage in which the tumor presents at the time of diagnosis. In stage I disease, the ten-year survival rate approaches 100 percent, whereas in stage four disease survival rates are often less than 50 percent. The younger the patient is when MTC is diagnosed, the better the prognosis. Males are considered to have a slightly worse outcome than females.

Poorly Differentiated Thyroid Carcinoma

Poorly differentiated thyroid carcinoma (PDTC), rarely encountered in pediatric age group patients,[135,136] occurs primarily in adults over 60 years of age. PDTC is an epithelial thyroid tumor that has microscopic and biologic features that fall between those of well differentiated carcinoma and anaplastic thyroid carcinoma.[137] Tumors usually present as a thyroid mass, without any specific anatomic site within the gland being most common. Females are more frequently affected than males, and tumors can measure up to 5 cm in diameter or greater. BRAF, p53 and B-catenin mutations have been identified in PDTC.[138,139]

The tumor has one distinct histologic appearance that consists of tumor nodules arranged in an insular pattern (Figure 18.50). Tumor nodules generally are surrounded by a delicate fibrovascular stroma. Tumors will tend to have a high mitotic index with necrosis (Figure 18.51). More rarely, tumors in children will demonstrate an anaplastic pattern.

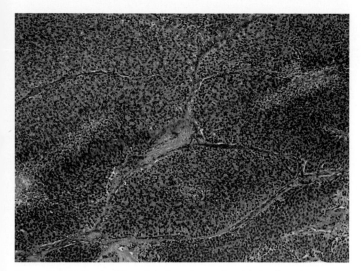

Figure 18.50 Poorly differentiated carcinoma showing insular pattern.

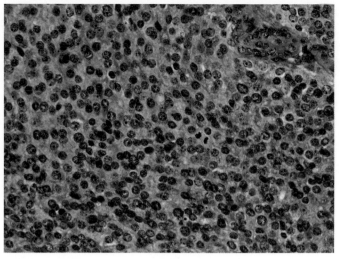

Figure 18.51 High power photomicrograph of a PDTC showing nuclei with dark stippled chromatin and significant mitoses.

Treatment and Prognosis

Treatment typically includes total thyroidectomy and postoperative radioactive iodine therapy and thyroxine supplement. Demeythylating agents have been employed as well. Five-year survival rates approach 50 percent.

Spindle Cell Tumor with Thymus-like Differentiation (SETTLE)

The spindle epithelial tumor with thymus-like differentiation is a rare biphasic tumor that is typically identified in patients less than 20 years of age.[140] Males are more often affected than females and most tumors present as a thyroid mass. The tumor will show a pattern of growth in which there is a spindle cell epithelial core, aggregated with glandular structures that show primitive thymus differentiation.[141,142] Tumors probably arise from ectopic thymic tissue trapped in the intrathyroid region or from branchial pouch remnants that retain thymic differentiation potential. Patients can have tracheal compression in rare instances, and patients often have a prolonged course. On thyroid scan, the tumor will usually present as a "cold" nodule. Tumors tend to have metastatic potential in which case they extend to the lungs, lymph nodes, kidney and associated head and neck soft tissues.[142]

Pathologic Features

Grossly, the tumor will present as a lobular soft tissue nodule that may show adhesion to the surrounding fat. Tumors are usually encapsulated or at least partially encapsulated. The vast majority of tumors will range in size from 1 to 4 cm in diameter. On cut section, the tumor tends to have a yellow color with a firm or gritty cut section. Histologically, the tumor will consist of lobular aggregates of tumors cells that are separated by fibrous connective tissue septa. Tumors will typically be biphasic, demonstrating short, interlacing streaming aggregates of epithelial fascicles that blend into glandular structures and structures that appear tubulo-papillary. The tumor can often have a storiform pattern. Individual tumor cells will have elongated nuclei, delicate nuclear chromatin and minimal pleomorphism. The glandular component of the tumor will be composed of large cystic spaces that are typically lined by respiratory-type epithelium. The glandular epithelium will show minimal mitotic activity and mucin may be seen entrapped within glandular spaces. Occasionally the glandular spaces can be marginated by squamous metaplasia. Calcifications are rare within the tumor. Rare monophasic forms of the tumor, in which the spindle cell epithelial component or the glandular component predominate, have been reported.[143]

On IHC examination, both the spindle cell and glandular component of the tumor will be EMA, AE1/AE3, CK7, vimentin and CD117 positive. Tumors will be negative for S-100 protein, calcitonin, CEA and CD5.

From a differential diagnostic standpoint, SETTLE can mimic undifferentiated carcinoma, synovial carcinoma, medullary carcinoma of the thyroid and ectopic thymoma. Synovial sarcoma can be distinguished from SETTLE on the basis of its SYT-SSX gene fusion. MTC will demonstrate significant amyloid accumulation, which will not be seen in SETTLE, and ectopic thymomas will typically show a lobulation that is jigsaw puzzle-like or mosaic-like, unlike SETTLE.

Treatment and Prognosis

Thyroidectomy is the treatment of choice for SETTLE. Neoadjuvant chemotherapy can be used to reduce tumor size, and radiotherapy is usually employed only to control local or regional recurrence.[144] Ninety percent of patients will survive over a five-year term. When lesions do metastasize, they metastasize to regional lymph nodes. Distant metastases occur in 50 to 70 percent of cases after lengthy periods, often up to 20 years. Lymph node metastasis typically occurs to lung lymph nodes, kidney and soft tissues.

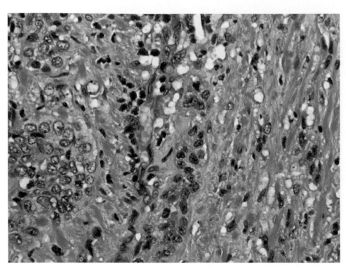

Figure 18.52 Sclerosing mucoepidermoid carcinoma with eosinophilia, characterized by mucous secreting cells epidermoid cells and eosinophiles.

Rare Additional Thyroid Tumors

Additional tumors can be encountered in the thyroid gland of pediatric patients including paragangliomas, teratomas, smooth muscle tumors, peripheral nerve sheath tumors, ectopic thymomas, smooth muscle tumors and solitary fibrous tumors.

Benign and malignant hematopoietic tumors, including Rosai–Dorfman disease, follicular dendritic cell tumor, Langerhans cell histiocytosis and lymphomas can be encountered in the thyroid gland. These tumors are discussed in other sections of this text.

Other significant malignant thyroid tumors including anaplastic carcinoma; mucoepidermoid carcinoma; sclerosing mucoepidermoid carcinoma with eosinophilia (Figure 18.52); squamous cell carcinoma and carcinoma showing thymus-like differentiation can also be encountered in the pediatric age patients.

Disorders of the Parathyroid Glands

Most individuals have four parathyroid glands that are generally located behind the back of the thyroid gland on the right and left sides in superior and inferior polar locations. Supernumerary glands can occur and occasionally only three glands are present. The normal parathyroid gland is ovoid to bean shaped, measures from 0.6 to 1.2 cm along its long axis and has an average weight of 30 to 40 grams. The principal role of these glands is to control calcium levels in the blood and in bone. When this control mechanism is altered or lost, individuals will develop either hypoparathyroidism or hyperparathyroidism, disorders that are characterized by an insufficient or excessive function of the parathyroid glands, and the over production or under production of parathyroid hormone (PTH).

Little was recorded about hyperparathyroidism in children and adolescents before 1984;[1,2] however, the introduction of multichannel blood chemistry analyzers in the 1970s followed by immunoassays for intact PTH have advanced our understanding of hyperparathyroidism.[140] Hyperparathyroidism can be caused by the following: 1) parathyroid adenoma, 2) prior radioactive iodine therapy, 3) radiation therapy to the neck, 4) long term use of lithium, 5) hereditary forms of hyperparathyroidism, 6) parathyroid hyperplasia and 7) multiple endocrine neoplasia syndromes.

Three types of hyperparathyroidism occur; primary, secondary and tertiary. *Primary hyperparathyroidism (PHPT)*, characterized by excess PTH secretion can be caused by genetic mutations that result in parathyroid hyperplasia, adenoma and carcinoma. PHPT is uncommon in infants and children with an incidence of 2 to 5 per 100,000. The disease shows no gender predilection.[1,2,3,4,5,6,7] Genetic syndromes, germline or somatic mutations and radiation exposure have all been advanced as causes of PHPT. *Secondary hyperparathyroidism* is a compensatory disease that occurs in response to hypocalcemia due to factors such as malnutrition, malabsorption, low vitamin D levels or chronic renal failure. *Tertiary hyperparathyroidism* is characterized by the excessive secretion of PTH and an increase in gland mass in response to chronic overstimulation of the parathyroid gland typically after a lengthy period of secondary hyperparathyroidism. This form of hyperparathyroidism occurs most often in renal transplant patients, patients on hemodialysis and in patients with x-linked hypophosphatemic rickets. Tertiary hyperparathyroidism is further characterized by the fact that after removal of the stimulating factor, the disease can persist.

While secondary and tertiary hyperparathyroidism in pediatric age group patients are primarily reactionary in nature, PHPT occurs due to primary conditions that affect the parathyroid gland, most often hyperplasia or a benign or malignant neoplasm.

Neonatal Hyperparathyroidism

The calcium-sensing receptor gene (CaSR) is responsible for sensing extracellular calcium ion levels. This class C, G-protein couple receptor regulates PTH release, and by doing so controls calcium homeostasis. When the CaSR gene is mutated, *familial hypocalciuric hypercalcemia* (FHH) can occur. FHH is an autosomal dominant disorder that is due to heterozygous loss of function mutations in the CaSR gene, which encodes a receptor that can sense calcium.[145] Individuals who are homozygous for CaSR mutations will develop not FHH, but instead develop neonatal severe hyperparathyroidism (NSHPT).[145,152,153] While FHH is typically benign and often asymptomatic, NSHPT can prove to be fatal.[154,155]

Hypocalcemia due to vitamin D deficiency and disorders such as lipid storage diseases can result in *transient neonatal hyperparathyroidism.*[156]

The clinical features of neonatal hyperparathyroidism include skeletal abnormalities with marked bone demineralization, and a tendency to develop fractures, hypotonia, failure to thrive and respiratory distress.[145,146,149,157,158] Elevated serum iPHT, elevated serum calcium concentration and low urinary calcium excretion will be observed in NSHPT and FHH. In both of these disorders all four parathyroid glands will show features of parathyroid hyperplasia pathologically, in which there will be an increase in parenchymal cell mass characterized histologically by a marked chief cell and water clear cell increase.

Treatment and Prognosis

Conventional treatment for neonatal hyperparathyroidism includes intravenous saline therapy, intravenous bisphospho-nate therapy and parathyroidectomy, and high dose vitamin D therapy or paricalcitol use, a vitamin analog. Cinacalcet, which activates allosteric to induce the CaSR, has recently been employed with success.[159]

Childhood/Adolescent Primary Hyperparathyroidism

PHPT in childhood and adolescence is quite rare, and is most often associated with single or multiple parathyroid adenomas, familial hypercalciuric hypercalcemia[160] or multiple endocrine neoplasia syndrome.

Individuals with multiple or single parathyroid adenomas, somatic mutations in MENIN or PRAD1, and HPRT2 germline or somatic mutations have been reported.[160] Most children will be asymptomatic and show only slightly elevated levels of PTH.

Multiple endocrine neoplasia syndromes, MENI and MENII, are most often related to an inherited form of PHPT in which diffuse parathyroid hyperplasia or multiple parathyroid adenomas are the common associated pathology. Additional tumors that may occur to a lesser degree in MENI include pancreatic islet cell tumor or hyperplasia, and pituitary tumors.

Hyperparathyroidism-jaw tumor syndrome (HPT-JT) is a rare autosomal disease caused by inactivating germ-line mutations of HRPT2 gene. The disorder is characterized by PHPT due to parathyroid adenomas and the development of ossifying fibromas of the jaws, renal tumors, renal cysts and uterine tumors, Wilms tumors and neuroblastomas. Parathyroid car-cinoma will develop in 15 percent of cases.[161,162] Children and adolescents typically present with vague symptoms that can include long bone, jaw and abdominal pain. Additional findings include serum hypercalcemia, elevated iPTH, hypopho-sphatemia and hypercalciuria.

Treatment and Prognosis

Selective parathyroidectomy is the treatment of choice for childhood/adolescent hyperparathyroidism. Jaw tumors in syndrome related disease are treated by surgical excision. Long term follow-up of the HPT-JT patient is mandatory, due to the recurrence risk and the risk for malignancy.

Parathyroid Pathology

Parathyroid Hyperplasia

Parathyroid hyperplasia is characterized by the enlargement of all four parathyroid glands. The hallmark of a hyperfunctioning parathyroid gland includes not only glandular enlargement but also hypercellularity of the gland. Typically, an enlarged parathyroid gland will weigh more than one gram and 20 percent of parathyroid hyperplasias will weigh 5 to 10 grams. There are no reliable histologic methods of differen-tiating a parathyroid adenoma from hyperplasia, particu-larly when only one gland is being available for histologic assessment.

Parathyroid hyperplasia is associated with one of the forms of multiple endocrine neoplasia syndrome in 15 to 20 percent of cases. Wermer syndrome (MEN1) is most often the associ-ated syndrome. All of the three types of hyperparathyroidism can be parathyroid hyperplasia associated and females are affected more often than males at a 3:1 ratio.

Patients can present with lethargy, weakness, arthralgia and bone pain. Laboratory tests will show elevated serum calcium, elevated PTH levels and typically decreased serum phosphorous.

Pathologic Findings

Parathyroid glands with minimal enlargement may be indis-tinguishable from normal glands. While glands may appear grossly asymmetrical, this feature alone will not allow one to distinguish parathyroid hyperplasia from an adenoma. Hyper-plastic glands, like adenomatous glands, will appear soft and tan to brown in color.

Microscopically, hyperplasias of the parathyroid gland will present as either 1) primary chief cell hyperplasia or 2) water-clear hyperplasia. A third histologic variant is sometimes included, *parathyromatosis*, characterized by nests of parathy-roid tissue, composed primarily of chief cell hyperplasia that occurs in the mediastinum, or the neck. *Primary chief cell hyperplasia* will be characterized histologically by an increase in the parachymal mass of the gland, with a marked increase in the number of chief cells.[163] The process can be either nodular or diffuse (Figure 18.53). Chief cells will be arranged in sheets,

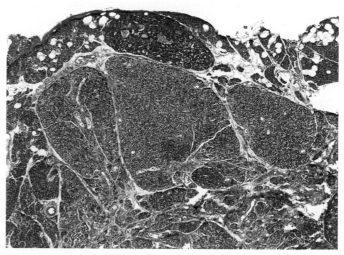

Figure 18.53 Parathyroid hyperplasia showing a nodular pattern of hyperplastic growth.

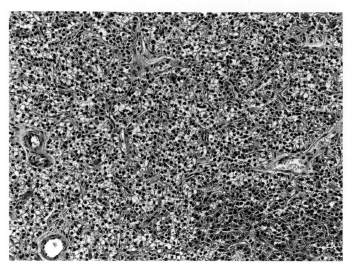

Figure 18.54 High power photomicrograph of chief cells in a hyperplastic parathyroid gland. No discernable difference can be seen between this field and similar fields in a parathyroid adenoma.

nests and cords and present as round or polyhedral cells that have centrally placed nuclei and coarse chromatin. (Figure 18.54) Occasionally, tumor cells will have eosinophilic granular cytoplasm and large nuclei, in which case the cells are often described as *oncocytic* in their appearance.

Stromal fat cells will tend to be sparse and lacking, however, fat cells can rarely dominate the stromal component of the gland. Mitotic figures can be seen, but are rare. *Water-clear cell hyperplasia* is characterized histologically by cells with clear cytoplasm and occasional cytoplasmic vacuolization.

In cases of *secondary hyperparathyroidism*, chief cells, oxyphilic cells and so-called transitional cells will dominate the histologic picture. Stromal fat cells will vary in number and fibrosis may be present. In *tertiary hyperparathyroidism* chief cells will be the most prominent cells seen. IHC evaluation of tissue samples in all forms of hyperplasia will demonstrate *chief cells* that will stain positively with cytokeratin stains and with the neuroendocrine markers chromogranin and synaptophysin. *Clear cells* will be cytokeratin reactive, chromogranin reactive and calcitonin reactive.[163,164] On electron microscopic assessment, chief cells will display characteristic secretory granules while clear cells will contain variable amounts of membrane bound vacuoles.

Differential Diagnoses

The most significant microscopic differential diagnosis will include parathyroid adenoma. Whereas parathyroid hyperplasia will generally involve more than one parathyroid gland, parathyroid adenomas typically affect one gland only. Parathyroid adenoma will also more often be encapsulated and display an absence of tumor stromal fat. Parathyroid carcinoma with which parathyroid hyperplasia can also be confused, will be characterized by enlargement of a single gland, and be associated with extremely high levels of serum calcium and PTH. In nearly 70 percent of cases, parathyroid carcinoma will invade surrounding anatomic structures and show vascular and neural invasion.

Rarely, parathyroid hyperplasia can resemble a follicular thyroid neoplasm, however, parathyroid hyperplasia will be PTH (cytoplasmic) positive and thyroglobulin negative.[1]

Treatment and Prognosis

If parathyroid hyperplasia is the cause of PHPT, it is most often is treated by subtotal parathyroidectomy, with complete removal of three glands. A fourth gland or gland remnant is routinely left. Secondary hyperparathyroidism, if caused by parathyroid hyperplasia, is treated in a similar manner. Recurrent hyperplasias can be associated with proliferation of parathyroid tissue ectopically, usually in muscle or fat. All forms of parathyroid hyperplasia associated hyperparathyroidism can recur. Recurrence is seen in 8 to 15 percent of patients even after subtotal parathyroidectomy. Such recurrences may not be recognized for many years.

Parathyroid Adenoma

Parathyroid adenomas are benign neoplasms of the parenchymal cells of the parathyroid gland. Their etiology is unknown; however, there is a known link to ionizing radiation exposure.[165,166] Parathyroid adenomas are the most frequent cause of PHPT, and most often a single parathyroid gland is involved. Parathyroid adenomas can be associated with the HPT-JT with its component renal cysts ossifying fibromas of the jaw, Wilms tumor and renal cell carcinoma.

Rare in pediatric age group patients, parathyroid adenomas nonetheless represent the primary cause of hyperparathyroidism in that demographic.[167] Pediatric age patients can present with a variety of tumor associated symptoms including growth retardation, pathologic fractures, mood swings, hypercalcemia, fatigue, depression, vomiting and polyuria.[168,169] Tumors generally will not be evident as a palpable mass, and females tend to be affected more often than males. Serum PTH levels will be elevated as will serum calcium levels. Radiographic assessment, which mandatorily includes Tc-99m studies, can localize the tumor mass in the vast majority of cases. Tumor associated loss of heterozygosity of the HRPT2 gene mapped to defined chromosomal region on 1q 25-q31 has been reported in syndrome associated hyperparathyroidism caused by a parathyroid adenoma.

Pathologic Features

On gross inspection, most parathyroid adenomas will present as a solitary nodular growth. Multiple lesions tend to be hyperplasias and not adenomas. Tumors will be brown to tan, sometimes lobulated and occasionally cystic. A thin marginating tumor capsule may or may not be grossly evident. (Figures 18.55 & 18.56). Tumors will generally weigh less than 1 gram.

Microscopically, the parathyroid adenoma will be composed predominantly of neoplastic chief cells. These cells will

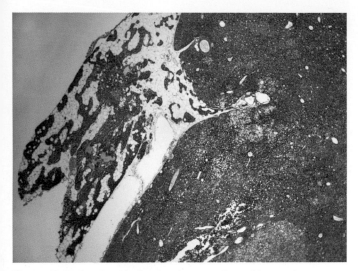

Figure 18.55 Parathyroid adenoma demonstrating a thin capsule surrounding the tumor.

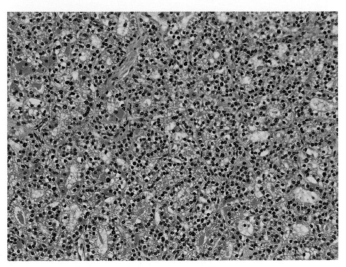

Figure 18.57 Chief cells in this parathyroid adenoma show faintly eosinophilic cytoplasm and central hyperchromatic dark round nuclei.

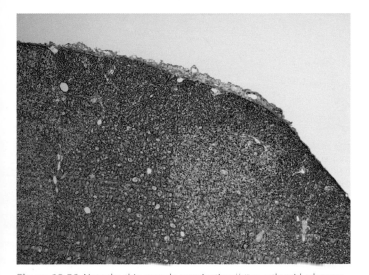

Figure 18.56 Note the thin capsule marginating this parathyroid adenoma and the associated adipose tissue.

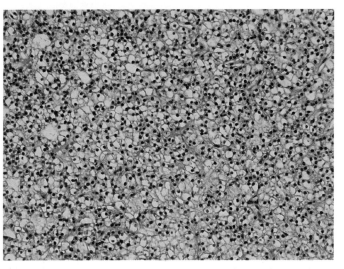

Figure 18.58 Parathyroid adenoma demonstrating clear chief cells with abundant glycogen content.

be larger than normal chief cells and will contain a centrally placed nuclei (Figure 18.57). The cytoplasm of tumor cells is typically eosinophilic. Enlarged hyperchromatic nuclei and cells with clear cytoplasm (Figure 18.58) may be seen distributed throughout the tumor. Cysts may be common as well (Figure 18.59). Tumors can sometimes appear rich in oncocytic cells, in which case they are subclassified as *oxiphilic adenomas*. (Figure 18.60) A second tumor variant, the *lipoadenoma*, which is characterized by a proliferation of parenchymal and fat cells, is exceedingly rare in pediatric age patients. The lipoadenoma can display follicular, solid or nesting patterns. Solid and follicular histologic patterns are common to parathyroid adenomas as well (Figures 18.61 & 18.62).

Parathyroid adenomas can also demonstrate a rare atypical adenomatous pattern in which case tumors are subclassified as *atypical adenomas*. This class of tumor will demonstrate atypical histologic features including a trabecular growth pattern, eccentric tumor cell nesting, increased mitotic activity and gigantiform chief cells (Figures 18.63 & 18.64).

On IHC examination, parathyroid adenomas will stain positively for PTH, cytoplasmically, and for neuroendocrine markers, including chronogranin and synaptophasin. Tumors will be reactive to low molecular weight cytokeratins (CK8, CK19, CK118) and to parafibromin, a HRPT-2 gene product.

Treatment and Prognosis

The parathyroid adenoma when identified as a single lesion in pediatric age group patients is treated by excision of the involved adenomatous gland via microinvasive parathyroidectomy in association with pre-operative and post-operative PTH assays in neonates, children and adolescents. At the time of surgery one additional gland is often biopsied to exclude

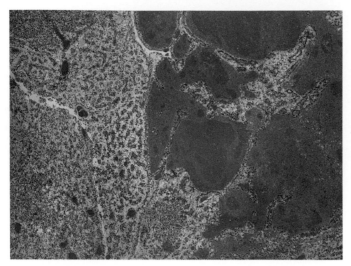

Figure 18.59 Parathyroid adenoma demonstrating cystic areas filled with hemorrhage.

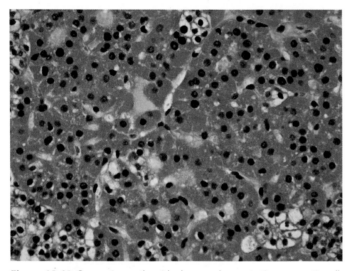

Figure 18.60 Oncocytic parathyroid adenoma demonstrating oncocytic cells with eosinophilic granular cytoplasm and a large central nucleus.

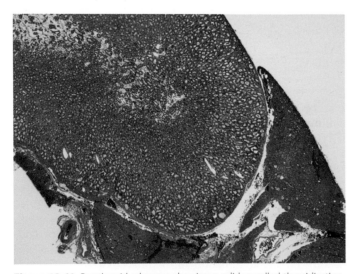

Figure 18.61 Parathyroid adenoma showing a solid so-called thyroidization pattern.

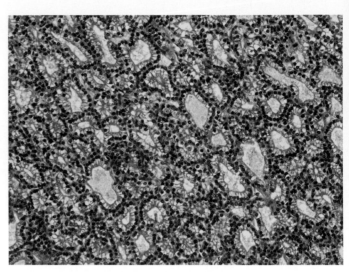

Figure 18.62 Parathyroid adenoma demonstrating a follicular histologic pattern.

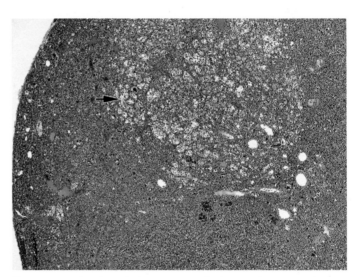

Figure 18.63 Parathyroid adenoma, atypical subtype at low power showing eccentric nesting of tumor cells (arrow).

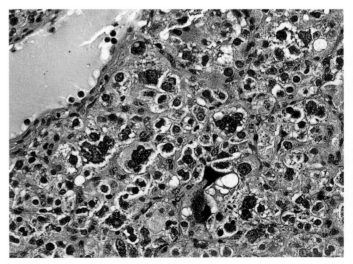

Figure 18.64 High power photomicrograph showing gigantiform chief cells with bizarre hyperchromatic nuclei in atypical parathyroid adenoma.

hyperplasia and carcinoma.[170,171,172,173,174] Hyperparathyroidism of recent onset occurs in 10 percent of cases. The "brown tumor" of hyperparathyroidism will affect bone, primarily the jaws in the head and neck region, in some individuals who have parathyroid adenomas. These lesions result in bone resorption in association with elevated serum calcium levels caused by the adenoma.

Histologically, "brown tumors" of hyperparathyroidism resemble central giant cell "granulomas" of bone and will be composed of multinucleated giant cells set in a loosely reticular, often hemorrhagic, fibrous stroma. Patients with parathyroid adenomas must be followed routinely over the long term for assessment of local recurrence or aggressive biologic behavior by the tumor.

Atypical parathyroid adenomas will demonstrate two or more of the following histologic features:

- Clinically adherent gland without tissue invasion
- Incomplete or equivocal capsular invasion
- Fibrous bands
- Back-to-back trabecular growth patterns
- Mitotic activity > 1/10HPF
- Tumor necrosis without secondary explanation

Atypical parathyroid adenomas will not demonstrate:

- Metastasis
- Angiolymphatic invasion
- Perineural invasion
- Unequivocal invasion

Malignant Neoplasms

Parathyroid Carcinoma

Parathyroid carcinoma, which is extremely rare in the pediatric population, is a PTH secreting neoplasm of parathyroid parenchyma that accounts for approximately 1 to 2 percent of the cases of hyperparathyroidism. Fewer than 150 cases of parathyroid carcinoma have been documented in pediatric age patients. The etiology of parathyroid carcinoma remains unknown; however, irradiation of the tissues of the neck represents a probable cause. Parathyroid carcinoma is also associated with certain rare inherited disorders, including familial isolated hyperparathyroidism, multiple endocrine neoplasia syndrome type 1 (MEN1), secondary parathyroid hyperplasia and HPT-JT.[175,176,177,178]

Tumors in adults affect males and females equally. There are too few reported cases in pediatric age group patients to state a gender predilection. Tumors tend to involve the lower parathyroid glands more often than the upper glands and individuals of Japanese descent have the greatest worldwide incidence.[175,176,177,178]

Patients can present with a host of symptoms that can range from a lump in the neck to symptoms of weakness, weight loss, nausea, vomiting, hoarseness, bone pain, recurrent laryngeal or nerve palsy.

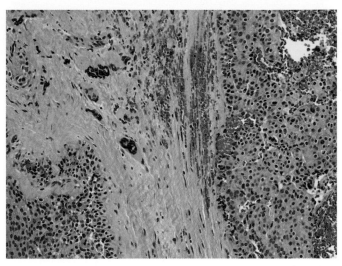

Figure 18.65 Parathyroid carcinoma showing infiltrating pattern of neoplastic chief cells and associated fibrosis.

Laboratory assessment will typically demonstrate exceedingly high serum calcium levels, high PTH levels of greater than 1000 ng/L and serum alkaline phosphatase elevation, Tc-99m studies will be strongly reactive, as will single photon emission CT scans, and both imaging studies are capable of pinpointing a tumor's location.

Pathologic Features

On gross inspection, parathyroid carcinoma will present as a firm gray-white to tan mass. Tumors commonly contain adherent adjacent fat, muscle, nerves or connective tissue and central tumor necrosis may be evident. Tumors in children rarely reach a size of greater than 3 cm in diameter.

Microscopically, parathyroid carcinoma will be composed of neoplastic aggregates of parathyroid chief cells infiltrating surrounding soft tissue (Figure 18.65). More rarely, the tumor will be composed of infiltrating oncocytic cells. Tumor cells will show capsular invasion and vascular invasion. Neoplastic chief and oncocytic cells may show high nuclear to cytoplasmic ratios, increased mitoses and spindling. There is no standard staging system for parathyroid carcinoma, and tumors are therefore classified as either localized or metastatic. Parathyroid carcinomas demonstrate recurrent losses of chromosome 13q, a chromosomal region that contains the retinoblastoma (RB1) and BRCA2 tumor suppressor genes.[179]

Immunohistochemically, parathyroid carcinoma will be chromogranin-A, PTH (Figure 18.66), pan cytokeratin cyclin D-1 and S-100 protein reactive, but parafibromin, TT-F-1 and thyroglobulin negative. Differential diagnoses include parathyroid adenoma, metastatic renal cell carcinoma and MTC. Parathyroid adenomas will not demonstrate cytologic atypia and will tend to stain Bcl-2 and mdm2 positively, unlike parathyroid carcinoma, which will more frequently stain negatively.[180] Renal cell carcinomas will demonstrate a sinusoidal growth pattern while parathyroid carcinoma will not. Thyroid

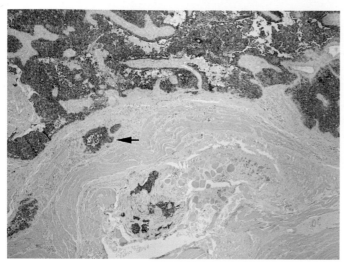

Figure 18.66 PTH stain in parathyroid carcinoma, highlighting groups of neoplastic chief cells infiltrating the surrounding soft tissue (arrow).

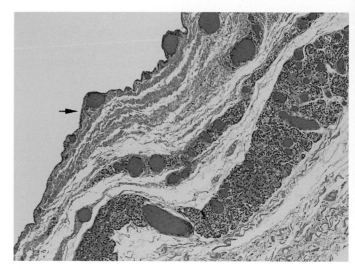

Figure 18.68 High power photomicrograph showing the thin cyst lining (arrow) above nests of parathyroid cells.

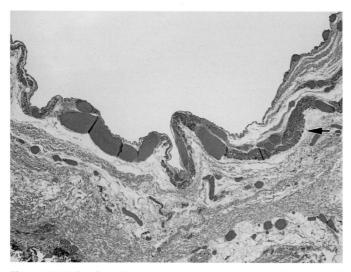

Figure 18.67 Parathyroid cyst. Low power photomicrograph of a parathyroid cyst showing nests of parathyroid tissue in the cyst wall and peri-cystic fibrosis (arrow).

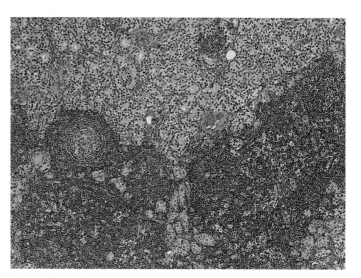

Figure 18.69 Chronic parathyroiditis demonstrating a lymphocytic infiltrate in the parathyroid gland with associated germinal center formation.

carcinomas, regardless of their histologic pattern will tend to be TTF-1 positive when stained immunohistochemically.

Treatment and Prognosis

Radical surgical resection is the treatment of choice for parathyroid carcinoma, although radiation therapy and chemotherapy are also employed. Control of the metabolic effects of elevated serum calcium and high levels of PTH are mandatory in patients with parathyroid carcinoma.

Rare Parathyroid Lesions in Children

Parathyroid Cysts

Parathyroid cysts can occur in children as lesions that are classified as either functioning or non-functioning.[181] On average these cysts will be 4 cm in diameter, but can be as large as 10 cm in diameter. Cystic contents tend to be clear and watery, and histologically the cyst will be lined by a flattened layer of cuboidal epithelium with a surrounding fibrous tissue wall that contains parathyroid tissue nests. (Figures 18.67 & 18.68). Aspiration of the cyst contents, sclerotherapy or surgical removal are the treatments of choice.[182,183]

Chronic Parathyroiditis

Chronic parathyroiditis (Figure 18.69) can occur in the context of autoimmune disease in children and can be associated with hyperparathyroidism.[184,185] In pediatric age patients it is important to separate this extremely rare form of parathyroid disease from Hashimoto's thyroiditis which might have a similar autoimmune mechanism and clinical presentation.

References

Thyroid Developmental and Inflammatory Disease

Lingual Thyroid, Thyroid Aplasia and Hypoplasia

1. Batsakis JG, El-Naggar AK, Luna MA. Thyroid gland ectopias. *Ann Otol Rhinol Laryngol* 1996; 105:1000.

2. Basaria S, Westra WH, Cooper DS. Ectopic lingual thyroid masquerading as thyroid cancer metastasis. *J Clin Endocrinol Metab* 2001; 86:392–395.

3. Toso A, Colombani F, Averno G, et al. Lingual thyroid causing dysphagia and dyspnea. Case reports and review of the literature. *Acta Otorhinolaryngol Italica* 2009; 29:213–217.

4. Peters P, Stark P, Essig G, et al. Lingual thyroid: an unusual and surgically curable cause of sleep apnea in a male. *Sleep and Breathing* 2010; 14:377–380.

5. Neinas FW, Gorman CA, Devine KD, Woolner LB. Lingual thyroid. Clinical characteristics of 15 cases. *Ann Int Med* 1973; 79:205–210.

6. Schoen EJ, Clapp W, To T, Fireman B. The key role of newborn thyroid scintography with isotopic iodide (123I) in defining and managing congenital hypothyroidism. *Pediatr* 2004; 114: e683–e688.

7. Baughman R. Lingual thyroid and lingual thyroglossal tract remnants. An oral clinicopathologic study and review of the literature. *Oral Surg Oral Med Oral Pathol* 1972; 34:781–799.

8. Huang TS, Cheng HY. Dual thyroid ectopic with a normally located pretracheal thyroid gland: case report and literature review. *Head and Neck* 2007, 29:885–888.

9. Ugar-Cankal D, Denizci S, Hocaoglu T. Prevalence of tongue lesions among Turkish school children. *Saudi Med J* 2005; 26:1962–1967.

10. Prasad KC, Bhat V. Surgical management of lingual thyroid: a report of four cases. *J Oral Maxillofac Surg* 2000; 58:223–227.

11. Eugene D, Djemli A, Van Vilet G. Sexual dimorphism of thyroid function in newborns with congenital hypothyroidism. *J Clin Endocrinol Metab* 2005; 90:2696–2700.

12. Capelli Gandossi E, Cumetti D, et al. Ectopic lingual thyroid tissue and acquired hypothyroidism: Case report. *Ann Endocrinol (Paris)* 2006; 67: 245–248.

13. Singhal P, Sharma KR, Singhal A. Lingual thyroid in children. *J Indian Soc of Pedodo and Preventive Dentistry* 2012; 29:270–272.

14. Klein R, Mitchell ML. Hypothyroidism in infants and children. In: Braverman LE, Utiger RO, eds. *Werner and Ingbar's The Thyroid*. Ed 8. Sidney: Lippincott Williams and Wilkins, 2000, 973–982.

15. Diaz-Arias AA, Bickel JT, Loy TS, et al. Follicular carcinoma with clear cell change arising in lingual thyroid. *Oral Surg Oral Med Oral Pathol* 1992; 74:206–211.

16. Toso A, Colombani F, Averono G., et al. Lingual thyroid causing dysphasia and dyspnea. Case reports and review of the literature. *Acta Otochinolaryngologia Ital* 2009; 29:213–217.

17. Seonane JM, Cameselle-Teijeiro J, Romero MA. Poorly differentiated oxyphilic (Hurthle cell) carcinoma arising in lingual thyroid: a case report and review of the literature. *Endocr Pathol* 2002; 13:353–360.

18. Chaabouni AM, Intidhar Labidi S, Kraiem T., et al. Papillary follicular carcinoma arising in a lingual thyroid. *Ann Otolaryngol Chircevicofac* 2006; 123:199–202.

19. Massinc RE, Durning SJ, Koroscil TM. Lingual thyroid carcinoma: a case report and review of the literature. *Thyroid* 2001; 11:1191–1196.

Thyroglossal Tract Cyst

20. Allard LH. The thyroglossal cyst. *Head Neck Surg* 1982; 5:134–146.

21. Dedivitis RA, Camargo DL, Peisoto GL, et al. Thyroglossal duct: a review of 55 cases. *J Am Coll Surg* 2002; 194:274–277.

22. Mondin V, Ferlito A, Muzzi E, Silver CE, et al. Thyroglossal duct cyst: personal experience and literature review. *Auris Nasus Larynx* 2008; 35:11–25.

23. Diaz MC, Stormorken A, Christopher NC. Thyroglossal duct causing apnea and cyanosis in a neonate. *Pediatr Emerg Care* 2005; 21(2): 35–37.

24. Soloman JR, Rangercroft L. Thyroglossal duct lesions in childhood. *J Pediatr Surg* 1984; 19:555–561.

25. Peretz A, Lieberman E, Kapelushnik J, Hershkovitz E. Thyroglossal duct carcinoma in children: case presentation and review of the literature. *Thyroid* 2004; 14:777–785.

26. Patel NN, Hartley BE, Howard DJ. Management of thyroglossal tract disease after failed Sistrunk procedure. *J Laryngol Otol* 2003; 117:710–712.

Ectopic Thyroid Tissue and Parasitic Thyroid Nodules (Thyroid Inclusions in Lymph Nodes)

27. Noussios G, Panaglotis A, Goults D, et al. Ectopic thyroid tissue: anatomical, clinical, and surgical implication of a rare entity. *Eur J Endocrinol* 2011; 165:375–382.

28. LiVolsi V. Thyroid lesions in unusual locations. In: Bennington JL, ed. *Surgical Pathology of the Thyroid. Major Problems in Pathology*. Vol. 22. Philadelphia: WB Saunders, 1990, 351–363.

29. Kumar R, Khullar S, Gupta R, et al. Dual thyroid ectopy: case report and review of the literature. *Clin Nucl Med* 2000; 25:253–254.

Thyroid Pigment and Crystals

30. Goldfischer S, Grotsky IIW, Chang CH, et al. Idiopathic neonatal iron storage involving the liver, pancreas, heart and endocrine and exocrine glands. *Hepatology* 1981; 1:58–64.

31. Alexander CB, Herrera GA, Jaffe K, et al. Black thyroid. Clinical manifestations, ultrastructural findings, and possible mechanisms. *Hum Pathol* 1985; 16:72–78.

32. Reid JD, Choi CH, Oldroyd N. Calcium oxalate crystals in the thyroid. Their identification, prevalence, origin, and possible significance. *Am J Clin Pathol* 1987; 87:443–454.

Autoimmune Thyroiditis

33. Lorini R, Gastaldi R, Traggiai C, et al. Hashimoto's thyroiditis. *Pediatr Endocrinol Rev* 2003; 1:205–211.

34. Tandon N, Zhang L, Weetman AP. HLA associations with Hashimoto's thyroiditis. *Clin Endocrinol (oxf)* 1991; 34:383–386.

35. Nicholson L, Wong F, Ewins D, et al. Susceptibility to autoimmune thyroiditis in Down's syndrome is associated with the major histocompatibility class II DQA 0301 allele. *Clin Endocrinol (oxf)* 1994; 41:381–383.

36. Goudie RB, Anderson JR, Gray KG, et al. Autoimmune associations of

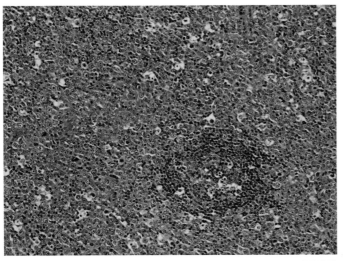

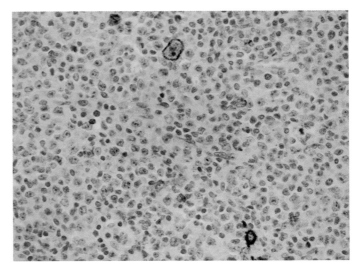

Figure 19.14 EBV lymphadenitis. LMP1 immunostain demonstrates EBV infection in scattered large cells and small lymphocytes.

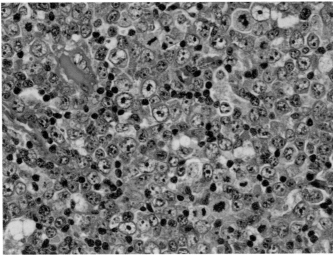

Figures 19.12 (top) & 19.13 (bottom) EBV lymphadenitis. The interfollicular regions contain mixed lymphocytes with many immunoblasts, which are large in size and have a round nucleus, vesicular chromatin and a large nucleolus.

Figure 19.15 CMV lymphadenitis. Florid follicular hyperplasia with interfollicular expansion.

in some cases, and cases of EBV lymphadenitis with sheets of reactive immunoblasts must be distinguished from diffuse large B cell lymphoma (DLBCL). Clinical findings (fever, pharyngitis and splenomegaly) and serum tests are also crucial in establishing an accurate diagnosis, in conjunction with careful microscopic observation. EBV lymphadenitis shows marked interfollicular expansion with at least partially preserved architecture, whereas in CHL and DLBCL the nodal architecture is typically effaced. EBV studies of the tissue sections are very helpful; in EBV lymphadenitis, the virus is present in a small subset of both large atypical and small lymphocytes. In cases of EBV-positive CHL and DLBCL, only the tumor cells are positive for virus infection with a diffuse staining pattern.

Cytomegalovirus Lymphadenitis

Cytomegalovirus (CMV) infection is a less common cause of childhood lymphadenopathy than EBV. The clinical and pathologic features of CMV infection may closely resemble those of EBV-related IM.[16] CMV infection is usually asymptomatic or only mildly symptomatic in immunocompetent hosts. Some patients have fever with pharyngitis and lymphadenopathy. The most common complications include hepatitis, encephalitis, pericarditis and pneumonia.

In immunocompetent pediatric patients, CMV lymphadenitis typically shows mixed follicular hyperplasia and paracortical expansion. Some cases may display distortion of nodal architecture with florid follicular hyperplasia (Figure 19.15), which is similar to human immunodeficiency virus related lymphadenopathy. The expanded interfollicular regions contain mixed lymphocytes, immunoblastic proliferation and perivascular monocytoid B cell proliferation (Figure 19.16). Rare large atypical cells with characteristic "owl's eye" intranuclear viral inclusions are unique to

CMV infection, and they are usually confined to areas of monocytoid B cell hyperplasia (Figure 19.17). Immunohistochemistry for CMV highlights infected cells in the lymph node.

EBV and CMV primary infections show similar clinical and pathologic presentations. Therefore, simultaneous serologic testing for these two viruses is necessary to provide a specific and efficient diagnosis. Careful microscopic examination at high power should be performed to search for the diagnostic large eosinophilic intranuclear inclusions, best seen in areas with monocytoid B cell hyperplasia. CMV lymphadenitis may mimic CHL in cases with marked nodal architectural distortion and large atypical cells containing prominent intranuclear inclusions. Lymphocytes with CMV inclusions may also stain positively with CD15.[17]

Cat Scratch Disease

Cat scratch disease (CSD) is a common cause of lymphadenopathy in pediatric populations. *Bartonella henselae*, a fastidious Gram-negative bacterium, is the major causative agent of CSD.[18,19] Patients are typically scratched or bitten by a young cat, and develop ipsilateral lymphadenopathy within one to three weeks. Lymphadenopathy is the most common clinical manifestation of CSD and is described in more than 80 percent of patients. Most individuals have a mild, self-limited clinical course; however, severe systemic manifestations may occur in immunocompromised patients.

The infected lymph nodes show necrotizing, suppurative granulomatous inflammation with reactive follicular hyperplasia (Figure 19.18). The granulomas are well defined, with central, neutrophil-rich necrosis and peripheral palisading histiocytes (Figure 19.19). Multinucleated giant cells may be

Figure 19.16 CMV lymphadenitis. Expanded paracortex (left side of image) with sheets of monocytoid B cell hyperplasia.

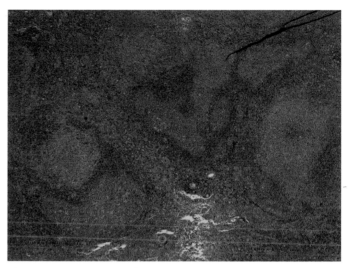

Figure 19.18 CSD. Reactive lymphoid hyperplasia with several well-defined granulomas.

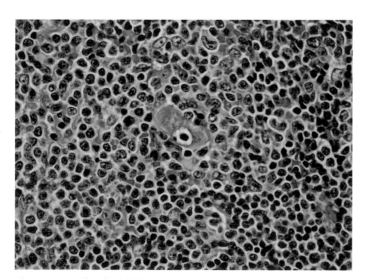

Figure 19.17 CMV lymphadenitis. A large cell with a prominent intranuclear viral inclusion is present among the monocytoid B cells.

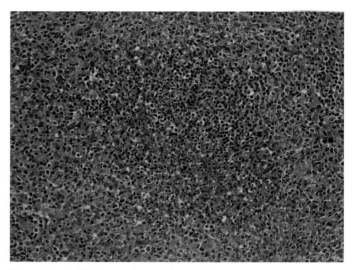

Figure 19.19 CSD. A granuloma with central suppurative necrosis and peripheral palisading histiocytes.

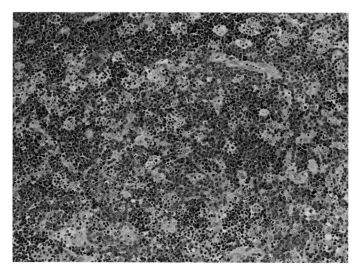

Figure 19.43 BL. Low power examination with "starry sky" appearance due to tingible body macrophages (clear spaces), as well as individual cell necrosis (pyknotic nuclei).

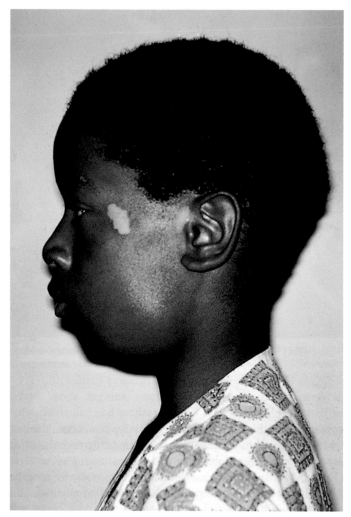

Figure 19.42 Endemic BL in a five-year-old child. (Reprinted from Marx R, Stern D. *Oral and Maxillofacial Pathology: A Rationale for Diagnosis and Treatment* with permission from Quintessence Publishing Company).

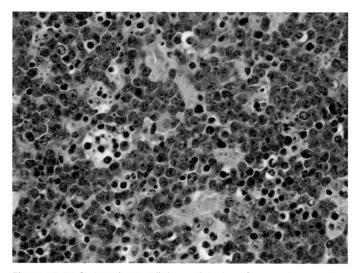

Figure 19.44 BL. Lymphoma cells have relatively uniform, medium-sized, round to oval nuclei with multiple nucleoli.

presents with an intra-abdominal mass, often involving the ileocecal region. Other commonly involved sites in BL include omentum, breasts, ovaries, kidneys and bone. Breast involvement is often bilateral and may be associated with pregnancy or lactation. Lymph nodes and bone marrow may be involved, especially in the immunodeficiency-associated variant. All variants have a tendency to involve the CNS. A minority of cases will present with prominent peripheral blood involvement. Rare cases where the blood and marrow represent the main involved sites are referred to as the leukemic variant of BL, or Burkitt leukemia.

Microscopy shows involved sites to be replaced by diffuse sheets of monotonous, medium-sized lymphoid cells. The appearance recapitulates the appearance of the zona densa in a reactive germinal center, with frequent mitotic figures, frequent individual cell necrosis and frequent tingible body macrophages admixed among the neoplastic lymphocytes, giving the lesion a classic "starry sky" appearance at low power examination (Figure 19.43). The nuclei of the lymphoma cells are round to oval, and usually contain multiple small- to medium-sized nucleoli (Figure 19.44). Wright–Giemsa stains of smears or touch imprints show the BL cells to have basophilic cytoplasm with frequent clear vacuoles (Figure 19.45); the vacuoles contain lipids and are thus highlighted on Oil Red O stains. Some cases of immunodeficiency-associated BL appear somewhat plasmacytoid.

Immunohistochemistry shows the cells of BL to be positive for markers of mature B cells (CD19, CD20, CD79a, PAX5) (Figure 19. 46), and for markers of germinal center B cells (CD10, bcl6) (Figures 19.47 & 19.48); they are negative, or at best focally and weakly positive, for bcl2 (Figure 19.49). MIB1 (Ki-67) shows a very high proliferation rate, with nuclear positivity seen in over 90 percent and usually nearly 100 percent of the lymphoma cells (Figure 19.50). A classic IHC finding in BL is the relative scarcity of reactive CD3-positive

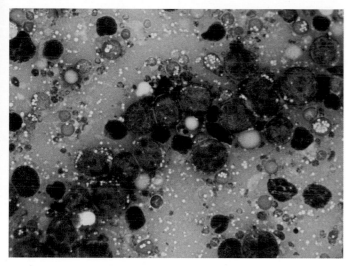

Figure 19.45 Touch imprint of BL shows cells with high nucleus to cytoplasm ratio, multiple nucleoli, scant basophilic cytoplasm and clear cytoplasmic vacuoles.

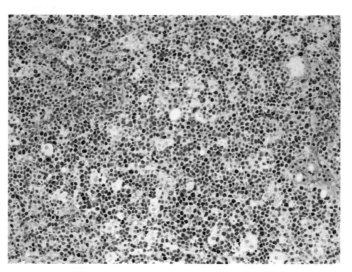

Figure 19.48 BL. Diffuse strong nuclear expression of BCL6, a marker of germinal center-type B cells.

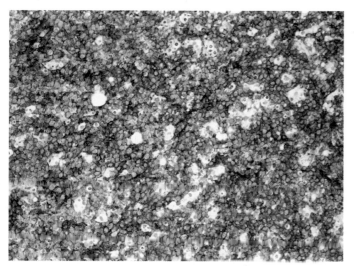

Figure 19.46 BL. Diffuse strong membranous expression of CD20.

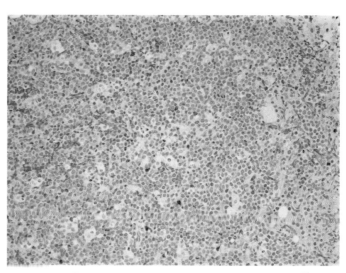

Figure 19.49 BL. The lymphoma cells should be negative for BCL2 (the rare positive cells are admixed T cells).

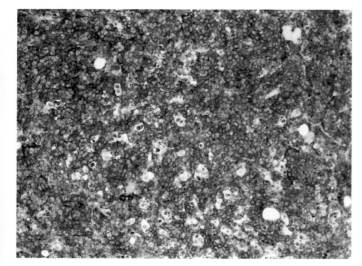

Figure 19.47 BL. Diffuse membranous expression of CD10, a marker of germinal center-type B cells.

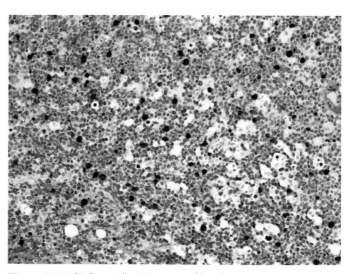

Figure 19.50 BL. Essentially 100 percent of lymphoma cells show nuclear expression of proliferation marker Ki-67.

T cells found admixed within the tumor in comparison to other B cell NHLs; this scarcity of T cells has been attributed to the rapid growth rate of the tumor. Markers of immaturity, such as TdT and CD34, should be negative.

Flow cytometry will show the presence of a CD10-positive population of B cells expressing monotypic surface light chain and mu surface heavy chain (thus, IgM-positive).

Molecular analysis usually identifies the presence of a monoclonal rearrangement of the *IGH* gene.

The large majority of cases have rearrangement of the *MYC* gene at 8q24. In most cases, the *MYC* gene is translocated to the *IGH* gene at 14q32, though in significant minorities of cases *MYC* will be translocated to the genes encoding either the kappa (2p12) or lambda (22q11) light chains. Around 10 percent of cases of BL will not have a demonstrable *MYC* rearrangement by FISH; if all other features are compatible with BL, the diagnosis is still allowable in such cases.

Treatment of BL involves the use of multiagent chemotherapy. Patients whose disease is amenable to complete surgical resection require less intense chemotherapy. More intense chemotherapy regimens are required for high stage disease, such as cases with CNS or bone marrow involvement.[45] Overall, BL has excellent cure rates of over 90 percent using modern treatment regimens, with cure rates approaching 100 percent in patients with early stage, surgically resectable disease. Relapses of BL usually occur within a few months of reaching remission, and have a poor prognosis.[45]

Diffuse Large B Cell Lymphoma

DLBCL is the most common type of NHL in adults. It is much less common in children, accounting for only around 20 percent of pediatric NHLs.[43,44] Rather than being a unique biological entity, such as BL, the diagnostic criteria for DLBCL encompass a relatively heterogeneous group of lymphomas that may differ from case to case with regards to molecular findings, cytogenetic findings and response to treatment. DLBCL may present as either nodal disease, extranodal disease or both.

Microscopic review of DLBCL shows significant replacement of much or all of the biopsied lymph node or extranodal tissue by a diffuse infiltrate of large, atypical lymphoid cells (Figure 19.51). Occasionally, lymph nodes may be only partially replaced by DLBCL, in which case an interfollicular pattern of involvement is commonly seen. Fibrosis may be variably present within the tumor, and is especially prominent in DLBCL involving bone. The definition of a "large cell," as provided by the WHO, is a lymphocyte with a nucleus that is as large or larger than an average macrophage nucleus, or more than twice as large as an average lymphocyte nucleus. Generally, the neoplastic cells in DLBCL have more prominently vesicular nuclei (i.e. more open appearing chromatin) with larger and more prominent nucleoli than is seen in BL.

DLBCL may be divided into different morphologic variants, based upon the appearance of the lymphoma cells. The most common variant is centroblastic, with the lymphoma cells resembling the activated centroblasts seen in reactive germinal centers, exhibiting round to oval vesicular nuclei with multiple irregular nucleoli that are often adherent to the nuclear membrane and interconnected to each other by strands (Figure 19.52). The centroblastic variant is the most common variant in adults, and is even more common in pediatric DLBCL, accounting for 75 percent or more of cases. The immunoblastic variant is rare in children, accounting for a much reduced proportion of DLBCL cases than in the adult population.[46] In this variant the large majority of lymphoma cells are immunoblasts, characterized by thick nuclear membranes, the presence of a single, prominent, round nucleolus located in the center of the nucleus and somewhat basophilic cytoplasm (Figure 19.53). The immunoblastic variant may

Figure 19.51 DLBCL. Diffuse replacement of lymph node tissue by atypical large lymphoid cells.

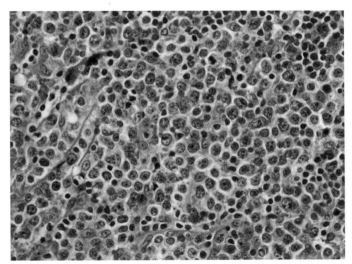

Figure 19.52 DLBCL, centroblastic type. The lymphoma cells resemble centroblasts, with round to oval nuclei with multiple stranded nucleoli.

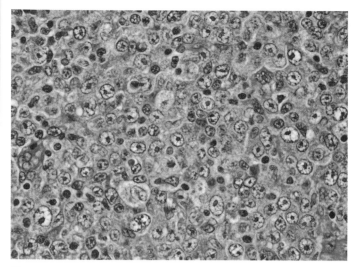

Figure 19.53 DLBCL, immunoblastic type. The lymphoma cells have more optically clear chromatin than the centroblastic variant, and usually have one prominent centrally located nucleolus.

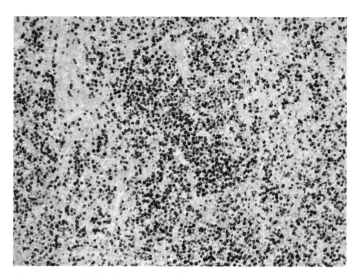

Figure 19.55 DLBCL. The majority of lymphoma cells are positive for proliferation marker Ki-67, albeit a lesser percentage than seen in the above pictured BL.

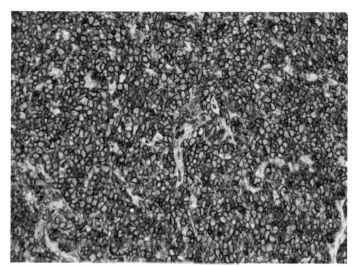

Figure 19.54 DLBCL. Diffuse strong membranous expression of CD20.

start to show morphologic and IHC evidence of plasmablastic differentiation, although this is uncommon in children. The anaplastic variant of DLBCL is characterized by markedly bizarre, exceedingly malignant-appearing lymphoma cells. The anaplastic variant accounts for only a small percentage of pediatric DLBCL. In this author's opinion, it is best to omit the word "anaplastic" from the pathology report and merely report these cases as DLBCL, in order to avoid clinical confusion with anaplastic large cell lymphoma (ALCL), which is an entirely different entity.

IHC analysis of DLBCL will show strong, diffuse expression of B cell antigens CD19, CD20, CD22, CD79a and PAX5 (Figure 19.54). Germinal center B cell (GCB)-type DLBCL tends to be positive for CD10 and bcl6 and negative for MUM.1, although some of these cases may lack CD10 expression. A GCB-type immunophenotype is seen in the large majority of pediatric DLBCL, being present much more frequently than in adult DLBCL. Activated B cell (ABC)-type DLBCL is usually positive for MUM.1, can be positive or negative for bcl6 and lacks CD10. Ki-67 usually shows a high but variable proliferation rate, with anywhere from 30 percent to nearly 100 percent of lymphoma cells labeling (Figure 19.55). If Ki-67 labels 90 percent or more of lymphoma cells, thought should be given to the possibility of BL or B cell NHL with features intermediate between BL and DLBCL, although standard DLBCL may show very high proliferation rates. Bcl2 is expressed in around 40 percent of pediatric DLBCL, both in GCB-type and ABC-type cases. Rare cases of DLBCL may show aberrant expression of CD3, or express ALK1. Cases showing plasmablastic differentiation may lose expression of CD45 and/or CD20 and gain expression of CD138, to varying degrees.

Cytogenetic analysis of pediatric DLBCL only rarely shows rearrangements of *BCL2* and/or *BCL6*, which are both much more frequent in adult DLBCL. Rearrangements of *MYC* may be seen in a minority of cases, and this finding warrants consideration of a diagnosis of BL or B cell NHL with features intermediate between DLBCL and BL, although a diagnosis of DLBCL with a *MYC* rearrangement is also an acceptable option.

Treatment for pediatric DLBCL is similar to the treatment for BL described above, typically including CNS prophylaxis, and shows similar outcomes.[46] This differs from the adult scenario, as diagnoses of DLBCL and BL in adults have been shown to require different treatment regimens. Thus, in children, the importance of differentiating between BL and DLBCL may not be as important, at least according to currently available data.

Anaplastic Large Cell Lymphoma

ALCL is by far the most common mature T cell neoplasm of children, and accounts for around 10 to 20 percent of cases of

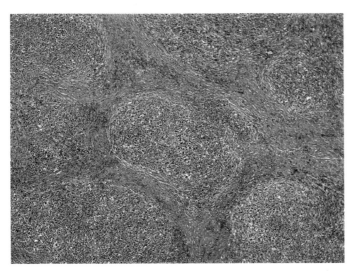

Figure 19.73 CHL, nodular sclerosis subtype. Cellular nodules of inflammatory cells and scattered HRS cells are separated by collagenous fibrous bands.

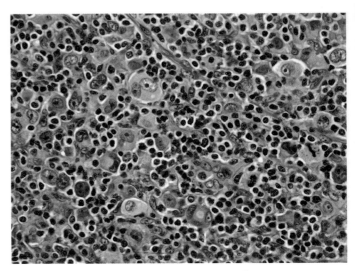

Figure 19.75 CHL, mixed cellularity subtype. HRS cells are present in a background of mixed inflammatory cells.

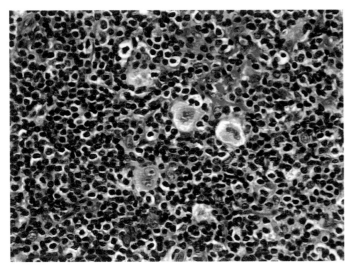

Figure 19.74 CHL, nodular sclerosis subtype. Examples of the lacunar variant of HRS cell, where cytoplasmic retraction has created a clear space around the malignant cells.

lymphocytes, histiocytes, plasma cells, neutrophils and/or eosinophils; one or more of these cell types can be absent from the infiltrate in any given case.

The most common subtype of CHL in pediatric patients is nodular sclerosing (NSCHL), which accounts for up to 80 percent of CHL cases in adolescents. The large majority of cases of NSCHL present with involvement of mediastinal lymph nodes; cervical lymph nodes are also frequently involved. NSCHL tends to spread to contiguous lymph node groups. On low power examination, the histology of NSCHL consists of cellular nodules containing a mixture of inflammatory cells, with intervening, relatively paucicellular, fibrous bands (Figure 19.73). Fibrous septa may project from the fibrous bands into the cellular nodules. The HRS cells in NSCHL frequently have a lacunar appearance, as retraction of the HRS cell cytoplasm

during processing results in a cell that appears to exist in the middle of a clear lacuna on histologic sections (Figure 19.74). NSCHL may vary in appearance from predominantly fibrotic to predominantly cellular. The pathologist should be aware of a cellular variant of NSCHL known as the syncytial variant, which consists of sheets and islands of contiguous HRS cells. In this variant, the HRS cells are frequently mononuclear, and necrosis is frequently present within the aggregates of HRS cells; thus, the histologic findings can mimic necrotizing granulomatous disease.

The mixed cellularity subtype (MCCHL) accounts for most of the remainder of pediatric CHL cases. MCCHL shows a male predominance, and is a frequent subtype in CHL patients with HIV/AIDS. MCCHL tends to involve peripheral lymph nodes and spare the mediastinum. On histologic review, MCCHL lacks the fibrous band formation that is seen in NSCHL, and usually involves the lymph node in a diffuse or, less commonly, interfollicular pattern (Figure 19.75).

The lymphocyte rich subtype (LRCHL) thankfully accounts for only a small minority of CHL cases, as it can be diagnostically difficult to distinguish from NLPHL or T cell/histiocyte-rich large B cell lymphoma (THRLBCL). In LRCHL, the lymph node is replaced by an infiltrate of small lymphocytes, with or without admixed histiocytes (Figure 19.76). HRS cells are scattered among the infiltrate, but are often rare and more difficult to locate than in other CHL subtypes (Figure 19.77). Immunohistochemistry usually shows the background lymphocytes to consist entirely of small T cells, mimicking THRLBCL, although in a minority of cases they consist predominantly of small T cells with admixed nodules of small B cells, mimicking NLPHL. In addition, the HRS cells in LRCHL may show a phenotype intermediate between a typical CHL phenotype (see below) and that of NLPHL, making the diagnosis even more difficult. Clinically, LRCHL presents similarly to NLPHL, usually involving peripheral lymph nodes, usually sparing the mediastinum and usually lacking B symptoms.

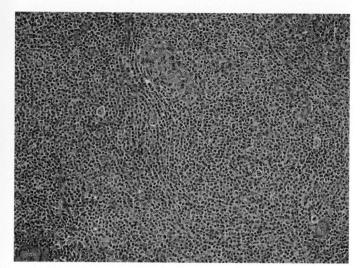

Figure 19.76 CHL, lymphocyte rich subtype. Low power view shows effacement of nodal architecture by small lymphocytes, with occasional admixed histiocytes (top center). Scattered larger cells are appreciable at low power in this case.

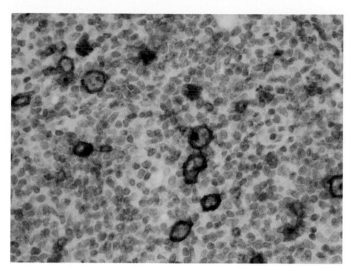

Figure 19.78 CHL. The HRS cells show strong cell membrane and Golgi apparatus expression of CD30 ("ring and dot" pattern).

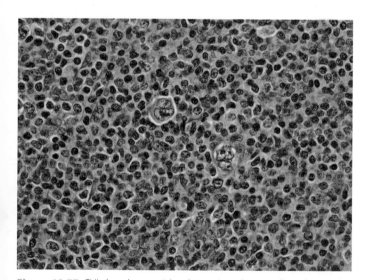

Figure 19.77 CHL, lymphocyte rich subtype. Lymphoma cells with typical features of HRS cells can usually be found, but may be scarce.

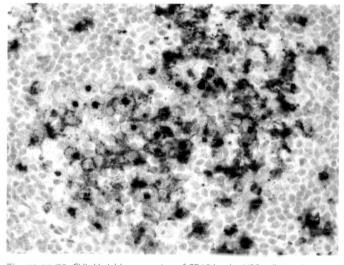

Figure 19.79 CHL. Variable expression of CD15 by the HRS cells in a "ring and dot" pattern.

The immunophenotype of HRS cells is usually very distinctive. The large majority of HRS cells in essentially all cases are strongly positive for CD30, which highlights the cell membrane and Golgi apparatus in a "ring and dot" pattern (Figure 19.78). In the majority of cases, there is also positivity for CD15 on the HRS cells, also in a "ring and dot" pattern, although expression of CD15 is often limited to a subset of the HRS cells in any one case (Figure 19.79). HRS cells are almost always negative for CD45 (leukocyte common antigen), although the dense background inflammatory infiltrate often makes interpreting IHC for CD45 difficult. HRS cells may show surface expression of CD20 in up to 40 percent of cases, although expression of this antigen is usually only seen on a subset of the HRS cells and is of weaker intensity than would

be expected for B cell NHL (Figure 19.80). Most cases lack expression of B cell markers CD79a, BOB.1 and OCT-2, although a majority will express PAX5, a nuclear marker of B cell lineage. If any of these four previous antigens are expressed, it is usually at a lesser intensity than that seen in background reactive B cells (Figure 19.81). EBV positivity, as assayed by ISH studies for EBV Early RNA (EBER), is variable, ranging from around a quarter of cases of NSCHL, to a majority of cases of MCCHL. HRS cells should be negative for ALK and for histiocytic markers such as CD68.

Although HRS cells do contain clonally rearranged *IGH* genes, molecular analysis of the *IGH* gene performed on tissue samples usually fails to identify a monoclonal B cell population, due to the scarcity of the HRS cells. Similarly, flow cytometry almost always fails to identify the HRS cells. Both of these assays are of some utility, however, in helping to exclude NHL.

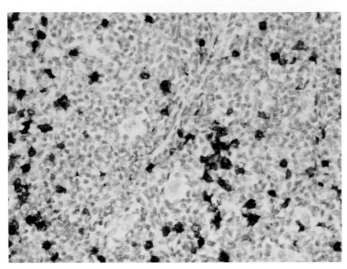

Figure 19.80 CHL. HRS cells are negative for CD20 expression. CD20 is strongly expressed by small reactive B lymphocytes in the background infiltrate.

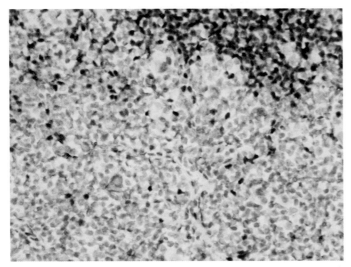

Figure 19.81 CHL. HRS cells (center and lower portion of image) show weak nuclear expression of PAX5 relative to the strong expression seen in background reactive B lymphocytes (top portion of image).

Cytogenetic analysis of CHL usually shows gains of chromosomes, consistent with the multinucleation of the cells, but there are no specific recurrent cytogenetic abnormalities useful for establishing a diagnosis of CHL. Comparative genomic hybridization may be useful if clinically available, as recurrent gains and losses of specific chromosomal regions have been documented by this method.

Pediatric CHL currently has excellent cure rates using a first line regimen of chemotherapy with or without involved field radiotherapy. For early stage disease, cure rates exceed 90 percent, and for advanced stage disease cure rates exceed 80 percent.[43,50] The main prognostic predictors are disease stage at presentation, and presence or absence of bulky disease. Cases that are refractory to primary therapy, or that relapse after primary therapy, still may obtain a cure via various salvage therapies, which may include autologous or allegeneic hematopoietic stem cell transplantion.[50]

Nodular Lymphocyte Predominant Hodgkin Lymphoma

Although categorized as a Hodgkin lymphoma by the WHO, NLPHL is significantly different in appearance and disease course than CHL, and also requires different treatment, and is thus best regarded as its own distinct entity. Thus, an effort should be made when reporting a diagnosis of NLPHL to convey that the diagnosis does not equate to a generic diagnosis of "Hodgkin disease."

Despite its uniqueness from CHL, NLPHL is often classified as a Hodgkin lymphoma for epidemiological purposes. NLPHL accounts for less than 10 percent of all cases classified as Hodgkin lymphoma in children, however is relatively more prevalent in pre-pubertal children, where it accounts for up to 20 percent of all cases classified as Hodgkin lymphoma.[52] The male predominance seen in adults with NLPHL is more prominent in children and teens, where up to 75 percent of NLPHL cases are in males. Patients present with painless localized lymphadenopathy, with the cervical region and the inguinal region being the most commonly involved locations. Extranodal sites and the mediastinum are almost never involved. The history of lymphadenopathy is often long established by the time NLPHL is diagnosed, although the majority of cases are still at an early stage at diagnosis.

The histology of NLPHL explains its historical relation to CHL, since similarly to CHL the neoplastic cells in NLPHL are large, atypical lymphoid cells that are scattered in a background of reactive inflammatory cells, and thus account for only a small minority of cells in the involved lymph nodes. The neoplastic cells in NLPHL are referred to variably as LP cells or L&H cells. The LP cells have scant cytoplasm and large nuclei that are characterized by strikingly clear, vesicular nuclei, usually with a convoluted nuclear membrane, giving many of the nuclei the appearance of popcorn and resulting in their colloquial name of "popcorn cells" (Figure 19.82). LP cells have indistinct nucleoli, which is one of the better ways of distinguishing them from CHL cells. The LP cells are present in a background of small lymphocytes and histiocytes, usually with a vaguely to prominently nodular growth pattern that is discernible on the H&E-stained sections. Eosinophils, neutrophils and plasma cells are not a significant part of the reactive background in NLPHL.

IHC studies show the LP cells to have a typical B cell phenotype, being strongly positive for both CD45 (leukocyte common antigen) and B cell markers CD19, CD20, CD79a, BOB.1, OCT2 and PAX5 (Figures 19. 83, 19.84 & 19.85). The LP cells are negative for CD15, and are usually negative for CD30, although a minority of cases may contain a subset of LP cells that are weakly positive for CD30 (Figure 19.86). EBV studies are negative. Studies for B cell and T cell markers show the nodules to be composed predominantly of small reactive

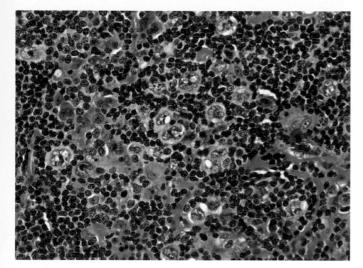

Figure 19.82 NLPHL. The LP cells have large, optically clear nuclei, with smaller nucleoli than HRS cells, and with hyperconvoluted nuclear shapes resembling popcorn.

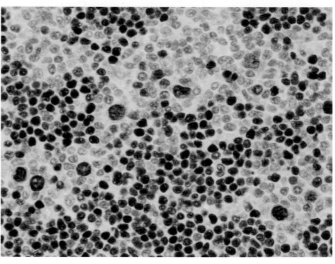

Figure 19.84 NLPHL. The LP cells express nuclear B cell marker OCT-2 at a similar intensity as the background reactive B lymphocytes.

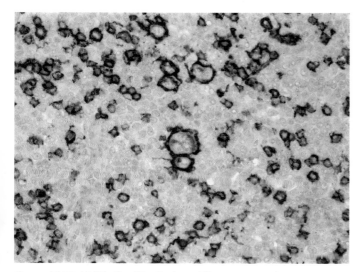

Figure 19.83 NLPHL. The LP cells show diffuse, strong nuclear expression of CD20.

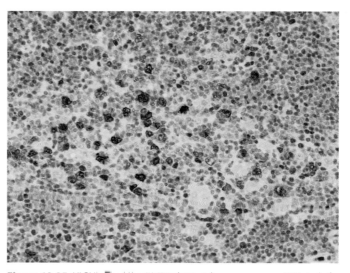

Figure 19.85 NLPHL. The LP cells stand out at low power on an IHC study for nuclear B cell marker BOB.1.

B cells, with the intervening areas composed largely of small reactive T cells. T cells with a follicular helper T cell phenotype (CD4+/bcl6+/CD57+/PD1+) may form rosettes around the LP cells (Figure 19.87). CD21, CD23 and CD35 highlight follicular dendritic cell networks within the nodules. Early in the disease course, the B cell nodules are prominent, whereas in more advanced disease, the T cells start to predominate and the nodules are less obvious. Eventually, the nodules may become inconspicuous or absent, and the disease may essentially overlap with the T cell-rich variant of DLBCL.

Flow cytometry almost always fails to identify the neoplastic B cells due to their scarcity, with results usually just reflecting the background populations of polyclonal B cells and T cells. For similar reasons, monoclonal rearrangement of the *IGH* gene is detectable by PCR in only a minority of cases.

Cytogenetic evaluation of NLPHL frequently detects karyotypic abnormalities; rearrangement of *BCL6* at 3q27 is seen in around half of cases, including some cases with *IGH/BCL6* translocation.

NLPHL has an indolent course and a very favorable prognosis. It requires less intense therapy than CHL. The large majority of cases of NLPHL are diagnosed at an early stage, and reports suggest that surgical resection followed by observation, or chemotherapy alone, may be appropriate initial therapies in these patients, though multimodal therapy (chemotherapy and radiation) is still commonly used.[52]

Neoplasms of Myeloid Lineage

Myeloid neoplasms include those hematopoietic neoplasms composed of cells of one or more of the myeloid lineages,

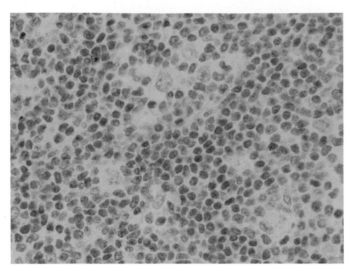

Figure 19.86 NLPHL. The LP cells are negative for CD30.

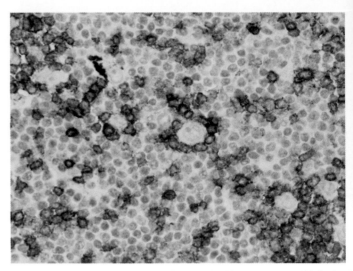

Figure 19.87 NLPHL. An IHC study for CD57 highlights a rosette of follicular helper T cells surrounding an LP cell.

which includes the granulocytic, monocytic, erythroid and megakaryocytic lineages. The neoplastic cells may be immature (myeloblasts, monoblasts and/or promonocytes) or mature, or a combination of both. These neoplasms usually present primarily with blood and marrow involvement. If they consist of more than 20 percent immature myeloid cells (as listed above) in either the blood or marrow, or if they contain certain recurrent cytogenetic abnormalities, they are classified as acute myeloid leukemia (AML). Otherwise, they are classified as a myeloproliferative neoplasm (MPN), myelodysplastic syndrome (MDS) or as an overlapping MDS/MPN. These neoplasms may present with or develop mass-forming involvement of solid tissues, and rarely may present with solid tissue involvement in the absence of significant blood and marrow involvement.

Myeloid Sarcoma

Myeloid sarcoma refers to a solid tissue mass formed by immature myeloid cells, with or without admixed mature myeloid cells. The immature cells may be myeloblasts or immature monocytic cells or both. Myeloid sarcoma may arise as the first manifestation of disease, or may arise in persons with a pre-existing diagnosis of AML in the blood or marrow. In addition, the occurrence of myeloid sarcoma in persons with pre-existing diagnoses of an MPN or MDS is considered to represent transformation of the pre-existing disease to AML. The WHO states that a diagnosis of myeloid sarcoma "should be considered equivalent to a diagnosis of AML."

AML accounts for only around 11 percent of childhood leukemias, though it accounts for up to one-third of leukemias in adolescents. Myeloid sarcoma occurs much less commonly than typical AML, although some types of AML, especially those with monocytic differentiation, have a higher propensity to result in myeloid sarcoma. Myeloid sarcoma can occur anywhere, with favored sites including bone, especially the skull and facial bones, as well as skin and lymph nodes.

If a myeloid sarcoma contains a significant component of maturing granulocytes, these granulocytes will contain cytoplasmic myeloperoxidase. This results in the tumor having a green color on gross examination upon sectioning, which will gradually fade over a few hours after exposure to air. This phenomenon resulted in such tumors being referred to historically as chloromas; however, this term should be avoided in the present because it is not specific, as it can be applied both to a subset of myeloid sarcomas as well as to tumors that lack a significant component of immature cells, such as in cases of soft tissue involvement by chronic myelogenous leukemia (CML).

Histologically, myeloid sarcoma at least partially replaces the involved tissue. Penetration of tissues by individual malignant cells, or with formation of only small aggregates of malignant cells, does not qualify for a diagnosis of myeloid sarcoma, and is better described as soft tissue infiltration by AML. Cytologically, myeloid sarcoma can show a wide range of appearances. The cells may appear predominantly blastic, with scant cytoplasm, high nucleus to cytoplasm ratio and open chromatin with one or more distinct nucleoli. They may appear predominantly promonocytic, with more abundant cytoplasm and convoluted, folded nuclei, though usually still with relatively open chromatin and distinct nucleoli (Figure 19.88). They may contain an admixture of more mature appearing monocytes and/or granulocytes, though the immature component should account for a significant percentage of cells (one might reasonably assume such a percentage to be 20 percent, but it is currently not explicitly stated by the WHO).

The above histologic appearance is not specific, and in the absence of a pre-existing diagnosis of hematologic malignancy, it might easily be mistaken for NHL. Thus, immunophenotyping, by immunohistochemistry, flow cytometry or preferably both, is the key for establishing a diagnosis of myeloid sarcoma. Useful antigens to assess on the immature-appearing cells include antigens commonly expressed on myeloblasts

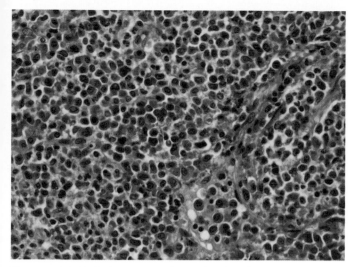

Figure 19.88 Myeloid sarcoma involving a lymph node. Distinction from lymphoma would be very difficult, if not impossible, without immunophenotyping.

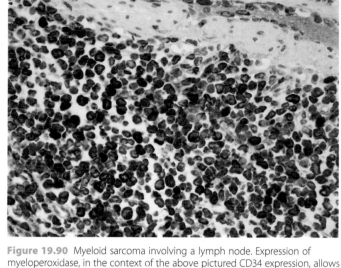

Figure 19.90 Myeloid sarcoma involving a lymph node. Expression of myeloperoxidase, in the context of the above pictured CD34 expression, allows for identification of the malignant cells as myeloid blasts.

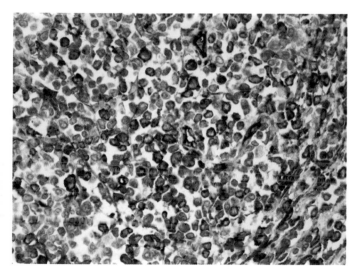

Figure 19.89 Myeloid sarcoma involving a lymph node. Diffuse expression of CD34 confirms the presence of a neoplasm of immature cells.

(CD13, CD33, CD34, CD117, myeloperoxidase) and antigens of monocytic differentiation (lysozyme, CD14, CD11b, bright CD64, CD68) (Figures 19.89 & 19.90). CD43 is particularly useful, as it usually expressed by both myeloblasts and monoblasts/promonocytes. CD56 may be expressed, especially by cases with monocytic differentiation. Up to half of cases of myeloid sarcoma may express CD99 and/or TdT. It should be remembered that the antigens listed above, other than myeloperoxidase, are not highly specific for myeloid lineage, and thus a panel of multiple antibodies should be employed, including antibodies against common T cell and B cell antigens to further exclude lymphoma.

Cytogenetic abnormalities are commonly detected in myeloid sarcoma, and mirror those known to be associated with AML. These abnormalities may be detectable in the blood or marrow of myeloid sarcoma patients even in the absence of morphologic evidence of blood or marrow involvement.

Myeloproliferative Neoplasms

The most common myeloproliferative neoplasms in children are CML, which accounts for around 3 percent of childhood leukemias, and juvenile myelomonocytic leukemia (JMML), which is actually classified as an overlapping myeloproliferative /myelodysplastic neoplasm, and accounts for around 3 percent or less of childhood leukemias.[41] Both of these diseases should have less than 20 percent immature myeloid cells in the blood and marrow. While their involvement is often limited to the blood and marrow, with possible enlargement of the liver and spleen, they may occasionally involve nodal or extranodal sites in the head and neck region.

Histology will show replacement of the involved tissue by the leukemic cells. In contrast to myeloid sarcoma, there is no significant component of immature-appearing cells. Thus, CML will show mainly mature granulocytes (myelocytes, metamyelocytes, bands and segmented granulocytes) and JMML will show mainly mature granulocytes and monocytes. As it may be difficult to histologically distinguish between mature cells and immature cells, especially with mononuclear mature cells such as myelocytes and monocytes, immunophenotyping can be performed. There should be a paucity of cells expressing markers of immaturity, such as CD99, CD117 and CD34. In addition, flow cytometry is useful for evaluating the presence or absence of blasts, and for assessing the maturational status of lesional monocytes.

In cases of CML, cytogenetics should usually detect a translocation (9;22) resulting in formation of the Philadelphia chromosome and transcription of a BCR-ABL1 mRNA transcript that can be detected by RT-PCR. Rare cases may have a variant translocation that may not be detectable by cytogenetic analysis. JMML is negative for t(9;22). Only a minority of cases of JMML have an identifiable cytogenetic abnormality, with monosomy 7 being the most common.

Histiocytic Neoplasms

Accumulations of histiocytes in the soft tissues and lymph nodes of the head and neck are much more commonly seen in reactive conditions, as histiocytic neoplasms are rare entities.[53] The histiocytic neoplasms include both neoplasms of the monocyte/macrophage cell lineage and neoplasms of dendritic cell lineages, such as Langerhans cells, interdigitating dendritic cells and indeterminate cells.

Neoplasms of cells with the appearance and phenotype of mature monocytes and/or macrophages are very rare, and are termed histiocytic sarcoma. The cytology of these tumors may range from bland to markedly atypical, though usually some features of histiocytic differentiation (oval nuclei, abundant cytoplasm) are maintained to a significant degree. The neoplastic cells typically express CD68, CD14 and lysozyme, and may express CD163.

Due to the rarity of histiocytic sarcoma, three alternative options should be considered before establishing such a diagnosis. First, a reactive condition should be excluded, especially if the cytologic features are relatively bland. Certain soft tissue infections, metabolic storage disorders, and other conditions may lead to accumulations of benign, non-clonal histiocytes, and these conditions should be excluded. Second, the possibility of histiocytic transdifferentiation of lymphoma should be considered, especially if there is previous history of lymphoma. In these cases, the histologic and immunophenotypic appearance of the tumor will be entirely histiocytic, and will not betray its lymphomatous origins, unless one is fortunate enough to have a biopsy that samples an adjacent area of lymphoma. Thus, cytogenetic and molecular analysis of these tumors is strongly recommended, as these studies may find typical findings of

NHL (such as *IGH-BCL2* gene fusion or clonal rearrangement of the *IGH* gene), which would support a diagnosis of histiocytic transdifferentiation of lymphoma.

Third, the possibility of an AML with monocytic differentiation involving tissues should be considered. This is especially important if the lesional cells have a morphologic appearance that is more reminiscent of monocytes than of histiocytes. In cases of AML with monocytic differentiation, there may be complete or partial absence of one or more mature macrophage markers, and there may be retention of markers of immaturity such as CD34 or CD117. Unfortunately, AML with monocytic differentiation may adopt a relatively mature phenotype when it involves solid tissues, and the resultant overlap between this entity and histiocytic sarcoma can be impossible to resolve by analysis of the biopsy alone. Thus, evaluation of blood and marrow is useful to assess for the possible presence of AML before establishing a diagnosis of histiocytic sarcoma.

LCH is much more common than histiocytic sarcoma. LCH is a disorder of Langerhans cells, which are bone marrow-derived antigen-presenting cells normally present in the skin and mucosal membranes. LCH is characterized by an extremely variable clinical course, ranging from indolent, localized disease to aggressive, systemic disease. Most if not all cases of LCH are now thought to represent neoplasms.[53]

Clinically, patients with more indolent versions of LCH tend to be older children and adults; they tend to have localized disease, which most often involves the lung, the skin or the diaphysis of a long bone. LCH may also be multifocal within one organ system; in such cases multifocal bone involvement is most common, and some cases of this type have been historically termed Hand–Schuller–Christian disease. The bony lesions in these cases have a predilection for the jaw and skull bones, and may result in such symptoms as splaying of teeth, tooth loss, diabetes insipidus (due to impingement upon the hypothalamus) and exophthalmos (Figures 19.91, 19.92 & 19.93).

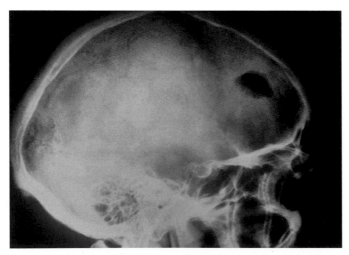

Figure 19.91 LCH. Skull radiolucency in a patient with multifocal disease. (Reprinted from Marx R, Stern D. *Oral and Maxillofacial Pathology: A Rationale for Diagnosis and Treatment* with permission from Quintessence Publishing Company).

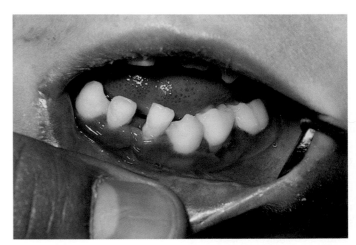

Figure 19.92 LCH. Mobile splayed teeth are a common finding when the mandible is involved. (Reprinted from Marx R, Stern D. *Oral and Maxillofacial Pathology: A Rationale for Diagnosis and Treatment* with permission from Quintessence Publishing Company).

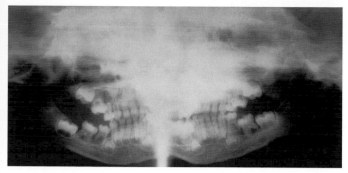

Figure 19.93 LCH. Severe alveolar bone loss around the primary molars in a child with LCH. (Reprinted from Marx R, Stern D. *Oral and Maxillofacial Pathology: A Rationale for Diagnosis and Treatment* with permission from Quintessence Publishing Company).

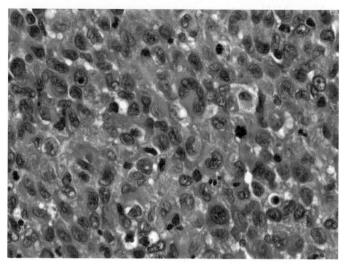

Figure 19.95 LCH. High power view of the neoplastic Langerhans cells.

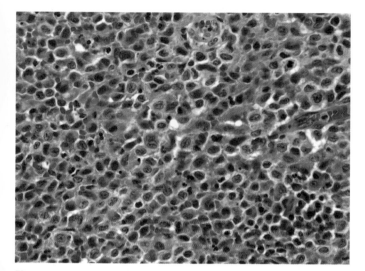

Figure 19.94 LCH. The neoplastic Langerhans cells contain abundant eosinophilic cytoplasm and mildly atypical nuclei with open chromatin and prominent nuclear grooves. Note the admixed eosinophils.

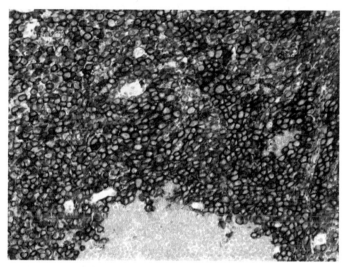

Figure 19.96 LCH. Strong membranous expression of CD1a by the neoplastic cells.

Aggressive systemic cases of LCH tend to be seen in infants and young children. They often present with systemic symptoms (fever, malaise), and often have widespread bone lesions with enlargement of the liver, spleen and/or lymph nodes. Cervical lymph nodes are most often involved, but lymphadenopathy may involve any site. Pancytopenia may be present, due either to bone marrow involvement by LCH or to hemophagocytic syndrome, which occurs in response to a minority of cases of LCH. Numerous other sites may be involved, resulting in numerous other possible signs and symptoms. A minority of cases of LCH occur in concert with a second hematologic malignancy, most frequently CHL.

Histologically, Langerhans cells are of relatively large size (10 to 15um). They have characteristic clear nuclei with folds and convolutions resulting in nuclear grooves. Nucleoli are inconspicuous if present (Figures 19.94 & 19.95). Cytologic atypia is usually absent to minimal, though in rare cases, termed Langerhans cell sarcoma, it may be striking. Often, the lesions of LCH include an infiltrate of one or more types of inflammatory cells; these infiltrates may be of eosinophils,

neutrophils, plasma cells and/or histiocytes, with eosinophilic infiltrates being particularly common (Figure 19.94). Plasma cells are usually not a prominent component of the lesions.

Immunophenotypically, Langerhans cells, both normal and neoplastic, are characterized by expression of CD1a, langerin and S-100 protein (Figure 19.96). The neoplastic cells in LCH usually show variable expression of CD68, and a subset of cases show weak positivity for CD4. They are negative for B cell and T cell markers (with the exception of CD1a, and of CD2, which is often expressed). LCH cells are negative for CD15 and CD30, and are negative for evidence of EBV infection.

LCH lacks recurrent cytogenetic abnormalities. Recently, it has been found that a majority of cases of LCH, though not all cases, harbor a V600E mutation of the *BRAF* gene, a mutation that has been found in other tumor types.[54] Specific IHC studies for the mutated BRAF protein are now commercially available, and may aid in diagnosis.

References

Introduction

1. Larsson LO, Bentzon MW, Berg K, Mellander L, Skoogh BE, Stranegård IL. Palpable lymph nodes of the neck in Swedish schoolchildren. *Acta Paediatrica*. 1994;83:1092–1094.

2. Park YW. Evaluation of neck masses in children. *Am Family Physician*. 1995; 51(8):1904–1912.

3. Yaris N, Cakir M, Sözen E, Cobanoglu U. Analysis of children with peripheral lymphadenopathy. *Clin Pediatr (Phila)*. 2006 Jul;45(6):544–549.

4. Twist CJ, Link MP. Assessment of lymphadenopathy in children. *Pediatric Clinics of North America*. 2000;49: 1009–1025.

5. Chau I, Kelleher MT, Cunningham D, Norman AR, Wotherspoon A, Trott P, Rhys-Evans P, Querci Della Rovere G, Brown G, Allen M, Waters JS, Haque S, Murray T, Bishop L. Rapid access multidisciplinary lymph node diagnostic clinic: analysis of 550 patients. *Br J Cancer*. 2003 Feb 10; 88(3):354–361.

6. Montgomery ND, Mathews SP, Coward WB, Rao KW, Fedoriw Y. Clonal karyotypic abnormalities associated with reactive lymphoid hyperplasia. *Cancer Cytogenetics*. 2013;206(4): 135–139.

Reactive Lymphadenopathy

7. Leung AK and Robson WL. Childhood cervical lymphadenopathy. *J Pediatr Health Care*. 2004;18:3–7.

8. Oguz A, Karadeniz C, Temel EA, Citak EC, Okur FV. Evaluation of peripheral lymphadenopathy in children. *Pediatr Hematol Oncol*. 2006;23:549–561.

9. Moore SW, Schneider JW, Schaaf HS. Diagnostic aspects of cervical lymphadenopathy in children in the developing world: a study of 1,877 surgical specimens. *Pediatr Surg Int*. 2003;19:240–244.

10. Papadopouli E, Michailidi E, Papadopoulou E, Paspalaki P, Vlahakis I, Kalmanti M. Cervical lymphadenopathy in childhood epidemiology and management. *Pediatr Hematol Oncol*. 2009;26:454–460.

Progressive Transformation of Germinal Centers

11. Ramsay AD. Reactive lymph nodes in pediatric practice. *Am J Clin Pathol*. 2004;122 (Suppl):S87–97.

12. Shaikh F, Ngan BY, Alexander S, Grant R. Progressive transformation of germinal centers in children and adolescents: an intriguing cause of lymphadenopathy. *Pediatr Blood Cancer*. 2013;60:26–30.

13. Sato Y, Inoue D, Asano N, et al. Association between IgG4-related disease and progressively transformed germinal centers of lymph nodes. *Mod Pathol*. 2012;25:956–967.

Epstein–Barr Virus Lymphadenitis

14. Kutok JL, Wang F. Spectrum of Epstein-Barr virus-associated diseases. *Annu Rev Pathol*. 2006;1:375–404.

15. Hurt C, Tammaro D. Diagnostic evaluation of mononucleosis-like illnesses. *Am J Med*. 2007;120: 911.e1–911.e8.

Cytomegalovirus Lymphadenitis

16. Ventura KC, Hudnall SD. Hematologic differences in heterophile-positive and heterophile-negative infectious mononucleosis. *Am J Hematol*. 2004;76:315–318.

17. Rushin JM, Riordan GP, Heaton RB, Sharpe RW, Cotelingam JD, Jaffe ES. Cytomegalovirus-infected cells express Leu-M1 antigen. A potential source of diagnostic error. *Am J Pathol*. 1990;136:989–995.

Cat Scratch Disease

18. Miller-Catchpole R, Variakojis D, Vardiman JW, Loew JM, Carter J. Cat scratch disease. Identification of bacteria in seven cases of lymphadenitis. *Am J Surg Pathol*. 1986;10:276–281.

19. Ridder GJ, Boedeker CC, Technau-Ihling K, Sander A. Cat-scratch disease: otolaryngologic manifestations and management. *Otolaryngol Head Neck Surg*. 2005;132:353–358.

20. Rolain JM, Gouriet F, Enea M, Aboud M, Raoult D. Detection by immunofluorescence assay of Bartonella henselae in lymph nodes from patients with cat scratch disease. *Clin Diagn Lab Immunol*. 2003;10:686–691.

21. Mouritsen CL, Litwin CM, Maiese RL, Segal SM, Segal GH. Rapid polymerase chain reaction-based detection of the causative agent of cat scratch disease (Bartonella henselae) in formalin-fixed, paraffin-embedded samples. *Hum Pathol*. 1997;28:820–826.

22. Hansmann Y, DeMartino S, Piemont Y, et al. Diagnosis of cat scratch disease with detection of Bartonella henselae by PCR: a study of patients with lymph node enlargement. *J Clin Microbiol*. 2005;43:3800–3806.

Toxoplasma Lymphadenitis

23. Eapen M, Mathew CF, Aravindan KP. Evidence based criteria for the histopathological diagnosis of toxoplasmic lymphadenopathy. *J Clin Pathol*. 2005;58:1143–1146.

24. Lin MH and Kuo TT. Specificity of the histopathological triad for the diagnosis of toxoplasmic lymphadenitis: polymerase chain reaction study. *Pathol Int*. 2001;51:619–623.

25. Montoya JG, Huffman HB, Remington JS. Evaluation of the immunoglobulin G avidity test for diagnosis of toxoplasmic lymphadenopathy. *J Clin Microbiol*. 2004;42:4627–4631.

26. Paul M. Immunoglobulin G avidity in diagnosis of toxoplasmic lymphadenopathy and ocular toxoplasmosis. *Clin Diagn Lab Immunol*. 1999;6:514–518.

Kikuchi–Fujimoto Lymphadenitis

27. Rivano MT, Falini B, Stein H, et al. Histiocytic necrotizing lymphadenitis without granulocytic infiltration (Kikuchi's lymphadenitis). Morphological and immunohistochemical study of eight cases. *Histopathology*. 1987;11:1013–1027.

28. Tsang WY, Chan JK, Ng CS. Kikuchi's lymphadenitis. A morphologic analysis of 75 cases with special reference to unusual features. *Am J Surg Pathol*. 1994;18:219–231.

Systemic Lupus Erythematosus Lymphadenopathy

29. Eisner MD, Amory J, Mullaney B, Tierney L,Jr, Browner WS. Necrotizing lymphadenitis associated with systemic lupus erythematosus. *Semin Arthritis Rheum*. 1996;26:477–482.

30. Biasi D, Caramaschi P, Carletto A, et al. Three clinical reports of Kikuchi's lymphadenitis combined with systemic lupus erythematosus. *Clin Rheumatol*. 1996;15:81–83.

31. el-Ramahi KM, Karrar A, Ali MA. Kikuchi disease and its association with systemic lupus erythematosus. *Lupus*. 1994;3:409–411.

Kimura Disease

32. Abuel-Haija M, Hurford MT. Kimura disease. *Arch Pathol Lab Med*. 2007;131:650–651.

33. Chen H, Thompson LD, Aguilera NS, Abbondanzo SL. Kimura disease: a clinicopathologic study of 21 cases. *Am J Surg Pathol.* 2004;28:505–513.

34. Kapoor NS, O'Neill JP, Katabi N, Wong RJ, Shah JP. Kimura disease: diagnostic challenges and clinical management. *Am J Otolaryngol.* 2012;33:259–262.

35. Schirren CG, Eckert F. Angiolymphoid hyperplasia with eosinophils. Case report and differentiation from Kimura disease. *Hautarzt.* 1991;42:107–111.

Rosai–Dorfman Disease

36. Carbone A, Passannante A, Gloghini A, Devaney KO, Rinaldo A, Ferlito A. Review of sinus histiocytosis with massive lymphadenopathy (Rosai-Dorfman disease) of head and neck. *Ann Otol Rhinol Laryngol.* 1999;108:1095–1104.

37. Foucar E, Rosai J, Dorfman R. Sinus histiocytosis with massive lymphadenopathy (Rosai-Dorfman disease): review of the entity. *Semin Diagn Pathol.* 1990;7:19–73.

Hematologic Malignancies

38. Swerdlow SH, Campo E, Harris NL, Jaffe ES, Pileri SA, Stein H, Thiele J, Varidman JW (Eds.), *WHO Classification of Tumours of Hematopoietic and Lymphoid Tissues*, 4th ed. Lyon: IARC, 2008.

39. Asselin BA (2011). Epidemiology of childhood and adolescent cancer In Kliegman RM (Ed.), *Nelson Textbook of Pediatrics*, 19th ed. (pp. 1725–1727). Philadelphia: Elsevier.

40. Howlader N, Noone AM, Krapcho M, Garshell J, Miller D, Altekruse SF, Kosary CL, Yu M, Ruhl J, Tatalovich Z, Mariotto A, Lewis DR, Chen HS, Feuer EJ, Cronin KA (Eds.), *SEER Cancer Statistics Review, 1975–2011*, Bethesda, MD: National Cancer Institute. http://seer.cancer.gov/csr/1975_2011/, based on November 2013 SEER data submission, posted to the SEER web site, April 2014.

Neoplasms of Immature Lymphoid Cells

41. Tubergen DG, Bleyer A, Ritchey AK (2011). The leukemias In Kliegman RM (Ed.), *Nelson Textbook of Pediatrics*, 19th ed. (pp. 1732–1739). Philadelphia: Elsevier.

42. Ohgami RS, Arber DA, Zehnder JL, Natkunam Y, and Warnke RA (2013), Indolent T-lymphoblastic proliferation (iT-LBP): a review of the clinical and pathologic features and distinction from malignant T-lymphoblastic lymphoma, Advances in Anatomic Pathology; 20(3):137–140

43. Waxman IM, Hochberg J, Cairo MS (2011). Lymphoma In Kliegman RM (Ed.), *Nelson Textbook of Pediatrics*, 19th ed. (pp. 1739–1746). Philadelphia: Elsevier.

Burkitt Lymphoma and Diffuse Large B Cell Lymphoma

44. Perkins SL (2007). Hematopoietic system, part 1: bone marrow, peripheral blood and lymphomas In Gilbert-Barnes E (Ed.), *Potter's Pathology of the Fetus, Infant and Child*, 2nd ed. Philadelphia: Mosby Elsevier.

45. Molyneux EM, Rochford R, Griffin B, Newton R, Jackson G, Mcnon G, Harrsion CJ, Israels T, Bailey S. Burkitt's lymphoma. *Lancet.* 2012;379:1234–1244.

46. Reiter A, Klapper W. Recent advances in the understanding and management of diffuse large B-cell lymphoma in children. *British Journal of Haematology.* 2008;142:329–347.

Rare Pediatric Non-Hodgkin Lymphomas

47. Swerdlow SH. Pediatric follicular lymphomas, marginal zone lymphomas, and marginal zone hyperplasia. *American Journal of Clinical Pathology.* 2004; 122(S1):S89–S109.

48. Gitelson E, Al-Saleem T, Robu V, Millenson MM, Smith MR. Pediatric nodal marginal zone lymphoma may develop in the adult population. *Leukemia and Lymphoma.* 2010; 51(1):89–94.

49. Claviez A, Meyer U, Dominick C, Beck JF, Rister M, Tiemann M. MALT lymphoma in children: a report from the NHL-BFM Study Group. *Pediatric Blood and Cancer.* 2006;47:210–214.

50. Bhuvana AS, Termuhlen AM. Rare pediatric non-Hodgkin lymphoma. *Current Hematologic Malignancy Reports.* 2010 5:163–168.

Hodgkin Lymphoma

51. Daw S, Wynn R, Wallace H. Management of relapsed and refractory classical Hodgkin lymphoma in children and adolescents. *British Journal of Haematology.* 2010;152: 249–260.

52. Shankar A, Daw S. Nodular lymphocyte predominant Hodgkin lymphoma in children and adolescents - a comprehensive review of biology, clinical course and treatment options. *British Journal of Haematology.* 2012;159:288–298.

Histiocytic Neoplasms

53. Onciu M. Histiocytic proliferations in childhood. *Am J Clin Pathol.* 2004; 122(S1):S128–S136.

54. Badalian-Very G, Vergilio JA, Degar BA, MacConaill LE, Brandner B, Calicchio ML, Kuo FC, Ligon AH, Stevenson KE, Kehoe SM, Garraway LA, Hahn WC, Meyerson M, Fleming MD, Rollins BJ. Recurrent BRAF mutations in Langerhans cell histiocytosis. *Blood.* 2010 Sep; 116(11):1919–1923.

20

Developmental and Syndromic Disturbances of the Craniofacial Region

Robert E. Marx and Robert O. Greer

Introduction

Developmental disorders and birth defects are common to the craniofacial complex in pediatric age patients. These disorders can affect the craniofacial soft tissues, the jaws, the teeth and associated structures, and they can be broadly defined as genetic in origin, inherited, environmental or of an unknown cause. The most common of these defects to occur at birth in the craniofacial are the encephalocele and complex cleft palate and cleft lip. A host of less commonly encountered developmental anomalies are discussed in this section of the chapter.

Some disturbances occur during a so-called window of opportunity period during embryogenesis while others develop later in life. Many disturbances are syndrome associated and their etiologies, although broadly defined as genetic, inherited, environmental or unknown, can be linked to hormonal imbalance, chromosomal abnormalities, lymphatic and vascular abnormalities, neurogenic abnormalities and localized alteration during intrauterine development.

Glial Choristoma

Clinical Findings

The glial choristoma is a rare, usually congenital, ectopic soft tissue tumor that, when it occurs in the head and neck region, is most often reported to involve the middle ear and the tongue.[1,2] Tongue lesions present as nodules that can be either painless or painful. Glial choristomas tend to be most common from birth to ten years of age. The lesions can be found in concert with nasal sinus gliomas and extranasal gliomas.[3] Only rarely will lesions reach a maximum size of 2 cm in diameter. Those lesions that involve the middle ear are commonly associated with pain, and a loss of hearing can result. Neither lesions of the tongue or middle ear tend to be associated with any form of generalized central nervous system pathology.

In an infant, glial choristoma should be considered in the differential diagnosis of any suspected congenital developmental malformation of the tongue, including lingual thyroid nodule, vascular or lymphatic malformations and teratoma. Glial choristomas occurring in the infratemporal fossa or the parapharyngeal space will require differentiation from a meningocele or encephalocele. CT scans can be quite helpful in differentiating a glial choristoma from lesions in which there is a true intracranial connection.

Pathologic Findings

The glial choristoma will present grossly as an unencapsulated submucosal nodule or mass. Histologically, the lesion will be composed of interlacing aggregates of loosely arranged neuroglial fibers and scattered neurons that are admixed with astrocytes, choroid plexuses and ependymal cells. Astrocytes can present as either mononuclear or multinucleated cells. Interlacing bands of fibrous connective tissue will make up the lesional stroma.

From a differential diagnostic standpoint, glial choristoma must be distinguished histologically from neurilemoma, or a metastatic anaplastic brain malignancy.[3] Glial choristoma can easily be differentiated from neurilemoma microscopically because the neurilemoma will lack glial elements and demonstrate significant cellular maturity. Neurilemoma will also be immunoreactive to S-100 protein, GFAP and occasionally vimentin, whereas the glial choristoma or an anaplastic brain neoplasm will not.

Treatment and Prognosis

Most glial choristomas will present at birth or manifest within the first few years of life,[4] and most lesions grow quite slowly, and certainly no faster than the tissue that surrounds them. Although dyspnea and dysphagia can occur as a result of a glial choristoma, these findings are rare. Tumors are generally treated by conservative surgical excision and the glial choristoma is not reported to have any malignant potential.[4,5,6]

Fordyce Granules (Fordyce Spots, Fordyce Disease)
Clinical Features

Fordyce granules, first reported in 1896,[7] represent ectopic normal sebaceous glands that occur on the lips, buccal mucosa, genital mucosa and esophagus rather than with their normal parent tissue skin.[8,9] Although most patients with Fordyce granules are adults, Fordyce granules have been reported in children.[8]

Fordyce granules in the head and neck region will typically appear as multicentric white to yellowish, elevated, often coalescent papules and plaques, or as cauliflower-like excrescences involving the oral mucous membranes. Individual plaques or papules usually range in size from 3 mm to 5 mm in diameter. The mucosa around Fordyce granules generally appears normal. In children as in adults, the lesions are most

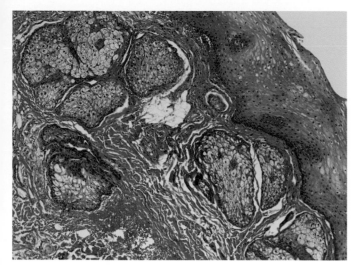

Figure 20.1 Medium power photomicrograph of Fordyce granules.

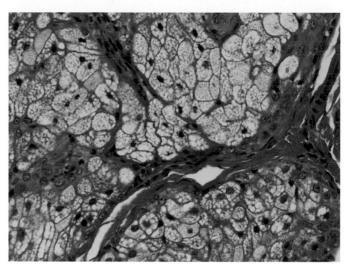

Figure 20.2 High power photomicrograph of Fordyce granules showing ectopically located sebaceous glands in the lamina propria of oral mucosa, with evidence of rudimentary excretory ducts.

often bilateral and involve the buccal mucosa, and hundreds of ectopically located glands can occur. Fordyce granules have been reported to occur in association with hereditary non-polyposis colorectal cancer[10] and rarely sebaceous gland adenomas of the buccal mucosa have reported to arise from pre-existing Fordyce disease.[11] Fordyce granules in children can become so coalescent, nodular and diffuse that they can resemble sebaceous hyperplasia of the skin.

Pathologic Features

Most often, Fordyce granules can be adequately diagnosed based upon clinical examination and evaluation. When biopsied, histologic findings will show normal appearing clusters of sebaceous glands in the lamina propria of the oral mucosa (Figure 20.1). Glands will display rudimentary excretory ducts that ramify throughout a collagenous stroma (Figure 20.2). Excretory ducts, however, may be entirely absent. Hair follicles, typical of sebaceous glands in the dermal layer of skin, will be lacking and the entire ductal apparatus is typically aberrant. Glands tend to occur superficially in the lamina propria of the oral mucosa. On occasion, inflammatory cells can be seen in the supporting glandular stroma, and pseudocysts may be identified. These pseudocysts can sometimes resemble neoplasms of salivary gland origin, most notably low grade mucoepidermoid carcinoma, but they will lack the epithelial proliferation, and cohesiveness of that neoplasm, and they will not be associated with a mucin product. Neoplastic transformation of Fordyce granules to sebaceous carcinoma has been reported.[10]

Treatment and Prognosis

Therapeutic intervention is not required for Fordyce granules except in very rare instances when inflammation occurs, and lesions, especially those involving the lips, become cosmetically problematic for the patient. In those instances in which long term or repetitive inflammation occurs, clindamycin has been employed as an effective therapy.[12] CO_2 Laser therapy and oral isotretinoin have been used to ablate Fordyce granules. However, the side effects of such therapy, which can include a persistent burning sensation involving the mucosa, post-operative inflammatory hyperpigmentation and scaring tends to limit the use of such therapies.[12]

De Felice et al.[10] have demonstrated germline mutations in mismatch repair (MMR) genes in children in families with non-polyposis colorectal cancer syndrome and syndrome associated gingival or buccal ectopic sebaceous glands. This finding may ultimately prove helpful in the early identification of gene carriers and affected families with the syndrome.[12]

Cleidocranial Dysplasia

Clinical Features

Cleidocranial dysplasia (CCD), first described by Siggers[13] in 1975 as cleidocranial dysostosis, is an uncommon, most often inherited, autosomal dominant skeletal dysplasia that affects both teeth and bone.[14] Individuals with CCD present clinically with skull deformities. They are characteristically of short stature and they will have hypoplasia or aplasia of one or both clavicles (Figure 20.3). Additional features include closure of the cranial fontanels and sutures, frontal and parietal bossing, widening of the pubic syntheses, underdevelopment of the premaxilla, pseudoanodontia, impaction of permanent teeth, supernumerary teeth and malocclusion.[14,15] (See Figure 20.4.) CCD is caused by mutations of the transcription factor RUNX2, a principal regulator of osteoblast differentiation. CCD is most often identified in childhood, and the disorder has been reported in children as young as 2 years of age.

Individuals from families that have a low frequency of CCD associated dental abnormalities have been shown to have no mutation in the RUNX2 gene or any mutations outside of the runt domain (Q292fs→X299).[15] However, patients from

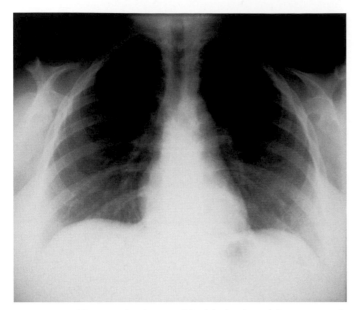

Figure 20.3 CCD. Note the absence of the left clavicle and the presence of only a rudimentary right clavicle on a chest radiograph. (Reprinted from Marx R, Stern D. *Oral and Maxillofacial Pathology: A Rationale for Diagnosis and Treatment* with permission from Quintessence Publishing Company).

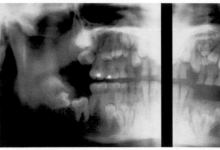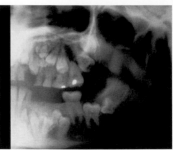

Figure 20.4 Teeth in the shape of premolars in a child with CCD. Unerupted, normal appearing premolar teeth are also present. (Reprinted from Marx R, Stern D. *Oral and Maxillofacial Pathology: A Rationale for Diagnosis and Treatment* with permission from Quintessence Publishing Company).

families who have severe dental alterations, including most often, multiple impacted and supernumerary teeth, tend to show heterozygous missense mutations of the R190Q and R225Q domains that in turn impair the runt domain,[15] and the domain associated down regulation necessary for full odontoblast differentiation.[16,17]

Radiographic imaging in patients with CCD will typically demonstrate radiolucent zones in the craniofacial complex that correspond to areas where there have been delayed cranial bone formation. The frontal and sphenoid sinuses are typically quite small or absent, as are the maxillary and ethmoid sinuses in CCD patients. Secondary calcification is often recognizable in skull suture lines and a small percentage of CCD patients will develop a so-called doubled dentition, in which a duplicate row of teeth form lingual and occlusal to the unerupted permanent premolars. Cephalographic analysis will generally show persistent open sutures in wormian bones, and chest films usually demonstrate aplasia or hypoplasia of the clavicles. Thirty-five percent of CCD patients will show no associated apparent inheritance pattern. Those patients more than likely represent spontaneous mutations disease induced.[17,18]

The multiple unerupted teeth that are seen in CCD are likely due to the absence of cellular cementum and the inter-delayed exfoliation of the primary dentition due to delayed root resorption.[18] The supernumerary teeth that are present in CCD are thought to be related to failure of the dental lamina to involute. Patients between the ages of two and a half and six years with CCD will usually show normal eruption and normal formation of the 20 primary teeth. However, CCD patients in the mixed dentition stage of tooth development, (6 to 12 years) will demonstrate numerous unerupted teeth. Since CCD is characterized by delayed root resorption and the normal physiologic exfoliation of the primary teeth, it is postulated that for every permanent tooth that should occur in the jaws, a concomitant supernumerary tooth can be expected in patients with CCD.[18]

Pathologic Findings

The clinical and radiographic appearance of CCD is usually pathognomonic of the disorder. Therefore, biopsies of tissue from affected individual are not indicated. Microscopic examination of affected primary and permanent teeth that have exfoliated will show a lack of root surface cellular cementum.[18]

Treatment and Prognosis

CCD is most effectively managed by minimizing or reducing the dental and facial deformities that occur in association with the disease, including the exceedingly common, malocclusion, which is generally treated by the removal of supernumerary teeth and orthodontic therapy. Individuals with CCD frequently develop dentigerous cysts or periapical cysts that become either symptomatic of interfere with orthodontic treatment. In such instances extraction of the involved tooth, teeth or cyst(s) is indicated. For CCD patients who have rare submandibular clefts, orthognathic surgery is often indicated. In some instances CCD patients will require extensive restorative dental treatment and or prosthetic replacement for missing or extracted teeth.

Guided eruption of teeth, a common management modality for patients who don't have CCD, is often fought with failure in CCD patients since these patients lack the cellular cementum necessary for tooth eruption. Therefore the teeth cannot effectively be guided into place orthodontically and stabilized. CCD should be suspected by the clinician in patients of short stature, who also have underdeveloped or absent clavicles, frontal bossing and multiple supernumerary and unerupted teeth. Timely recognition of the disease and hereditary tendency counseling can be quite beneficial in CCD patients because of the possibility of covert transmissibility.[19,20,21]

Idiopathic Bone Cavity

Idiopathic bone cavities (IBC) are uncommon cavitary lesions that when encountered in children and adolescents are most

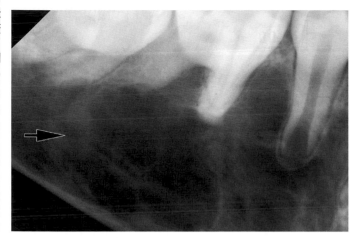

Figure 20.5 Idiopathic bone cavity in the body of the mandible of a child.

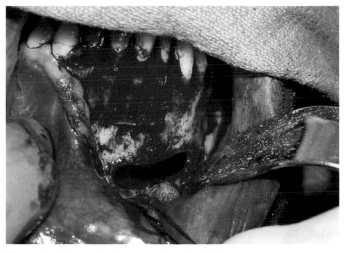

Figure 20.6 Surgical exploration of an IBC will demonstrate an empty cavity within bone. (Reprinted from Marx R, Stern D. *Oral and Maxillofacial Pathology: A Rationale for Diagnosis and Treatment* with permission from Quintessence Publishing Company).

often located in the posterior mandible. Maxillary lesions and lesions involving long bones, primarily the humerus, also occur.[22,23,24,25] Perdigao et al.[22] reviewed a series of 43 mandibular IBC and found the median age in their sample to be 16 years for boys and 18 years for girls.

Sometimes referred to as *traumatic bone cysts*, or *simple bone cysts*, the idiopathic bone cavity is not a true cyst since it is not lined by epithelium.[24] Most IBC are identified as an ancillary finding during routine radiographic screenings of the jaws. The IBC can resemble an odontogenic keratocyst, radicular cyst, ameloblastoma, ameloblastic fibroma or a central giant cell lesion (granuloma) radiographically.[23] Lesions are typically well defined and often bilateral radiolucencies that demonstrate a rather characteristic scalloped pattern as they extend between the roots of teeth and into the inter-radicular bone (Figure 20.5).[25] Pseudocysts of the auricle are considered to be the equivalent of IBC in that site.[26]

At one time, investigators thought that IBC occurred as a result of trauma to the jaws. Most authorities now suggest however, that the IBC is if in fact the result of some alteration or disturbance in the remodeling and recontouring of trabecular bone. An alteration that is driven by hormonal, biochemical or molecular events that tend to show a peak effect during adolescence.[27]

Although the most common radiographic appearance of the idiopathic bone cavity is that of a radiolucency interdigitating or undulating between the roots of teeth, not all lesions will demonstrate this appearance,[28] and the IBC may present as an isolated unilocular radiolucency, or even as a multilocular one. The lesions can, on occasion, expand bone, but they do not displace the mandibular canal, which will course through the lesion normally, regardless of the IBCs size.

Differential Diagnosis

It may be difficult to distinguish an idiopathic bone cavity from a vascular lesion of the jaw, such as arterial venous malformation or hemangiomas, or from certain odontogenic cysts. One way of distinguishing an idiopathic bone cavity from a vascular

lesion is via aspiration. An aspirated idiopathic bone cavity will return a few air bubbles, or a small amount of straw colored fluid within the syringe before blood appears. Any blood, within an IBC will quickly decrease in flow. Hemangiomas and other vascular lesions will, on the other hand, demonstrate a continual flow or oozing of blood after initial aspiration.

Pathologic Findings

IBC are relatively innocuous lesions that nonetheless are often surgically explored, largely because the clinical differential diagnosis for an IBC can include, odontogenic tumors and cysts, giant cell lesions of the jaw or fibro-osseous lesions such as ossifying fibroma or fibrous dysplasia. None of the aforementioned lesions, when explored surgically, will be devoid of contents as will the IBC (Figure 20.6). Tissue curetted from an IBC, when examined microscopically, will consist of an accumulation of proteinaceous debris, serosanguineous fluid and normal or reactive bone that may be marginated by osteoclasts and osteoblasts (Figure 20.7). A true epithelial cyst lining will not be seen.

Treatment and Prognosis

The most appropriate initial treatment for an idiopathic bone cavity is aspiration of the lesion, although radiographic monitoring of the lesion can also be employed. Since the IBC will typically be devoid of contents, aspiration with 1 ml of saline in the syringe will yield only air bubbles and a minimal amount of straw colored fluid, rather than blood or tumor cells. Most traumatic bone cysts will resolve after surgical intervention or remodel themselves without intervention.[28,29] On occasion, large lesions have to be explored more than once in order to initiate bony remodeling and repair of the osseous void. Surgical exploration is curative. Implanting foreign material such as hydroxylapatite into the lesion in order to help resolve it is contraindicated.

with DI, but the dentin/enamel junction tends to be fragile in these patients. The occlusal forces that are generated in mastication can easily fracture away any residual enamel and dentin, resulting in crown or root fracture. Patients with dentin dysplasia are also commonly treated with full crown coverage of the affected teeth, with dental implants or with removable or fixed dental appliances. However, patients with dentin dysplasia type 1 have extremely short roots, and the affected teeth often become so periodontally involved that the teeth exfoliate on their own.

Osteogenesis Imperfecta

Clinical Features

OI is a congenital disorder of bone that is most often causally attributed to a defect in the gene that produces type I collagen (collagen 1A and 1B), a product that is mandatory for the normal development of bone. OI is most often an inherited autosomal dominant disease.[79,80] Rarely, however, genetic mutations can also cause OI, including rare instances of autosomal recessive inheritance, spontaneous inheritance and instances in which there have been disease triggering gene point mutations that affect procollagen synthesis. Instances of OI have also been reported in which collagen synthesis is not truly altered, but instead the collagen molecule itself is aggregated improperly.[81] Thus OI is currently considered to be a disorder that develops in multiple alternate ways. OI must therefore be seen as a multifactorial and multiscale connective tissue disorder that develops due to alterations at the genetic, nano, microscopic and gross anatomic levels, to affect not simply bone but other connective tissue derivatives as well[81]

Also known as brittle bone disease, OI results in the production of bone that fails to have the elasticity of normal bone. The resulting bone is prone to fracture, a classic hallmark of OI.

OI occurs as a result of abnormal collagen that is composed of fibers that are less thick and round than normal collagen fibers. This aberrant collagen allows the underlying choroidal veins uveal vessels and pigment of the eye to show through the normally white sclerae of the eye.

In addition to being characterized by bone fractures, OI is also characterized by bruising, joint hypermobility, bowing of the long bones and aortic dilations. DI, a disorder of dentin that is also associated with abnormal collagen synthesis, can occur in concert with OI, or as a genetically induced non-DI associated dental abnormality of its own.

The incidence of OI is estimated to be 1 per 20,000 live births. Sillence et al.[80] investigated the heterogenicity of the disease extensively, ultimately classifying DI into four distinct subtypes.[79,80,81,82]

Since that group's original 1979 classification of DI, five additional rare types of OI have been identified. However, these rare OI subtypes subdesignated as types 5 through 8 have not been identified in the bones of the jaws or facial skeleton.

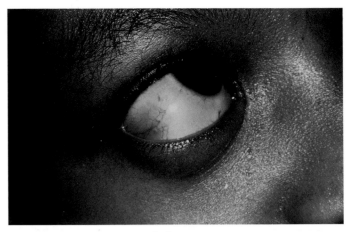

Figure 20.17 Blue sclerae typical of OI. (Reprinted from Marx R, Stern D. *Oral and Maxillofacial Pathology: A Rationale for Diagnosis and Treatment* with permission from Quintessence Publishing Company).

OI types 1A and B, which are considered to be mild forms of the disease, are most often encountered in the oral and maxillofacial region and in the bones of the skull. Fractures are common in these individuals and fracture frequency increases with age. Affected individuals can also have blue sclera (Figure 20.17), and bowing of the long bones. Ninety percent of patients with OI will have some form of hearing loss before the age of 30. Classically, individuals with type 1B OI will develop varying degrees of DI in addition to their skeletal abnormalities, and it is type 1B O1 in which well vascularized pulpal tissue within teeth will tend to show through aberrant poorly formed dentin, to cause teeth to have an opalescent or brown hue.[81] Ultimately, the pulps of affected teeth may become obliterated. The enamel in the teeth of such patients will be normal, but the dentin and the linkage between dentin and enamel will be altered such that the enamel will often flake away from the dentin.[81]

Individuals with type 2A, B and C OI, a prenatal and lethal form of the disease, will have poor overall cranial mineralization, and incomplete skeletal development. Autopsies on these individuals have shown that they tend to have enlarged dental pulps and constricted dental tubules in their teeth.[80] Patients with type 3 OI tend not to show significant head and neck pathology and they will lack blue sclera.[80] Approximately, 50 percent of type 3 OI patients will also have dentinogenesis imperfect as part of their disease. Patients with type 4 OI tend to be short statured with fragile bones and normal appearing sclera. Type 4 OI patients tend to have a high incidence of associated DI with concomitant enamel loss, opalescent discoloration of the teeth, pulp chamber obliteration and deposition of gnarled secondary dentin in the teeth.[82,83,84,85] Hearing loss is common in type 4 OI patients as well.

Pathologic Findings

Bony ossification does not occur in OI and the cortical bone is typically thin, with minimal or little associated medullary trabecular bone and marrow. The bone is thus undermineralized,

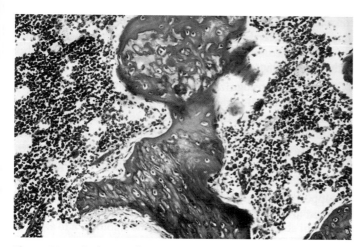

Figure 20.18 Undermineralized and highly cellular bone in OI. (Reprinted from Marx R, Stern D. *Oral and Maxillofacial Pathology: A Rationale for Diagnosis and Treatment* with permission from Quintessence Publishing Company).

(Figure 20.18) and prone to fracture. Indeed, one of the hallmarks of OI will be the histologic presence of a fractured callus. It is possible, especially in infants, with OI, for the entire skull to be composed predominantly of fibrous connective tissue with only minimal amounts of bone. In adults, the bone will be wormian in nature with less evidence of fibrous connective tissue and the presence of numerous aberrant or irregular sutures.

From a differential diagnostic perspective, the most frequent disorder to be considered when a diagnosis of OI is entertained is the battered child syndrome. This syndrome may be difficult to distinguish from OI. Thus, examination of dental structures, and evaluation of the patient for DI and blue sclera, is mandatory in order to exclude battered child syndrome as a diagnosis. The presence of OI associated blue sclera along with DI can prove helpful in establishing a diagnosis of OI, however, DI can occur as a distinct entity of its own, unassociated with OI. A host of other syndromes can result in multiple bone fractures, including CCD, mandibuloacral dysplasia, progeria, Marfan syndrome and Ehlers–Danlos syndrome. Therefore an appropriate diagnostic evaluation of any individual suspected of having OI will necessitate the exclusion of the aforementioned disorders.

Treatment and Prognosis

Since the major management consideration in patients with OI is fracture, the treatment of fractures is of paramount importance. Treatment with bisphosphonates has been effective in reducing the incidence of facial, jawbone and cranial fractures in OI patients. The most commonly used bisphosphonates have been Aredia and Novartis.[82] When DI is a component of OI, extensive dental therapy may be required, including full crown coverage of the teeth or the placement of implants. Malocclusion is common in individuals with OI and must be managed.[86] Since patients with OI associated DI have very short roots, management of any malocclusion can prove difficult. OI is not a disease that can be cured. It rather, has to be

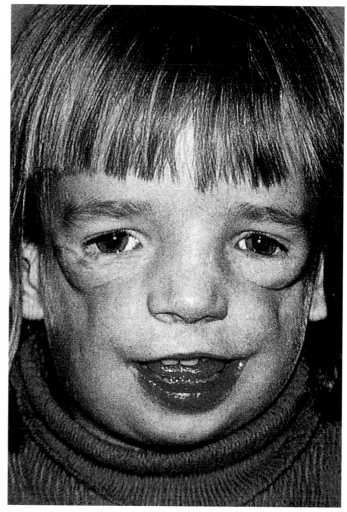

Figure 20.19 Child with TCS. Note the classic "bird-like" or "fish-like" facial appearance. (Reprinted from Marx R, Stern D. *Oral and Maxillofacial Pathology: A Rationale for Diagnosis and Treatment* with permission from Quintessence Publishing Company).

managed effectively. The outcome for the OI patient is dependent upon how fully the disease is expressed, and on which of the eight various types of OI that patient has.

Mandibulofacial Dysostosis (Treacher Collins Syndrome)

Mandibulofacial dysostosis, also known as, TCS, is an autosomal dominant disorder that affects the cranial facial apparatus, and most often is characterized by mid-face hypoplasia, atresia of the auditory canals, external ear abnormalities, conductive hearing loss, cleft palate and microdontia. Individuals who have TCS will characteristically have a convex mid-face with underdevelopment of the mandible, maxilla and zygoma, such that they will tend to have a bird or fish-like facial appearance[87] (Figure 20.19). Individuals with TCS may also have a prominent cross-bite (Figure 20.20).

TCS occurs in approximately 1 in 50,000 live births[88] and more than 60 percent of individuals with TCS do not appear to

The inflammatory response is more than likely mediated by cytokines. The most likely expressed cytokines are matrix metalloproteinase, cyclooxygenases or tumor necrosis factor alpha.

Treatment and Prognosis

The disease, associated facial edema will resolve without treatment. A gluten-free diet using grains such as corn and rice instead of gluten containing grains such as wheat, barley, oats and rye has been effective in one author's (REM) limited experience with the disease. This management is based on our knowledge of the associated humeral and cellular immune responses to gluten in the gastrointestinal tract of susceptible individuals known to have sprue or Celiac disease.

Lip edema may also respond to intralesional steroids using triamcinolone 10 mg/ml with 2% xylocaine and injecting 2 to 5 ml in each lip every month. As an alternative, systemic oral prednisone may be used. However, in children the dosage should be given on a per weight basis of, 1 mg/kg for two week courses and the patient should be monitored carefully.[141,142]

Surgery in the form of a reduction cheiloplasty may also help with the lip swellings but requires removing the internal lesional substance within the lip and advancing the mucosa orally to reposition the vermillion skin junction to a symmetrical position in order to correct the excessive lip eversion that the Melkersson–Rosenthal syndrome creates.

Multiple Endocrine Neoplasia Syndrome Type 2B (Multiple Mucosal Neoplasia Type 3)

Clinical Presentation and Pathogenesis

MENS 2B, is a disease of autosomal dominant inheritance in which there is a mutation in the RET proto-oncogene on chromosome 10q 11.2.[143,144,145] Fifty percent of these mutations occur intrautero with normal parents. This mutation is similar to that seen in MENS II known as Sipple syndrome which produces familial medullary thyroid carcinoma, along with Hirschsprung Megacolon and primary hyperparathyroidism. MENS IIb results in mucosal neuromas, pheochromocytomas and medullary thyroid carcinoma.[146] Additionally, a Marfinoid habitus also known as long face syndrome is often seen as well.

The most aggressive expressions develop signs and symptoms in infancy and less aggressive forms primarily before puberty. The recognition of multiple non-painful nodules in the substance of the tongue and/or the lips should alert the clinician to this syndrome and prompt life-saving action should be taken, as the medullary thyroid carcinomas seen in the syndrome occur early, are very aggressive and metastasize early.[147]

The neuromas seen in MEN2B syndrome most often occur in children and present in the body of the tongue and lower lip and/or the upper eye lids (Figure 20.36). These may be the first sign of this syndrome. The syndrome associated Pheochromocytomas occur in 50 percent of cases and are usually first seen later in life than childhood. Symptoms of hypertension,

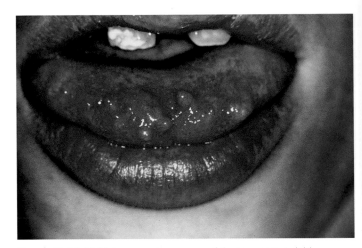

Figure 20.36 Multiple mucosal neuromas of the tongue in a child with MEN2B. (Reprinted from Marx R, Stern D. *Oral and Maxillofacial Pathology: A Rationale for Diagnosis and Treatment* with permission from Quintessence Publishing Company).

tachycardia, sweating and flushing are the well known manifestations of a Pheochromocytoma. The syndrome associated medullary thyroid carcinomas are the most life threatening component of MEN 2B due to aggressiveness and metastasizing potential. Most tumors are asymptomatic and most often only is noted as a suspicious neck mass.

Differential Diagnosis

Oral mucosal neuromas and schwannomas may develop in a child unrelated to MEN2B but they are usually single isolated tumors as compared to the clustered and multifocal neuromas seen in MEN2B. Mucosal cysts or mucoceles may mimic mucosal neuromas, as can the focal epithelial thickenings seen in Heck's disease.[148] However, neither of these processes are identical to the small firm nodules with a normal overlying mucosal surface seen in MEN2B.

Diagnostic Workup

Multiple nodules within the substance of the tongue require an excisional biopsy of two or more nodules. If a neuroma is confirmed a CT scan or MRI of thyroid area and abdomen is recommended. In addition, serum thyroid function tests are needed to assess thyroid function. Tests for urinary vanillymandelic acid, a metabolic product of catecholamine degradation can prove useful in pointing toward a Pheochromocytoma.

Pathologic Features

The mucosal tumors in MEN type III syndrome are characterized by a proliferation of nerve bundles that are hyperplastic. These nerve aggregates will be set in a collagenous stroma, and they will show a tendency to be surrounded by a thickened perineurium. Thyroid tumors are medullary in type and demonstrate amyloid and calcifications (Figure 20.37).

Treatment and Prognosis

The mucosal neuromas seen in MEN2B do not require specific treatment. They may be excised if bothersome to the patient.

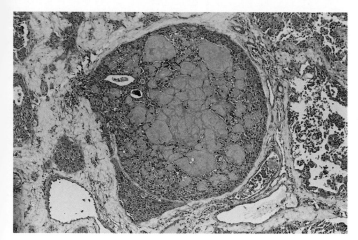

Figure 20.37 Medullary thyroid carcinoma in a patient with MENS IIb. Note the abundant amyloid product. (Reprinted from Marx R, Stern D. *Oral and Maxillofacial Pathology: A Rationale for Diagnosis and Treatment* with permission from Quintessence Publishing Company).

However, a total thyroidectomy is indicated due to the nearly universal development of medullary thyroid carcinoma in patients. Because a Pheochromocytoma, a functionally benign tumor, only develops in 50 percent cases, and occurs later into adulthood, further workup and surgery is typically deferred until signs and symptoms of the tumor occur.

If the thyroid is removed in a MENS patient prior to the development of a medullary thyroid carcinoma, the prognosis is good and radiotherapy is not usually recommended. However, if the thyroidectomy is performed with an already developed medullary thyroid carcinoma, post surgical radiotherapy is recommended and the prognosis declines to a 50 percent survival potential. If a Pheochromocytoma develops later (teenage years to early twenties), the prognosis for the patient if an adrenalectomy is performed is good. Vandetanib has been employed to treat the associated medullary thyroid carcinomas.[7] However, if an adrenal hypertensive crisis occurs, a 10 percent death rate ensues.

Fabry Syndrome

Clinical Presentation and Pathogenesis

Fabry syndrome is an x-linked genetic lysosomal storage defect in the production of the enzyme alpha galactosidase A (alpha GAL).[149] Therefore, the syndrome occurs predominantly in boys and men. However, some girls/women with one defective alpha GAL gene are not mere "carriers" but develop some of the signs and symptoms of the disorder as boys and men, by virtue of a variable normal x-chromosome inactivation which allows the defective x-chromosome to be more phenotypically expressed.

The disease is inherited with a prevalence range between 1/40,000 and 1/200,000 live births.[150] Fabry syndrome will usually show clinical signs and symptoms in early childhood. The signs and symptoms are a result of the buildup of globotriaosylceramide, a type of glycolipid known as GL-3. As this glycolipid deposits and accumulates in blood vessels, patients develop a variety of signs and symptoms of varying severity. Mild cases often go unrecognized while more severe cases create significant morbidity.[151]

The most recognizable sign of the syndrome will be multiple red vascular nodules that do not blanch referred to as angiokeratomas. The most common symptom will be a set of parasthesias of the hands and feet which may also be painful. The GL-3 deposits may also affect major organs and can result in arrhythmias, shortness of breath and proteinuria leading to renal failure and stoke. Additional signs that may be observed in children include a whorled cornea and anhydrosis.

Differential Diagnosis

Fabry syndrome often goes without consideration in the differential diagnosis, especially in early childhood. The angiokeratomas seen in the syndrome may resemble the hemangiomas of Maffuci syndrome or be confused with keratoacanthoma syndromes, especially the Ferguson–Smith type which is common to children and/or the Grybowski type that is more often seen in adults.

Diagnosis

The confirmatory test for Fabry syndrome is a blood alpha GAL activity assay.

Treatment and Prognosis

There is no cure for Fabry syndrome. Most patients are managed with non-steroidal analgesics or anticonvulsants if pain and parasthesias are the prominent symptoms. The syndrome associated angiokeratomas are not usually removed surgically because they recur and their numbers increase over time.

Enzyme replacement therapy with beta agalsidase (Fabrazyme ® GENETEC) can reduce symptoms but is not a cure for the disorder.[152] Most individuals contend with their disease and manage symptoms while leading otherwise normal lives.[153] However, disability and even mortality may result in severely expressed cases.

Hereditary Gingival Fibromatosis and Related Syndromes

Clinical Presentation and Pathogeneses

Hereditary gingival fibromatosis is an autosomal dominant hereditary disorder that results in a firm enlargement of the gingiva. Gingival fibromatosis alone is the most common presentation of gingival fibromatosis. However, five syndromic entities can have gingival fibromatosis as one part of their syndrome complex components.[154,155,156,157] Those disorders are outlined below:

1. Ramon Syndrome: Gingival fibromatosis together with Cherubism, mental retardation, seizure disorders and variable neuromuscular weakness.
2. Laband Syndrome: gingival fibromatosis with developmental defects of nose, nails, ear and bones as well as hepatosplenomegaly.

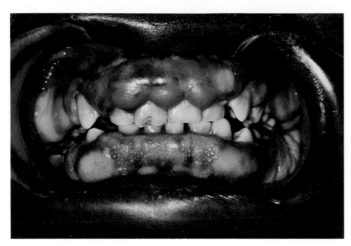

Figure 20.38 Moderate hereditary gingival fibromatosis in a teenager. Most of the crowns of the teeth are enveloped by the hyperplastic gingiva. (Reprinted from Marx R, Stern D. *Oral and Maxillofacial Pathology: A Rationale for Diagnosis and Treatment* with permission from Quintessence Publishing Company).

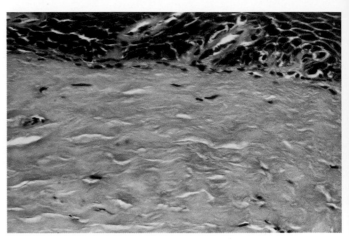

Figure 20.39 Hereditary gingival fibromatosis demonstrating dense fibrosis of the lamina propria just below the oral epithelial surface. (Reprinted from Marx R, Stern D. *Oral and Maxillofacial Pathology: A Rationale for Diagnosis and Treatment* with permission from Quintessence Publishing Company).

3. Rutherford Syndrome: Gingival fibromatosis and corneal opacities.
4. Cross Syndrome: gingival fibromatosis with microphthalmia, mental retardation, corneal opacities and skin hypopigmentation.
5. Murray–Puretic–Drescher Syndrome: Gingival fibromatosis with multiple hyaline fibromas of the skin and scalp which display marked recurrence if excised.

Although hereditary, the clinical gingival enlargement seen in the disorder does not usually begin until the age of three or four years, and sometimes not until the early teenage years. (Figure 20.38) The degree of enlargement does not seem to be related to the length of time of its presence, but to the degree of genetic expression. That is, younger patients may have more severe clinical enlargements than older adults and if left untreated the fibromatosis will gain a certain size and then become stable. Rare cases may also be associated with mental retardation, seizures and hypertrichosis resembling what can be seen clinically in Ramon syndrome without the Cherubism component.

Differential Diagnosis

Gingival enlargement is well known to be induced by certain drugs, i.e. dilantin, cyclosporine, nifedipine and verapamil, which should be ruled out causally by history. Other causes of diffuse gingival enlargements include hereditary NF and a gingival leukemic infiltrate. However, a gingival leukemic infiltrate will create a soft friable and hemorrhagic gingiva rather than the firm gingival enlargements seen in hereditary gingival fibromatosis.

Additionally, the practitioner is wise to assess the patient for the components of the five syndromes that include gingival fibromatosis and rule out each with a knowledge of each syndrome's components.

Pathologic Features

The lesions of hereditary gingival fibromatosis will present as dense fibro collagen that will be covered by oral mucosal surface epithelium. The collagen will be avascular, relatively acellular and spiral in all directions.[156,157,158] (Figure 20.39) The overlying epithelium may demonstrate pseudoepitheliomatous hyperplasia. Inflammation of the collagenous tissue is generally mild. Rare dystrophic calcific foci may be seen.

Diagnosis

The diagnosis of gingival fibromatosis is usually one of clinical recognition, an appropriate history and the ruling out syndromes in which gingival fibromatosis can be present. A biopsy maybe required to rule out hereditary NF or a leukemic infiltrate.

Treatment and Prognosis

Mild cases of hereditary gingival fibromatosis require only a dental prophylaxis and periodontal maintenance to eliminate any inflammatory contribution to the enlargement, or to reduce pain. Many cases require no treatment once the enlargement attains its stable size. Excessive gingival enlargements can interfere with jaw closure, lip competence and swallowing. In such cases, surgical excision may be indicated. Such excisions usually require general anesthesia and electrocautery to excise through the dense disease associated tissue. The outcome can be a dramatic improvement and will expose teeth that may have been completely covered by the disease process. However, informed consent should include the fact that there is a tendency for recurrence of and the possibility of a reoperation in the future.

The prognosis is good and patients largely adapt to their condition. Some undergo repeated surgeries. However, tooth loss due to caries and/or periodontal bone loss is common due to the gingival enlargement that inhabits appropriate plaque control.

Ehlers–Danlos Syndrome

Clinical Features

Ehlers–Danlos syndrome is a disorder caused by an inherited defect in the synthesis of type III collagen.[159] The disorder is likely due to deletions of the enzymes pro-collagen peptidase and/or lysine hydroxylase, which normally cause cross linking of collagen to form mature insoluble collagen.[160] A weak, pliable and excessively stretchable collagen results to produce the eight known genetic variants of Ehlers–Danlos syndrome. There are four autosomal dominant forms of the disorder including the rare periodontal form, which results in early tooth mobility and tooth loss. There is an x-linked form of the disease and three autosomal recessive and severe forms.[161]

Other than the periodontal form of the disorder, most cases of Ehlers–Danlos syndrome are notable because of the patient's for hyperstrechable skin and hyperextensible joints. It should be noted that the skin is hyperstretchable, not hyperelastic. The term hyperelastic requires that the skin recoil to its original form, which does not happen in Ehlers–Danlos syndrome. Additional signs may include ecchymosis, poor wound healing, a peculiar scarring of the skin known as cigarette paper skin blue scleras, tarsal plate eversion due to protrusion and eversion of the upper eyelids known as metenier sign and tendon rupture. These findings are all related to the defect in the collagen's tertiary structure and therefore its strength.

Differential Diagnosis

Most cases of Ehlers–Danlos syndrome can be recognized based on clinical findings and patient symptoms along with family history. However, some cases of Marfan syndrome and even OI will exhibit joint hyperextensibility. Neither disorder will produce a hyperstretchable skin. Additionally, a rare condition known as Marfanoid hypermobility syndrome, which is unrelated to either Marfan syndrome or Ehlers–Danlos syndrome also produces hyperextensible joints but not hyperstretchable skin. This entity probably represents a mild and as yet unknown collagen defect.

Pathologic Features

Routine light microscopy will show a somewhat altered dermal contour with ectatic vessels in the reticular and papillary dermis. Irregular and loosely arranged collagen bundles will be present. Electron microscopy will demonstrate disorganized collagen fibers that are poorly aggregated to give a cauliflower-like appearance.

Treatment and Prognosis

There is no known effective treatment for Ehlers–Danlos syndrome. However, due to the associated known poor wound healing and vascular friability, elective surgeries are discouraged.[162] Required surgeries carry a greater risk of bleeding and wound dehiscence. Therefore, most surgeries require local hemostatic measures, a plan for possible transfusion and use of long term non-resorbable sutures.

Individuals with mild forms of Ehlers–Danlos syndrome live a normal life span.[163] Patients with the ecchymotic forms and more severe forms of the disease are at risk for gastrointestinal bleeds and great vessel rupture, most of which tend to occur in the teenage years.

Peutz–Jegher's Syndrome

Clinical Features

Peutz–Jegher's syndrome is an autosomal dominant disorder caused by inheritance of a mutation in the tumor suppressor serine threonine kinase-11 (STK-11) gene on chromosome 19p (19q13.4).[164,165,166,167] The inherited form of the disease accounts for 65 percent of cases with as much as 35 percent representing new mutations. These mutations result in the general clinical findings of melanotic macules of skin and mucus membranes and intestinal polyposis. Although it was once thought that the disease associated intestinal polyposis was benign and limited to the small intestines, it has since been shown that two types of polyps develop. A benign hamartomatous polyp that merely represents an intestinal wall overgrowth and an adenomatous polyp, which has a malignant transformation rate of more than 20 percent. Both types of polyps may also be found in the stomach, large intestines and even in the rectum. In rare cases, nasal, pharyngeal and esophageal polyps have even been noted.

Syndrome associated skin and mucosal melanotic macules appear in infancy and early childhood, whereas the intestinal polyps usually do not develop until the late teenage years and twenties.

Differential Diagnosis

Subtle or incomplete cases where only melanotic macules develop may be difficult to separate from a normal variation of pigment deposition. However, Addison's disease patients may develop numerous melanotic macules that can resemble those of Peutz–Jegher's syndrome. Juvenile polyposis, familial polyposis coli and even Gardner syndrome may feature similar polyps but these disorders will not exhibit melanotic macules. Fibrous dysplasia associated Albrights syndrome and hereditary neurofibromatosis type I (NF1) will feature Café-au-Lait macules which are similar to the melanotic macules of Peutz–Jegher's syndrome. However, such macules are usually larger and will not be associated with intestinal polyps.

Pathologic Features

The pigmented lesions seen in the head and neck region in Peutz–Jegher's syndrome will show increased melanin pigmentation along the basal layer of the mucosal or cutaneous epithelium. Melanocytes and melanophages will drop off prominently into the supporting collagen.[168]

Diagnosis

Peutz–Jegher's syndrome can be diagnosed on the basis of patient history and clinical recognition. However, once diagnosed or suspected, upper and lower gastrointestinal endoscopy with biopsy is recommended.

Treatment and Prognosis

There is no specific treatment for the disorder other than close follow-up and repeated fiber optic studies with removal of large or ulcerated polyps suspicious for malignant transformation, and close long term follow-up of the patient.[169]

Marfan Syndrome
Clinical Features

Marfan syndrome is a disorder that is characterized by set of clinical signs and symptoms that are created by an autosomal dominant trait whereby defective collagen is produced resulting in reduced collagen strength. The mutation arises as a result of mutations in the fibrillin (FBN1) gene located on chromosome 15 and actually occurs in the sperm or the oocyte prior to fertilization.[170,171,172,173] The resultant defective protein is not collagen itself, but a protein responsible for the tertiary structure of collagen. The resulting malformed collagen is more soluble in body fluids and more elastic. About 85 percent of Marfan's syndrome cases are inherited with the remaining 15 percent being sporadic mutations. Recent investigators have suggested that abnormalities in the transforming growth factor beta (TGF-B) pathway may contribute to the marfanoid phenotype.[170]

The clinical signs of Marfan's syndrome are:

1. The well known Marfanoid appearance i.e. slender build, long vertical face, long arms and legs
2. High arched palate
3. Aranchnodactyly
4. Blue scleras
5. Vertical maxillary excess
6. Constricted dental arches with malocclusion
7. Dislocated eye lenses
8. Higher frequency of detached retinas
9. Hyperextensible joints
10. Elastic skin

A young boy with classic "marfanoid" features is seen in Figure 20.40.

A particular concern in the marfanoid patient relates to the defective collagen in heart valves, which produces mitral valve prolapse in 80 percent of individuals. Involvement of the ascending aorta creates aortic regurgitation and prevents adequate refilling of the coronary arteries, frequently resulting in angina and ischemic EKG changes. In severe cases, aortic aneurysms form, which can rupture, lead to sudden death, most often in the latter teen years.[171]

Differential Diagnosis

The blue scleras seen in Marfan's syndrome may also be seen in OI, homocystinuria and Ehlers–Danlos syndrome. The long face appearance common to Marfan's syndrome is also common to patients with MEN2B, Klinefelter syndrome and

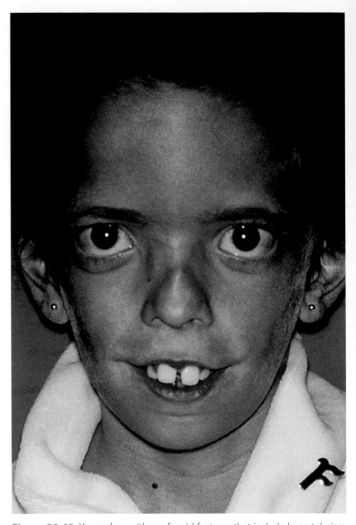

Figure 20.40 Young boy with marfanoid features that include hypertelorism, blue sclera, dolichocephaly and a characteristically long face. (Reprinted from Marx R, Stern D, *Oral and Maxillofacial Pathology: A Rationale for Diagnosis and Treatment* with permission from Quintessence Publishing Company).

homocystinuria. Additionally, a long face appearance may be unrelated to any syndrome.[174]

Pathologic Features

Microscopic findings are non-specific and range from microfibril degeneration to vascular smooth muscle apoptosis. These histologic abnormalities lead to hemodynamic sequellae such as aortic stiffness and reduced opening.

Diagnosis

Most cases of Marfan syndrome are diagnosed on the basis of history and recognition of the disorder's clinical features. However, a complete cardiovascular workup and ophthalmologic examination is needed to assess the degree of organ system involvement in an effort to reduce the risks and complications seen later in life.

Treatment and Prognosis

Cardiovascular defects associated with aortic regurgitation due to valvular incompetence are often treated with beta blockers to reduce intra-aortic pressures if the symptoms are mild. More severe cases of valvular incompetence are treated with aortic valve replacement.

Malocclusion can be improved somewhat with orthodontic care. However, most cases involve a skeletal deformity that requires orthognathic surgery as well. In such cases, the cardiovascular disease component must be stable and the patient's ejection fraction must be compatible with general anesthesia. Such surgery also requires the American Heart Association IE antibiotic prophylaxis regimen.

Despite the availability of aortic valve replacements and even with thorough medical management, the long term prognosis for Marfan syndrome patients remains poor. This poor prognosis is largely due to the continued disease associated collagen breakdown and re-synthesis which affects almost all tissues in the body including heart itself, heart vessels and other major organs.

Proteus Syndrome

Clinical Features

Proteus syndrome, also known as Wiedemann syndrome, is an extremely rare mosaic genetic mutation disorder arising from an aberrancy in the gene coding for AKT1 kinase.[176,177,178,179,180,181] This mutation is usually sporadic so that an inheritance pattern is not known. The mutation occurs intrautero and thus clinical manifestations appear early in life. Most clinical manifestations become apparent by the late first decade. The rarity of this syndrome is underscored by the fact that there were less than 120 known cases in the United States as of 2011.

The clinical manifestations of the disorder occur as a result of uncontrolled growth of skin, subcutaneous fat, blood vessels and lymphatics, which occur unilaterally. Therefore, irregular pendulous overgrowth of one side of the body is the major feature of the disorder. The bones of the skull and chest are usually enlarged and irregular as well. In addition to its peculiar unilateral involvement the syndrome is associated with an overgrowth of soft tissue over an involved foot. This finding is known as the *moccasin foot* characteristic of Proteus syndrome. The syndrome also includes an increased incidence of basal cell adenomas of the parotid gland, meningiomas, testicular tumors and ovarian cystadenomas.

It is now certain that the celebrated "Elephant man," Joseph (John) Merrick actually suffered from Proteus syndrome rather than hereditary NF1, as conjectured in the Hollywood movie about him, and that he died from the most common complication of Proteus syndrome, a pulmonary embolus, rather than an upper airway obstruction.

Differential Diagnosis

Proteus syndrome can be distinguished from hereditary NF1 by its lack of bilateral involvement and the presence of separate nodular neurofibromas in NF1, as opposed to the pendulous overgrowth of one side of the body that is characteristic of Proteus syndrome. If doubt remains, a biopsy of the tissue under local anesthesia is straightforward and will enable one to distinguish between the hyalinized connective tissue of Proteus syndrome and the neurofibromas of hereditary NF1.

Pathologic Features

Microscopic findings of tissue examined from patients with proteus syndrome are not uniform. Lesions range from lipomatous swellings to vascular malformations to harmatomatous tissue overgrowths in which the native tissue for the site is disorganized with an associated abnormal distribution and architecture.[177]

Treatment and Prognosis

There is no universally accepted treatment for Proteus syndrome. On rare occasion, excision of the excessive tissue mass may be warranted but regrowth should be expected. One author has related a good response to Rapamycin therapy, but too few cases have been assessed to be certain of a treatment's effect.[178]

The prognosis remains poor as the excessive tissue proliferations continue throughout the teenage years. A shortened life span is expected, usually from pulmonary emboli leading to sudden death.[178]

Ramsay Hunt Syndrome

Ramsay Hunt syndrome is a disorder that results as a complication of latent varicella viral infection (VCV). The disorder is seen world-wide and is thought to account for 16 percent of all causes of unilateral facial palsies in children.[182,183,184,185,186] A high percentage of Bells palsy cases are thought to be associated with the syndrome. Ramsay Hunt syndrome in fact accounts for 15 percent of unilateral facial palsies in children. The disease is quite rare in patients younger than six years of age.[185] Patients with the disease will have acute peripheral facial neuropathy that can be accompanied by a skin rash that is vesicular, and often extends into the ear canal or involves mucous membranes. VCV can cause not only palsy, but deafness, tinnitus, nystagmus and ataxia, vertigo or complete facial paralysis.

The patients can ultimately develop cellulitis or complete facial paralysis. The vesicular/bullous eruptions that are seen in Ramsay Hunt syndrome can simulate those of Bells palsy, trigeminal neuralgia and post-therapeutic neuralgia, however, lesions present in such a classic manner that the clinical findings of an eruptive vesicular bullous disease in the appropriate anatomic site is generally diagnostic. However, to definitively diagnose the disease, VCV isolation using cell culture techniques will be required. VCV antigen detection by direct immunofluorescence assay can also be diagnostic.[187] Tzanck tests can be useful in identifying a viral cytopathic affect in which ballooning giant cells are in evidence microscopically (Figure 20.41). The virus can also be identified using PCR techniques. MRI imaging techniques have been used to show

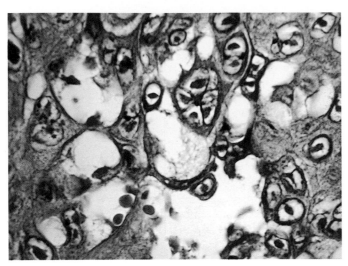

Figure 40.41 Ballooned and edematous gasserian ganglions cells infected by VCV. (Reprinted from Marx R, Stern D. *Oral and Maxillofacial Pathology: A Rationale for Diagnosis and Treatment* with permission from Quintessence Publishing Company).

alterations in the level of the blood labyrinthine barrier.[188] However, these findings are not fully diagnostic of the disorder.

Ramsay Hunt disease can be staged clinically, such that the disease can be rated on a scale that ranges from one to five. Patients who are judged to be at level 1 will appear essentially clinically normal whereas patients who are at the fifth phase of disease progression typically show complete fascial paralysis. The stages in between stage 1 and 5 can show mild dysfunction, in which patients have slight facial muscle weakness, to moderately severe dysfunction, in which patients have facial muscle weakness and disfigurement.

Treatment and Prognosis

Most cases of Ramsay Hunt syndrome are treated with oral acyclovir and cortical steroid therapy.[189] Patients must also be protected from corneal irritation and injury if they have Bells palsy-type symptomatology. Ramsay Hunt syndrome is generally self-limiting. The recovery rate for the disease is less than 50 percent and patients may have symptoms of long term facial weakness.[190]

Albers–Shonberg Syndrome

Albers–Schonberg disease or syndrome, first described in 1904,[191] is a clinical syndrome that becomes manifest when osteoclasts fail to resorb bone. When this important biologic activity fails or is impeded, patients will have a resultant increase in bone mass that is associated with skeletal fragility. Three forms of the disease are recognized, 1) an infantile form, 2) a rare intermediate form and 3) an adult form. The adult form of the disease is typically autosomal dominant with a good prognosis, while the infantile form of the disease is typically autosomal recessive with a poor prognosis. Also known as osteopetrosis, the Albers–Schonberg syndrome is reported to occur in one patient per 100,000 to 500,000 of the population.[192] The etiology of Albers–Schonberg disease is

clearly related to an osteoclast aberrancy in which osteoclasts fail to mature. The inability of these cells to mature is largely related to a cell signaling error in which RNKL, a ligand that stimulates osteoclasts activity is bound and unable to function normally.[193,194] Rare forms of osteopetrosis have also been linked to mutations of the CLCN7 chloride channel gene as well.[195]

Adult osteopetrosis (benign osteopetrosis) is generally diagnosed in adulthood, while infantile osteopetrosis (malignant osteopetrosis) occurs early in life and can be associated with patients who show a failure to thrive, and develop growth retardation symptoms.

Clinically, individuals with infantile osteoporosis will demonstrate a host of clinical findings including 1) nasal stuffiness that is related to mastoid sinus malformations and paranasal sinus malformations, 2) neuropathies associated with cranial nerve entrapment, 3) deafness, 4) delayed eruption of teeth, 5) fragile bones that are prone to fracture, 6) osteomyelitis, 7) defective but abundant osseous tissue with lack of bone marrow, 8) anemia and 9) extreme craniofacial bone density. Patients with infantile Albers–Schonberg syndrome will typically be short in stature, demonstrate frontal bossing and an enlarged head and frequently have hepatosplenomegaly.[196]

Several disorders can resemble osteopetrosis, including hyperparathyroidism, hypoparathyroidism and pseudohyperparathyroidism in children. Paget's disease can resemble osteopetrosis as well, but is typically a consideration only in adults. Rarely malignancies such as leukemia can simulate osteopetrosis and on rare occasions sickle cell disease will simulate osteopetrosis as well.

Patients with infantile osteopetrosis may show elevation of parathyroid hormone, acid phosphatase, hypocalcemia and elevated levels of creatinine kinase. Biopsies of the disease process can be helpful in rendering a diagnosis for patients; however, biopsy is not absolutely necessary. Radiographically, osteopetrosis can be quite diagnostic. Patients will tend to show densely sclerotic bone and the bones may be club-like. Fractures are common to the involved bones. The most dramatic finding in the head and neck region is a thickening of the bone of the entire skull, including its base. Sinuses will be compressed and sometimes obliterated and the involved bone may show alternating radiolucent and radiosclerotic bands.

Pathologic Features

In infantile osteopetrosis the bone will grossly be dense and appear to be over-mineralized. Osseous trabeculae will show zones of heavily calcified, cartilaginous-like material that will often be surrounded by irregular woven bone. Bony trabeculae may or may not show thickening in the early disease stage, but in the later disease stage the individual trabeculae become confluent and massive and bone marrow will be absent. Osteoclasts can be normal, increased in number or decreased in number in any one tissue sample that is examined. Osteoclasts have been shown to lack the ruffled borders that are typically

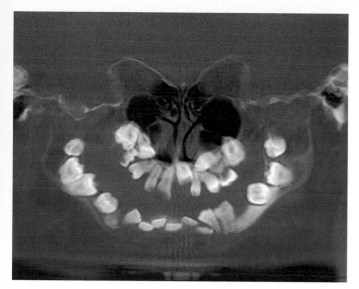

Figure 20.42 Resorption of the mandibular ramus, inferior border and condyle in a patient with Gorham–Stout syndrome. (Reprinted from Marx R, Stern D. *Oral and Maxillofacial Pathology: A Rationale for Diagnosis and Treatment* with permission from Quintessence Publishing Company).

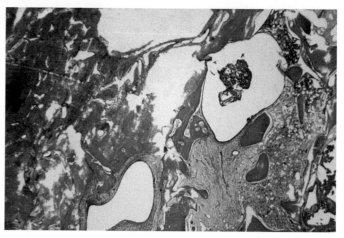

Figure 20.43 Back-to-back anastomosing endothelially lined vascular and lymphatic channels in a biopsy from a patient with Gorham–Stout syndrome. (Reprinted from Marx R, Stern D. *Oral and Maxillofacial Pathology: A Rationale for Diagnosis and Treatment* with permission from Quintessence Publishing Company).

seen ultrastructurally with that cell. In addition to appearing trabecular, involved bone can appear globular or have an osteophytic pattern. In the maxilla and mandible where teeth are present, the teeth will often show enamel hypoplasia and defects in dentin, mineralization and attenuated or resorbed pulpal chambers. Unerupted teeth may demonstrate ankylosis.[197]

Treatment and Prognosis

Infantile osteopetrosis can be treated using vitamin D, which can stimulate dormant osteoclasts.[198] However, any gains in managing the disease will end if the vitamin D therapy is discontinued. Patients with infantile osteopetrosis have also been treated with gamma interferon, in association with vitamin D with success. Patients often have anemia for which erythropoietin can be used. In cases of pediatric osteopetrosis, surgery is sometimes employed because of multiple fractures.[199]

For those instances in which teeth have to be extracted and the associated alveolar bone managed, rough or sharp bony edges should be smoothed by the surgeon. Clorhexidin gluconate oral rinses can be used to reduce the number of disease associated micro-organisms when there is maxillary, mandibular or oral cavity involvement. The most common infections that are associated with osteopetrosis tend to be actinomyces infections. There is a close association between osteopetrosis and the recently described entity *bisphosphonate induced osteonecrosis of the jaws*. Both diseases are related to a defect in the osteoclast/osteoblast bone renewal cycle. Bone marrow failure can occur in infantile osteopetrosis and if untreated, death will ensue, generally within the first decade of life. Patients generally succumb to severe anemia, infections or a bleeding diathesis. Bone marrow transplantation has been used to treat infantile osteopetrosis with some success.[196] Bone marrow transplantation, however, is fought with significant risk because of the marked immunosuppression that can occur and the associated risk of a host versus graft reaction.

Gorham–Stout Syndrome

Gorham–Stout disease is a rare bone disease that is also known as phantom bone disease or vanishing bone disease. The disorder is rarely seen in children. Lesions most often affect the shoulder, skull, jaw, ribs or spine. The disorder is characterized by a proliferation of thin walled vascular channels associated with regional osteolysis.[201] In a review of 67 cases seen in mainland China, Hu et al. found that men with the disorder significantly outnumbered women and found that the mean age at the time of diagnosis was 28 years, with an age range of 1.5 to 71 years. The most common clinical symptoms in the patients studied were pain, functional impairment and swelling.

Gorham–Stout syndrome is a disease of exclusion and typically the diagnosis is based on combined histological radiographic and clinical features.[203] Radiographs will typically show a disappearance of bone in the affected area with an associated progressive resorption of regional bone (Figure 20.42). Dong et al.[204] report that only 50 cases of the disorder have been reported in the maxillofacial region in the entire world literature.[205] Although patients can present with an abrupt onset of pain, swelling or pathologic fracture, patients can also present without any symptomatology except slight swelling. In most cases, the bone resorption will end spontaneously and, thus the disease has a good prognosis.

The histologic findings in the disorder will depend on the clinical stage in which disease is being observed microscopically. In early phases of the disease, the histopathology will be that of a high concentration of blood vessels or lymphatic appearing vessels[205] (Figure 20.43). In late stages of the disorder only fibrous connective tissue or fibro adipose tissue of fibro fatty marrow may be seen. From a differential diagnostic perspective, skeletal angiomas and infections should be considered. The extreme rarity of the disorder in children makes Gorham–Stout syndrome a disease of exclusion when a radiographic osteolytic lesion in the craniofacial region of a child cannot otherwise be explained.

Treatment and Prognosis

The prognosis for Gorham–Stout syndrome is quite good. In some instances patients must be treated with antiresorptive bisphosphonate therapy.[206,207,208] Nir et al. have reported successful treatment of Gorham–Stout syndrome in which there had been progressive angiomatosis in a child who had had the syndrome since the age of 13 using propranolol.[209]

References

Glial Choristoma

1. Baldwin DJ, Thayalan K, Amrita J, et al. Glial choristoma of the tongue: report of a case and clinicopathological features. *Int J of Pediatr Dent*, 2009, 19: 219–221.

2. Martinez-Peñuela A, Quer S, Beloqui, R. Glial choristoma of the middle ear: report of 2 cases. *Otology and Neurology*, 2011, 32: e26–e27.

3. Strome SE, McClatchey K, Kileny PR, et al. Neonatal choristoma of the tongue containing glial tissue. Diagnostic and surgical considerations. *Int J Pediatr Otorhino Laryngol*, 1995, 33: 265–273.

4. Sun LS, Zhi-Peng S, Xu-Chen MA. Glial choristoma in the oral and maxillofacial region. A clinicopathologic study of 6 cases. *Arch Pathol Lab Med*, 2008, 132: 984–998.

5. Fan SQ, Ou YM, Liang QC. Glial choristoma of the tongue: report of a case and review of the literature. *Pediatr Surg Int*, 2008, 24: 515–519.

6. Takamizawa S, Inoue T, Ono Y, et al. A case report of glial choristoma of the tongue. *J Pediatr Surg*, 2006, 41: e13–e15.

Fordyce Granules

7. Fordyce JA. A peculiar affection of the mucous membrane of the lips and oral cavity. *J Cutan Dis*, 1896, 14: 413–419.

8. Lee JH, Lee JH, NA HK: Clinicopathologic manifestations of patients with Fordyce's spots. *Ann Dermatol*, 2012, 24: 103–106.

9. Oliver JH. Fordyce granules on the prolabia and oral mucous membranes of a selected population. *SADJ*, 2006, 61: 72–74.

10. DeFelice C, Patrini S, Chitano G. et al. Fordyce granules and hereditary non-polyposis colorectal cancer syndrome. *Gut*, 2005, 41: 1279–1282.

11. Miller AS, McCrea MW. Sebaceous gland adenoma of the buccal mucosa. *J Oral Surg*, 1968, 26: 593–595.

12. Miller ML, Harford RR, Yeager JK. Fox Fordyce disease treated with topical clindamycin solution. *Arch Dermatol*, 1995, 131: 1112–1113.

Cleidocranial Dysplasia

13. Siggers DC. Cleidocranial dysostosis. *Dev Med Child Neurol*, 1975, 4: 522–524.

14. Shen Z, Chio C, Chun Z, et al. Cleidocranial dysplasia: Report of 3 cases and literature review. *Clinical Pediatrics*, 2009, 2: 194–198.

15. Bufalino A, Paranaiba LMR, Gouvêa AF, et al. Cleidocranial dysplasia: oral features and genetic analysis of 11 patients. *Oral Diseases*, 2012, 18: 184–190.

16. Ducy P, Zhang R, Geoffroy V, et al. Osf2/Cbfa1: a transcriptional activator of osteoblast differentiation. *Cell*, 1997, 89: 747–754.

17. Komori T. Regulation of bone development and extracellular matrix protein genes by RUNX2. *Cell Tissue Res*, 2010, 339: 189–195.

18. Marx RE, Stern D. *Oral and Maxillofacial Pathology: A Rationale for Diagnosis and Treatment*. Ed 2, Chicago: Quintessence Publishing Company, 2012, 231–232.

19. Suda N, Hattori M, Kosaki K, et al. Correlation between genotype and supernumerary tooth formation in cleidocranial dysplasia. *Orthod Craniofac Res*, 2010, 13: 197–202.

20. Gorlin RJ, Cohen MN, Levin LS. *Syndromes of the Head and Neck*. Ed 3, New York NY, Oxford University Press; 1990: 249–253.

21. Jarvis JL, Keats TE. Cleidocranial dysostosis: a review of 40 new cases. *Am J Roentgenol Radium Ther Nucl Med*, 1974, 121: 5–16.

Idiopathic Bone Cavity

22. Perdigao PF, Silva ED, Sakurai E, et al. Idiopathic bone cavity: a clinical, radiographic and histological study. *Brit J Oral MG*, 2003, 41: 407–409.

23. Shigematsu K, Fujita W. Atypical simple bone cyst of the mandible. *J Oral Maxillofac Surg*, 1994, 23: 298–299.

24. Manor E, Kachko L, Puterman MB. Cystic lesions of the jaws: a clinicopathological study of 322 cases and review of the literature. *Int J Med Sci*, 2012, 9: 20–26.

25. Patrikiou A, Sepheriadouo-Mauropulou G, Zambelis G. Bilateral traumatic bone cysts of the mandible. *Oral Surg*, 1981, 51: 131–133.

26. Zhu L, Wang X. Histological examination of the auricular cartilage and pseudocyst of the auricle. *J Laryngol Otol*, 1999, 106: 103–104.

27. Marx RE, Stern D. *Oral and Maxillofacial Pathology: A Rationale for Diagnosis and Treatment*. Ed 2, Chicago: Quintessence Publishing Company, 2012, 216–217.

28. Velez I, Siegel MA, Mintz SM et al. The relationship between idiopathic bone cavity and orthodontic tooth movement: analysis of 44 cases. *Dentomaxillofac Radiol*, 2010, 39: 162–166.

29. Cortell-Ballester I, Figueiredo R, Berini-Aytes L, et al. Traumatic bone cyst: a retrospective study of 21 cases. *Med Oral Patol Oral Cir Bucal* 2009, 14: E239–E243.

Lingual Mandibular Salivary Gland Depressions

30. Kaffe I, Littner MM, Arensburg B. The anterior buccal mandibular depression. Physical and radiologic features. *Oral Surg Oral Med Oral Pathol*, 1990, 69: 647–654.

31. Apruzzese D, Longoni S. Stafne cyst in an anterior location. *Oral Maxillofac Surg*, 1999, 57: 333–338.

32. Stafne EC. Bone cavities situated near the angle of the mandible. *J Am Dent Assoc*, 1942, 29: 1969–1972.

33. Buchner A, Carpenter WM, Merrell PW, et al. Anterior lingual salivary gland defect. Evaluation of twenty-four cases. *Oral Surg Oral Med Oral Pathol*, 1991, 71: 131–136.

34. Shimizu M, Osa N, Okamura K, et al. CT analysis of the Stafne's bone defects of the mandible. *Dentomaxillofac Radiol*, 2006, 35: 95–102.

35. Baughman R. Testing your diagnostic skills. Case No. 2. Lingual mandibular salivary gland depression. *Todays FDA*, 2006, 18: 20–23.

36. Sisman Y, Miloglu O, Sekerci AE, et al. Radiographic evaluation of the prevalence of Stafne bone defect: a study from two centres in Turkey. *Dentomaxillofacial Radiol*, 2011, 35: 1–7.

Fibrous Hamartoma of Infancy

37. Reye RDK. A consideration of certain subdermal fibromatous tumors of infancy. *J Pathol*, 1956, 72: 149–154.

38. Sotelo-Avilla C, Bale PM. Subdermal fibrous hamartomas of infancy: pathology of 40 cases and differential diagnosis. *Pediatr Path*, 1994, 14: 39–52.

39. Paller AS, Gonzalez-Grussi F, Sherman JO. Fibrous hamartomas of infancy: eight additional cases and a review of the literature. *Arch Dermatol*, 1989, 125: 88–91.

40. Scott DM, Pena JR, Omura E. Fibrous hamartomas of infancy. *J Am Acad Dermatol*, 1999, 41: 857–858.

41. Westphal SL, Bancila E, Milgraum SS. Fibrous hamartomas of infancy presenting as an inflamed epidermoid cyst. *Pediatr Dermatol*, 1990, 7: 157.

Median Rhomboid Glossitis

42. Boquot JE, Gundlach KKH. Odd tongues: the prevalence of common tongue lesions in 23,616 white Americans over 35 years of age. *Quintessence Int*, 1986, 17: 719–730.

43. Ugar-Cankel D, Denizci S, Hocaoglu J. Prevalence of tongue lesions among Turkish school children, *Sandi Med*, 2005, 26: 1962–1967.

44. Marx RE, Stern D. *Oral and Maxillofacial Pathology: A Rationale for Diagnosis and Treatment*. Ed 2, Chicago: Quintessence Publishing Company, 2012, 99.

45. Mathew AL, Pai KM, Sholapurkar AA, et al. The prevalence of oral mucosal lesions in patients visiting a dental school in Southern India. *Indian J Dent Res*, 2008, 19: 99–103.

46. Koay CL, Lim JA, Siar CH. The prevalence of tongue lesions in Malaysian dental out-patients from the Klang valley area. *Oral Dis*, 2011, 17: 210–216.

Hemifacial Microsomia

47. Ohtani J, Hoffman WY, Vargevik K. Team management and treatment outcomes for patients with hemifacial microsomia. *Am J Orthodontics and Dentofacial Orthopedies*, 2012, 141: 574–581.

48. Poswillo D. The pathogenesis of first and second bronchial arch syndrome. *Oral Surg, Oral Med, Oral Pathol*, 1973, 35: 301–328.

49. Kelberman D, Tyson DC, Chandler AM, et al. Hemifacial microsomia: progress to understanding the genetic basis of a complex malformation syndrome. *Hum Genet* 2001, 109: 638–645.

50. Pruzansky S. Not all dwarfed mandibles are alike. *Birth Defects*, 1969, 4: 120–129.

51. Cousley RR A comparison of two classification systems for hemifacial microsomia. *Br J Oral Maxillof Surg*, 1993, 31: 78–82.

52. Zanardi G, Parente EV, Esteves LS. Orthodontic and surgical treatment of a patient with hemifacial microsomia. *Am J Orthodontics and Dentofacial Orthopedics*, 2012, 141: 5130–5139.

Hemifacial Hyperplasia

53. Miranda R, Barros LM, Nogueira dos Santos LA, et al. Clinical and imaging features in a patient with hemifacial hyperplasia. *J Oral Sci*, 2010, 52: 509 512.

54. Bergman JA. Primary hemifacial hypertrophy. Review and report of a case. *Arch Otolaryngol*, 1973, 97: 490–494.

55. Yashimoto H, Hano H, Kobayashi K, et al. Increased proliferative activity of osteoblasts in congenital hemifacial hypertrophy. *Plast Reconstr Surg*, 1998, 102: 1605–1610.

56. Marx RE, Stern D. *Oral and Maxillofacial Pathology: A Rationale for Diagnosis and Treatment*. Ed 2, Quintessence Publishing Company, 2012, 240

57. Islam MN, Bhattacharyya I, Ojha J, et al. Comparison between true and partial hemifacial hypertrophy. *Oral Surg Oral Med Oral Pathol Oral Radiol Endod*, 2007, 104: 501–509.

58. Azevedo RA, Veronica FS, Sarmento VA, et al. Hemifacial hyperplasia. A case report. *Quintessence Int*, 2005, 36: 483–486.

Ectodermal Dysplasia (Hypohidrotic Ectodermal Dysplasia)

59. Wisniewski SA, Trzeciak WH. A new mutation resulting in the truncation of the TRAF6-interacting domain of XEDAR: a possible novel cause of hypohidrotic ectodermal dysplasia. *J Med Genet*, 2012, 49: 499–501.

60. Clarke A. Hypohidrotic ectodermal dysplasia. *J Med Genet*, 1987, 24: 659–663.

61. Subramaniam P, Neeraja G. Witkop's tooth and nail syndrome: a multifaceted approach to dental management. *J Indian Soc Pedod Prev Dent*, 2008, 26: 22–25.

62. Lamartine J. Towards a new classification of ectodermal dysplasias. *Cin Exp Dermatol*, 2003, 28: 351–355.

63. Priolo M, Lagana C. Ectodermal dysplasia a new clinical-genetic classification. *J Med Genet*, 2001, 38: 579–585.

64. Guckes AD, Brahim JS, McCarthy GR, et al. Using endosseous dental implants for patients with ectodermal dysplasia. *JADA*, 1991, 122: 59–62.

65. Ekstrand K, Thomsson M. Ectodermal dysplasia with partial anodontia: prosthetic treatment with implant prosthesis. *J Dent Child*, 1988, 4: 282–284.

66. Smith RA, Vargervik K, Kearns G, et al. Placement of an endosseous implant in a growing child with ectodermal dysplasia. *Oral Surg Oral Med Oral Pathol*, 1993, 75: 669–673.

Amelogenesis Imperfecta

67. Urzua B, Ortega-Pento, Morales-Bozo et al. Defining a new candidate gene for amelogenesis imperfecta: from molecular genetics to biochemistry. *Biochem Genet*, 2011, 49: 104–121.

68. Stephanopoulos G, Garefalaki E, Lyroudia K. Genes and related proteins involved in amelogenesis imperfect. *J Dent Res*, 2005, 84: 1117–1126.

69. Weinmann JP, Svobcda JF, Woods RW. Hereditary disturbances of enamel formation and calcification. *J Am Dent Assoc*, 1945, 32: 397–418.

70. Chaudhary M, Dixit S, Singh A. Amelogenesis imperfecta: reporting of a

case and review of the literature. *J Oral Maxillofac Pathol*, 2009, 13: 70–77.

71. Witkop CJ, Jr. Amelogenesis imperfecta, dentinogenesis imperfecta and dentin dysplasia revisited: problems in classification. *J Oral Pathol Med*, 1989, 17: 547–543.

72. Schulze C. Erbbedingte strukturanomalicin menschlicher zahne. *Acta Genet Med Gemellol*, 1957, 7: 231–235.

Dentinogenesis Imperfecta

73. Kinney H, Pople JA, Driessen CH, et al. Intrafibrillar mineral may be absent in dentinogenesis imperfecta type II. *J Dental Res*, 2001, 1:80: 1555–1559.

74. Thofakura SR, Mah J, Srinivasan R, et al. The non collagenous dentin matrix proteins are involved in dentinogenesis imperfecta type II. *J Dent Res* 2000, 79: 835–839.

75. Bhandari S, Pannu K. Dentinogenesis imperfecta: a review and case report of a family over four generations. *Indian J Dent Res*, 2008, 19: 357–361.

76. Shields ED, Bixler D, El-Kafrawy AM. A proposed classification of heritable human dentin defect with a description of a new entity. *Arch Oral Biol*, 1973, 18: 543–553.

77. Levin LS, Leaf SH, Jemini RJ, et al. Dentinogenesis imperfecta in the Brandywine isolate hereditary opalescent dentin in an Ashkenazic Jewish family. *Oral Surg Oral Med Oral Pathol*, 1985, 59: 608–615.

78. Von Marschall Z, Mok S, Phillips MD. Rough endoplasmic reticulum trafficking errors by different classes of mutant dentin sialophosphorprotein (DSPP) causes dominant negative effects in both dentinogenesis imperfecta and dentin dysplasia by encapping normal DSPP. *J Bone Miner Res*, 2012, 27: 1309–1321.

Osteogenesis Imperfecta

79. Buday K. *Beiträge zar Lehre der osteogenesis imperfect*, 1895.

80. Sillence DO, Senn A, Danks DM. Genetic heterogenicity in osteogenesis imperfecta. *J Med Genet*, 1979, 16: 101–116.

81. Rosen A, Modig M, Larson O. Orthognathic bimaxillary surgery in two patients with osteogenesis imperfecta and a review of the literature. *Int J Oral Surg*, 2011, 40: 866–873.

82. Marx RE, Stern D. *Oral and Maxillofacial Pathology: A Rationale for Diagnosis and Treatment*. Ed 2, Chicago: Quintessence Publishing Company, 2012, 232–236.

83. Huber MA. Osteogenesis imperfect. *Oral Surg Oral Med Oral Pathol Oral Radiol Endod*, 2007, 103: 314–320.

84. Bergstrom L. Osteogenesis imperfecta: otologic and maxillofacial aspects. *Laryngoscope*, 1977, 87: 1–42.

85. O'Connel AC, Marini JC. Evaluation of oral problems in an osteogenesis imperfect population. *Oral SLurg Oral Med Oral Pathol Oral Radiol Endod*, 1999, 87: 189–196.

86. Kindelan J, Tobin M, Robert-Harry RA. Orthodontic and orthognatic management of a patient with osteogenesis imperfect and dentinogenesis imperfect. A case report. *J Orthod* 2003, 30: 291–296.

Mandibulofacial Dysostosis (Treacher Collins Syndrome)

87. Marszalek B, Wyojcicki P, Kobus K, et al. Clinical features, treatment and genetic background of Treacher Collins syndrome. *J Appl Genet*, 2002, 43: 223–233.

88. Dixon J, Edwards SJ, Anderson L. Identification of the complete coding sequence and genetic organization of the Treacher Collins syndrome gene. *Genome Res*, 1997, 7: 223–234.

89. Rovin S, Dachi SF, Borenstein DB, et al. Mandibulofacial dysostosis, a familial study of five generations. *J Pediat*, 1964, 65: 215–221.

90. Jones KL, Smith DW, Harvey MA, et al. Mandibulofacial dysostosis older paternal age and fresh gene mutation: data on additional disorders. *J Pediat*, 1975, 86: 84–88.

91. LeMerrer M, Cikuli M, Ribier J, et al. Acrofacial dysostosis. *Am J Med Genet*, 1989, 33: 318–322.

92. Dixon J, Trainor MJ, Dixon MJ. Treacher Collins syndrome. *Orthodontics and Craniofacial Research*, 2007, 10: 88–95.

93. Horiuchi K, Ariga T, Fujioka H, et al. Mutational analysis of the TCOF1 gene in 11 Japanese patients with Treacher Collins syndrome and mechanism of mutagenesis. *J Med Genet*, 2005, 134:363: 367.

94. Cohen J, Ghezzi F, Goncalves L, et al. Prenatal sonographic diagnosis of

Treacher Collins Syndrome: A case and review of the literature. *Am J Perinatol*, 1995, 12: 416–419.

White Sponge Nevus

95. Cannon AB. White nevus of the mucosa (naevus spongiosus albus mucosa) *Arch Derm Syphiol*, 1935, 31: 365–373.

96. Hernandez-Martin A, Fernandez-Lopez E, deUnamuno M. Diffuse whitening of the oral mucosa in a child. *Pediatr Dermatol* 1997, 14: 316–320.

97. Naseem S, Brady R, McDonald J. Diffuse white oral plaques. *Clinical Infectious Diseases* 2003, 36: 519–520.

98. Jorgenson RJ, Levin LS. White sponge nevus. *Arch Dermatol* 1981, 117: 73–76.

99. Allingham RR, Seo B, Rapersaud E, et al. A duplication in chromosome 4q35 is associated with hereditary benign intraepithelial dyskeratosis. *Am J Hum Genet* 2001, 68: 491–494.

100. Chao SC, Tsai Y-M, Yang MH, et al. A novel mutation in the keratin 4 gene causing white sponge naevus. *Br J Dermatol* 2003, 184: 1125–1128.

101. Sadeghi EM, Witkop CJ. The presence of *Candida albicans* in hereditary benign intraepithelial dyskeratosis. An ultrastructural observation. *Oral Surg Oral Med Oral Pathol* 1979, 48: 342–346.

102. Greer RO, Jr. Oral manifestations of smokeless tobacco use. *Otolaryngologic Clinics of North America*, 2010, 44: 31–56.

103. Lim J, Ng S. Oral tetracycline rinse improves symptoms of white sponge nevus. *J Am Acad Dermatol*, 1992, 26: 1003–1005.

Beckwith–Wiedemann Syndrome

104. Elliott M, Bayly R, Cole T, Temple IK, Maher ER. Clinical features and natural history of Beckwith-Wiedemann syndrome: presentation of 74 new cases. *Clinical Genetics*, 1994, 46, 168–174.

105. Thorburn MJ, Wright ES, Miller CG, Smith-Read EHL. Exomphalos-macroglossia-gigantism syndrome in Jamaican infants. *American J Diseases of Children*, 1970, 119: 316–321.

106. Pettenati MJ, Haines JL, Higgins RR, Wappner RS, Palmer CG, Weaver DD. Wiedemann-Beckwith syndrome: presentation of clinical and cytogenetic data on 22 new cases and review of the

literature. *Human Genetics*, 1986, 74: 143–154.

107. DeBaun MR, Niemitz EL, McNeil DE, Brandenburg SA, Lee MP, Feinberg AP. Epigenetic alterations of H19 and L1T1 distinguish patients with Beckwith-Wiedemann syndrome with cancer and birth defects. *Am J Human Genetics*, 2002, 70: 604–611.

Papillon–Lefévre Syndrome

108. Ullbro C, Crossner CG, Nederfors T, Alfadley A, Thestrup-Pedersen K. Dermatological and oral findings in a cohort of 47 patients with Papillon-Lefevre syndrome. *J Am Acad Dermatol*, 2003, 48: 345–351.

109. Cagli NA, Hakki SS, Darsun R, et al. Clinical genetic, and biochemical findings in two siblings with Papillon-Lefévre syndrome. *J Periodontal*, 2005, 76: 2322–2329.

110. Wani A, Devkar N, Patole M, Shouche Y. Description of two new cathespin C gene mutations in patients with Papillon-Lefévre syndrome. *J Peridontol*, 2005, 76: 2322–2329.

Reactive Arthritis

111. Zadik Y, Drucker S, Pallmon S. Migratory stomatitis (ectopic geographic tongue) on the floor of the mouth. *J Am Acad Dermatol*, 2011, 6: 459–460.

112. Kvien T, Glennas A, Melby K, Granfors K, et al. Reactive arthritis: incidence, triggering agents and clinical presentation. *J Rheumatology*, 1994, 21: 115–122.

113. Hill Gaston JS, Lillicrap MS. Arthritis associated with enteric infection. *Clinical Rheumatology*, 2003, 17: 219–239.

Ramon Syndrome

114. Suhanga J, Chakshu A, Mohideen K, et al. Cherubism combined with epilepsy, mental retardation and gingival fibromatosis. (Ramon syndrome): a case report. *Head and Neck Pathol*, 2010, 4: 12–131.

115. Ramon Y, Berman, W, Bubus JJ. Gingival fibromatosis combined with Cherubism. *Oral Surg, Oral Med, Oral Pathol*, 1967, 24: 436–448.

Kasabach–Merritt Syndrome

116. Hall G. Kasabach-Merritt syndrome: pathogenesis and management. *Br J Haematol*, 2001, 112: 851–862.

117. Kasabach HH, Merritt KK. Capillary hemangioma with extensive purpura:

report of a case. *Am J Dis Child*, 1940, 59: 1063.

118. el-Dessouky M, Azmy A, Raine P, Young D. Kasabach-Merritt syndrome. *J Pediatr Surg*, 1998, 23: 109–111.

119. Enjolras O, Mulliken J, Wassef M, Frieden I, Rieu P, Burrows P, Salhi A, Léauté-Labrèze C, Kozakewich H. Residual lesions after Kasabach-Merritt phenomenon in 41 patients. *J Am Acad Dermatol*, 2000, 42: 224–235.

Parry–Romberg Syndrome

120. Stone J. Neurological rarity: Parry-Romberg syndrome. *Practical Neurology*, 2006, 6: 185–188.

121. Leao M, da Silva ML. Progressive hemifacial atrophy with agenesis of the head and the caudate nucleus. *J Med Genetics*, 1994, 31: 969–971.

122. Muchnik RS, Aston SJ, Rees TD. Ocular manifestations and treatment of hemifacial atrophy. *Am J Ophthalmology*, 1979, 88: 889–897.

123. Lewkonia RM, Lowry RB, Opitz JM. Progressive hemifacial atrophy (Parry-Romberg syndrome): report with review of genetics and nosology. *Am J Med Genetics*, 1983, 14: 385–390.

124. Inigo F, Jimenez-Murat Y, Arroyo O, Fernandez M, Ysunza A. Restoration of facial contour in Romberg's disease and hemifacial microsomia. Experience with 118 cases. *Microsurgery*, 2000, 20: 167–172.

Encephalotrigeminal Angiomatosis, (Sturge Weber Anomaly)

125. Shirley MD, Tang H, Gallione CJ, et al. Sturge-Weber syndrome and Port wine stains caused by somatic mutations in GNAQ. *New England J Med*, 2013, 368: 1971–1979.

126. Sturge WA. A case of partial epilepsy, apparently due to a lesion of one of the vasomotor centres of the brain. *Transactions of the Clinical Society of London*, 1879, 12: 162.

127. Greenwood M, Meechan JG. General medicine and surgery for dental practitioners Part 4: Neurological disorders. *Br Dent*, 2003, 195: 19–25.

128. Weber FP. Right-sided hemi-hypertrophy resulting from right-sided congenital spastic hemiplegia, with a morbid condition of the left side of the brain, revealed by radiograms. *J Neurology and Psychopathology (London)*, 1922, 3: 134–139.

Kawasaki Disease

129. Kubota M, Usami I, Yamakawa M, Tomita Y, Haruta T. Kawasaki disease with lymphadenopathy and fever as sole initial manifestations. *J Paediatrics and Child Health*, 2008, 44: 359–362.

130. Scardina GA, Fucà G, Carini F, et al. Oral necrotizing microvasculitis in a patient affected by Kawasaki disease. *Medicina Oral, Patologia Oral Y Cirugia Buc*, 2007, 12: E560–E564.

131. Do JH, Baek JG, Kim HJ, et al. Kawasaki disease presenting as parotitis in a 3 month old infant. *Korean Circulation Journal*, 2009, 39: 502–504.

132. Michie C, Kinsler V, Tulloh R, Davidson S. Recurrent skin peeling following Kawasaki disease. *Archives of Disease in Childhood*, 2000, 83: 353–355.

Gardner Syndrome

133. Gardner EJ, Richards RC. Multiple cutaneous and subcutaneous lesions occurring simultaneously with hereditary polyposis and osteomatosis. *Am J Hum Genet*, 1953, 5: 139–147.

134. Knudsen AL, Bisguard ML, Bůlow S. Attenuated familial adenomatous polyposis (AFAP). A review of the literature. *Fam Cancer*, 2003, 2: 43–55.

135. Miyoshi Y, Nagase H, Ando H, et al. Somatic mutations of the APC gene in colorectal tumors. Mutation in the cluster region in the APC gene. *Hum Mol Genet*, 1992, 1: 229–233.

136. Saurin JC, Chayvialle JA, Ponchon T. Management of duodenal adenomas in familial adenomatous polyposis. *Fam Cancer*, 2008, 7: 173–177.

Melkersson–Rosenthal Syndrome

137. Lourenco SV, Boggio P, Suquyama K, et al. Severe and relapsing upper lip enlargement in a 10 year old boy. *Acta Paediatr*, 2010, 99: 1958.

138. Rogers RS. Melkersson-Rosenthal syndrome and orofacial granulomatosis. *Dermatol Clin*, 1996, 14: 371–379.

139. Khouri JM, Bohane TD, Day AS. Is orofacial granulomatosis in children a feature of Crohn's disease. *Acta Paediatr*, 2005, 94: 501–504.

140. Scully C. *Oral and Maxillofacial Medicine: The Basis of Diagnosis and Treatment*. Ed 3, Edinburgh: Churchill Livingstone, 2013, 298–301.

141. Saalman R, Sundell S, Kullberg-Lindhc C, et al. Long standing oral mucosal lesions in solid organ transplanted children – a novel clinical entity. *Transplantation*, 2010, 89: 606.

142. Williams PM, Greenberg MS. Management of cheilitis granulomatosa. *Oral Surg, Oral Med, Oral Pathol*, 1991, 72: 436–439.

143. Kano Y, Shiohara T, Yagita A, et al. Treatment of recalcitrant cheilitis granulomatosa with metronid. *J. Am Acad Dermatol*, 1992, 27: 629–630 (a3.1).

Multiple Endocrine Neoplasia Syndrome

144. Haverman CW, Sloan TB, Sloan RT. Multiple endocrine neoplasia syndrome type III: review and case report. *Spec Care Dentist*, 1995, 15: 102–106.

145. Pasquali D, Matteo FM, Renzullo A, et al. Multiple endocrine neoplasia of the old and the new: mini review. *G Ghir*, 2012, 33: 370–373.

146. Kahn MA, Cote J, Gagel RE. RET proto-oncogene mutation analysis in multiple endocrine neoplasia syndrome type 2B. Case report and review of the literature. *Oral Surg Oral Med Oral Pathol Oral Radiol Endod*, 1996, 82: 288–294.

147. Raue F, Frank-Raue K. Multiple endocrine neoplasia type 2. *Fam Cancer*, 2010, 9: 449–457.

148. Camacho CP, Huff AO, Lindsey SC. Early diagnosis of multiple endocrine neoplasia syndrome type 2B. A challenge for physicians. *Arq Bras Endocrine Metabol*, 2008, 52: 1393–1398.

149. Fox E, Widemann BC, Ckuk MK, et al. Vandetanib in children and adolescents with multiple endocrine neoplasia type 2B associated medullary thyroid carcinoma. *Clin Ca Res*, 2013, 19: 4239–4248.

Fabry Syndrome

150. Mehta A, Ricci R, Widmer U, et al. Fabry disease defined: baseline clinical manifestations of 366 patients in the Fabry outcome survey. *European J Clinic Invest*, 2004, 34: 236–242.

151. Gutierrez-Solana LG. Advances in the treatment of lysosomal diseases in infancy. *Rev Neural*, 2006, 5:suppl 1: 137–144.

152. Gorlin RJ, Sedano HO. Stomatologic aspects of cutaneous diseases: angiokeratoma corporis diffusum (Fabry syndrome). *J Dermatol Surg Oncol*, 1979, 5: 180–181.

153. Altarescu G, Berri R, Eiges R, et al. Prevention of lysosomal storage diseases and derivation of mutant stem cell liner by preimplantation genetic diagnosis. *Mol Biol Int*, 2012, doi 10.1155/2012/97342 Epub 2012, Dec 26.

154. Surjushe A, Jindal S, Sao P, et al. Anderson-Fabrys disease with marfanoid features. *Indian J Dermatol Venereol*, 2008, 74: 389–391.

Hereditary Gingival Fibromatoses

155. Prasad SS, Radharani C, Sinna S, et al. Hereditary gingival fibromatosis with distinctive facies. *J Contemp Dent Pract*, 2012, 1: 892–896.

156. Shi J, Lin W, Li X, et al. Hereditary gingival fibromatous a true generation case and pathologic mechanism research on progress of the disease. *J Periodontol*, 2011, 82: 1089–1095.

157. Avelar RL, deLana Campos GJ, deCarvalho-Bezerra Falcao PG, et al. Hereditary gingival fibromatosis: a report of four cases in the same family. *Quintessence Int*, 2010, 41: 99–102.

158. Breen GH, Adante R, Black CC. Early onset of hereditary gingival fibromatosis in a 28-month-old. *Pediatr Dent*, 2009, 31: 286–288.

159. Martelli H, Jr, Santos SM, Guimaraes AL, et al. Idiopathic gingival fibromatosis: description of two cases. *Minerva Stomatol*, 2010, 59: 143–148.

Ehlers–Danlos Syndrome

160. Byers PH, Murray ML, et al. Heritable collagen disorders. The paradigm of Ehlers Danlos syndrome. *J Invest Dermatol*, 2012, 15: E6–E11. doi: 10.1038/skinbio.2012.3.

161. Eder J, Laccone F, Rohbach M, et al. A new COL3A1 mutation in Ehlers-Danlos syndrome type IV. *Exp Dermatol*, 2013, 22: 231–234.

162. Mao JR, Bristow J. The Ehlers-Danlos syndrome: on beyond collagens. *J Clin Invest*, 2001, 107: 1063–1069.

163. Pinto YM, Pals G, Ziglstra JG, et al. Ehlers-Danlos syndrome type IV. *N Eng J Med*, 2000, 343: 366–368.

164. Yassin OM, Rihani FB. Multiple developmental dental anomalies and hypermobility type Ehlers-Danlos syndrome. *J Clin Pediatr Dent*, 2006, 30: 337–341.

Peutz–Jegher's Syndrome

165. Calva D, Howe JR. Hamartomatous polyposis syndromes. *Surg Clin North Am*, 2008, 88: 779–817.

166. Brosens LA, Van Hatley WA, Jansen M, et al. Gastrointestinal polyposis syndromes. *Current Mol Med*, 2007, 7: 29–46.

167. Hinds R, Philp C, Hyer W, et al. Complications of childhood Peutz-Jegher's syndrome. Implications for pediatric screening. *J Pediatr Gastroenteral Nutr*, 2004, 39: 219–220.

168. Mehenni H, Blouin JL, Radhakrishna U, et al. Peutz-Jeghers syndrome: confirmation of a linkage to chromosome 19p13.3 and identification of a potential second locus on 19p13.4. *Am J Hum Genet*, 1997, 61: 1327–1334.

169. McCarity TJ, Amos C. Peutz-Jegher's syndrome: clinicopathology and molecular alterations. *Cell Mol Life Sci*, 2006, 63: 2135–2144.

170. Tovar JA, Eizaquirre I, Albert A, et al. Peutz-Jegher's syndroms in children: report of two cases and review of the literature. *J Pediatr Surg*, 1983, 18: 1–6.

Marfan Syndrome

171. Loeys BL, Chen J, Neptuine ER. A syndroms of altered cardiovascular, craniofacial, neurocognitive and skeletal development caused by mutations in TGFBR1 and TGFBR2. *Nat Genet*, 2005, 37: 275–281.

172. Dean JG. Marfan syndromes. Clinical diagnosis and management. *European J Hum Genetics*, 2007, 15: 724–733.

173. deVries BB, Pals G, Odink R, et al. Homozygosity for a FBN1 missence mutation clinical and molecular evidence for recessive Marfan syndrome. *Eur J Hum Genet*, 2007, 15: 930–935.

174. Faivre L, Gorlin FJ, Wirtz MK, et al. In frame fibrillin-1 gene deletion in autosomal dominant weill-marchesani syndrome. *J Med Genet*, 2003, 40: 34–36.

175. Pyeitz RE. The Marfan syndrome in childhood. Features, natural history and differential diagnosis. *Prog Pediatric Cariol*, 1996, 5: 151–157.

176. Bolar N, Van Laer, Loeys BL. Marfan syndrome: from gene to therapy. *Curr Opin Pediatr*, 2012, 24: 498–504.

Proteus Syndrome

177. Cohen MM, Jr. Proteus syndrome: an update. *Am J Med Genet C Seminar Med Genet*, 2005, 137: 38–52.

178. Hoey SE, Eastwood D, Monsell, et al. Histopathological features of proteus syndrome. *Clin Exp Dermatol*, 2008, 33: 234–238.

179. Happle R. The manifold faces of proteus syndrome. *Arch Dermatol*, 2004, 140: 1001–1002.

180. Twede JV, Turner JT, Biesecker LG, et al. Evolution of skin lesions in proteus syndrome. *J Am Acad Dermatol*, 2005, 52: 834–838.

181. Cardoso MT, deCarvalho TB, Casulari LA, et al. Proteus syndrome and somatic mosaicism of the chromosome 16. *Panminerva Med*, 2003, 45: 267–271.

182. Lindhurst MJ, Sapp JC, Teer JK, et al. A mosaic activating mutation in AKT1 associated with proteus syndrome. *N Engl J Med*, 2011, 365: 611–619.

Ramsay Hunt Syndrome

183. Bhupal HK. Ramsay Hunt syndrome presenting in primary care. *Practitioner*, 2010, 254: 33–35.

184. Kleinschmidt-DeMasters BK, Gilden DH. The expanding spectrum of herpes virus infections of the nervous system. *Brainn Pthol*, 2001, 11: 440–451.

185. Sandoval CC, Nunez FA, Lizama CM, et al. Ramsay Hunt syndrome in children: four cases and review. *Rev Chilena Infectol*, 2008, 25: 458–464.

186. Ryer EW, Lee HY, Lee SY, et al. Clinical manifestations and prognosis of patients with Ramsay Hunt syndrome. *Am J Otolaryngol*, 2011, 33: 313–318.

187. Furuta Y, Aizawa H, Ohtani F, et al. Varicella-Zoster virus reactivation on Ramsay Hunt syndrome. *Ann Otol Rhinol Laryngol*, 2004, 113: 700–705.

188. Coffin SE, Hodkinka RL. Utility of direct immunofluorescence and virus culture for detection of varicella-zoster virus in skin lesions. *J Clin Microiol*, 1995, 33: 2792–2795.

189. Naganawa S, Nakashima T. Cutting edge of inner ear MRI. *Acta Otolaryngol Supp*, 2009, 560: 15–21.

190. Uscategui T, Doree C, Chamberlain IJ, et al. Antiviral therapy for Ramsay Hunt syndrome (herpes zoster oticus with facial palsy) in adults. *Cochrane Data Base System Review*, Oct 8 2008, doi: 10.1002/14651858.

191. deRu JA, VanBenthem PP. Combination therapy is preferable for patients with Ramsay Hunt syndrome. *Oto Neurotol*, 2011, 32: 852–855.

Albers–Schonberg Syndrome

192. Albers–Schonberg H. Roetgenbilder einer seltenen knochennerkrankung. *Muuch Med Wochenschr*, 1904, 51: 365.

193. Start Z, Savarirayan R. Osteopetrosis. *Orphanet J Rare Dis*, 2009, 4: 5.

194. Tritelbaum SL. Bone resorption by osteoclasts. *Science*, 2000, 289: 1504–1508.

195. Wada T, Nakashima T, Oliveria-dos-Santos, et al. The molecular scatfold Bag 2 is a critical component of RANK signaling and osteoclastogenesis. *Nat Med*, 2005, 11: 394–399.

196. Cleiren E, Benichou O, VanHul E, et al. Albers-Schonberg disease (autosomal dominant osteopetrosis, type II) results from mutations in CICN7 chloride channel gene. *Hum Mol Genet*, 2001, 10: 2861–2667.

197. Mazzolari E, Forino C, Razza A, et al. A single-center experience in 20 patients with infantile malignant osteopetrosis. *Am J Hematol*, 2009, 84: 473–479.

198. Marx RE, Stern D. *Oral and Maxillofacial Pathology: A Rationale for Diagnosis and Treatment.* Chicago: Quintessence Publishing Company, 2012.

199. Symposium on osteopetrosis: proceedings and abstracts of the first interactive symposium on osteopetrosis: Biology and therapy. Oct 23–24, 2003, Bethesda Maryland. USA J Bone Miner Res, 2004, 19: 1356–1375.

200. Armstrong DG, Newfield JY, Gillespie R. Orthopedic management of osteopetrosis: results of a survey and review of the literature. *J Pediatr Orthop*, 1999, 19: 122–132.

Gorham–Stout Syndrome

201. Lata PHJ, Sharma R, Parmar M. Massive osteolysis of hemimandible: a case report. *J Maxillofac Oral Surg*, 2009, 8: 381–383.

202. Lee S, Finn L, Sze RW. Gorham Stout syndrome (disappearing bone disease): two additional case reports and a review of the literature. *Arch Otolaryngol Head Neck Surg*, 2003, 129: 1340–1343.

203. Hu P, Yuan XG, Chan XY, et al. Gorham-Stout syndrome in mainland China: a case series of 67 patients and review of the literature. *J Zhejiang Univ Sci B*, 2013, 14: 729–735.

204. Ruggieri P, Montalti M, Angelini A, et al. Gorham-Stout disease: the experience of the Rizzoli Institute and review of the literature. *Skeletal Radiol*, 2011, 40: 1391–1397.

205. Dong Q, Yafei Z, Chuankong S. Gorham-Stout syndrome affecting the left mandible: a case report. *Exp Ther Med*, 2013, 5: 162–164.

206. Escande C, Schouman T, Francoise G, et al. Histological features and management of a mandibular Gorham-Stout disease: a case report and review of maxillofacial cases in the literature. *Oral Surg Oral Med Oral Pathol Oral Radiol Endod*, 2008, 106: e30–e37.

207. Silva S. Gorham-Stout disease affecting both hands: stabilization during bisphosphonate treatment. *Hand (NY)*, 2011, 6: 85–89.

208. Zheng MW, Yang M, Qiu JX, et al. Gorham-Stout syndrome presenting in a 5-year-old girl with successful bisphosphonate therapeutic effect. *Exp Ther Med*, 2012, 4: 449–451.

209. Nir V, Guralnik L, Livnat G. Propranolol as a treatment option in Gorham-Stout syndrome. A case report. *Pediatr Pulmonol*, 2014, 49: 417–419.